P9-BYW-137

Clinical manual of
HEALTH ASSESSMENT

Clinical manual of

# HEALTH ASSESSMENT

## Arden C. Bowers, R.N., M.S.

Instructor, College of Nursing;
Instructor, Department of Psychiatry,
College of Medicine,
Ohio State University,
Columbus, Ohio

## June M. Thompson, R.N., M.S.

Assistant Professor of Nursing,
School of Nursing,
The University of Texas,
Houston, Texas

**SECOND EDITION**

*with 588 illustrations*

## THE C. V. MOSBY COMPANY

ST. LOUIS • TORONTO • PRINCETON    1984

**MOSBY**

**A TRADITION OF PUBLISHING EXCELLENCE**

*Editor:* Barbara Ellen Norwitz
*Assistant editors:* Terry Young, Sally Adkisson
*Manuscript editor:* Carlotta Seely
*Book design:* Jeanne Bush
*Cover design:* Diane Beasley
*Production:* Mary Stueck, Judy England, Susan Trail

SECOND EDITION

Previous edition copyrighted 1980

Printed in the United States of America

The C.V. Mosby Company
11830 Westline Industrial Drive, St. Louis, Missouri 63146

**Library of Congress Cataloging in Publication Data**

Thompson, June M., 1946-
    Clinical manual of health assessment.

    Authors' names in reverse order on earlier ed.
    Includes bibliographical references and index.
    1.  Physical diagnosis.  2.  Nursing.  I.  Bowers, Arden C.
II.  Title.  [DNLM: 1.  Diagnosis.  2.  Health.  3.  Health
status. WB 200 T473c]
RT48.T48   1984        616.07'54        84-3353
ISBN 0-8016-4955-2

GW/VH/VH   9   8   7   6   5   4   3   2   1        01/A/048

# Preface

This manual has been designed to be used in a clinical or laboratory setting as a procedural guide for students who are learning health assessment. Each chapter outlines the knowledge necessary to proceed with a given portion of assessment, the explicit skills for the student to perform, and the expected findings that result from individual assessment efforts. Because of the procedural nature of the content, the knowledge base related to assessment is not offered. The student should refer to the suggested readings as advance preparation for skill practice and refinement.

Each chapter includes integrated information concerning the adult, the child, and the elderly client. Clinical and behavioral differences and similarities are presented in separate sections of each chapter for the reader's convenience. Some of the information is repeated in the separate age-related sections so that the student can extract a specific portion for immediate clinical reference. Although this approach is somewhat redundant, it allows each section to stand alone.

The manual is divided into three major areas: the health data base chapter, 14 clinical chapters that present specific systems or body regions for study, and the integration chapter, which offers a detailed outline of the entire health assessment process. Each chapter can be used as a single unit of study. The 14 clinical chapters follow a consistent format, comprising the following sections:

1. *Vocabulary.* A list of defined terms associated with the system or region of study.
2. *Cognitive objectives.* An outline of defined learning needs.
3. *Clinical objectives.* An outline of clinical entities that must be assessed.
4. *Health history additional to screening history.* An in-depth systemic or regional history that investigates common problems, complaints, and client risk potential.
5. *Clinical guidelines.* A procedural outline that includes (a) examiner behaviors and clinical entities to be assessed, (b) expected nor-

mal findings, and (c) common deviations from normal findings. Throughout the manual this section is supported with illustrations.

6. *Clinical strategies.* Notes and helpful hints for the beginning student regarding examination techniques and client behaviors.

7. *Sample recording.* An example of a written description of normal findings.

8. *History and clinical strategies: the pediatric client.* A discussion of approaches to the child and additional history data.

9. *Clinical variations: the pediatric client.* A detailed outline of the examination procedure for the child, anticipated normal findings, and commonly identified deviations.

10. *History and clinical strategies: the geriatric client.* A discussion of approaches to the older adult and additional history data.

11. *Clinical variations: the geriatric client.* A detailed outline of the examination procedure for the older adult, anticipated normal findings, and commonly identified deviations.

12. *Cognitive self-assessment.* A quiz section that demonstrates the student's understanding of related textbook and manual material and monitors progress. Answers are provided at the end of the book.

13. *Suggested readings.* Because of the procedural nature of this text, additional reading is necessary. This list complements the information in each chapter.

The assessment procedures are elaborate and detailed. The format of the book guides the student through cognitive application, a sequence of skill maneuvers and detailed descriptors of common findings within normal limits and findings that extend beyond normal. The illustrations, photographs, and careful description of findings assist students in being accountable for the results of their assessment efforts. However, this text does not attempt to lead students to diagnoses. Giving meaning to the findings requires clinical practice, preceptorship, and further study.

We have found that the clinical guidelines are extremely useful in the laboratory setting. We suggest to our students that they read aloud and discuss procedures while following along with a fellow student. The students are asked to describe the procedure, their rationale for their behaviors, and the characteristics of the findings as they progress. They frequently complete a practice session by writing out their actual findings for one another to critique.

**Arden C. Bowers**
**June M. Thompson**

# Contents

# Introduction

Assessment of an individual begins with careful, deliberate, and concrete observations of the whole person. Textbooks traditionally divide the remainder of the examination process into parts composed of body systems or regions. This division is convenient for the learner, who functions cognitively and clinically in logically sequenced segments, gradually coordinating the segments to form a total process of assessment.

This manual proceeds in a logical fashion. The whole person is assessed, from a personal viewpoint, through the use of the data base chapter (Chapter 1). Simultaneously, the examiner must be aware of the information provided in the chapter on general and mental status assessment (Chapter 2). The examiner begins collecting objective data as soon as the client is encountered and throughout the history-taking session. Dress, mannerisms, general body movement, and behavior are observed and noted as contributions to the final summary. Thereafter the student can proceed through the remaining clinical chapters, segment by segment, gradually using and synthesizing knowledge until all the parts are fitted together. The final chapter offers a detailed outline for fitting examiner behavior and clinical findings into a coordinated procedure and total summary.

We have used this manual in the laboratory setting for several years and have noted that predictable levels of learning are exhibited by the student. These phases must be acknowledged by both learner and teacher in designing and evaluating student progress.

A knowledge base is essential to the learner before psychomotor skills can be practiced. Anatomy and physiology supply the rationale for performing an examination and for the presence of normal findings. A cognitive introduction to the use of instruments and the practices of observation, palpation, auscultation, and percussion prepares the student for laboratory performance. Interviewing skills and analytical thinking are necessary prerequisites for acquiring an accurate and effective data base.

Much of the laboratory time is devoted to the mechanical aspects of the examination. Students need to concentrate on how to position the client (usually a fellow student) and how to maneuver their own bodies during the examination. They need to practice the skills of percussion, auscultation, and palpation. The use of equipment and the sequence of maneuvers are frequently the focus of attention before any cognitive application can occur.

Some body systems require a great deal of psychomotor skill. For example, use of the ophthalmoscope is difficult, and much time is consumed in manipulating the instrument and the client's and examiner's bodies. We have found that deep palpation of the abdomen is a new experience for many students and that tactile awareness is an acquired skill. Giving *meaning* to the findings that result from the process of examination may not occur until after several practice sessions.

When the learner is comfortable with the physical maneuvers, attention can then be given to the findings and their significance. Learners must be encouraged to describe findings in concrete terms rather than to simply label a part as "normal" or "OK." Normal findings have variations, with many gray areas between normal and abnormal. Examiners must be precise about what they have found and be able to clearly convey descriptions to others. We have found that beginning students have a difficult time accounting for their findings. They benefit greatly by verbally describing their findings as they examine and by writing up the results of the examination in each laboratory session.

Simulated abnormal findings can be taught in a laboratory. For example, audiovisual equipment can demonstrate skin lesions or abnormal heart sounds. However, the real application of performing a full assessment and sorting the resultant data does not usually occur until the student practices in a clinical setting with a preceptor. It is our feeling that knowing the significance of findings and responding to them with direct intervention or referral to others is a lifelong learning process.

We certainly acknowledge that human beings are more than the sum of their parts. They are dynamic entities interacting with the environment to attain or maintain a state of maximum well-being. As the student begins to pool information about a person, the development of a problem list, a client profile, and a risk profile should take place. The therapeutic application of the information in that final summary requires further professional knowledge beyond the scope and intent of this book. Recognizing client strengths, setting priorities with the client for seeking solutions to problems, and taking into account all the environmental variables that alter the client's state of well-being involve additional professional preparation.

This manual is designed to provide the student with an orderly, thorough method of collecting and categorizing accurate and well-defined data in preparation for subsequent professional care.

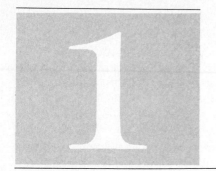

# Total health data base

## VOCABULARY

**active listening** State of selective attention and alertness that encompasses the skill of observation so that verbal and nonverbal cues are registered and clarified in an interaction; involves data absorption, retention, and exchange for clarification of meaning.

**assessment** Process of gathering and analyzing subjective and objective client data for summarization of a client's status.

**data base** Collection or store of information.

*subjective* Portion of the client data that is supplied by the client; the client's perceptions of himself.

*objective* Portion of the client data that is perceived by the examiner through physical examination or obtained from other external sources (such as laboratory studies).

**empathic response** State of mind that enables one to view another as that person views himself; coupled with interviewing skills that enable an examiner to verbally or nonverbally respond to a client statement without coloring or altering the client's intended meaning.

**exacerbation** Increase in intensity of signs or symptoms.

**hypothesis** Formation of an idea that relates available information to a probable cause. (*Note:* In the context of research *hypothesis* has a broader meaning.)

**incidence** The number of times an event occurs.

**precipitating factor** Event or entity that hastens the onset of another event. EXAMPLE: Chronic overeating is a precipitating factor for obesity.

**predisposing factor (risk factor)** Event or entity that contributes to the cause of another event. EXAMPLE: A family history of obesity increases the risk for obesity.

**problem list** Compilation of findings that appear at the end of the data base; may be diagnoses (medical or nursing), clusters of interrelated findings, or isolated findings that the examiner wishes to pursue but cannot label or attach to other findings. EXAMPLE: *diagnoses*—herpes simplex, knowledge deficit; *clusters*—polydipsia, polyuria, polyphagia; *finding*—lower back pain.

**questions**

*closed* Question posed in such a way that the respondent is directed toward a brief answer or a "yes" or "no"; does not encourage the respondent to elaborate. EXAMPLE: "Has your back pain improved since the last visit?"

*open* A broadly stated question that encourages a free-flowing, open response. EXAMPLE: "How has your back been feeling since your last visit?"

*directive* General term for a question or series of questions that leads the client in the questioner's channel of thinking. (*Note:* Most of the questions in the review of systems are directive.) EXAMPLES: "Have you ever noticed blurred vision?" "Double vision?" "Do you see spots or floaters?"

*probing* Form of directive questioning that enables the examiner to pursue a line of thinking to prove or disprove a hypothesis.

*leading* A question worded in such a way that it suggests the answer to the respondent. EXAMPLE: "Do you find that your chest pain radiates to your left arm or shoulder?" versus "Does your chest pain ever move around or locate in another area?"

**remission** Disappearance or diminishment of signs or symptoms.

**sign** Objective finding; one perceived by the examiner.

**significant negative** Absence of a finding that is often significant in clarifying the client's status. EXAMPLE: A client with diagnosed congestive heart failure shows no sign of ankle edema. (This is significant and should be reported as negative, or not present, because it clarifies the client's physical status for the reader.)

**symptom** Subjective indicator or sensation perceived by the client.

## Cognitive objectives

At the end of this chapter the learner will demonstrate knowledge of the effective techniques and components of the health history by the ability to do the following:

1. Apply the terms in the vocabulary section.
2. Discuss the rationale and options for examiner behaviors when gathering and analyzing health data for the:
   a. Well adult
   b. Well child
   c. Well elderly adult
   d. Ill (or symptomatic) client
3. Define the 10 components of the adult data base.
4. List the sections and provide at least one example of relevant information gathered in each section of the social history.
5. List and define the 11 components of the analysis of a symptom.
6. Recognize the characteristics of the pediatric data base that are collected in addition to or as substitution for the adult data base.
7. Recognize the characteristics of the geriatric data base that are collected in addition to or as substitution for the adult data base.

## Clinical objectives

At the end of this chapter the learner will be able to do the following:

1. Demonstrate the application of effective nurse behaviors for establishing a nurse-client relationship during the data base collection session.
2. Conduct a systematic and accurate assessment of an individual's health status (adult, pediatric, geriatric) using a predesignated format.
3. Organize health assessment data to establish a preliminary problem list that accurately reflects the client's priorities, concerns, and physiological state.
4. Systematically record a full data base and subsequent problem list using a predesignated format.
5. Create a client profile that summarizes the life-style and the client's assessment of the ability to provide self-care.

## Data base overview

The data base format presented in this text is known as the *long form*. It covers everything that an examiner could want to know about a client. Practitioners who use this format can spend anywhere from 1 to 3 hours collecting, compiling, and collating client data. The long form is also known as the *exhaustive method* for problem solving because its framework incorporates nonjudgmental descriptors of every aspect of the human condition. It does not urge the user to hypothesize about symptoms or to veer from the format to pursue an idea or a suspected diagnosis. The long form discourages straying from pure data collection and encourages the examiner to remain in a state of suspended judgment until all the facts have been gathered for sifting and analysis. The components of this format are presented in the box below.

When students attempt to use the exhaustive method in some clinical situations, they find that time and space constraints negate this format. Seasoned preceptors may role-model a questioning mode that quickly launches into specific probing questions. For example, if a client has presenting symptoms of weight loss, thirst, polyuria, and excessive hunger, the experienced examiner might immediately ask about a family history of diabetes, vaginal irritation, and skin infections. The exhaustive style would pursue a detailed symptom analysis (see box, p. 15) to clarify each symptom; family history and review of specific systems would come later. There are advantages to each approach, depending on the (1) intent of the interview, (2) condition of the client, (3) knowledge base and experience of the examiner, (4) constraints of the clinical setting, and (5) expectations of the client.

**Intent of the interview.** Medical inquiry has traditionally focused on exploration of *effects* (symptoms), which leads to *cause* (diagnosis), which leads to *cure*. The intent is to spend a minimum amount of time lingering on the effects and to quickly check hunches (hypotheses) about causes (suspected diseases), which leads to prescriptions for treatment. This can sometimes be accomplished if the symptoms are localized (e.g., earache). If the client has broad or vague presenting symptoms (e.g., fatigue or weight loss), the examiner remains longer in a state of suspended judg-

---

### DATA BASE OUTLINE

1. Biographical data
2. Reason for visit (chief complaint)
3. Present health status (general summary and symptom analysis; also known as history of present illness [HOPI])
4. Current health data
5. Past health status
6. Family history
7. Review of physiological systems
8. Psychosocial history
9. Health maintenance efforts
10. Environmental health

ment to clarify such factors as onset and duration, before asking probing, directive questions. The physician will branch off into an area of questioning to prove or disprove a hypothesis. If probing in this fashion disproves the hunch, the physician returns to nonjudgmental inquiry to get more information until another hypothesis forms, which leads to further probing.

Nursing inquiry frequently elicits more information about the effects. The nurse is interested in how the client functions within his environment. Pathological factors are relevant, but nurses recognize that causes may stem from such conditions as environmental influences, family relationships, or the client's coping skills. Nurses tend to inquire more closely and broadly about effects and to remain in suspended judgment for a longer period of time to gather this information.

Traditional medical and nursing modes are becoming blurred. Physicians, especially those in primary care settings, are being taught and urged to gather a broad data base and to give more attention to the client effects. Nurses have extended into some of the medical functions and are posing questions in the traditional medical mode to uncover disease. Many professional people are becoming more holistically oriented. The holistic philosophy demands that the examiner acquire complete information about each client because it holds that illness cannot be separated from wellness and both are entrenched in the client's environment and life-style.

Some practitioners have a completely nondirective approach, which is often used in a psychological interview. The client is asked the reason for the visit and is encouraged to give information in whatever order and pace he devises. Probing and confrontation are deliberately delayed to give the client total freedom of expression.

Whichever approach is chosen, it is extremely important that the examiner understand the *purpose* of the interview. The history format is intended to be flexible and to be used as a vehicle for effective, efficient information gathering.

**Condition of the client.** Urgency dictates expediency. A client with severe pain should not be subjected to a prolonged history. Biographical data may be delayed to pursue the chief complaint, with a symptom analysis and selected system reviews done to enable the examiner to hypothesize quickly and identify the cause, which leads to prompt alleviation of pain. A client with depression might be given more time to freely divulge feelings and surrounding circumstances without interference from the examiner. An elderly client with multiple symptoms, a long history of illness

and hospitalizations, and numerous problems at home would benefit from a full data base (exhaustive) approach.

**Knowledge base and experience of the examiner.** In order to hypothesize about causes, one must have a storage of knowledge to draw from, since human perceptions are narrowed by lack of knowledge and experience. A beginner cannot invent directive questions that lead to diagnosis. Therefore, students are urged to prolong the state of suspended judgment and to get full details about clients. The process of hypothesizing channels one's thinking and perceptions into a specific area and shuts out extraneous information. Lack of knowledge blurs the difference between what is extraneous and what is significant. It is important that students have experience with gathering a full data base. In this way they learn the value of each component of the history, and they give themselves and the client more time to sift through the facts to arrive at a series of findings.

**Constraints of the clinical setting.** Practitioners with nondirective approaches or holistic beliefs can become very frustrated (and ineffective) in a clinic setting that allocates 30 minutes for each client appointment! Time and space can dictate a philosophy and practice mode regardless of examiner intent or client condition. If cost-effectiveness is related to rapid patient turnover, the examiner must either function accordingly within that value system, change the system, or become creative in accomplishing his intent. A full data base can be gathered over a period of time. In some instances clients can complete portions of the history at home or in the waiting room. It is important to remember that it is pointless to record a full data base if no one is going to read it or make use of the information. Gathering such data is misleading to the client if no one has the time (or intention) to follow up with identified problems. Students sometimes become frustrated when they cannot use a full data base in a real-life setting. Yet it is a valuable lesson to be knowledgeable about the potential for a complete history and to have to relinquish portions of it for expediency. The student is very aware of what is missing and may choose to question the value of expediency.

**Expectations of the client.** A client with a painful ingrown toenail wants relief. He does not expect to discuss the condition of his neighborhood or his relationship with significant others. Because many clinics have an episodic care modality, clients have been conditioned to present tangible symptoms for diagnosis and treatment. They do not expect a 3-hour interview, even if they have multiple problems, and they may be confused or annoyed by a long interview. Other clients do expect adequate time for relaying all of their circumstances and benefit from such attention. Some clients expect a leisurely interview session and have difficulty with efficient conveyance of information. It is extremely important that the examiner, the client, and the health agency are clear about *why* the history is being taken. If an examiner has only 15 minutes, this information should be shared with the client at the onset. People generally become more efficient when they know that time is limited. If the interview will be lengthy, the client needs to be prepared and accepting of this.

With most histories both the examiner and the client benefit if the examiner is nondirective for the first 5 to 10 minutes of the interview. The client is asked the reason for the visit and allowed to freely convey information in his own fashion. This requires active listening, observing, and empathic skills on the part of the questioner. The practitioner can make observations about the client's behaviors and verbal styles in addition to getting unfettered facts from the client. This approach also establishes a condition of trust between client and professional. At the same time the client is observing the examiner. He needs to know that he has the examiner's full attention and concern. A state of suspended judgment broadens the examiner's perceptions and increases openness for inflow of data; it allows for patient priorities to be identified. It is human nature to hypothesize and to probe. The examiner must be aware when he is doing this and acknowledge that directive questions are being posed. Otherwise the client can easily be steered into a thinking channel that diverts from his original one.

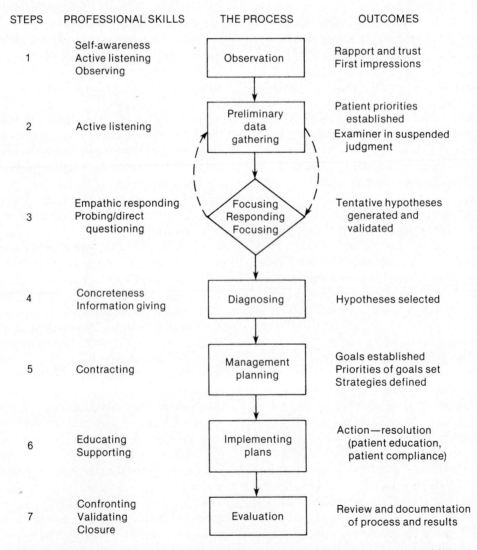

| STEPS | PROFESSIONAL SKILLS | THE PROCESS | OUTCOMES |
|---|---|---|---|
| 1 | Self-awareness<br>Active listening<br>Observing | Observation | Rapport and trust<br>First impressions |
| 2 | Active listening | Preliminary data gathering | Patient priorities established<br>Examiner in suspended judgment |
| 3 | Empathic responding<br>Probing/direct questioning | Focusing<br>Responding<br>Focusing | Tentative hypotheses generated and validated |
| 4 | Concreteness<br>Information giving | Diagnosing | Hypotheses selected |
| 5 | Contracting | Management planning | Goals established<br>Priorities of goals set<br>Strategies defined |
| 6 | Educating<br>Supporting | Implementing plans | Action—resolution (patient education, patient compliance) |
| 7 | Confronting<br>Validating<br>Closure | Evaluation | Review and documentation of process and results |

**FIG. 1-1.** Clinical problem solving. (Modified from Comprehensive humanistic health care, The Ohio State University, Grant No. 713297, Health Resources Administration, Department of Health and Human Services, Cherry McPherson, chief investigator, 1980-1983.)

At some point the history moves into a probing style (hypothesis generation and follow-up). It may go back and forth between probing, asking nonjudgmental questions, allowing free flow of conversation, and more probing. The questioner must judge the importance of being nondirective versus redirecting the client to answer specific questions. Sometimes practitioners with nondirective styles need to learn to interrupt and retrace a line of thinking. Directive people must concentrate and develop a facilitative style to permit client expression. This practice is both an art and a science.

A model for clinical problem solving is shown in Fig. 1-1. Note that the history-taking aspect of problem solving is contained in the first four steps of the process. Step 3 denotes the shift from nonjudgmental to directive questioning. This may precede step 2 in certain situations or may not occur until the entire history has been taken.

The expanded data base outline that follows provides a method for collecting data about the client's physiological, psychological, and sociocultural health. It also includes questions about the client's past health and the health of the family. When integrated, the information becomes the client's *health data base*. The practitioner must analyze and organize the data base to formulate the following:

1. A subjective data problem list (including physiological symptoms and psychological, social, or environmental factors that concern the client and/or the examiner). This will later be combined with the physical assessment problem list to develop a total problem list in the final write-up.
2. A risk profile (risk factors related to certain body systems are listed in subsequent chapters).
3. A client profile (a summary, from the *client's* viewpoint, of his life-style and ability to cope with self-care).

These data will serve as a constant resource for comparison as the client changes and provides new information in future assessments.

## Expanded data base outline for the adult client

### BIOGRAPHICAL DATA

1. Name
2. Age
3. Race
4. Culture
5. Address
6. Marital status
7. Children and family in home (if not family, significant others)
8. Occupation

9. Means of transportation to health care facility, if pertinent
10. Description of home; size and type of community

### REASON FOR VISIT

One statement that describes the reason for the client's visit or the chief complaint. State in the client's own words.

### PRESENT HEALTH STATUS

1. Summary of client's current major health concerns
2. If illness is present, include symptom analysis (box, p. 15)
   a. When was client last well
   b. Date of problem onset
   c. Character of complaint
   d. Nature of problem onset
   e. Course of problem
   f. Client's hunch of precipitating factors
   g. Location of problem
   h. Relation to other body symptoms, body positions, and activity
   i. Patterns of problem
   j. Efforts of client to treat
   k. Coping ability

### CURRENT HEALTH DATA

1. Current medications
   a. Type (prescription, over-the-counter drugs, vitamins, etc.)
   b. Prescribed by whom
   c. Amount per day
   d. Problems
2. Allergies (describe agent and reactions)
   a. Drugs
   b. Foods
   c. Contact substances
   d. Environmental factors
3. Last examinations (note physician/clinic, findings, advice, and/or instructions)
   a. Physical
   b. Dental
   c. Vision
   d. Hearing
   e. ECG
   f. Chest radiograph
   g. Pap smear (females)
4. Immunization status (note dates or year of last immunization)
   a. Tetanus, diphtheria
   b. Mumps
   c. Rubella
   d. Polio
   e. Tuberculosis tine test
   f. Influenza

**PAST HEALTH STATUS**

Although each of the following is asked separately, the examiner must summarize and record the data *chronologically*.

1. Childhood illnesses: rubeola, rubella, mumps, pertussis, scarlet fever, chickenpox, strep throat
2. Serious or chronic illnesses: scarlet fever, diabetes, kidney problems, hypertension, sickle cell anemia, seizure disorders, blood infections
3. Serious accidents or injuries: head injuries, fractures, burns, other trauma
4. Hospitalizations: elaborate upon, giving reason for, location, primary care providers, duration
5. Operations: what, where, when, why, by whom
6. Emotional health: past problems, help sought, support persons
7. Obstetrical history
   a. Complete pregnancies: number, pregnancy course, postpartum course, and condition, weight, and sex of each child
   b. Incomplete pregnancies: duration, termination, circumstances (including abortions and stillbirths)
   c. Summary of complications

**FAMILY HISTORY**

Family members include the client's blood relatives, spouse, and children. Specifically the interviewer should inquire about the client's maternal and paternal grandparents, parents, aunts, uncles, spouse, and children, as well as about the general health, stress factors, and illnesses of other family members. Questions should include a survey of the following:

| | |
|---|---|
| Cancer | Retardation |
| Diabetes | Alcoholism |
| Heart disease | Endocrine diseases |
| Hypertension | Sickle cell anemia |
| Epilepsy (or seizure disorder) | Kidney disease |
| Emotional stresses | Unusual limitations |
| Mental illness | Other chronic problems |

The most concise method to record these data is by a family tree. Fig. 1-2 is an example.

**REVIEW OF PHYSIOLOGICAL SYSTEMS**

The purpose of this component of the data base is to collect information about the body regions or systems and their function.

1. General—reflect from client's previous description of current health status.
   a. Fatigue patterns
   b. Exercise and exercise tolerance
   c. Weakness episodes
   d. Fever, sweats
   e. Frequent colds, infections, or illnesses
   f. Ability to carry out activities of daily living
2. Nutritional
   a. Client's average, maximum, and minimum weights during past month, 1 year, 5 years
   b. History of weight gains or losses (time element; specific efforts to change weight)
   c. Twenty-four-hour diet recall (helpful to mail client chart to fill in before visit) (Fig. 1-3)
   d. Current appetite
   e. Who buys, prepares food?
   f. Who does client normally eat with?
   g. Is client able to afford preferred food?
   h. Does client wear dentures? Is chewing a problem?
   i. Client's self-evaluation of nutritional status
3. Integumentary
   a. Skin
      (1) Skin disease or skin problems or lesions (wounds, sores, ulcers)
      (2) Skin growths, tumors, masses
      (3) Excessive dryness, sweating, odors
      (4) Pigmentation changes or discolorations
      (5) Pruritus (itching)
      (6) Texture changes
      (7) Temperature changes
   b. Hair
      (1) Changes in amount, texture, character
      (2) Alopecia (loss of hair)
      (3) Use of dyes
   c. Nails
      (1) Changes in appearance, texture
4. Head
   a. Headache (characteristics, including frequency, type, location, duration, care for)
   b. Past significant trauma
   c. Dizziness
   d. Syncope
5. Eyes
   a. Discharge (characteristics)
   b. History of infections, frequency, treatment
   c. Pruritus (itching)
   d. Lacrimation, excessive tearing
   e. Pain in eyeball
   f. Spots (floaters)
   g. Swelling around eyes
   h. Cataracts, glaucoma
   i. Unusual sensations or twitching
   j. Vision changes (generalized or vision field)
   k. Use of corrective or prosthetic devices
   l. Diplopia (double vision)
   m. Blurring
   n. Photophobia
   o. Difficulty reading
   p. Interference with activities of daily living

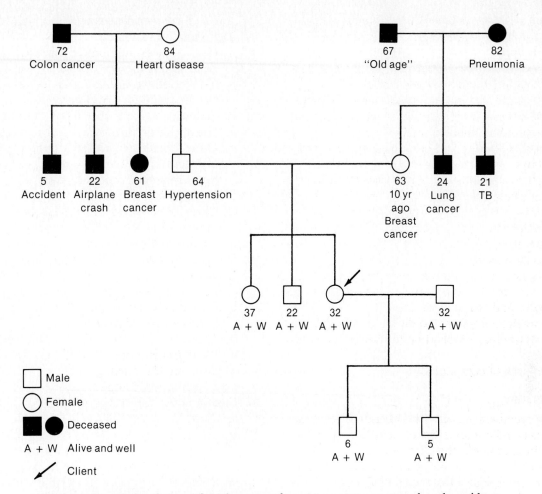

**FIG. 1-2.** Sample family tree (identifying grandparents, parents, aunts and uncles, siblings, spouse, and children).

| | Food eaten | Amount | Calories |
|---|---|---|---|
| Breakfast | | | |
| Lunch | | | |
| Dinner | | | |
| Snacks | | | |
| Total | | | |

**FIG. 1-3.** Twenty-four-hour diet record.

6. Ears
   a. Pain (characteristics)
   b. Cerumen (wax)
   c. Infection
   d. Hearing changes (describe)
   e. Use of prosthetic devices
   f. Increased sensitivity to environmental noise
   g. Vertigo
   h. Ringing and cracking
   i. Care habits
   j. Interference with activities of daily living
7. Nose, nasopharynx, and paranasal sinuses
   a. Discharge (characteristics)
   b. Epistaxis
   c. Allergies
   d. Pain over sinuses
   e. Postnasal drip
   f. Sneezing
   g. General olfactory ability
8. Mouth and throat
   a. Sore throats (characteristics)
   b. Lesions of tongue or mouth (abscesses, sores, ulcers)
   c. Bleeding gums
   d. Hoarseness
   e. Voice changes
   f. Use of prosthetic devices (dentures, bridges)
   g. Altered taste
   h. Chewing difficulty
   i. Swallowing difficulty
   j. Pattern of dental hygiene
9. Neck
   a. Node enlargement
   b. Swellings, masses
   c. Tenderness
   d. Limitation of movement
   e. Stiffness
10. Breast
    a. Pain or tenderness
    b. Swelling
    c. Nipple discharge
    d. Changes in nipples
    e. Lumps, dimples
    f. Unusual characteristics
    g. Breast examination (pattern, frequency)
11. Cardiovascular
    a. Cardiovascular
       (1) Palpitations
       (2) Heart murmur
       (3) Varicose veins
       (4) History of heart disease
       (5) Hypertension
       (6) Chest pain (character and frequency)
       (7) Shortness of breath
       (8) Orthopnea
       (9) Paroxysmal nocturnal dyspnea
    b. Peripheral vascular
       (1) Coldness, numbness
       (2) Discoloration
       (3) Peripheral edema
       (4) Intermittent claudication
12. Respiratory
    a. History of asthma
    b. Other breathing problems (when, precipitating factors)
    c. Sputum production
    d. Hemoptysis
    e. Chronic cough (characteristics)
    f. Shortness of breath (precipitating factors)
    g. Night sweats
    h. Wheezing or noise with breathing
13. Hematolymphatic
    a. Lymph node swelling
    b. Excessive bleeding or easy bruising
    c. Petechiae, ecchymoses
    d. Anemia
    e. Blood transfusions
    f. Excessive fatigue
    g. Radiation exposure
14. Gastrointestinal
    a. Food idiosyncrasies
    b. Change in taste
    c. Dysphagia (inability or difficulty in swallowing)
    d. Indigestion or pain (associated with eating?)
    e. Pyrosis (burning sensation in esophagus and stomach with sour eructation)
    f. Ulcer history
    g. Nausea/vomiting (time, degree, precipitating and/or associated factors)
    h. Hematemesis
    i. Jaundice
    j. Ascites
    k. Bowel habits (diarrhea/constipation)
    l. Stool characteristics
    m. Change in bowel habits
    n. Hemorrhoids (pain, bleeding, amount)
    o. Dyschezia (constipation resulting from habitual neglect in responding to stimulus to defecate)
    p. Use of digestive or evacuation aids (what, how often)
15. Urinary
    a. Characteristics of urine
    b. History of renal stones
    c. Hesitancy
    d. Urinary frequency (in 24-hour period)
    e. Change in stream of urination

f. Nocturia (excessive urination at night)
g. History of urinary tract infection, dysuria (painful urination, urgency, flank pain)
h. Suprapubic pain
i. Dribbling or incontinence
j. Stress incontinence
k. Polyuria (excessive excretion of urine)
l. Oliguria (decrease in urinary output)
m. Pyuria

16. Genital
   a. General
      (1) Lesions
      (2) Discharges
      (3) Odors
      (4) Pain, burning, pruritus (itching)
      (5) Venereal disease history
      (6) Satisfaction with sexual activity
      (7) Birth control methods practiced
      (8) Sterility
   b. Males
      (1) Prostate problems
      (2) Penis and scrotum self-examination practices
   c. Females
      (1) Menstrual history (age of onset, last menstrual period [LMP], duration, amount of flow, problems)
      (2) Amenorrhea (absence of menses)
      (3) Menorrhagia (excessive menstruation)
      (4) Dysmenorrhea (painful menses); treatment method
      (5) Metrorrhagia (uterine bleeding at times other than during menses)
      (6) Dyspareunia (pain with intercourse)

17. Musculoskeletal
   a. Muscles
      (1) Twitching
      (2) Cramping
      (3) Pain
      (4) Weakness
   b. Extremities
      (1) Deformity
      (2) Gait or coordination difficulties
      (3) Interference with activities of daily living
      (4) Walking (amount per day)
   c. Bones and joints
      (1) Joint swelling
      (2) Joint pain
      (3) Redness
      (4) Stiffness (time of day related)
      (5) Joint deformity
      (6) Noise with joint movement
      (7) Limitations of movement
      (8) Interference with activities of daily living

   d. Back
      (1) History of back injury (characteristics of problems, corrective measures)
      (2) Interference with activities of daily living

18. Central nervous system
   a. History of central nervous system disease
   b. Fainting episodes
   c. Seizures
      (1) Characteristics
      (2) Medications
   d. Cognitive changes
      (1) Inability to remember (recent vs. distant)
      (2) Disorientation
      (3) Phobias
      (4) Hallucinations
      (5) Interference with activities of daily living
   e. Motor-gait
      (1) Coordinated movement
      (2) Ataxia, balance problems
      (3) Paralysis (partial vs. complete)
      (4) Tic, tremor, spasm
      (5) Interference with activities of daily living
   f. Sensory
      (1) Paresthesia (patterns)
      (2) Tingling sensations
      (3) Other changes

19. Endocrine
   a. Diagnosis of disease states (thyroid, diabetes)
   b. Changes in skin pigmentation or texture
   c. Changes in or abnormal hair distribution
   d. Sudden or unexplained changes in height and weight
   e. Intolerance of heat or cold
   f. Exophthalmos
   g. Goiter
   h. Hormone therapy
   i. Polydipsia (increased thirst)
   j. Polyphagia (increased food intake)
   k. Polyuria (increased urination)
   l. Anorexia (decreased appetite)
   m. Weakness

20. Allergic and immunological (Optional; use if client indicates allergic history. Note precipitating factors in each case.)
   a. Dermatitis (inflammation or irritation of skin)
   b. Eczema
   c. Pruritus (itching)
   d. Urticaria (hives)
   e. Sneezing
   f. Vasomotor rhinitis (inflammation and swelling of mucous membrane of nose; nasal discharge)
   g. Conjunctivitis (inflammation of conjunctiva)
   h. Interference with activities of daily living
   i. Environmental and seasonal correlation
   j. Treatment techniques

21. Does client have any other physiological problems or disease states not specifically discussed. If so, explore in detail (e.g., fatigue, insomnia, nervousness).

## PSYCHOSOCIAL HISTORY

1. General statement of client's feelings about self
2. Feelings of satisfaction or frustration in interpersonal relationships
   a. Home; occupants
   b. Client's position in home relationships
   c. Most significant relationship (in and out of home)
   d. Community activities
   e. Work or school relationships
   f. Family cohesiveness patterns
3. Activities of daily living
   a. General description of work, leisure, and rest distribution
   b. Significant hobbies or methods of relaxation
   c. Family demands
   d. Community activities and involvement
   e. During period of day/week is client able to accomplish all that is desired?
4. General statement about client's ability to cope with activities of daily living
5. Occupational history
   a. Jobs held in past
   b. Current employer
   c. Educational preparation
   d. Satisfaction with present and past employment
   e. Time spent at work versus time spent at play
6. Recent changes or stresses in client's life-style (e.g., divorce, moving, new job, family illness, new baby, financial stresses)
7. Patterns in which client copes with situations of stress
8. Response to illness
   a. Does the client cope satisfactorily during own or others' illness?
   b. Do the client's family and friends respond satisfactorily during periods of illness?
9. History of psychiatric care or counseling
10. Feelings of anxiety or nervousness (characteristics and coping mechanisms)
11. Feelings of depression (symptoms such as insomnia, crying, fearfulness, marked irritability or anger)
12. Changes in personality, behavior, or mood
13. Use of medications or other techniques during times of anxiety, stress, or depression
14. Habits
    a. Alcohol
       (1) Kinds (beer, wine, mixed drinks)
       (2) Frequency per week
       (3) Pattern over past 5 years, 1 year
       (4) Drinking companions
       (5) Alcohol consumption increased when anxious or stressed?
    b. Smoking
       (1) Kind (pipe, cigarette, cigar)
       (2) Amount per week/day
       (3) Pattern over past 5 years, 1 year
       (4) Smoking with others
       (5) Smoking increased when anxious or stressed?
       (6) Desire to quit smoking? (method, attempts)
    c. Coffee and tea
       (1) Amount per day
       (2) Pattern over past 5 years, 1 year
       (3) Consumption increased when anxious or stressed?
       (4) Physiological effects
    d. Other
       (1) Overeating or sporadic eating (e.g., always in refrigerator, soft drink abuse, cookie jar syndrome)
       (2) Nail biting
       (3) "Street drug" usage
       (4) Nervous noneating
15. Financial status
    a. Sources
    b. Adequacy
    c. Recent changes in resources and expenditures

## HEALTH MAINTENANCE EFFORTS

1. General statement of client's own physical fitness
2. Exercise (amount, type, frequency)
3. Dietary regulations; special efforts (describe in detail)
4. Mental health; special efforts such as group therapy, meditation, yoga (describe in detail)
5. Cultural or religious practices
6. Frequency of physical, dental, and vision health assessment

## ENVIRONMENTAL HEALTH

1. General statement of client's assessment of environmental safety and comfort
2. Hazards of employment (inhalants, noise, heavy lifting, psychological stress, machinery)
3. Hazards in the home (concern about fire, stairs to climb, inadequate heat, open gas heaters, inadequate toilet facilities, concern about pest control, inadequate space)
4. Hazards in neighborhood (noise, water, and air pollution, inadequate police protection, heavy traffic

on surrounding streets, isolation from neighbors, overcrowding)
5. Community hazards (unavailability of stores, market, laundry facilities, drugstore; no access to bus line)

## Clinical strategies: the adult client

1. Complete data base collection and symptom analysis take practice and constant validation with an experienced practitioner. Complete your problem list *before* checking with your clinical resource advisor. Use *all* the steps; each is important.
2. Write up as many histories for review by an experienced practitioner as possible. It takes practice to write successfully.
3. The examiner needs ample time to formulate an accurate and complete data base. Negotiate for time and space with your employer. Next, contract for an extended time period with your client. Collecting a full data base from an individual may take an hour or more.
4. Frequently the client may come to see the examiner because of an episodic care problem. It may not be appropriate for the examiner to collect a complete data base, so a systematic and routine manner of collecting episodic care data must be developed. Following is a list of data that should be collected about every episodic care problem:
   a. Chief complaint
   b. Analysis of the symptom or complaint (see box, p. 15 for details)
   c. Interrelationship of current problem to other body systems (would include a review of associated body systems; vague symptoms such as weakness or fatigue must be thoroughly explored by reviewing all body systems)
   d. Relation of current problem to past health and health maintenance
5. Following are several "nuggets" of interviewing that facilitate data collection:
   a. Pose questions without suggesting answers: "Tell me about your pain," not "Does your pain travel down your arm?"
   b. Begin questioning with the most *recent* episode (if client has experienced a number of "attacks" over a period of time), then move on to preceding episodes. The client is most likely to remember specific details of the most recent episode.
   c. Begin questioning with the most *urgent* problem (if client presents a number of complaints that are worrying him): "What brought you to the clinic today?"
   d. Chronology is the anchor of the history: request calendar dates and clock times.
   e. Use simple language (e.g., instead of saying *void*, use *urinate* or *pass your water*).
   f. Pose one question at a time.
   g. Keep the client politely on track: "Before we go on to that, I would like to hear more about. . . ."
   h. Clarify the client's responses: What do these really mean to the client? Do they mean the same to you?
      (1) Quasimedical terms
         (a) Tumor
         (b) Nervous breakdown
         (c) Sick-to-the-stomach
         (d) Pneumonia
         (e) Sciatica
         (f) Dizziness
         (g) Heart attack
         (h) Diarrhea
      (2) Quantities (unclear)
         (a) A lot
         (b) Often
         (c) Once in a while
   i. If you accept a diagnosis from a client, record it in quotations. Follow up with a summary of the symptoms that prompted diagnosis (e.g., *hemorrhoids*—involves five or six droplets of bright red blood on tissue; associated with once-a-week constipation; pain localized at anus with each daily bowel movement; palpable tags at anal area).
   j. At the end of the interview, summarize (aloud) what the client has said.
6. Following are several hazards of interviewing that will hinder data collection.
   a. The need to hurry. Clients will sense this, and thus incomplete data may be collected.
   b. Nonverbal cues. If the examiner is uninterested, the client may sense this and provide incomplete data.
   c. Environment. The examiner and client need a quiet, private environment with adequate chairs and writing space. If the facility or environment is busy, noisy, nonprivate, or confusing, incomplete data may be collected.
   d. "Nonhuman" techniques. This includes the "just the facts" approach. The examiner rapidly moves from one question to the next without taking time to build a relationship with the client.
   e. "Aha!" This technique is more of a hazard for the experienced practitioner. The temptation is to leap to a "diagnosis" without collecting ample information; incorrect assessment can be based on incomplete data.

f. "Oh, my!" This response allows the examiner to indicate disapproval, which could stifle examiner-client communication. For example, the client admits that he has not taken his hypertension medication for 4 months because he "felt so good." The examiner responds with "oh, my."

g. "Halo effect." This hazard might prohibit the examiner from collecting all relevant data about a client. For example, the client is a 42-year-old new widow, and the examiner neglects to ask if the client is sexually active.

h. Use of *normal, negative, healthy,* or *well.* Each of these terms has a different meaning to individual examiners with different levels of expertise. The beginning practitioner is encouraged to use descriptive terminology to define significant findings or significant negatives to describe "normal" states.

i. Limited knowledge is perhaps the biggest hazard of all. The beginning examiner must be disciplined enough to use the suggested data collection tools and to continue to study and learn.

7. Write an outline of the data collection format on small cards to use as a reference while taking histories. The beginning examiner cannot memorize all the data categories.

8. Use a clipboard or a small notebook for taking notes during the interview. The examiner will need a portable, hard surface to write on. This will permit seating comfort with maintenance of eye contact.

9. During progression of data base collection skills, monitor efficiency in terms of collecting, organizing, and recording a data base. Cost-effectiveness is an issue in most employment settings.

10. *Note:* The client often does not present a tidy package of symptoms for analysis at the onset of the interview. Symptoms will be uncovered as the examiner pursues information in the review of systems. The examiner *must* stop and analyze these problems as thoroughly as those presented initially.

## Analysis of a symptom

In addition to the health data base, the examiner must be prepared to collect in-depth information about a symptom. The following format is a data collection tool that can be used for physiological, psychological, or sociological symptoms.

### CHIEF COMPLAINT

A one-sentence or brief statement using the client's words to describe the reason for the visit. Details about the complaint are included in the *Present health status* section or the symptom analysis (box on p. 15).

### ANALYSIS APPROACH

Reconstruction from the client's own words the body or mental processes underlying the symptom.

# SYMPTOM ANALYSIS

1. Last time client was entirely well
   a. Patient may confuse onset of symptom with the first time he was *concerned* about it.
   b. Major symptom may have been preceded by other less alarming ones (e.g., fatigue) that the client will not recall unless questioned.
2. Date of current problem onset
   a. Name specific date and time if possible.
   b. Inquiry about the setting at the time of onset may help establish chronology (time of day, month).
   c. How was client feeling before symptom onset?
3. Character (describe the qualities of the problem)
   a. Move back to quoting the client: What is the pain like? "Like being stabbed?" "Squeezed in a vise?"
   b. Severity (Does it interfere with activities of daily living?)
4. Nature of problem onset
   Was the onset slow? Abrupt? Noticeable to others? Use quotes if possible.
5. Client's hunch of precipitating factors
   In determining aggravating or alleviating factors, word questions to avoid influencing answers. For example, angina: "What effect does walking have?" or vertigo: "What happens if you move your head?"
6. Course of problem (Did client continue with normal activity during episode?)
   a. Consistent
   b. Intermittent
   c. Duration
7. Location of problem
   a. Pinpoint
   b. Generalized, vague
   c. Radiation patterns
8. Effect on other systems and activities
   a. Symptoms, signs
   b. Body functions or positions
   c. Activities (body movement, exercise)
   d. Eating
9. Patterns
   The client may exhibit a symptom that has been occurring intermittently over a period of time. Most previous questions have elicited data about the quantity and quality of *one* episode. This section concerns multiple episodes, identifies patterns, and provides an overview of chronology.
   a. *Timing.* Relate incidences to number of times per hour, day, week, month; inquire about client's well-being during the intervals.
   b. *Duration* and quality variations. May indicate a stepping up or increase in intensity over a period of time. ("Has it been getting any better? Worse? Staying the same?")
   c. If there have been exacerbations or remission, try to associate with other symptoms, activities, or precipitating factors.
10. Efforts to treat
    a. Home remedies (what and when)
    b. Body positions (e.g., bed rest)
    c. Over-the-counter medications
    d. Prescription medications and physician visits (give details)
11. In-depth exploration of client's life-style and coping ability as related to the symptom
    a. Pose questions to discover an association between daily activities and the symptom.
       (1) What mandatory activities make the symptom worse? For example, if stair climbing causes chest pain, does the client have to use stairs at home or at work?
       (2) What activities are altered or curtailed because of the symptom? For example, if the client complains of nocturnal urination, how much sleep is lost? Is fatigue a problem? Possible to sleep during the day?
       (3) Do altered activities pose a threat to the client? If client complains of diminished vision or glare, is driving hazardous? Is reading part of job?
    b. Pose questions that indicate an association between client's ability to deal with current life-style and the symptom. For example, if a mother complains of marked fatigue, does this interfere with child-rearing activities or management of the home?
    c. A general question such as, "What does this problem *mean* to you?" might help to summarize the previous questions. It also permits the client to voice an emotional response to changes or problems. It may help the examiner to grasp more fully the impact or severity of the symptom.

## SAMPLE ADULT DATA BASE WRITE-UP

Once the data base is collected, it must be organized, synthesized, and documented. Following is a sample data base write-up. Refer to the pediatric and geriatric sections of this chapter to make the appropriate changes.

### Biographical data

Cynthia M. Stoner; 32 years old; white; female; married; two sons, ages 6 and 7; 3792 Hedge Creek Lane, Maysville, Ohio; lives in single-family dwelling owned by family; described as three-bedroom "comfortable" home in midst of rural community.

### Reason for visit

Time for Pap smear; "lower abdominal discomfort off and on"; desire to lose weight.

### Present health status

Health during past 5 years has been good; during past year has noted 15-pound weight gain and periods of not feeling "up to par"; complains of being "tired" much of the time; no fatigue pattern identified; currently most significant concern is lower abdominal discomfort.

Initial problem onset 8 months ago; since then increased episodes and severity; increased discomfort before menses, with increased flatus and full bladder; discomfort described as nonradiating, sharp, and stabbing; pinpoint location in LLQ; client perceives problem associated with uterus or left ovary; coping methods: client aware of discomfort but problem not interfering with activities of daily living.

Currently taking no medications.

### Current health statistics

Immunizations
  Polio: 1972
  Diphtheria, tetanus: 1978
  Tuberculosis tine test: 1978
  Influenza, mumps, rubella: none
Allergies
  Seasonal and environmental: pollen, dust, grass; no treatment
Last examination
  Physical, Pap smear, chest x-ray examination: Sept. 1979
  Dental: June 1979
  Vision: Oct. 1978
  Hearing: high school
  ECG: 1972

### Past health status

**1946 to 1956** Childhood diseases: measles, mumps, chickenpox
**1958** Tonsillectomy: Marion, Ohio, Dr. Harris
**1961** Appendectomy: Marion, Ohio, Dr. Spencer
**1962** Hospitalized for hepatitis
**1964** Fracture of left tibia from riding accident; uncomplicated
**1970** Surgery: benign left breast cyst removed, Delaware, Ohio, Dr. Southwood
**1972** Pregnancy: delivered healthy 7 lb 2 oz boy; vaginal delivery, uncomplicated
**1973** Pregnancy: delivered healthy 7 lb, 9 oz boy; vaginal delivery; complications—high blood pressure, fluid retention, hospitalized 3 weeks before induced delivery; recovered to healthy state within 2 weeks following delivery
**1973** Tubal ligation, Delaware, Ohio, Dr. Southwood

### Family history

See Fig. 1-2.

### Review of physiological systems

1. General: Client considers herself in "good health" but has periods of fatigue with physical and emotional stress. Feels rested following sleep periods. Client states she would feel better if she could lose 20 pounds and exercise more regularly.
2. Nutritional
   Current weight: 142 lb; height: 5 feet, 4 in
   Weight past year: 138 to 140 lb
   Weight past 5 years: 120 to 138 lb
   Client considers the accompanying dietary recall to be typical. She states, "I know better than to eat all that junk." Dietary efforts have been sporadic; major methods involved skipping meals (breakfast and lunch) and protein (meat and salad) diets; no efforts in past 8 months.
   Client considers current appetite "too good." She enjoys eating and eats more when nervous or worried. Client does grocery shopping. States she buys foods that her children and husband like. Money or transportation not a problem.
3. Integumentary
   a. Skin: denies lesions, masses, discolorations. Some pruritus during winter; clears with lotion.
   b. Hair: denies texture changes or loss; uses color rinse monthly to maintain lightened color; no scalp irritation reported from the rinse.
   c. Nails: states she has always had brittle nails.
4. Head: periodic headaches in occipital area and back of neck usually follow tension period and are relieved by aspirin and rest (no more than four aspirin tablets/week consumed).
5. Eyes: denies infections or discharge from eyes; seasonal periorbital swelling associated with pollen allergy. Denies visual changes, diplopia, blurring, photophobia, pain in eyeball, or excessive

tearing. Client wears glasses for reading (past 3 years).

6. Ears: complains of chronic hearing problem (multiple ear infections as child); states hearing difficulty does not interfere with activities of daily living; "just certain sounds are not clear." Denies pain, infections, or vertigo; frequent complaints of ringing and cracking in ears. Cares for ears with cotton-tipped swabs.

7. Nose, nasopharynx, and paranasal sinuses: denies epistaxis, sinus problems, postnasal drip, or olfactory deficit; seasonal sneezing and discharge associated with allergies.

8. Mouth and throat: denies sore throats, lesions, gum irritation, chewing or swallowing difficulties, hoarseness, or voice changes. Brushes teeth two times a day and uses dental floss.

9. Neck: denies tenderness or range of motion difficulties.

10. Breast: breast tenderness before menses; breasts "feel lumpy"; "small amount of yellow" bilateral nipple discharge present since birth of second child. Examines own breasts each month following menstrual period. Breast biopsy with cyst removed in 1970. Client considers breasts to be "cystic, lumpy."

## Twenty-four-hour dietary recall

| Food eaten | Amount | Calories |
|---|---|---|
| **Breakfast** | | |
| Toast with peanut butter and butter | 1 slice | 214 |
| Coffee with cream | 8 oz | 30 |
| Orange juice | 4 oz | 100 |
| | | 344 |
| **Lunch** | | |
| Hamburger sandwich | 1 | 250 |
| Salad with ranch dressing | 6 oz | 105 |
| Coffee with cream | 8 oz | 30 |
| | | 385 |
| **Dinner** | | |
| Swiss steak | 3 oz | 300 |
| Baked potato | 1 | 230 |
| Green beans | 4 oz | 27 |
| Bread | 2 slices | 228 |
| Water | | |
| | | 785 |
| **Snacks** | | |
| Iced cupcake | 1 | 200 |
| Carbonated beverage | 8 oz | 105 |
| | | 305 |
| TOTAL | | 1819 |

11. Cardiovascular: denies chest pain, shortness of breath, or palpitations. No known history of heart murmurs, heart disease, or hypertension. Feet always feel cold. Denies discoloration or peripheral edema.

12. Respiratory: denies any breathing difficulties, chronic cough, or shortness of breath.

13. Hematolymphatic: describes periods of fatigue related to stress or excessive work. Denies lymphatic swelling, excessive bleeding, or bruising. Never tested for anemia.

14. Gastrointestinal: denies eating or digestion problems. Periodic pyrosis usually follows rapid food ingestion or occurs during stressful period. Denies hematemesis, jaundice, or ascites. Bowel movement once each day. Stools are soft and brown. Denies difficulty with diarrhea or constipation. No known hemorrhoids.

15. Urinary: describes urine as yellow and clear. Voiding frequency four to five times in 24 hours. Denies voiding difficulties, dysuria, urgency, or flank pain. Infrequent nocturia. Denies polyuria or oliguria. Complains of frequent episodes of stress incontinence since birth of second child. Condition becoming no worse but does present problem during laughing, running, or lifting heavy objects.

16. Genital: LMP, 6-14-84. Periods normally 28 to 30 days apart; regular intervals; heavy flow with clotting and cramps in first 24 hours. Cramps controlled by aspirin. LLQ pain increases just before menses. Denies genital lesions, discharges, or VD history. Sexually active, satisfied with sexual activity.

17. Musculoskeletal and extremities: denies muscular weakness, twitching, or pain; gait difficulties or extremity deformities; joint swelling, pain, stiffness, or noise; history of back injury problems.

18. Central nervous system: denies changes in cognitive function, coordination, or sensory defects.

19. Endocrine: denies endocrine disease, history of skin changes, polydipsia, polyuria, polyphagia, anorexia, or weakness.

20. Allergic: describes allergy problems as seasonal (August to October). Treatment consists of symptomatic relief by by a "cortisone shot" and an unidentified prescription. During allergic season client reports sneezing, vasomotor rhinitis, conjunctivitis; no interference with activities of daily living.

### Psychosocial history

Client states she feels good about herself most of the time. She experiences episodes of depression and fatigue and expresses a feeling that she should "do more" with her life.

Client expresses feelings of satisfaction with family members and friends. She considers her husband her

*Continued.*

## SAMPLE ADULT DATA BASE WRITE-UP—cont'd

**Psychosocial history—cont'd**

best friend but also speaks of two other very close female friends. She counts on her friends to help her "talk through" stress periods. Considers family very close; communication channels are open.

Client's energies revolve around maintaining home, raising two small sons, and working part-time (12 hours/week) at a local flower shop. Denies membership in clubs or church. Spends weekends just relaxing with family. Feels stress and at times "angry" when husband's business keeps him away on weekends. Client states that much of her time is spent meeting the needs of others. States she would like more time for herself.

As soon as children are older, client hopes to return to college to complete degree in horticulture (5 terms to go). Client loves work at flower shop and would like to either take a college course or two or work a few more hours at the flower shop. Husband supports career goals but for now believes client's job is at home with the children (seems to be a stress point).

Husband just accepted job promotion. Now travels approximately 12 days out of the month. This seems to cause direct stress and creates child care problems during client's working hours.

Client denies previous psychiatric counseling or feelings of anxiety or nervousness that she could not cope with. Methods of coping most frequently are (1) easy and sometimes inappropriate expression of anger, (2) increased sleeping, and (3) eating. To relax, client enjoys reading, playing with children, and going out with husband.

Client denies use of drugs or medications.

Alcohol: 3 or 4 glasses of wine a week

Smoking: none

Coffee: 4 or 5 cups a day. No increase over the past 5 years. Increased consumption with stress (6 to 8 cups/day).

Overeating: increased with stress; eats most when alone and after children go to bed.

Financial status: client feels they could do more as a family if there were more money but states there are no serious financial problems.

**Health maintenance efforts**

No specific health maintenance efforts. Health care patterns inconsistent, as previously stated.

**Environmental health**

Client believes her home and neighborhood environment are safe and without hazards. Client is exposed to fertilizer fumes at flower shop, but ventilation is adequate.

**Subjective problem list**

1. Periods of fatigue
2. LLQ pain: cyclical with menses? does not interfere with activities of daily living; increased severity and frequency past 8 months
3. Stress incontinence past 5 years, not increased in severity
4. Seasonal allergies: symptomatically treated; do not interfere with activities of daily living
5. Feet cold "most of time"
6. Long-standing hearing difficulty (since childhood); does not interfere with activities of daily living
7. Overweight for height and build; 22 lb weight gain in past 5 years; 4 lb in past year
8. Poor dietary habits
9. Needs Pap smear
10. Feels trapped at times by home and child-raising responsibilities; husband travels approximately 12 days a month

Final problem list is developed, and priorities are established following physical assessment.

**Risk profile**

1. Family cancer history
   Maternal: mother, breast cancer; uncle, lung cancer
   Paternal: aunt, breast cancer; grandfather, colon cancer
   Client: cystic breasts; already has had one cyst removed (1970); client performs breast examination regularly
2. Weight: Steady weight gain since 1972; attempts at regular dieting and exercise programs have failed
3. Irregular health maintenance program: health care visits, diet, exercise
4. At times client does not feel self-fulfilled; believes she is always meeting needs of others and neglecting self

**Client profile**

Client views herself as a healthy and resourceful 32-year-old female. Physiologically she is bothered by (1) LLQ discomfort, (2) overweight state, and (3) periodic fatigue.

Psychologically and sociologically, stresses viewed by client are (1) husband traveling too often, (2) feeling burdened periodically by family and household responsibilities, (3) a desire to return to college or become more actively involved in outside activities, and (4) fear of breast cancer. In summary, client views coping skills as adequate to meet present stresses.

## Total health data base for the pediatric client

Data base collection for the pediatric client is basically similar to that for the adult. Exceptions include prenatal, growth and development, behavioral, and school status histories. The following format parallels the adult history but includes the significant pediatric data.

### INFORMANT

Who is giving the history (relation to client)?

### BIOGRAPHICAL DATA

1. Name
2. Age
3. Race
4. Culture
5. Address and telephone
6. Children and family in home
7. Means of transportation to health care facility, if pertinent
8. Description of home; size and type of community

### REASON FOR VISIT

One statement that describes the reason for the client's visit, preferably in the client's own words.

### PRESENT HEALTH STATUS

1. Summary of client's major health concerns
2. If illness is present, record symptom analysis (box, p. 15).
   a. When was client last well
   b. Date of problem onset
   c. Character of complaint
   d. Nature of problem onset
   e. Course of problem
   f. Client's hunch of precipitating factors
   g. Location of problem
   h. Relation to
      (1) Other body symptoms
      (2) Body positions
      (3) Activity
      (4) Eating
   i. Patterns of problem
   j. Efforts of client to treat
   k. Coping ability
3. *Current* development of the child
   The examiner must develop a profile of the child's current developmental status. It is expected that the examiner will have a working knowledge of the appropriate developmental progression for the child's age. Developmental screening questions should reflect the following areas:

   a. Children from 1 month through preschool age*
      (1) *Motor development,* including rolling over, sitting, standing, walking, skipping, climbing, etc.
      (2) *Prehension,* including playing with hands, using pincer grip, using cup and spoon to feed self, stacking blocks, drawing with crayon, buttoning, drawing multiple-part persons, etc.
      (3) *Vision and hearing,* including ability to follow movement with eyes to midline and past midline, turn head to follow sound, smile at mirror image, recognize name when spoken to, etc.
      (4) *Cognitive development,* including ability to bring hands to mouth, suck thumb, recognize that actions can cause personal pleasure, search for object that has fallen, play peek-a-boo, drop object from chair to watch where it falls, remember solutions to simple problems, understand different points of view to conflicting problems, etc.
      (5) *Vocalization,* including ability to coo, smile, produce different tones, gurgle, and generate multiple verbal tones, single words, multiple words, and sentences.
   b. School-age children
      (1) *Gross motor development,* including assessment of running, jumping, climbing, general and eye-hand coordination, awkwardness, ability to ride a bicycle, etc.
      (2) *Fine motor development,* including assessment of ability to tie shoes, use scissors, draw with detail, print name, numbers, etc.
      (3) *Vocalization,* including assessment of child's verbal communication ability, vocabulary, ability to read and tell time, etc.
4. Common behaviors
   General statement about child's behavior pattern.

| | |
|---|---|
| Wants too little or too much attention | Bangs head |
| | Rocks |
| Accident prone | Encopresis (bowel incontinence) |
| Unsure of self | |
| Bites nails | Enuresis (wets bed) |
| Sucks thumb | Has temper tantrums |
| Stutters | Has breath-holding spells |
| Fearful | Smokes |
| Lies | Takes drugs, sniffs glue |
| Masturbates | Sets fires |
| Eats paint or dirt (pica) | |

*In addition to this list, refer to Appendix A for a complete developmental profile guide, The Washington Guide to Promoting Development in Young Children. It provides screening criteria as well as suggested activities for promotion of developmental tasks.

**TABLE 1-1.** Recommended schedule for active immunizations for infants and children

| Age | Immunization recommended |
|---|---|
| 2 mo | DPT (diphtheria, pertussis, and tetanus) and TOPV (trivalent Sabin) |
| 4 mo | DPT and TOPV |
| 6 mo | DPT (a third dose of TOPV is optional) |
| 1 yr | Tuberculin test |
| 15 mo | Measles, mumps, and rubella |
| 18 mo | DPT and TOPV |
| 4-6 yr | DPT and TOPV |
| 14-16 yr | TD (combined tetanus and diphtheria tox-oid, adult type) |

Modified from American Academy of Pediatrics Report of the Committee on Infectious Diseases, ed. 19, Chicago, 1982, copyright American Academy of Pediatrics.

**CURRENT HEALTH DATA**

1. Current medications: type (prescription, over-the-counter drugs, vitamins, etc.), prescribed by whom, amount per day, problems
2. Allergies
   a. Drugs
   b. Foods
   c. Contact substances
   d. Environmental factors
3. Last examinations (note physician/clinic, findings, advice, and/or instructions)
   a. Physical
   b. Dental
   c. Vision
   d. Hearing
   e. Developmental assessment such as Denver Developmental Screening Test
4. Immunization status (note dates administered)—see Table 1-1
5. Is there a public or visiting health nurse working with client?

**PAST HEALTH STATUS**

1. Perinatal history
   a. General health of mother during pregnancy
   b. Complications of pregnancy: bleeding, falls, swelling of hands and feet, high blood pressure, unusual weight gain
   c. Medications taken during pregnancy
   d. Radiographs taken
   e. Emotional state of mother during pregnancy: crying or depression states
   f. Pregnancy planned?
   g. Father's attitude
   h. Pregnancy history (para, gravida, abortions, miscarriages)
2. Labor and delivery
   a. Date and place of birth
   b. Complications
   c. Anesthesia used for delivery
   d. Number of weeks of gestation
   e. Type of delivery (breech, vertex, cesarean section)
   f. Weight
   g. Length
   h. Did baby cry immediately?
   i. Was there cyanosis, jaundice, or respiratory problems?
   j. Did baby go to the regular nursery?
   k. Was any special equipment used for the baby?
   l. Was baby discharged from hospital with mother?
3. Newborn
   a. Initial problems with feeding, formula, colic, diarrhea
   b. Choking spells
   c. Blue spells
   d. Excessive crying
4. Growth and development
   Unlike the developmental data collected under current health status, this section includes a survey of significant developmental milestones.
   a. General statement as to how this child compares with siblings
   b. Does parent feel that the child's growth and development have been normal?
   c. Note age: rolled over, sat up, walked, first tooth, first words, toilet trained
5. State age and complications of each: chickenpox, rubella, measles, mumps, whooping cough, hay fever
6. State age and complications of each serious or chronic illness: meningitis or encephalitis, pneumonia or chronic lung problems, rheumatic fever, asthma, hay fever, scarlet fever, diabetes, kidney problems, hypertension, sickle cell anemia, seizure disorders, blood infections, etc.
7. State age and extent of each serious accident or injury: head injuries, fractures, burns, traumas, poisonings, etc.
8. Hospitalizations: list reason, location, primary care providers, duration, and how child reacted to hospitalization
9. Operations: what, where, when, why, by whom
10. Emotional health: past behavior problems, help sought, support persons, how child reacted to stress

**FAMILY HISTORY**

Family members include the client's blood relatives. Specifically the interviewer should inquire about the client's maternal and paternal grandparents, parents, aunts, uncles, and siblings. The interviewer should inquire about the general health, stress factors, and illnesses of family members. Questions should include a survey of the following:

| | |
|---|---|
| Cancer | Hypertension |
| Diabetes | Sickle cell anemia |
| Heart problems | Blindness |
| Mental retardation | Endocrine diseases |
| Learning problems | Kidney diseases |
| Cystic fibrosis | Birth defects |
| Asthma | Infant deaths |
| Other allergies | Other chronic problems |
| Seizure disorders | |

**REVIEW OF PHYSIOLOGICAL SYSTEMS**

1. General
   a. Frequent colds, infections, or illnesses
   b. Frequent fevers, sweats
   c. Fatigue patterns
   d. Energetic or overactive patterns
2. Nutritional
   a. Recent weight gain or loss (describe)
   b. Appetite
   c. Twenty-four-hour diet recall, including types, amount of food eaten (formula, breast milk, meat, fruits, vegetables, cereals, juices, eggs, sweets, milk, snacks), and frequency (i.g., how many times a day or week)
   d. Child feeding self?
   e. Where does child eat?
   f. Who does child eat with?
   g. Parent's perception of child's nutritional status (note problems)
   h. Vitamins?
   i. Junk food consumption (amount and kinds)
3. Integumentary
   a. Skin
      (1) Chronic rashes
      (2) Easy bruising or petechiae
      (3) Easy bleeding
      (4) Acne (treatment pattern)
      (5) Excessive sweating
      (6) Skin diseases, problems, or lesions
      (7) Itching
      (8) Pigmentation changes, discolorations, mottling
      (9) Excessive dryness
      (10) Skin growths or tumors
   b. Hair
      (1) Changes in amount, texture, characteristics
      (2) Infections, lice
      (3) Alopecia
   c. Nails
      (1) Changes in appearance
      (2) Cyanosis
      (3) Texture
4. Head
   a. Headache (frequency, type, location, duration, care for)
   b. Past significant trauma
   c. Dizziness
   d. Syncope
5. Eyes
   a. Crossed eyes
   b. Strabismus
   c. Discharge
   d. Complaint of vision changes
   e. Reading difficulty
   f. Sitting close to television
   g. History of infections
   h. Pruritus
   i. Excessive tearing
   j. Pain in eyeball
   k. Swelling around eyes
   l. Cataracts
   m. Unusual sensations or twitching
   n. Excessive blinking
   o. Eye injury history
   p. Currently wears glasses
   q. Diplopia
   r. Blurring
   s. Gives history of inability to see distant images
6. Ears
   a. Multiple infections or earaches
   b. Myringotomy tubes in ears
   c. Discharge
   d. Cerumen
   e. Care habits
   f. Cracking or ringing
   g. Parent perceives problem in child's hearing
7. Nose, nasopharynx, and paranasal sinuses
   a. Discharge (character of)
   b. Epistaxis
   c. Allergies
   d. General olfactory ability
   e. Pain over sinuses
   f. Postnasal drip
   g. Sneezing
   h. Nasal stuffiness
8. Mouth and throat
   a. Sore throats (frequent)

    b. Tonsils present
    c. Mouth sores
    d. Toothaches, caries
    e. Voice changes
    f. Hoarseness
    g. Mouth breathing
    h. Chewing difficulties
    i. Swallowing difficulties
    j. Teeth brushing pattern

9. Neck
    a. Swollen glands
    b. Tenderness
    c. Limitations of movement
    d. Stiffness

10. Breast: applicable only with teenagers; refer to adult data base

11. Cardiovascular
    a. History of murmur
    b. History of heart problem
    c. Palpitations
    d. Hypertension
    e. Postural hypotension
    f. Cyanosis (what precipitates)
    g. Dyspnea on exertion
    h. Limitation of activities
    i. Frequent complaints of extremity coldness

12. Respiratory
    a. Breathing trouble
    b. Chronic cough
    c. Wheezing (precipitating factors)
    d. Croup history
    e. Noisy breathing
    f. Shortness of breath

13. Hematolymphatic
    a. Lymph node swelling (note frequency and location)
    b. Excessive bleeding or easy bruising
    c. Anemia
    d. Blood dyscrasias
    e. Lead exposures; deleading in past

14. Gastrointestinal
    a. Ulcer history
    b. Previously diagnosed problem
    c. Vomiting
    d. Diarrhea
    e. Constipation or stool-holding problems
    f. Rectal bleeding
    g. Stool color change
    h. Abdominal pains
    i. Pinworms by history
    j. Perianal pruritus
    k. Use of evacuation aids
    l. Toilet trained? If not, is it planned? Any problems?

15. Urinary
    a. Urinary tract infections during past year
    b. Previously diagnosed problems
    c. Characteristics of urine (cloudy, dark)
    d. Suprapubic pains
    e. Steadiness and force of urination stream
    f. Dysuria
    g. Nocturia
    h. Bed wetting (Associated with emotional upsets? Family history of bed wetting?)
    i. Urinary frequency
    j. Dribbling or incontinence
    k. Polyuria/oliguria
    l. Bubble bath used?

16. Genital
    a. Birth defects
    b. Discharges
    c. Odors
    d. Rashes, irritation
    e. Pruritus
    f. How is sexuality education handled in the home?
    g. Areas of concern
    h. If client is female and menstruating, refer to adult data base for appropriate questioning

17. Musculoskeletal
    a. Muscles
       (1) Twitching
       (2) Cramping
       (3) Pain
       (4) Weakness
       (5) Pain with use
    b. Extremities
       (1) General complaints of pain, weakness, deformity
       (2) Night pains in legs
       (3) Gait ability—strength and coordination
    c. Bones and joints
       (1) Joint swelling
       (2) Joint pain
       (3) Redness, stiffness
       (4) Joint deformity
       (5) Fracture or dislocation history
    d. Back
       (1) History of back injury
       (2) Curvature of spine
       (3) Characteristics of problems and corrective measures

18. Central nervous system
    a. General
       (1) Unusual episodic behaviors
       (2) History of central nervous system diseases
       (3) Birth injury
    b. Seizure: febrile versus afebrile

    c.  Speech
        (1) Stuttering
        (2) Speech misarticulations
        (3) Language delay
    d.  Cognitive changes
        (1) Hallucinations
        (2) Passing out episodes
        (3) Staring spells
        (4) Learning difficulties
    e.  Motor-gait
        (1) Coordination
        (2) Developmental clumsiness
        (3) Balance problems
        (4) Tic
        (5) Tremor, spasms
    f.  Sensory
        (1) Pain patterns
        (2) Tingling sensations
19. Endocrine
    a.  Diagnosis of disease states (e.g., thyroid, diabetes)
    b.  Changes in skin texture (e.g., increased or decreased dryness or perspiration)
    c.  Pigmentation
    d.  Abnormal hair distribution
    e.  Sudden or unexplained changes in height and weight
    f.  Intolerance to heat or cold
    g.  Exophthalmos
    h.  Goiter
    i.  Polydipsia (increased thirst)
    j.  Polyphagia (increased food intake)
    k.  Polyuria (increased urination)
    l.  Anorexia (decreased appetite)
    m.  Weakness
    n.  Precocious puberty
20. Allergic and immunological
    a.  Dermatitis (inflammation or irritation of the skin)
    b.  Eczema
    c.  Pruritus (itching)
    d.  Urticaria (hives)
    e.  Sneezing
    f.  Vasomotor rhinitis (inflammation and swelling of mucous membrane of nose; nasal discharge)
    g.  Conjunctivitis (inflammation of conjunctiva)
    h.  Interference with activities of daily living
    i.  Environmental and seasonal causes
    j.  Treatment techniques

**PSYCHOSOCIAL HISTORY**

1.  General status
    a.  General statement of child's feeling about self
    b.  Parents' observations of child's feelings of self

2.  Caretakers and family
    a.  Who lives in the child's home
    b.  Primary care provider for child
    c.  Child's position in home environment
    d.  Relationships among members
3.  Friends
    a.  How does child get along with friends, classmates, siblings?
    b.  Plays with older, younger, same age children?
    c.  Does child make friends easily?
4.  Activities of daily living
    a.  General
        (1) General description of typical day
        (2) Sleep patterns and naps: sound sleeper or fretful; numbers of hours per 24 hours; nightmares; other nighttime activity (e.g., wakes up at night); how does parent respond?
        (3) Kinds of play: amount of active and quiet play per 24 hours; television time per 24 hours
        (4) Significant hobbies or methods of relaxation (for older child)
    b.  Family
        (1) Does family do things as unit?
        (2) What are methods of discipline within family?
        (3) Is discipline effective?
        (4) Who disciplines child?
        (5) How does child react to discipline?
        (6) Parents or providers: type of employment; type of child care provided if both parents work
        (7) Does mother have emotional support for her care of child as well as time away from child?
    c.  School
        (1) Present grade in school or level of nursery care
        (2) School performance
        (3) Behavior problems
        (4) Grades skipped
        (5) Learning problems; in special class?
        (6) Attitude about school
        (7) Rate of absenteeism
5.  Ability to cope with stress
    a.  General statement: activities of daily living, family, school
    b.  How does child adapt to new situations?
    c.  Have there been any recent changes or stresses in child's life-style (home, school)?
    d.  Behavior patterns child uses to cope with stress
    e.  Change in personality, behavior, or mood
    f.  History of psychiatric care or counseling

**HEALTH MAINTENANCE EFFORTS**

1. General statement about physical fitness (parent attitudes and child opinion)
2. Dietary regulations to maintain health
3. Frequency of physical, dental, and vision health assessment
4. Statement reflecting parents' attitude about the importance of health maintenance education, including:
   a. Self-care techniques
   b. Poison control safety
   c. First aid
   d. Toy safety
   e. Environmental safety

**ENVIRONMENTAL HEALTH***

1. General statement of parents' assessment of environmental safety and comfort
2. Hazards in the home, to include survey of the following:
   a. Toys appropriate for age
   b. Special protection from poisons, household products, or medications
   c. Stairway protection (e.g., use of gates for toddlers or handrails for older children)
   d. Yard equipment for play and safety
   e. Type of bed (protection device to prevent falling)
   f. Pest control problems
   g. Unsafe building (e.g., no heat, poor toilet facilities, open gas heaters)
3. Hazards in neighborhood
   a. Unsafe play area
   b. Heavily traveled streets
   c. No sidewalks
   d. Water or air pollution
   e. Noise factor
   f. Isolation or overcrowding from neighbors

## Clinical strategies: the pediatric client

1. Depending on the age of the child, it might be helpful to set a time that the examiner may collect information from the parent without the child's presence. It would be quite disappointing to collect an inadequate or incomplete profile because of the child's impatience.
2. A second option facilitating complete data base collection is to divide the content to be collected into several visits. Once the total information is collected, it should be documented as a single entry.

---

*In addition to the following lists, tools such as the ones found in Appendix B may provide objective analysis regarding observations of parent and the child and the child's home environment.

3. It is undesirable to try to collect a complete data base when the child is ill. The examiner, child, and parent are all likely to become frustrated. The most likely solution is to schedule a well visit specifically for data collection.
4. If the child is old enough to participate in the interview, be sure to include his information.
5. For older children and adolescents the child and parent may conflict on details of the problem or concern. The examiner should collect separate accounts from each source, record each one, and at the end analyze all the data. During the examination the examiner should ask the client if the parent's presence is desirable or not.
6. It is also appropriate to excuse the parent from the room while recording the history from the child or teenager. Our experience has been that most children or teenagers are direct with their information when not stressed by the presence of their parent. This is particularly true when discussing sexual, social, or psychological screening questions.
7. It has long been debated at what age to terminate using the pediatric data base tool and to begin using the adult data base tool. Although there is no easy solution to this question, the ages 12 to 14 seem to be a fairly common break-off point. Other examiners desire to make minor adjustments to the pediatric tool and to continue using it through adolescence. The choice is yours.
8. For additional strategies, refer to *Clinical strategies* in the adult data base.

## Total health data base for the geriatric client

Geriatric clients are not different from other adults. There is no specific age when concerns related to the aging process warrant additional screening questions to complete an accurate data base.

The following questions and concerns are directed toward elderly adults. Many of the questions concern problems of disability, chronic illness, or normal changes that take place with aging. There are many older people who do not have chronic illnesses, disabilities, or marked aging changes that affect their daily lives. The practitioner can use the following format when it seems to be appropriate.

**BIOGRAPHICAL DATA**

1. Name
2. Age
3. Race
4. Culture
5. Address

6. Marital status
7. Children and family in home
8. Occupation/retirement status
9. Means of transportation to health care facility, if pertinent
10. Description of home and size and type of community

## REASON FOR VISIT

Some elderly clients present a multitude of problems. Some complaints are long-standing (e.g., stiff joints, hypertension, dry skin, chronic constipation), and others are more acute. Certain problems are not easily identified and, with skilled questioning, emerge as the assessment progresses (e.g., depression, weight loss, weakness, difficulty caring for self at home).

Other clients tend to minimize pain or other symptoms. Older individuals may not manifest fever associated with infection to the extent that younger clients do. Some elderly individuals complain less of pain (e.g., cholecystitis, angina) or seem to experience less pain. New symptoms may be attributed to "getting old" and therefore are not reported as significant.

It takes time and patience to identify the *priorities* of the client's concerns (which may be different from the examiner's priorities). It often takes time and patience to establish the actual reason for the visit.

The final statement describing the reason(s) should be brief, stated in the client's own words, and limited to the *client's* immediate concerns. The final problem list, risk profile, and client profile can absorb (identify) the multiplicity of concerns that are not directly related to the chief complaint.

## PRESENT HEALTH STATUS

1. Summary of client's current major health concerns
2. If illness is present, record symptom analysis (box, p. 15)
   a. When was client last well
   b. Date of problem onset
   c. Character of complaint
   d. Nature of problem onset
   e. Course of problem
   f. Client's hunch of precipitating factors
   g. Location of problem
   h. Relation to
      (1) Other body symptoms
      (2) Body positions
      (3) Activity
   i. Patterns of problem
   j. Efforts of client to treat
   k. Coping ability

## CURRENT HEALTH DATA

1. Current medications (include prescriptions, over-the-counter drugs, vitamins, home remedies)
   a. Name of drug
   b. Prescribed when and by whom
   c. Amount prescribed per day
   d. Amount taken per day
   e. Problems with compliance: complicated or inconvenient dosage schedule, large number and variety of drugs prescribed, visual difficulty (unable to read label), unpleasant side effects, inability to afford drugs, difficulty swallowing or administering, inability to get to pharmacy, client fearful of addiction, client considers drug ineffective, client overdosing to relieve symptoms. If the client is taking a large number of prescribed drugs (often prescribed by different physicians), request that all medications be brought in for review. Clients are often unaware of the names or the purposes of all their drugs.
2. Allergies (describe agent and reactions)
   a. Drugs
   b. Foods
   c. Contact substances
   d. Environmental factors
3. Last examination (note physician/clinic, findings, advice, and/or instructions)
   a. Physical
   b. Dental
   c. Vision
   d. Hearing
   e. ECG
   f. Chest radiograph
   g. Pap smear (females)
   h. Proctoscopic
   i. Tonometry
4. Immunization status (note dates or year of last immunization)
   a. Tetanus, diphtheria
   b. Mumps
   c. Rubella
   d. Polio
   e. Tuberculosis tine test
   f. Influenza

## PAST HEALTH STATUS

1. Childhood illnesses: rubeola, rubella, mumps, pertussis, scarlet fever, chickenpox, strep throat
2. Serious or chronic illnesses: Parkinson disease, diabetes, hypertension, arthritis, bone diseases, cardiovascular disease, stroke, respiratory disease, kidney or urinary problems, nervous or seizure disorders, blood diseases or infections, gastrointestinal

dysfunction, gynecological disorders, cancer, thyroid problems, diseases of eyes or ears

If client offers a diagnosis that is not confirmed by health records, record it in quotes.

3. Serious accidents or injuries: head injuries, fractures, burns, other trauma
4. Hospitalizations: elaborate upon, listing reason, location, primary care providers, duration
5. Operations: what, where, when, why, by whom
6. Emotional health: past problems, help sought, support persons
7. Obstetrical history
   a. Complete pregnancies: number, pregnancy course, postpartum course, condition, weight, and sex of each
   b. Incomplete pregnancies: duration, termination, circumstances, including abortions and stillbirths
   c. Summary of complications

An elderly individual's past health history may be quite lengthy, complicated, and time-consuming to amass and organize. If the individual has no difficulty with vision or writing skills, it is helpful to have this portion completed at home in advance of the assessment.

**FAMILY HISTORY**

Family members include the client's blood relatives, spouse, and children. Specifically the interviewer should inquire about the client's maternal and paternal grandparents, parents, aunts, uncles, spouse, and children, as well as the general health, stress factors, and illnesses of family members. Questions should include a survey of the following:

| | |
|---|---|
| Cancer | Retardation |
| Diabetes | Alcoholism |
| Heart disease | Endocrine diseases |
| Hypertension | Sickle cell anemia |
| Epilepsy (or seizure disorder) | Kidney disease |
| Emotional stresses | Unusual limitations |
| Mental illness | Other chronic problems |

The most concise method to record these data is by a family tree. An elaborate family history may be less meaningful with the geriatric client, in terms of serving as a predictor of potential medical problems, since many familial diseases are contracted at an earlier age. Cancer and diabetes are exceptions. However, the family tree serves as a reference for knowing what past experiences (perhaps fears) the client has had with diseases, disabilities, and causes of death.

**REVIEW OF PHYSIOLOGICAL SYSTEMS**

1. General—reflect from client's previous description of current health status.
   a. Fatigue patterns
   b. Exercise and exercise tolerance
   c. Weakness episodes
   d. Fevers, sweats
   e. Frequent colds, infections, or illnesses
   f. Activities of daily living assessment (optional package; to be used if the client has multiple complaints or disabilities, such as visual loss, limited energy, motor skill deficits, mental difficulties, arthritic changes); see opposite page. When the multiplicity of diseases, symptoms, and side effects strikes an individual, the general health status is sometimes best assessed in terms of the *impact of disability* on one's daily life. This tool is particularly helpful if the client is living alone or with an elderly companion or spouse.
2. Nutritional
   a. Client's average, maximum, and minimum weights during past month, year, 5 years
   b. History of weight gain or loss (time element); specific efforts to change weight—if dieting, describe efforts and type of diet used
   c. If client is on a special diet, describe
   d. Current appetite patterns—food type preferences (e.g., sweets, fruits, convenience foods), amounts consumed at one time, hunger more marked at certain times of day or night, loss or gain in appetite recently or over past year
   e. Food consumption patterns (e.g., three meals a day, smaller meals five or six times a day, eating at night). Does client have a similar eating pattern from day to day? Does client eat with others or alone? A 24-hour recall may not be indicative of client's real eating pattern, which may vary greatly from day to day.
   f. Specific foods and amounts consumed; a 24-hour recall, if appropriate, or foods consumed over a week's or a month's time
   g. Fluid intake (24-hour estimate)
   h. Who buys, prepares food?
   i. If someone else prepares and buys food, is it to the client's liking? Ability to maintain special diet?
   j. If client buys own food, ask about access to market, walking (clarify distance), bus, driving, taxi, frequency of trips to market
   k. If client prepares food in own home, is preparation a problem (e.g., fatigue, eating alone, decreased vision, refrigerator, stove, water in rural area)?
   l. Problem with chewing (dentures fit or loose, teeth loose or painful, edentulous)
   m. Problem with swallowing, choking
   n. Is client able to afford the food desired and needed?

**Activities of daily living (ADL) assessment**

A. Self-care
  1. Dressing, undressing, clothing
     a. Keeping clothes in good repair (mending)
     b. Access to clothes
     c. Getting into and out of underwear (bra, girdle, underpants, pantyhose, stockings, garter belt)
     d. Putting on and removing pants
     e. Getting arms in sleeves
     f. Managing zippers, buttons, snaps (especially in back), ties
     g. Putting on socks, shoes, tying laces
     h. Applying prostheses (e.g., glasses, hearing aids)
  2. Grooming and hygiene
     a. Washing, drying, brushing hair
     b. Brushing teeth
     c. Cleaning and putting in dentures
     d. Shaving
     e. Nail care (feet and hands)
     f. Applying makeup
     g. Preparing bath water and testing temperature
     h. Getting into and out of tub, shower
     i. Reaching and cleaning all body parts
  3. Elimination
     a. Position altered for urination or sitting on toilet
     b. Ability to wipe self
     c. Lowering onto and rising from toilet
B. Mobility
  1. Difficulty climbing or descending stairs (Is bedroom/bathroom on upper level? How many stairs/flights to apartment or house?)
  2. Sitting up, rising from bed
  3. Lowering to or rising from chair
  4. Walking (short and long distances); describe necessity for walking
  5. Opening doors
  6. Reaching items in cupboards
  7. Necessity for lifting (and any difficulty)
C. Communication
  1. Dialing telephone
  2. Reading numbers
  3. Hearing over telephone
  4. Answering door
  5. Immediate access to neighbors, help
D. Eating (see nutritional section that follows for details about appetite, weight, food consumption)
  1. Access to market
  2. Preparing food (opening cans, packages, using stove, reaching dishes, pots, utensils)
  3. Handling knife, fork, spoon (cutting meat)
  4. Getting food to mouth
  5. Chewing, swallowing
E. Housekeeping, laundry, house upkeep
  1. Making bed
  2. Sweeping, mopping floors
  3. Dusting
  4. Cleaning dishes
  5. Cleaning tub, bathroom
  6. Picking up clutter (to client's satisfaction)
  7. Taking out trash, garbage
  8. Use of basement (stairs, cleaning)
  9. Laundry facilities (in home or near residence, washtub, clothesline)
  10. Yard care (garden, bushes, grass)
  11. Other home maintenance concerns (e.g., access to fuse box, storm windows, furnace filters, painting)
F. Medications
  1. Large number of prescriptions
  2. Difficulty remembering
  3. Ability to see labels/directions
  4. Medications kept in one area
G. Access to community
  1. Busline
  2. Walking
  3. Driving (self or service from others)
  4. Church, dry cleaning, drugstore, bank, health care facility, dentist, other community agencies
H. Other
  1. Caring for spouse/relative/companion
  2. Financial management (able to write checks, make payments, cash checks)
  3. Care of pet(s)

    o. Client's summary of own nutritional status
3. Integumentary
  a. Skin
    (1) Skin disease or skin problems or lesions (wounds, sores, ulcers)
    (2) Growths, tumors, masses
    (3) Excessive dryness, sweating, odors
    (4) Pigmentation changes or discolorations
    (5) Pruritus (itching), scratching
    (6) Texture changes
    (7) Temperature changes
    (8) Increased or excessive bruises, excoriations (especially in skinfolds), redness, or trauma marks
    (9) Healing pattern of bruises, cuts, etc. (time element)
    (10) Decreased sensation to pain, heat
    (11) Increased sensation to pain, heat, cold, itching
    (12) History of chronic sun exposure
  b. Hair
    (1) Thinning, falling out, dulling
    (2) Texture changes
    (3) Brittleness, breaking
    (4) Use of dyes, permanents
  c. Nails
    (1) Brittleness, peeling, breaking
    (2) Changes in appearance, texture
    (3) Toenails: thickening, difficulty cutting

4. Head
   a. Headache (do full symptom analysis)
   b. Past significant trauma
   c. Dizziness (associated with body position or change—sitting up, standing, or head/neck movement)
   d. Syncope
5. Eyes
   a. History of glaucoma
   b. Cataracts, infections (frequency, treatment)
   c. Discharge characteristics
   d. Itching
   e. Lacrimation, excessive tearing
   f. Loss (or decrease) of tears
   g. Pain in eyeball
   h. Swelling around eyes
   i. Spots, floaters
   j. Unusual visual effects (e.g., light flashes, halos or rainbows around lights)
   k. General vision changes
   l. Loss of lateral vision (narrowing fields, tunnel vision)
   m. Double vision
   n. Sensitivity to glare
   o. Difficulty with night vision
   p. Difficulty distinguishing colors (e.g., traffic lights)
   q. Photophobia
   r. Blurring
   s. Difficulty reading
   t. Use of corrective or prosthetic devices (bifocals)
   u. Unusual sensations, twitching
   v. If bifocals, any problems with adjusting to far vision (e.g., stepping up on a curb)
   w. Do vision changes interfere with activities of daily living?
6. Ears
   a. Pain (pattern, position related?)
   b. Cerumen (wax)
   c. Infection
   d. Vertigo
   e. Ringing and cracking
   f. Care habits
   g. Hearing changes
   h. Use of prosthetic devices
   i. Increased sensitivity to environmental noise
   j. Interference with activities of daily living
   k. Does conversation (of others) sound garbled or distorted?
   l. If hearing aid is used, does client feel it is effective? Who prescribed it? How long ago? Does client wear it all the time?

7. Nose, nasopharynx, paranasal sinuses
   a. Discharge (characteristics)
   b. Epistaxis
   c. Allergies
   d. Pain over sinuses
   e. Postnasal drip
   f. Sneezing
   g. Dry nasal passages/crusting
   h. Painful nose breathing
   i. Mouth breathing
   j. General olfactory ability
8. Mouth and throat
   a. Sore throats
   b. Sore mouth
   c. Dry mouth
   d. Lesions (sores, ulcers, bumps on tongue, mouth, gums)
   e. Bleeding gums
   f. Burning mouth, palate, tongue
   g. Toothache
   h. Loose teeth
   i. Missing teeth
   j. Altered taste
   k. Chewing difficulty
   l. Swallowing difficulty
   m. Prosthetic devices (dentures, bridges)
   n. If client has dentures:
      (1) Wearing habits (e.g., for meals only, for appearance only, always, seldom, or never wears)
      (2) Wearing problems (e.g., rubbing or tenderness, looseness, clicking noises, talking difficulty, whistling dentures)
      (3) Cleaning habits and problems
   o. Sores at corner of mouth (associated with edentulous patients or ill-fitting dentures)
   p. Bad breath
   q. Bad taste in mouth
   r. Hoarseness
   s. Voice changes
   t. Pattern of dental hygiene
9. Neck
   a. Node enlargement
   b. Swellings, masses
   c. Tenderness
   d. Limitation of movement
   e. Stiffness
10. Breast
    a. Pain or tenderness
    b. Swelling
    c. Nipple discharge
    d. Changes in nipples
    e. Lumps, dimples

f. Unusual characteristics

g. Irritated skin under pendulous breasts, rubbing bra

h. Breast examination pattern, frequency

11. Cardiovascular
   a. Cardiovascular—chest pain may be reduced, even absent, in elderly. Dyspnea on exertion may be a primary symptom.
      (1) Chest pain (do full symptom analysis)
      (2) Dyspnea on exertion (specify *amount* of exertion, e.g., three stairs vs. one flight with 2-minute rest at landing; walking one block vs. walking from bed to bath)
      (3) Palpitations
      (4) Unusual breathing patterns (e.g., Cheyne-Stokes)
      (5) Orthopnea
      (6) Paroxysmal nocturnal dyspnea
      (7) Episodes of confusion
   b. Peripheral vascular
      (1) Coldness
      (2) Loss of sensation to pain, touch
      (3) Exaggerated response to cold (pain)
      (4) Pain associated with exercise
      (5) Color changes (especially feet and ankles: bluish-red or ruddy, mottling, pallor, associated with position)
      (6) Swelling (specify time of day; do full symptom analysis)
      (7) Varicosities
      (8) Does client wear constrictive clothing (e.g., girdles, garters, or stockings rolled at knees)?
   c. Heart and hypertension medications: toxicity symptoms
      The examiner need not pose questions about all these symptoms but should be alert to symptom groupings or patterns of drug reactions. Many clients take digitalis preparations, diuretics, and/or antihypertensive medications. The box opposite shows the major side effects and chief symptoms associated with toxicity.

12. Respiratory
   a. History of wheezing, bronchitis, other breathing problems
   b. Painful breathing (on deep or regular inspiration)
   c. Smoking (detailed questions covered under habits)
   d. Chronic cough (do full symptom analysis—specify time of day or night that cough is bothersome)
   e. Sputum production (amount, color, time element)

f. Hemoptysis

g. Night sweats

h. Exertional capacity (report present status and any recent change)
   (1) Shortness of breath (SOB) with heavy, sustained work (e.g., lifting, digging, snow shoveling)
   (2) SOB with sudden high-speed exercise (e.g., jogging, brisk walking, bicycling)
   (3) SOB with exertion at slower pace (e.g., slow walk around the block, light housekeeping)
   (4) SOB with slight exertion (e.g., rising from chair, walking from one room to another)

i. Has client been less active or immobilized recently or in past year for reasons other than respiratory (e.g., foot problems, fractured hip, arthritic pain)?

13. Hematolymphatic
   a. Lymph node swelling
   b. Excessive bleeding or easy bruising
   c. Petechiae, ecchymoses
   d. Anemia
   e. Blood transfusions
   f. Excessive fatigue
   g. Radiation exposure

14. Gastrointestinal
   a. Abdominal pain (heartburn, indigestion, pain in lower abdomen; specify if pain is associated with eating, before or after; do full symptom analysis)
   b. Excessive belching (sour taste, associated with pain?)
   c. Anorexia

| Digitalis | Diuretics | Anti-hypertensives |
|---|---|---|
| Anorexia | Fatigue | Lethargy |
| Nausea, vomiting, diarrhea | Weakness | Mood disturbances |
| Headache | Muscle cramps | Sedation |
| Drowsiness | Gastrointestinal distress | Postural syncope |
| Vision changes (yellow, brown, green vision, halos around lights) | Confusion | Dizziness |
|  |  | Nausea |
|  |  | Diarrhea |
| Arrhythmias (all varieties) |  | Fluid retention |
| Confusion |  | Drug rash |

d. Nausea, vomiting
e. Food idiosyncrasies (long-standing or recent)
f. Bloating
g. Flatulence
h. Grumbling bowel
i. Diarrhea
j. Swollen abdomen
k. Jaundice
l. Hemorrhoids (pain, bleeding, amount)
m. Bowel habits (frequency, defecation difficulty, straining)
n. Change in bowel habits
o. Describe stool (color, size, consistency)
p. Constipation (describe client's concern in detail, including use of digestive or evacuation aids)

15. Urinary
    a. Characteristics of urine; note changes (color, odor, clarity)
    b. Voiding pattern (in 24-hour period); note number of times client is up at night; note any recent change in pattern
    c. Characteristics of urine
    d. Urination pattern/problems (retention, incomplete emptying, straining to void, change in force of stream—does man have to stand closer to toilet?—hesitancy, dribbling, incontinence with stress, sneezing, coughing)
    e. Painful urination
    f. Urgency, frequency
    g. Oliguria (decrease in output)
    h. Polyuria (increase in output)
    i. Pyuria
    j. Hematuria
    k. Flank, groin, low back, or suprapubic pain

16. Genital
    a. General
       (1) Lesions
       (2) Discharges
       (3) Odors
       (4) Pain, burning, pruritus (itching)
       (5) Venereal disease history
       (6) Sexually active? If so, satisfaction with sexual activity
    b. Males
       (1) History of prostate trouble
       (2) Scrotal lumps, masses, surface changes
       (3) If uncircumcised, difficulty retracting foreskin
       (4) Scrotum self-examination practices
       (5) Does client have full erection, can he maintain erection to his satisfaction, complete ejaculation?
       (6) Pain preceding, during, or following erection

    c. Females
       (1) Menopause history (onset, course, LMP, associated problems, residual problems, any bleeding since LMP)
       (2) Any severe problems with menstrual history
       (3) Soreness or tenderness of vagina
       (4) Pressure sensation within vagina
       (5) Dyspareunia (pain with intercourse)

17. Musculoskeletal—history of injuries, fractures, dislocations, whiplash
    a. Muscles
       (1) Twitching
       (2) Cramping
       (3) Weakness or pain with use (location of weakness; activity such as stair climbing altered by weakness)
       (4) Manual dexterity problems
       (5) Other interferences with activities of daily living
    b. Extremities
       (1) Deformity or coordination difficulties
       (2) Problems with shoes (fit, rubbing)
       (3) Restless legs
       (4) Transient paresthesia—need to move legs at night
    c. Gait
       (1) Any alterations noted by client (e.g., weakness, balance, difficulty with steps, fear of falling)
       (2) Walking aids (cane, walker, special shoes; does client feel that aids are effective; any difficulty maneuvering aid?)
    d. Bones and joints
       (1) Joint swelling, pain, redness, deformity
       (2) Stiffness (pronounced at certain times of day, associated with or following activity or inactivity)
       (3) Limited movement (specify location, which joint)
       (4) Crepitation (creaking noise on movement)
       (5) Interference with activities of daily living
    e. Back
       (1) Pain (do full symptom analysis)
       (2) Stiffness
       (3) Corrective measures (use of bed board, special mattress, prosthetic devices)
       (4) Interference with activities of daily living
       (5) Client's assessment of effectiveness of prosthetic devices; any difficulty applying?

18. Central nervous system—history of any disease
    a. Seizure (characteristics, medications for)
    b. Speech

(1) Unusual speech patterns
(2) Aphasia
(3) Dysarthria (stammering)
c. Cognitive changes
(1) Inability to remember (recent vs. remote)
(2) Disorientation
(3) Phobias
(4) Hallucinations
(5) Passing out episodes
(6) Interference with activities of daily living
d. Motor-gait
(1) Coordinated movement
(2) Ataxia, balance problems
(3) Paralysis (partial vs. complete)
(4) Tic
(5) Tremor, spasm
(6) Interference with activities of daily living
e. Sensory
(1) Tingling sensations
(2) Areas of paresthesia (patterns)
(3) Other changes
19. Endocrine
a. Diagnosis of disease states (e.g., thyroid, diabetes)
b. Changes in skin pigmentation or texture
c. Changes in or abnormal hair distribution
d. Sudden or unexplained changes in height and weight
e. Intolerance of heat or cold
f. Exophthalmos
g. Goiter
h. Hormone therapy
i. Polydipsia (increased thirst)
j. Polyphagia (increased food intake)
k. Polyuria (increased urination)
l. Anorexia (decreased appetite)
m. Weakness
20. Allergic and immunological (Optional; use if client indicates allergic history. Note precipitating factors in each case.)
a. Dermatitis (inflammation or irritation of skin)
b. Eczema
c. Pruritus (itching)
d. Urticaria (hives)
e. Sneezing
f. Vasomotor rhinitis (inflammation and swelling of mucous membrane of nose; nasal discharge)
g. Conjunctivitis (inflammation of conjunctiva)
h. Interference with activities of daily living
i. Environmental and seasonal causes
j. Treatment techniques
21. Does client have any other physiological problems or disease states not specifically discussed? If so, explore in detail.

## PSYCHOSOCIAL HISTORY

1. General statement of client's feelings about self
2. Relatives and friends, in home, or nearby (sexual needs, affection, support). If individual lives alone: (a) to what extent is being alone tolerated; (b) does client have sufficient and satisfactory access to family and friends; (c) does client have a pet? If client lives with family: (a) are relationships satisfactory (with spouse, children, grandchildren); (b) does client participate in activities (meals, recreation) with family; (c) does client participate in family decisions; is there conflict?
3. Environment: is it adequately warm, sufficiently and conveniently spacious, sufficiently private, comfortable, safe, affordable?
4. Time/energy: too much or too little time to carry out daily life; does client have sufficient energy to meet needs?
5. Activities of daily living (see pp. 26-27 for details)
a. General description of work, leisure, and rest distribution
b. Significant hobbies or methods of relaxation
c. Family demands
d. Community activities and involvement (e.g., church, club)
e. Transportation
(1) Automobile: estimate amount of driving; does client consider himself safe (last driving test); financial problems with gas, upkeep, insurance
(2) Bus: easy access; availability to necessary and desired destinations; problems getting onto bus, tolerating wait
(3) Taxi: estimate amount used (financial burden)
(4) Driving services from others: availability, convenience
(5) Walking: problems with distance, carrying packages, using curbs and stairs, bad weather, fear of traffic
f. Occupational/volunteer history
(1) Major jobs held in past
(2) Current employment
(3) Volunteer and community activities
(4) Satisfaction with present activities
g. Work/retirement concerns
(1) Reduced/fixed income
(2) Moving or selling home
(3) Role change/time adjustment
(4) Problems in relationship with spouse because of retirement
6. General statement about client's ability to cope with activities of daily living
7. Recent changes or stresses in life-style: illness of

self or family member; death of spouse, close friend, or family member; retirement, moving, financial changes

8. Patterns in which client copes with stress: use of resources, worry pattern
9. Is there any history of psychiatric care or counseling?
10. Feelings of anxiety or nervousness; describe characteristics and coping mechanisms
11. Feelings of depression (consider symptoms such as insomnia, crying, fearfulness, marked irritability, or anger; review medication intake)
12. Changes in personality, behavior, or mood
13. Specific feelings of satisfaction/or frustration: aging changes, setting goals and meeting them, work activities, use of leisure time, mental capacity, intellectual capacity, aspirations
14. Use of drugs or other techniques during times of anxiety or stress
15. Response to illness
    a. Does the client cope satisfactorily during times of own or others' illness?
    b. Do the client's family and friends respond satisfactorily during periods of illness?
16. Physical well-being, particular fears and concerns about death
17. Habits
    a. Alcohol
       (1) Kinds (beer, wine, mixed drinks)
       (2) Frequency per week
       (3) Pattern over past 5 years, 1 year
       (4) Drinking companions?
       (5) Drinks when anxious?
    b. Smoking
       (1) Kind (pipe, cigarette, cigar)
       (2) Amount per week/day
       (3) Pattern over past 5 years, 1 year
       (4) Smokes with whom?
       (5) Smokes when anxious?
       (6) Desire to quit smoking? (method of attempts)
    c. Coffee and tea
       (1) Amount per day
       (2) Pattern over past 5 years, 1 year
       (3) Drinks more coffee when anxious?
       (4) Physiological effects
    d. Sleep
       (1) Has sleep pattern altered recently or in past year?
       (2) Sleep needs being met (fatigue)?
       (3) Concerns about interruptions at night (e.g., pain, SOB, nocturia, light sleeping, insomnia—specify difficulty falling asleep, staying asleep, awakening too early in morning)

(4) Excessive napping during day
(5) Inability to stay awake
(6) Describe *all* client efforts to regulate sleep (e.g., drugs, prescriptions, alcohol, warm milk, reading)

    e. Other
       (1) Overeating, sporadic eating
       (2) Nail biting
       (3) Withdrawal (e.g., sleeping)
18. Financial status
    a. Sources
    b. Adequacy
    c. Recent changes in resources/expenditures

## HEALTH MAINTENANCE EFFORTS

1. General statement of client's own physical fitness
2. Exercise: amount, type, frequency
3. Dietary regulations: special efforts (describe in detail)
4. Mental health: special efforts, such as group therapy, meditation, yoga
5. Cultural or religious practices
6. How often does the client seek:
   (a) Physical health assessment
   (b) Dental health assessment
   (c) Vision health assessment

## ENVIRONMENTAL HEALTH

1. General statement of client's assessment of environmental safety and comfort. Is client's community safe?
2. Hazards of employment: inhalants, noise, heavy lifting, psychological stress, machinery
3. Hazards in the home: concern about fire, stairs to climb, inadequate heat, open gas heaters, inadequate toilet facilities, concern about pest control, inadequate space
4. Hazards in neighborhood: noise, water pollution, air pollution, inadequate police protection, heavy traffic on surrounding streets, isolation from neighbors, overcrowding
5. Community hazards: unavailability of grocery stores, laundry facilities, drugstore; no access to bus line
6. Safety assessment (Optional; to be used if client is disabled or has difficulty with activities of daily living. This section suggests some major hazards.)
    a. Gait and balance problems
       (1) Slippery or irregular surfaces (floors, icy sidewalks, rug edges, small rugs, risers on stairs not fastened down)
       (2) Obstructions or clutter (on stairs, extension cords)
       (3) Steep, dark stairs (cellar)

(4) Bathtub slippery (oil in bath water)

(5) Shoes without support, laces untied

(6) Climbing: use of ladders to paint, make home repairs, replace light bulb, etc.

(7) Clothing too long

(8) Walking in heavy traffic areas

b. Decreased vision

(1) Insufficient illumination in home (dark hallways, stairways, no night light)

(2) Glare from polished floors, excess lighting

(3) Missing the bottom step

(4) Bifocals (client has difficulty with far vision, descending stairs, curb)

(5) Medication errors

c. Decreased sensation to pain and heat

(1) Hot bath water

(2) Heating pads, hot water bottles

d. Other

(1) Fire hazards: loose sleeves over stove burner, electric cords frayed, open heaters, stove burners left on, smoking (especially in bed)

(2) Driving and traffic accidents: slow reaction time, decreased vision, difficulty turning head with upper torso (arthritis), walking too slow for traffic signals

## Clinical strategies: the geriatric client

1. Many older people don't seem to "fit" into traditional clinics. If there is a tight appointment schedule, the examiner and client have time for little other than assessing immediate, acute problems.

a. Older clients often have a long story to tell (especially medical history)

b. Their reaction time may be slower. It takes longer for them to reflect and respond to questions.

c. Many of them have had unpleasant experiences being hurried or pressured (in department stores, heavy traffic, etc.). They may enter the health care facility with a reluctance to take up your time.

d. It takes *time* to develop trust with clients so that they will be willing to share their concerns.

2. If clinic (or employer) policies cannot be altered to meet geriatric client needs, some alternatives might be helpful.

a. Gather and organize all available history data from other sources before interviewing the client.

b. Ask the client to complete the medical history at home (if no vision or writing problems exist).

c. Spread out the data base collection over several appointments.

d. Supplement clinic visits with a home visit.

e. Set aside 1 day a week or month for prolonged appointments to collect initial data base from new clients.

f. Insist that time be made available! Otherwise, the client's needs are not being fully assessed.

3. Visual and hearing losses can distort information exchange. The examiner may believe the client is confused; the client may merely have difficulty hearing the examiner. Limitations of hearing and sight must be assessed early in the interview.

4. Do not shout. This rarely helps in communicating with those who have diminished hearing. It often further distorts conversation.

5. Directly face the client for a full view of your face. Speak slowly and distinctly.

6. Refer to *Clinical strategies* in the adult data base section for further suggestions.

## SUGGESTED READINGS

### General

Barsky, A.J., and others: Evaluating the interview in primary care medicine, Soc. Sci. Med. (Med. Psychol. Med. Sociol.) **14A**(6):653-658, 1980.

Bates, B.: A guide to physical examination, ed. 3, Philadelphia, 1983, J.B. Lippincott Co., pp. 1-27, 513-525.

Ber, R., and Alroy, G.: The teaching of history-taking and diagnostic thinking: description of a method, Med. Educ. **15**:97-99, 1981.

Cutler, P.: Problem solving in clinical medicine: from data to diagnosis, Baltimore, 1979, Williams & Wilkins.

Diekelmann, N.: Primary health care of the well adult, New York, 1977, McGraw-Hill Book Co., pp. 213-235.

Engle, G.L., and Morgan, W.L.: Interviewing the patient, London, 1973, W.B. Saunders Co., Ltd.

Gordon, M.: Nursing diagnosis: process and application, New York, 1982, McGraw-Hill Book Co.

Mahoney, E.A., Verdisco, L., and Shortridge, L.: How to collect and record a health history, Philadelphia, 1976, J.B. Lippincott Co.

Malasanos, L., and others: Health assessment, ed. 2, St. Louis, 1981, The C.V. Mosby Co., pp. 1-14, 25-57.

Patient assessment: taking a patient history, Programmed instruction, Am. J. Nurs. **74**(2):293-324, 1974.

Platt, F.W., and McMath, J.C.: Clinical hypocompetence: the interview, Ann. Intern. Med. **91**(6):898-900, 1979.

Prior, J.A., Silberstein, J.S., and Stang, J.M.: Physical diagnosis: the history and examination of the patient, ed. 6, St. Louis, 1981, The C.V. Mosby Co., pp. 2-35.

### Pediatric

Alexander, M., and Brown, M.S.: Pediatric history taking and physical diagnosis for nurses, ed. 2, New York, 1979, McGraw-Hill Book Co., pp. 1-54.

DeAngelis, C.: Basic pediatrics for the primary health care provider, Boston, 1975, Little, Brown & Co., pp. 1-14.

Malasanos, L., and others: Health assessment, ed. 2, St. Louis, 1981, The C.V. Mosby Co., pp. 559-590.

Pillitteri, A.: Nursing care of the growing family: a child health text, Boston, 1977, Little, Brown & Co., pp. 121-141, 163-169, 187-193, 213-224, 241-249.

Powell, M.L.: Assessment and management of developmental changes and problems in children, ed. 2, St. Louis, 1981, The C.V. Mosby Co.

Whaley, L.F., and Wong, D.L.: Nursing care of infants and children, ed. 2, St. Louis, 1983, The C.V. Mosby Co., pp. 87-99.

### Geriatric

Brown, M.: Readings in gerontology, ed. 2, St. Louis, 1978, The C.V. Mosby Co.

Burnside, I.M., editor: Nursing and the aged, ed. 2, New York, 1981, McGraw-Hill Book Co., pp. 325-347, 350-359, 428-436, 438-449.

Combs, K.L.: Preventative care in the elderly, Am. J. Nurs. **78**(8):1339-1341, 1978.

Diekelmann, N.: Pre-retirement counseling, Am. J. Nurs. **78** (8):1337-1338, 1978.

Dresen, S.E.: Autonomy: a continuing developmental task, Am. J. Nurs. **78**(8):1334-1346, 1978.

Gotz, B.E.: Drugs and the elderly, Am. J. Nurs. **78**(8):1347-1351, 1978.

Hogstel, M.: How do the elderly view their world? Am. J. Nurs. **78**(8):1335-1336, 1978.

Kalish, R.: Late adulthood: perspectives on human development, Monterey, Calif., 1975, Brooks/Cole Publishing Co., pp. 22-46.

Katz, S., and others: Studies of illness in the aged. The index of ADL: a standardized measure of biological and psychosocial function, J.A.M.A. **185**:94-99, 1963.

Kerzner, L.J., Greb, L., and Steel, K.: History-taking forms and the care of geriatric patients, J. Med. Educ. **57**(5):376-379, 1982.

Storz, R.R.: The role of a professional nurse in a health maintenance program, Nurs. Clin. North Am. **7**(2): 207-223, 1972.

# General and mental status assessment

## VOCABULARY

**affect** Observable behaviors indicating an individual's feelings or emotions.

**blocking** Interruption in a train of thought, loss of an idea, or repression of a feeling or idea from conscious awareness; can be a normal behavior or, in extreme form, indicative of abnormality.

**catatonia** Extreme physical immobility and rigidity; often associated with a schizophrenic state.

**compulsive behavior** A repetitive act that usually originates from an obsession; extreme anxiety emerges if the act is not completed.

**confabulation** The fabrication of events or sequential experiences often recounted to cover up memory gaps.

**conversion reaction** Conversion of emotional disturbances into motor or sensory symptoms. EXAMPLES: blindness, paralysis.

**delusion** Persistent belief or perception that is illogical or improbable.

**dementia** A broad term that indicates impairment of intellectual functioning, memory, and judgment.

**depersonalization** Sense of being out of touch with one's environment; loss of a sense of reality and association with personal events.

**dysarthria** Speech disorder involving difficulty with articulation and pronunciation of specific sounds; results from loss of control over muscles of speech.

**dysphasia** Speech disorder involving difficulty with use of language and words to convey meaning to others; often associated with cerebral vascular accidents.

**dysphonia** Difficulty in controlling laryngeal speech sounds; can be a normal event such as male vocal changes occurring at puberty.

**echolalia** Meaningless repetition of another person's words; may be associated with schizophrenia.

**euphoria** Sense of elation or well-being; can be a normal feeling or may be exaggerated to unrelated to reality.

**hallucination** Sensory perception that does not arise from an external stimulus; can be auditory, visual, tactile, gustatory, or olfactory.

**illusion** Perceptual distortion of an external stimulus. EXAMPLE: mirage in a desert.

**neologism** Newly invented word or phrase that has meaning understood only by the person who coins it; often accompanies psychotic states.

**neurosis** Ineffective or troubled coping mechanism stemming from anxiety or emotional conflict.

**obsession** Persistent thought or idea that preoccupies the mind; not always realistic and may result in compulsive behavior.

**perseveration** The persistent repetition of words or phrases; may be associated with a psychotic state or organic brain syndrome.

**phobia** Uncontrollable, often unreasonable, and intense fear of a specific object or event.

**psychosis** Any major mental disorder characterized by greatly distorted perceptions and severe disorganization of personality.

**sensorium** Status of level of consciousness and orientation to surroundings.

**schizoid** Exhibiting behaviors or having characteristics that resemble schizophrenia.

**schizophrenia** Any one of a large group of psychotic disorders characterized by marked distortion of reality and disorganization of personality characteristics.

When a practitioner first encounters a client (perhaps from across the room), a steady stream of data can be observed. Some of it may not operate at a conscious level. The examiner may quickly decide that the client looks "ill," "depressed," "alert," or "pleasant." Many of those observations cannot be classified under body systems, but they are vitally important and must be reported in concrete terms. The word *ill* does not convey a clear message to the reader. The following description does:

Skin is ashen, cool to touch, and moist. The client is slumped in a chair, and body and extremities appear limp. Client does not establish eye contact and responds to all questions in a monotone "yes" or "no."

Observation skills are enhanced through practice and a concentrated awareness of incoming perceptions. Every element of the examiner's behavior should be deliberate and focused on the client. A simple handshake indicates the client's ability to extend the arm, to firmly grip the hand, to respond with a smile or facial expression acknowledging an introduction, and to establish and maintain eye contact. It also permits the examiner to feel the coolness, warmth, dryness, or moisture of the palm.

The purpose of this chapter is to clarify and organize specific, observable behaviors that are valid indications of the client's general state as well as emotional and mental well-being. Note that it is impossible to include all possible behaviors that a client might exhibit. This chapter contains descriptions representative of some more commonly found behaviors.

## Cognitive objectives

At the end of this chapter the learner will demonstrate knowledge of assessment of the client's general and mental status by the ability to do the following:
1. Identify meanings associated with the holistic concept.
2. Identify major components of the general assessment.
3. Point out some common behaviors associated with mild to moderate anxiety.
4. Identify some common behaviors associated with moderate to severe anxiety.
5. Distinguish some common behaviors associated with depression.
6. Identify methods by which an examiner can validate the suspicion that a client is disoriented.
7. Point out characteristics of behaviors associated with hallucinations.
8. Identify some disorders that can disrupt thought content.

9. Identify selected pediatric and geriatric variations of behaviors associated with general and mental status.
10. Use the terms in the vocabulary section.

## Clinical objectives

At the end of this chapter the learner will perform a systematic assessment of the general and mental status of the client, demonstrating the ability to do the following:
1. Describe specific behaviors related to observation of the client:
   a. Initial response to examiner
   b. Body appearance
   c. Posture
   d. Body movements
   e. Gait
   f. Facial expression
   g. Vocal tones
   h. Speech patterns: pace, clarity, word and sentence delivery, volume, accent, or foreign language
   i. Apparel
   j. Grooming/hygiene
   k. Odors
   l. General mannerisms
2. Describe specific behaviors indicating the client's cognitive functions:
   a. Orientation to person, place, time
   b. Attention span and concentration ability
   c. Memory—recent and remote
   d. Ability to make judgments
   e. Abstract reasoning ⎫
   f. Underlying intelligence ⎪
      (1) Access to basic information ⎬ Optional history questions
      (2) Vocabulary ⎪
      (3) Similarities ⎪
   g. Ability to read and write ⎭
3. Describe specific behaviors indicating the client's emotional status.
4. Describe specific behaviors that show the client's ability to sustain a clear thinking process: coherency, thought content, clarity of perceptions.
5. Summarize results of the assessment with a written description of findings.

## Health history additional to screening history

Most of the information needed for the assessment of the "normal" client's mental status can be obtained through the use of the general questions in the *Psychosocial history* in Chapter 1. Basically, these questions ask the client: How do you feel about yourself?

Are you living in a relatively low-stress environment? Are your coping abilities adequate to meet the stressors that you encounter in your daily living?

The answers to these questions can become more apparent by observing the client's general behavior (described subsequently). If the client's self-assessment and the examiner's assessment are congruent and if the results indicate that the client is coping adequately to meet personal needs, it is not necessary to pursue further quesitoning. However, if there is an incongruity between what the client states and the behavior displayed, if behavior disturbances are noted, or if activities of daily living are interrupted, the following detailed questions are helpful.

1.  Anxiety or depressive states
    a.  Do you have difficulty falling asleep, staying asleep, or being wakeful early in the morning?
    b.  Describe your general mood in the morning.
    c.  Have you noticed any marked changes in appetite or eating habits?
    d.  Have you recently lost or gained weight?
    e.  Do you have periods of despondency or nervousness to the extent that you feel unable to cope? If so, how do you treat yourself? Is it effective?
    f.  Do you ever have crying spells?
    g.  Have there been any marked changes in your sexual habits or desires?
    h.  Have you noticed any change in the amount of energy you have to accomplish daily functions?
    i.  Do you have any difficulty making decisions?
    j.  Have you noticed any increase in irritability? Restlessness? Listlessness?
    k.  Do you ever feel as though you do not care about anything?
    l.  Do you spend much of your time alone? (Estimate number of waking hours per day, per week.)
    m.  Who are your significant friends, that is, individuals you trust and who are available when you need them?
    n.  If you had a crisis in the middle of the night, is there a resource you could seek; someone whom you know would be available?
    o.  Have you ever thought of hurting yourself or ending your life? (If so, describe past methods and any specific plans for future attempts.)
    p.  History of psychiatric counseling and use of medications have already been inquired about in the original data base, but they need to be carefully reviewed.
2.  Orientation
    a.  Person: Can you give me your full name, address, and telephone number? Do you recall what my name is? Can you give me the full name of your closest relative?
    b.  Place: Do you recall the name of this health agency? What part of town do you live in? What is the name of this town? This county?
    c.  Time: Do you recall what day it is? The month? What year is it?
3.  Attention span/concentration
    This can best be tested by giving the client a series of directions to follow, a sequence of behaviors. For example, "I would like you to reach into your purse, pull out your billfold, find an identification card, and show it to me. Then I would like you to empty your change purse on the table and put all the dimes and nickels in one stack and the quarters and pennies in another stack." Assuming there is no hearing, vision, or motor dysfunction, the client can be observed (and timed) going through the sequence of behaviors. If immobilized, the client can repeat a short story that you have related or describe a personal story. The examiner should be alert for (a) a total shift in direction of subject matter or sequence of behavior midway through the process, or (b) conversation or sequenced behavior dwindling into silence or inactivity before being completed.
4.  Memory
    a.  Recent: What did you have for breakfast this morning? What time did you arrive at the agency today? What time was your appointment? Ask client to repeat a series of three to six numbers.
    b.  Remote: Can best be tested by having the client describe past medical history, high school graduation, first job, when married, etc. (provided the examiner is able to verify the information).
5.  Ability to make judgments (offering solutions to hypothetical situations)
    a.  What would you do if you saw a man picking someone's pocket right in front of you?
    b.  What would you do if the newspaper deliverer came to the door to collect and you discovered you had no available change?
6.  Abstract reasoning
    Ask the client to describe what the following proverbs mean:
    a.  A bird in the hand is worth two in the bush.
    b.  Not to decide is to decide.
    c.  Every cloud has a silver lining.
7.  Emotional status alterations (previous questions

related to anxiety and depression are relevant in this area)

   a. Inquire again about stressors (e.g., money, intimate relationship, death or illness in family or friends, employment problems).

   b. How are you feeling right now?

   c. Do you consider your present feelings to be a problem in your daily life? If so, do you feel the problem is temporary or curable?

   d. Describe a typical day at home (and/or at school, work), and tell which times or experiences are easiest for you and which are difficult.

   e. Do you think you need help with your problem?

8. If underlying intelligence appears to be minimal, the following questions or tests will be helpful.

   a. Client's access to basic information. In what direction does the sun set? How many months are in a year? What month follows July? In what state is Philadelphia?

   b. Client's vocabulary level. Ask the client to define a list of words. The list should begin with simple words and progress to more difficult ones, for example, chair, trouble, tender, posture, maximum.

   c. Ability to see similarities. Ask the client to describe how the following words are alike: a carrot and a potato, a dog and a cat, a lantern and a candle, a rose and perfume, an automobile and a train, etc.

   d. Ability to read and write. Ask the client to write his name and address on a sheet of paper. Ask the client to read newsprint (also a test for near vision). *Note:* The inability to read and write is not always a measure of intelligence; however, this is useful information for a practitioner when devising a care plan.

9. Coherence and relevance dysfunction.

   *Incoherency* is a broad term indicating that an individual is unable to convey his intentions or perceptions clearly to another person. It can present itself in the form of a flight of ideas that is often characterized by rapid speech and sentences and ideas that run into one another and seem to have no connection. Incoherency can also manifest itself in extreme anxiety. The individual is easily distracted and preoccupied; word and sentence fragments do not proceed in an orderly sequence. Incoherency can also be observed in extreme forms through jibberish, neologisms, and utterance of unintelligible sounds. It is best tested by listening to the client talk. A detailed account of an event will usually not be completed if the client is incoherent.

10. Thought content disruptions

   a. Do you have certain thoughts or feelings that consistently return or disrupt your thinking? Are you able to control them?

   b. Do you ever lose control of your thoughts?

   c. Is your thinking the same as, as good as, or better than it was 5 years ago?

   d. Do you ever have trouble making decisions about everyday events?

   e. Do you have any dreadful or uncontrollable fears that keep returning?

   f. Do you ever have the feeling that something dreadful is going to happen?

   g. Do you feel that you have enemies? Is anyone trying to harm you, discredit you, or control you?

   h. Are you being watched or followed?

   i. Do you ever feel guilty about your behavior or your feelings?

   j. Do you ever have the feeling that you are losing touch with what is happening around you?

11. Perception distortion

   Do you ever hear voices or strange noises? Do you ever see visions, lights, or people that others cannot see? Do you ever experience strange odors or tastes? Have you ever experienced strange sensations (warm, cold, or pressure) on your skin?

# Clinical guidelines

| THE STUDENT WILL: | TO IDENTIFY: | |
|---|---|---|
| | NORMAL | DEVIATIONS FROM NORMAL |
| **1.** Observe the whole client and the client's interaction with the environment for:<br>**a.** Client's initial response to examiner<br> 1. Examiner introduces self, clarifies client's name, offers hand in greeting, and sits down to be at eye level with client | Client responds with smile or facial expression acknowledging examiner's presence<br>Establishes eye contact<br>Offers own name<br>Extends hand in greeting | Client does not attain or maintain eye contact; does not acknowledge presence of examiner with facial expression, body gesture, or extension of hand<br>Client may jump up, interrupt, or talk through examiner<br>May be tearful or grimacing with pain |
|     2. Examiner explains own role to client and begins interview with broad, open question | Client attentive, nodding head, maintaining eye contact, leaning toward examiner | Client looking away, eyes closed, eyes wandering around room<br>Body pulled back in chair or leaning forward, tense posture |
| **2.** Make more specific observations regarding:<br>**a.** Body appearance | (Height and weight measured with scale and results compared with standards [Tables 2-1 and 2-2]) | Excessively tall or short |

**TABLE 2-1.** Weights* for men (according to frame, ages 25-59) for greatest longevity†

| HEIGHT (in shoes)‡ | | SMALL FRAME | MEDIUM FRAME | LARGE FRAME |
|---|---|---|---|---|
| Feet | Inches | | | |
| 5 | 2 | 128-134 | 131-141 | 138-150 |
| 5 | 3 | 130-136 | 133-143 | 140-153 |
| 5 | 4 | 132-138 | 135-145 | 142-156 |
| 5 | 5 | 134-140 | 137-148 | 144-160 |
| 5 | 6 | 136-142 | 139-151 | 146-164 |
| 5 | 7 | 138-145 | 142-154 | 149-168 |
| 5 | 8 | 140-148 | 145-157 | 152-172 |
| 5 | 9 | 142-151 | 148-160 | 155-176 |
| 5 | 10 | 144-154 | 151-163 | 158-180 |
| 5 | 11 | 146-157 | 154-166 | 161-184 |
| 6 | 0 | 149-160 | 157-170 | 164-188 |
| 6 | 1 | 152-164 | 160-174 | 168-192 |
| 6 | 2 | 155-168 | 164-178 | 172-197 |
| 6 | 3 | 158-172 | 167-182 | 176-202 |
| 6 | 4 | 162-176 | 171-187 | 181-207 |

Courtesy Metropolitan Life Insurance Company, copyright 1983.
*Weight in pounds (in indoor clothing weighing 5 pounds).
†Metropolitan no longer labels these weights "ideal" or "desirable" because these adjectives mean different things to different people.
‡Shoes with 1-inch heels.

**TABLE 2-2.** Weights* for women (according to frame, ages 25-59) for greatest longevity†

| HEIGHT (in shoes)‡ | | SMALL FRAME | MEDIUM FRAME | LARGE FRAME |
|---|---|---|---|---|
| Feet | Inches | | | |
| 4 | 10 | 102-111 | 109-121 | 118-131 |
| 4 | 11 | 103-113 | 111-123 | 120-134 |
| 5 | 0 | 104-115 | 113-126 | 122-137 |
| 5 | 1 | 106-118 | 115-129 | 125-140 |
| 5 | 2 | 108-121 | 118-132 | 128-143 |
| 5 | 3 | 111-124 | 121-135 | 131-147 |
| 5 | 4 | 114-127 | 124-138 | 134-151 |
| 5 | 5 | 117-130 | 127-141 | 137-155 |
| 5 | 6 | 120-133 | 130-144 | 140-159 |
| 5 | 7 | 123-136 | 133-147 | 143-163 |
| 5 | 8 | 126-139 | 136-150 | 146-167 |
| 5 | 9 | 129-142 | 139-153 | 149-170 |
| 5 | 10 | 132-145 | 142-156 | 152-173 |
| 5 | 11 | 135-148 | 145-159 | 155-176 |
| 6 | 0 | 138-151 | 148-162 | 158-179 |

Courtesy Metropolitan Life Insurance Company, copyright 1983.
*Weight in pounds (in indoor clothing weighing 3 pounds).
†Metropolitan no longer labels these weights "ideal" or "desirable" because these adjectives mean different things to different people.
‡Shoes with 1-inch heels.

## Clinical guidelines—cont'd

| THE STUDENT WILL: | TO IDENTIFY: | |
| --- | --- | --- |
| | NORMAL | DEVIATIONS FROM NORMAL |
| | Body appears symmetrical in terms of size and placement of parts | Unilateral wasting or hypertrophy |
| | | Asymmetrical body alignment |
| | Body fat is sparse or moderate and evenly distributed | Wasted, cachectic appearance; obesity, odd fat cushion distribution (e.g., confined to abdomen, hips, or buttocks) |
| | Body parts present and in proportion | Arms or legs exceptionally short |
| | Arm span equals height; distance between crown and pubis nearly equal to distance between pubis and soles of feet | Extremities missing |
| | | Arm span exceeds body height |
| | | Prognathism |
| | Skin color evenly distributed; skin smooth | Sallow, pale, flushed |
| | | Patchy discoloration |
| | | Marked wrinkling (localized or general) |
| | Muscles well or moderately developed or defined | Muscle wasting (localized or general) |
| | Hair evenly distributed over scalp, present in brows, lashes; moderate to light distribution over extremities, torso | Hirsutism |
| | | Absence of scalp or body hair or excessive thinning |
| **b.** Posture | Shoulders back and relaxed; arms resting at sides or on chair; feet resting on floor; body relaxed in chair or on examining table | Asymmetrical posture (e.g., guarding or contractures) |
| | | Tense posture, client at edge of chair, curled up in bed; back/neck rigid (client must move torso to view side) |
| | | Rigid posture with extremities held in flexion (Fig. 2-1) |
| | | Slumped in chair |

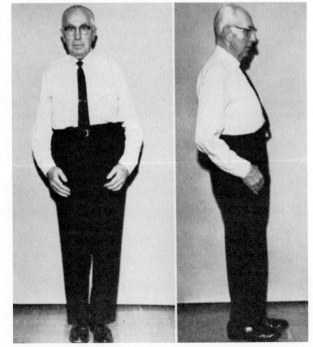

**FIG. 2-1.** Parkinson disease may be manifested in a series of different behaviors. Note staring, fixed facial expression and posture rigidity with arms held close to sides in semiflexed position. (From Prior, J.A., Silberstein, J.S., and Stang, J.M.: Physical diagnosis: the history and examination of the patient, ed. 6, St. Louis, 1981, The C.V. Mosby Co.)

| THE STUDENT WILL: | TO IDENTIFY: | |
|---|---|---|
| | NORMAL | DEVIATIONS FROM NORMAL |
| **c.** Body movements | Deliberate, smooth, and coordinated<br>Client sits motionless for brief periods, alternating with body position shifts and gestures<br>Client able to sit up in bed, swing legs to side; able to rise to standing position from sitting position with smooth even movements | Jerky, fidgety, constant movement; tremors (localized or general)<br>Movements very slow or very fast; client fails to move certain parts (e.g., may be splinting or guarding a painful area)<br>Hemiplegia or paraplegia<br>Total absence or paucity of movement of arms, torso, or legs<br>Movement uncoordinated (e.g., client slips when trying to rise; falls into chair rather than easing into it) |
| **d.** Gait | Steps even and smooth<br>Heel-strike, midstance, push-off, and swing phases easily executed | Client watches feet while moving<br>Stumbles, shuffles, staggers, limps (midstance phase shortened with painful leg or foot)<br>Steps uneven<br>One leg not functioning, lurching or propulsive, spastic or scissors gait |
| **e.** Facial expression | Eye contact maintained good part of time<br><br>Smile alternating with serious or thoughtful expressions appropriate to conversation<br><br><br><br>Facial features symmetrical | No eye contact<br>Staring fixedly (*Note:* A fixed gaze may indicate an effort to lip-read.)<br>Face immobile, expressionless<br>Constant smile<br>Grimacing (pain associated)<br>Face puffy, flushed, pale; excessive perspiration on forehead, upper lip<br>Dark circles under eyes (may be normal)<br>Asymmetrical features (Fig. 2-2)<br>Tearful expression<br>Brow constantly furrowed<br>Eyes darting around or constantly wandering about room<br>Tics, tremors, lip biting or licking<br>Squinting (inability to see) |

**FIG. 2-2.** Asymmetrical features. Note that flaccid left face flattens nasolabial fold, deepens line at left corner of mouth, shows marked discrepancy of eyebrow levels, and diminishes lines on left forehead. (From Prior, J.A., Silberstein, J.S., and Stang, J.M.: Physical diagnosis: the history and examination of the patient, ed. 6, St. Louis, 1981, The C.V. Mosby Co.)

| THE STUDENT WILL: | NORMAL | DEVIATIONS FROM NORMAL |
|---|---|---|
| **f.** Vocal tones | Moderate in pitch and volume; voice clear, firm, and audible; plentiful and varied inflections of tone in conversation | Very high pitched, loud, weak, inaudible<br>Hoarseness<br>Monotone (*Note:* Depression, drug usage, and Parkinson disease are common causes.) |

## Clinical guidelines—cont'd

| THE STUDENT WILL: | TO IDENTIFY: | |
| --- | --- | --- |
| | NORMAL | DEVIATIONS FROM NORMAL |
| **g.** Speech | | |
|    1. Pace | Moderate; may slow down with difficult or serious topic; may accelerate with excitement | Constantly rapid or very slow |
|    2. Clarity | Words easily understood | Slurred, garbled |
| | Enunciation of vowels and consonants clear | Client misses particular consonants at beginning of words or mispronounces vowels |
|    3. Word and sentence pattern | Style of verbal response may be brief or loquacious; client pauses to think | Paucity of words (e.g., confined to yes/no responses) |
| | | Constant flow of words and sentences |
| | | Stammering |
| | | Injection of numerous pauses (e.g., uhs, umms) |
|    4. Accent or foreign language | Varies according to origin | Accent very heavy (determine whether client able to use English language sufficiently to convey and receive messages) |
| **h.** Apparel | Clothing fits body | Clothing too tight, too small, too large (*Note:* May indicate recent weight loss or gain.) |
| | Shoes are intact and appear to fit snugly over feet | Skin bulges over top of shoes (may indicate edema or weight gain) |
| | | Shoes have holes or slits cut or worn in them (often done to minimize discomfort related to foot lesions, weight gain, or edema) |
| | Clothing clean, pressed, and "appropriate" for occasion (*Note:* Appropriate must be *broadly* defined; dress varies with age, life-style, financial resources, culture, climate) | Clothing dirty, rumpled |
| | | Distinctly bizarre dress or combination of colors |
| **i.** Grooming/hygiene | Hair brushed, shiny | Hair disheveled, dull, broken ends |
| | Men: shaved or trimmed facial hair | Unshaved |
| | Nails clean (*Note:* Some employment leaves nails chronically dirty.) | Dirty, ragged nails |
| | Women: moderate or no makeup | Bizarre makeup |
| | Shoes fitted and clean (*Note:* Cleanliness is subjective and may or may not be an indication of normalcy.) | Shoes ill fitted, dirty |
| **j.** Odors | Absent (*Note:* Some cultures do not promote use of deodorants.) | Pungent ammonia or fetid breath odors |
| | | Foul body odors |
| **k.** General mannerisms | Client may be quiet, thoughtful, somewhat passive (frightened) or active, moderately talkative, and demonstrative with body language | Tearful, angry, suspicious, questioning, evasive |
| | | Constant laughter and inappropriate joking |
| | | Noticeably subdued |
| | Mild to moderate anxiety (may be normal in a health alteration state; following are some common behaviors) | Moderate to severe anxiety (common signs and symptoms) |
| |    1. Client able to focus on conversation and respond appropriately |    1. Client either very limited or totally unable to focus on present situation |
| |    2. Increased alertness |    2. Skin cold, clammy; pallor |

| THE STUDENT WILL: | TO IDENTIFY: | |
| --- | --- | --- |
| | NORMAL | DEVIATIONS FROM NORMAL |
| | 3. Some muscle tension (leaning forward, listening intensely)<br>4. Some fidgeting, restlessness<br>5. Speech more rapid, voice pitch higher<br>6. Rapid-fire questions and responses<br>7. Increased eye contact<br>8. Moderately increased perspiration | 3. Frequent wetting of lips, tongue<br>4. Palpitations<br>5. Breathlessness<br>6. Dizziness<br>7. Trembling<br>8. Chills<br>9. Urinary frequency<br>10. Diarrhea<br>11. Abdominal cramp<br>12. Tires easily<br>13. Chest pain<br>Depression (some common behaviors, symptoms, signs)<br>1. Diminished body movements<br>2. Slow movements<br>3. Slouched posture<br>4. Voice often subdued, low in pitch and volume, monotone<br>5. Eye contact decreased<br>6. Smile absent or diminished<br>7. Sighing respirations<br>8. Tearfulness<br>9. Indecisive responses<br>10. Reports appetite change (anorexia, weight loss, increased appetite, weight gain)<br>11. Reports lack of energy<br>12. Reports loss of interest in daily activities<br>13. Reports insomnia (may take various forms: inability to fall asleep, awakening in middle of night, awakening very early in morning)<br>14. Reports constipation<br>15. Reports nagging muscular pains, backache<br>(*Note:* Some depression is manifested by increased motor activity, agitation, tachycardia, or constant smile.) |
| | Client shows no acute distress signs<br>Breathing even and moderately slow<br>Facial expression relaxed | Shows acute distress signs, such as dyspnea, pain (client splints, guards a part, limits movement), grimacing, moaning, writhing, coughing, wheezing, marked lethargy, drowsiness |
| **3.** Observe mental status<br>  **a.** Cognitive functions<br>    1. Orientation to person, place, and time | Client can indicate orientation to person, place, and time through discussion of history | Client unable to deliver accurate biographical data (e.g., address, name)<br>Client unable to name the agency that he is currently in |

## Clinical guidelines—cont'd

| THE STUDENT WILL: | TO IDENTIFY: | |
| --- | --- | --- |
| | NORMAL | DEVIATIONS FROM NORMAL |
| | Specific questions should be used only if examiner cannot assess orientation through conversation and general health interview | Client unable to identify year, month (*Note:* Many "normal" people cannot recall the day of the month!) |
| 2. Attention span and concentration | Client able to complete entire thought process (e.g., when describing a pain, client can recall location, duration, onset, character, etc. without wandering off subject) | Client unable to complete a thought; may digress in middle of sentence |
| 3. Recent memory | Accurate responses to questions about very recent events (e.g., How did you get to the clinic this morning? What did you have for breakfast?) | Client unable to recall very recent events (*Note:* Client's laugh may indicate embarrassment, may be an attempt to change subject or distract examiner.) |
| 4. Remote memory | Client's past medical history delivered accurately | Client unable to recall remote events |
| 5. Ability to make judgments | Client usually indicates ability to make judgments when describing personal health care practices and decisions made about maintaining or following health care routines | No indication that client can perceive a particular situation accurately and follow through with appropriate decisions |
| 6. Abstract reasoning (usually tested by asking client to explain proverbs) | Client offers appropriate explanation | Client unable to explain meaning |
| **b.** Emotional status, affect, mood | Client responds with smiles alternating with thoughtful or serious facial expressions appropriate to conversation<br><br>Body behaviors indicate relaxation or mild to moderate anxiety<br><br>Client describes self as well adjusted, generally happy, or appropriately concerned about present health alteration | Client demonstrates behavior indicating depression or moderate to severe anxiety or indicates through general questions that activities of daily living impeded or altered by mood, that coping capacity inadequate |
| **c.** Thought processes and perceptions | | |
|   1. Coherency and relevance | Client can complete entire thought (e.g., full symptom analysis description) without losing track of ideas or digressing<br><br>Answers to examiner's questions direct and appropriate | Ideas run together within sentence or stream of thought<br>Illogical ideas associated |
|   2. Thought content | Consistent, logical, and free-flowing thinking demonstrated as client describes history and self | Thought process interrupted with signs of compulsive or obsessive ideas (going off on a tangent); marked doubting and indecisiveness; phobias; free-floating anxieties; ideas of persecution, delusion; ideas of reference; feelings of unreality |
|   3. Perceptions | Client indicates to examiner, through descriptions of self, a consistent awareness of reality | Illusions<br>Hallucinations interfere with client's flow of perceptions |

| THE STUDENT WILL: | TO IDENTIFY: | |
| --- | --- | --- |
| | NORMAL | DEVIATIONS FROM NORMAL |
| | Client's perceptions of objects and surroundings consistent with those of examiner | |
| | Client able to accurately follow all directions: breathe deeply, sit up, walk to the other end of the room, tell me about your last hospitalization, etc. | Psychotic client may demonstrate preoccupation with self and little or no interest in examiner's activity |
| | | Affect may be inappropriate, (euphoric, flat, depersonalized, erratic or easily distracted) |
| | | Ritualistic, repetitive posturing or gestures may be evident |
| | | Periods of complete immobility |

## Clinical strategies

1. The first 5 to 10 minutes of the interview belong to the client. The examiner can begin with a very broad question, such as "What brings you to the clinic today?" This enables the client to talk freely about concerns and priorities and enables the practitioner to observe the client's verbal, nonverbal, and general behavior patterns.

2. Remember that the client is probably observing the examiner with equal intensity. The examiner must be acutely aware of personal behavior so that feelings of concern, caring, concentration, and confidence are conveyed, as well as curiosity.

3. Remember that many clients are anxious when being examined. Normal mild to moderate anxiety

may create a number of unusual behaviors—hyperactivity, stammering, excessive perspiration, excessive giggling, or listlessness. All these behaviors are worth noting in the final summary, but the examiner should be cautious about labeling behaviors as abnormal.

## History and clinical strategies: the pediatric client

1. The general and mental assessment of the child is patterned after that of the adult. The examiner must carefully observe the child interacting with the environment, the parents, and the examiner. Depending on the child's age and development, the examiner should observe for various normal behaviors. Following is an initial summary. Other areas are further detailed in the data base in Chapter 1 and in subsequent clinical chapters.

   The *newborn* should not mind being undressed or examined but will lie quietly on the examination table or the parent's lap (if not tired or cold) and will cooperatively allow the examiner to collect the appropriate assessment data.

   The examiner should collect history data before undressing the infant. During the history collection, observe the interaction between parent and child and how the child responds to the parent's techniques. Chapter 1 further describes specific information regarding parenting stresses and infant responses to stress.

   The *6-month-old to 2-year-old child* is acutely aware of the environment, viewing the parent as protector and the examiner as the enemy. The examiner must evaluate the child with the assistance

---

### SAMPLE RECORDING

The client is a neatly attired, clean-shaven, 42-year-old man. Facial expressions are alert, appropriate to the conversation, and coupled with frequent eye contact with examiner. Varied vocal tones are well modulated, and speech is audible and articulate. Body movements are smooth and coordinated.

General mood is one of seriousness accompanied by mild postural tension and intense listening behaviors while symptoms are discussed. Conversation indicates orientation to time, person, place. Client is able to offer logical and reasonable contributions to the problem and past attempts at dealing with the difficulty.

of the parent in eliciting various responses. During this time, observe the parent-child interaction. If the child does not cooperate, how does the parent respond? Does the child have eye contact with the examiner? Does the child separate with difficulty from the parent?

It is anticipated that the child will respond most favorably if examined while sitting on the parent's lap.

The *child from ages 2 to 4 years* is curious to find out who the examiner is and what will take place but still clings to the parent for security. After becoming familiar with the examiner, the child should relax and enter into game playing, conversation, and free expression of giggles and smiles. The examiner should again observe parent-child interactions and the child's ability to communicate and cooperate with the examiner.

The preschool *child from 4 to 6 years of age* will generally cooperate with the examiner and separate with ease from the parent. The examiner should evaluate the child's maturity, eye contact, attention span, and interaction with the parent.

In general, as the child matures, developmental progression, increased attention span, the ability to cooperate with the examiner, and decreased dependence on the parent should be observed. Any deviation from this should stimulate the examiner to develop a thorough behavioral profile for the child based on history and physical data.

2. The examiner must be alert to common behavioral problems in children and common behavioral concerns of parents. Although the actual mental status examination follows the same guidelines as for the adult client, other common problems or concerns that the examiner should screen for follow. In each of these situations the examiner should employ the elements of symptom analysis to develop a situational profile.

   a. Intellectual limitations of the child: the parent may feel the child is not performing up to capacity.
   b. Short attention span: the parent may feel that the child is unable to maintain concentration appropriate for age.
   c. Inability to problem-solve: the parent may express concern that the child is unable to perform tasks or solve problems appropriate for age.
   d. Communication difficulties: the child may have difficulty with speech development, eye contact, or communication with parents or peers.
   e. Variability: the child's mood is unpredictable; one moment happy or organized, the next minute unhappy or disorganized.
   f. Emotional immaturity: the child may lag in development, acting impulsively without thinking through the consequences, even though there has been previous experience with a similar problem.
   g. Hyperactivity: the child demonstrates an inappropriate amount of activity for age; the parent may state that the child has a difficult time sitting still or following through with an activity; may demonstrate a repetitive activity such as finger tapping.
   h. Perception difficulties: the child may demonstrate a pattern of inappropriate behaviors that might be a sign of difficulties with perception. Common difficult concepts are the differences between right and left, up and down, in and out, before and after. The child may also demonstrate an inability to complete a puzzle appropriate for age, difficulty learning to tie a shoe, or difficulty screwing or unscrewing the cap on a jar.
   i. Aloneness: the preschool or school-age child does not interact with or play with other children.
   j. Change in routine: the child may have difficulty with or react violently to a change in routine.
   k. Personal contact: the infant or child might not like to be cuddled; does not extend the arms to be picked up; or does not like to be held.

3. Other common stress behaviors that the examiner must note are thumb sucking, nail biting, teeth grinding, rocking, or stuttering.

4. In general, the examiner must assess how the child is developing and coping with the environment. As the examiner collects developmental, psychological, and physical data, patterns or collective signs that indicate how the child is coping with the environment and how the parent is coping with the child must be observed. Areas of the text most likely to facilitate this collective analysis are the *Psychosocial history* and pediatric areas of the data base, musculoskeletal, and neurological chapters (Chapters 1, 14, and 15).

## History and clinical strategies: the geriatric client

Elderly clients can be observed and assessed in the same manner as adult clients.

1. It is helpful to remember that elderly individuals are frequently subject to a greater number and intensity of stressors than are many younger people. They invariably suffer losses: loss of friends and loved ones through death, loss of occupation through retirement, and loss of a youthful body and

energy. They are frequently subject to changes in living conditions, financial status, and positions of authority and impact previously ensured in work, parenting, and social environments. There is no indication that the number and intensity of stressors can predict the individual's responses; in terms of depression, withdrawal, anxiety, or grieving, however, the examiner must be alert for signals indicating a maladaptive response.

2. The examiner should also be alert for signs of confusion. Many elderly people are confused as a result of physical illness. Confusion may be the first indicator of an altered health state, and its onset is usually sudden. Early indicators of confusion are:
   a. Limited attention span (losing track of thought in midsentence or indicating loss of attention through nonverbal behavior such as breaking eye contact during a conversation)
   b. Loss of recent memory (remote memory may remain intact)
   c. Emotion lability (sudden episodes of tearfulness)
   d. Decreased use of judgment (inability to think through a situation and make decisions)
   e. Confusion that is exaggerated at night (wandering or sleeplessness) and diminishes or disappears during the day
3. Some physiological states that might be associated with confusion follow:
   a. Infectious process
   b. Cardiorespiratory disturbances
   c. Metabolism disorders
   d. Trauma
   e. Alcohol or drug abuse
   f. Neoplasms

Most often, confusion associated with altered health states is reversible. This kind of confusion is usually compounded when elderly individuals are admitted to hospitals. Loss of a familiar environment and daily routines creates complex problems.

Mild confusion can sometimes be masked in clients who have well-preserved social skills. They can participate in polite conversations and skirt issues or direct questions that they are unsure of.

Hearing loss or visual impairment can be mistaken for confusion. The examiner should assess early in the interview the client's ability to receive communications.

4. Organic brain syndrome is not a disease. The term describes brain changes that result in a variety of altered client behaviors. The onset is usually slow and can be manifested in an intermittent or progressive fashion. A stable environment and a limited number of stressors can be therapeutic. Altered behaviors associated with this syndrome vary greatly according to the individual clients. Some common behaviors are:
   a. Diminished emotional responsiveness
   b. Disorientation (especially to time and place)
   c. Depression (often in the form of apathy or withdrawal)
   d. Confabulation
   e. Agitation
   f. Paranoic beliefs
   g. Loss of interest in appearance
   h. Shortened attention span
   i. Decreased intellectual skills
   j. Decreased ability to make judgments
5. The examiner must assess the client's use of drugs (over the counter and prescribed) and alcohol if confusion or disorientation is suspected.

---

**Cognitive self-assessment**

1. The holistic nature of humans means:
   - ☐ a. that they are the sum of all their parts
   - ☐ b. that they are dynamic and ever-changing
   - ☐ c. that they constantly interact with their environment
   - ☐ d. that they are sentient beings
   - ☐ e. that they are fluctuating energy fields
   - ☐ f. all the above
   - ☐ g. all except e
   - ☐ h. a, b, and c
   - ☐ i. all except a
2. Name eight general areas of behavior that you would look for while performing a general assessment, beginning with:
   a. posture

   b.

c.

d.

e.

f.

g.

h.

3. A symptom that a client might exhibit if mildly anxious is:
   - ☐ a. breathlessness
   - ☐ b. dizziness
   - ☐ c. increased alertness
   - ☐ d. abdominal cramps
   - ☐ e. none of the above

4. A sign of severe anxiety is:
   - ☐ a. intense listening
   - ☐ b. increased alertness
   - ☐ c. constipation
   - ☐ d. inability to clearly focus on present situation
   - ☐ e. none of the above

5. Which of the following behavior(s) might be seen with depression?
   - ☐ a. slow body movements
   - ☐ b. indecisive responses
   - ☐ c. constipation
   - ☐ d. b and c
   - ☐ e. a, b, and c

6. When an individual appears to be disoriented, the examiner can validate this suspicion by:
   - ☐ a. asking the client to name the present date
   - ☐ b. asking the client to describe personal feelings
   - ☐ c. asking the client to define words on a vocabulary list
   - ☐ d. all the above
   - ☐ e. none of the above

7. If an individual can follow a series of brief, simple directions without prompting, you know that the client is:
   - ☐ a. intelligent
   - ☐ b. able to control attention span
   - ☐ c. not depressed
   - ☐ d. not hallucinating
   - ☐ e. none of the above

8. Hallucinations:
   - ☐ a. are most often auditory
   - ☐ b. can be visual
   - ☐ c. can be experienced through taste
   - ☐ d. are not always obvious to the observer
   - ☐ e. are always obvious to the careful observer
   - ☐ f. all except e
   - ☐ g. a, b, and e
   - ☐ h. a, b, and d
   - ☐ i. b and d
   - ☐ j. all except d

9. Thought content can be disrupted by:
   ☐ a.  free-floating anxiety
   ☐ b.  phobia
   ☐ c.  obsessive ideas
   ☐ d.  ideas of persecution
   ☐ e.  ideas of reference
   ☐ f.  b, c, and d
   ☐ g.  all except a
   ☐ h.  all the above
   ☐ i.  none of the above
   ☐ j.  a, d, and e

## SUGGESTED READINGS
### General

Anxiety: Programmed instruction, recognition and intervention, Am. J. Nurs. **65**:9, 1965.

Bates, B.: A guide to physical examination, ed. 3, Philadelphia, 1983, J.B. Lippincott Co., pp. 428-446.

Jones, D.A., Dunbar, C.F., and Jirovec, M.M.: Medical-surgical nursing, New York, 1978, McGraw-Hill Book Co., pp. 3-22.

Malasanos, L., and others: Health assessment, ed. 2, St. Louis, 1981, The C.V. Mosby Co., pp. 161-179.

Prior, J.A., Silberstein, J.S., and Stang, J.M.: Physical diagnosis: the history and examination of the patient, ed. 6, St. Louis, 1981, The C.V. Mosby Co., pp. 36-63.

Snyder, J.C., and Wilson, M.F.: Elements of a psychological assessment, Am. J. Nurs. **77**(2):235-239, 1977.

### Pediatric

Alexander, M., and Brown, M.S.: Pediatric history taking and physical diagnosis for nurses, ed. 2, New York, 1979, McGraw-Hill Book Co., pp. 34-41.

Alexander, M., and Brown, M.S.: Physical examination: the why and how of examination, Nursing '73 **3**:25-28, 1973.

DeAngelis, C.: Basic pediatrics for the primary health care provider, Boston, 1975, Little, Brown & Co., pp. 337-378.

Pillitteri, A.: Nursing care of the growing family: a child health text, Boston, 1977, Little, Brown & Co., pp. 17-22, 710-713, 777-782.

Powell, M.L.: Assessment and management of developmental changes and problems in children, ed. 2, St. Louis, 1981, The C.V. Mosby Co., pp. 1-19.

### Geriatric

Burnside, I.M.: Nursing and the aged, ed. 2, New York, 1981, McGraw-Hill Book Co., pp. 41-69.

Caird, F.I., and Judge, T.G.: Assessment of the elderly patient, London, 1977, Pitman Medical Publishing Co., Ltd., pp. 87-98.

Comfort, A.: Non-threatening mental testing of the elderly, J. Am. Geriatr. Soc. **26**(6):216-262, 1978.

Dodd, M.J.: The confused patient: assessing mental status, Am. J. Nurs. **78**(9):1500-1503, 1978.

Steinberg, F.U., editor: Care of the geriatric patient, ed. 6, St. Louis, 1983, The C.V. Mosby Co., pp. 417-449.

Wolanin, M.O., and Phillips, L.R.: Confusion: prevention and care, St. Louis, 1981, The C.V. Mosby Co., pp. 58-87.

## ASSESSMENT OF THE

# Integumentary system

### VOCABULARY

**annular** Describes a lesion that forms a ring around a clear center of normal skin.

**atrophy** Diminution of size or wasting; can also refer to loss of elastic tissue resulting in a slightly sunken epidermis that wrinkles easily when pulled to the side.

**bulla** An elevated, circumscribed, fluid-filled lesion greater than 1 cm in diameter.

**circinate** Circular.

**circumscribed** Encircled, limited, and well defined.

**confluent** Describes lesions that run together.

**contusion (bruise)** Swelling, discoloration, and pain without a break in the skin; caused by a blow to the area.

**crust** Dried serum, blood, or purulent exudate on the skin surface.

**desquamation** Sloughing process of the cornified layer of the epidermis; when accelerated, the process can cause peeling, scaling, and loss of the deeper layers of skin.

**diffuse** Spread out, widely disbursed, copious.

**ecchymosis** Discoloration of skin or the mucous membrane caused by leakage of blood into the subcutaneous tissue; can also be a bruise.

**eczematous** Describes a superficial inflammation characterized by scaling, thickening, crusting, weeping, and redness.

**erosion** Wearing away or destruction of the mucosal or epidermal surface; often develops into an ulcer.

**erythematous** Reddish.

**excoriation** Scratch or abrasion on the skin surface.

**fissure** Linear crack in the skin.

**herpetiform** Describes a cluster of vesicles resembling herpes lesions.

**induration** Hardening of the skin, usually caused by edema or infiltration by a neoplasm.

**ischemia** Diminished supply of blood to a body organ or surface; characterized by pallor, coolness, and pain.

**keloid** Hypertrophic scar tissue; prevalent in non-Caucasian races.

**keratosis** Overgrowth and thickening of the cornified epithelium.

**lichenification** Thickening of the skin characterized by accentuated skin markings; often the result of chronic scratching.

**macule** Flat, circumscribed lesion of the skin or mucous membrane; 1 cm or less in diameter.

**necrosis** Localized death of tissue.

**nevus** Congenital, pigmented area on the skin. EXAMPLES: mole, birthmark.

**nodule** Solid skin elevation that extends into the dermal layer; 1 cm or less in diameter.

**papule** Solid, elevated, circumscribed, superficial lesion; 1 cm or less in diameter.

**paronychia** Inflammation of the fold of skin that adjoins the nail bed; characterized by redness, swelling, and pain; may be pustular.

**patch** Flat, circumscribed lesion of the skin or mucous membrane; more than 1 cm in diameter.

**petechiae** Tiny, flat, purple or red spots on the surface of the skin resulting from minute hemorrhages within the dermal or submucosal layers.

**plaque** Solid, elevated, circumscribed superficial lesion; more than 1 cm in diameter.

**pruritus** Itching.

**purpura** Hemorrhage into the tissue, usually circumscribed; lesions may be described as petechiae, ecchymoses, or hematomas, according to size.

**pustule** Vesicle or bulla that contains pus.

**reticular** Describes a netlike pattern or structure of veins on a tissue surface.

**scale** Small, thin flakes of epithelial cells.

**seborrhea** Group of skin conditions characterized by noninflammatory, excessively dry scales or by excessive oiliness.

**telangiectasia** Dilatation of a superficial capillary or network of small capillaries that produces fine, irregular red lines on the skin surface.

**tumor** Solid skin elevation extending into the dermal layer; more than 1 cm in diameter.

**turgor** Normal resiliency of the skin.

**ulcer** Circumscribed crater on the surface of the skin or mucous membrane that leaves an uncovered wound.

**urticaria (hives)** Pruritic wheals, often transient and allergic in origin.

**vesicle** Fluid-filled, elevated, superficial lesion; 1 cm or less in diameter.

**wheal** Elevated, solid, transient lesion; often irregularly shaped but well demarcated; an edematous response.

## Cognitive objectives

At the end of this chapter the learner will demonstrate knowledge of assessment of the integument by the ability to do the following:

1. Identify relationships and primary functions of these integumentary components:
   a. Stratum corneum
   b. Epidermis
   c. Dermis
   d. Sebaceous gland
   e. Eccrine sweat gland
   f. Apocrine sweat gland
   g. Subcutaneous tissue
   h. Keratin
   i. Melanin
2. Point out differentiating characteristics of 10 common primary lesions:
   a. Macule
   b. Papule
   c. Nodule
   d. Vesicle
   e. Patch
   f. Plaque
   g. Tumor
   h. Bulla
   i. Pustule
   j. Wheal
3. Identify client conditions or situations that increase the importance of periodic skin assessment.
4. Identify pressure points for assessment of an immobilized, recumbent, or chair-bound client.
5. Point out the characteristics of sequential skin alterations in response to continued pressure.
6. Identify some systemic or local conditions that affect the skin, hair, and nails.
7. Apply the terms in the vocabulary section.
8. Identify selected pediatric characteristics of the integumentary examination, including:
   a. Newborn characteristics
   b. Common alterations in pigmentation
   c. Common lesions
   d. Common developmental changes
9. Identify selected common integumentary characteristics of the geriatric client.

## Clinical objectives

At the end of this chapter the learner will perform a systematic assessment of the integumentary system, demonstrating the ability to do the following:

1. Obtain a pertinent health history from a client.
2. Demonstrate and describe the results of inspection and palpation of the following skin characteristics:
   a. Color
   b. Moisture
   c. Temperature
   d. Texture
   e. Thickness variations
   f. Mobility and turgor
   g. Hygiene
   h. Lesions
3. Show and describe the results of inspection and palpation of nails for:
   a. Configuration
   b. Consistency
   c. Color
   d. Adherence to nail bed
4. Demonstrate and describe the results of inspection of hair for:
   a. Distribution and configuration
   b. Texture
   c. Color
   d. Quantity
   e. Parasites
5. Summarize results of the assessment with a written description of findings.

## Health history additional to screening history

1. Is there a family history of skin problems (chronic, allergic, intermittent, or acute in nature)?
2. Does anyone at home (or closely associated with client) have any skin lesions, itching, or infections?

3. Does the client use any lotions, home remedies, or local applications of any kind on the skin?
4. Inquire about the client's assessment of the "delicacy" or "sensitivity" of the skin. Do cuts, bruises, or minor injuries heal fast enough and without complications? Does the client feel diminished or heightened skin sensitivity to discomfort?
5. What are the client's sun-exposure circumstances (outdoor work) or sunbathing habits?
6. Facial care: What cosmetics, soaps, or cleansing agents are used? How does the client manage pimples or minor lesions (by squeezing or picking)?
7. Hair care: What shampoos, rinses, coloring, or lubricating agents are used? Have there been any recent changes in hair care patterns?
8. Does the client have difficulty cutting or clipping fingernails or toenails? What instruments are used?
9. Itching (sometimes unaccompanied by rash or redness) should be located. Is it generalized or more intense in certain areas? Is it intermittent? More pronounced at certain times of the day (or night)? How severe is it? Does it interfere with daily activities (especially sleep)? Does the client have problems with scratching?
10. Dry skin: Is it more intense in certain areas of the body or generalized? Does the client use bath oils or powder? How would the client estimate the degree of humidity at home or at work (especially in the winter)? Is the skin dryness seasonal, intermittent, constant? Is it associated with itching?
11. If a client has a skin problem, these additional questions are warranted:
    a. Is the problem seasonal?
    b. Is it associated with stress?
    c. Are there occupational hazards (e.g., skin contact materials, radiation, abnormal lighting)?
    d. Inquire again about drugs being taken (prescribed and over the counter), especially recent changes.
    e. Is the problem associated with leisure activities (e.g., weekends, hiking, swimming, yard work, hobbies involving use of special materials)?
    f. How is the client adjusting to the problem (e.g., use of wig or excessive cosmetics to cover up the problem, fear of rejection, fear of infecting others)?
12. Multiple cuts or bruises need to be followed by careful inquiry. The examiner should consider the possibility of abuse. Posing direct or indirect questions about the source of injury will depend on the situation, the condition of the client, the relationship between practitioner and client, and information gathered previously regarding the client and the family.
13. Multiple cuts or bruises might also indicate frequent falls. The underlying cause for the falls should be considered (e.g., dizziness, alcohol or drug abuse, sensorium disturbances).

## Clinical guidelines

| THE STUDENT WILL: | TO IDENTIFY: | |
| --- | --- | --- |
| | NORMAL | DEVIATIONS FROM NORMAL |
| **1.** Be certain that there is adequate light available | | |
| **2.** Inspect and palpate the skin for: | | |
| **a.** Color | | |
| 1. General tone (best determined in areas of body not exposed to sun) | Deep to light brown, whitish pink to ruddy pink, olive, and yellow overtones | Diffuse, marked hyperpigmentation<br>General pallor (loss of underlying red tones in dark skin)<br>Ashen gray appearance<br>Yellow tone (jaundice)<br>General redness or flush |
| 2. Uniformity | Sun-darkened areas | Localized hyperpigmentation (especially in skinfolds, nail beds, old scars) |
| | Areas of lighter pigmentation in dark-skinned individuals (palms, nail beds, lips) (Fig. 3-1) | Pigmentation around ankles (Fig. 3-2)<br>Patchy or localized hypopigmentation (associated with inflammation, scaling, atrophy, scarring) |

| THE STUDENT WILL: | TO IDENTIFY: | |
| --- | --- | --- |
| | NORMAL | DEVIATIONS FROM NORMAL |

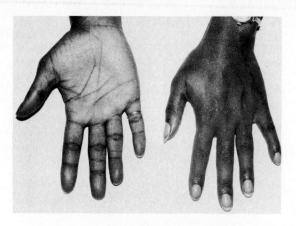

FIG. 3-1. Area of light pigmentation on black skin.

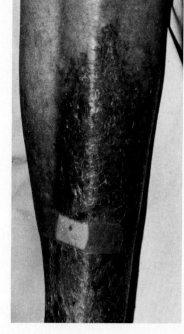

FIG. 3-2. Stasis dermatosis pigmentation.

| THE STUDENT WILL: | NORMAL | DEVIATIONS FROM NORMAL |
| --- | --- | --- |
| | Labile pigment areas often associated with use of birth control pills or pregnancy (cheeks, forehead, axillae, linea alba, areolae, flexor surface of wrist, genital area)<br>Crinkled skin areas appear darker (knees, elbows)<br>Calloused areas appear yellowish (palms, soles) | |
| 3. Examine extremities at heart level | | Marked pallor or mottling of extremities (especially when elevated)<br>Deep, dusky red color of dependent extremities |
| | Dark-skinned (Mediterranean origin) individual may have lips with bluish hue<br>Vascular flush areas (cheeks, neck, upper chest, genital area) may appear red, especially with excitement or anxiety<br>Skin color masking incurred through use of cosmetics, tanning agents | Cyanosis (dusky, bluish pallor), especially lips, area around mouth, nail beds, extremities |
| b. Moisture | Dampness in skinfolds<br>Increased perspiration associated with warm environs or activity<br>Wet palms, scalp, forehead, axillae often associated with anxiety | Excessive dryness and flaking<br>Excessive perspiration<br>Onset of excessive oiliness |
| c. Surface temperature (examiner's hands should be warm) | | Excessive coolness (general or localized), especially extremities<br>Excessive heat (general or localized) |
| d. Texture: stroke inner aspect of client's arms with finger pads | Smooth, even, soft | Rough, dry, coarse<br>Velvety smooth |

## Clinical guidelines—cont'd

| THE STUDENT WILL: | TO IDENTIFY: | |
| --- | --- | --- |
| | NORMAL | DEVIATIONS FROM NORMAL |
| **e.** Thickness | Wide body variation<br>Thickness increases in response to pressure and rubbing (e.g., calluses) | Excessive thickness (generalized change in condition or localized, especially extremities) |
| **f.** Mobility and turgor: pick up skin under clavicle where there is usually no excess (Fig. 3-3) | Skin moves easily when lifted and returns to place immediately when released | Skin remains in pinched position and returns slowly to place (tenting) (Fig. 3-4)<br>Decreased mobility with edema (skin appears shiny, taut)<br>Edema present (legs, feet, fingers, eyelids) |

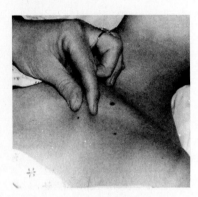

FIG. 3-3. Testing for skin turgor.

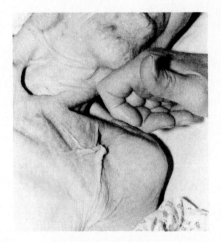

FIG. 3-4. Tenting associated with loss of skin turgor.

| THE STUDENT WILL: | NORMAL | DEVIATIONS FROM NORMAL |
| --- | --- | --- |
| **g.** Hygiene | Skin clean, free of odor | Crusted, dirty<br>Marked body odor |
| **h.** Surface alterations or lesions | Striae (stretch marks, usually silver or pinkish) (Fig. 3-5) | Macules, papules, nodules, vesicles, patches, plaque, tumors, bullae, pustules, wheals (Fig. 3-6) |

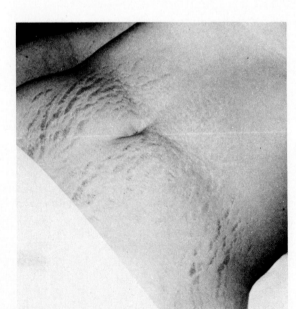

FIG. 3-5. Abdominal striae.

| THE STUDENT WILL: | TO IDENTIFY: | |
|---|---|---|
| | NORMAL | DEVIATIONS FROM NORMAL |

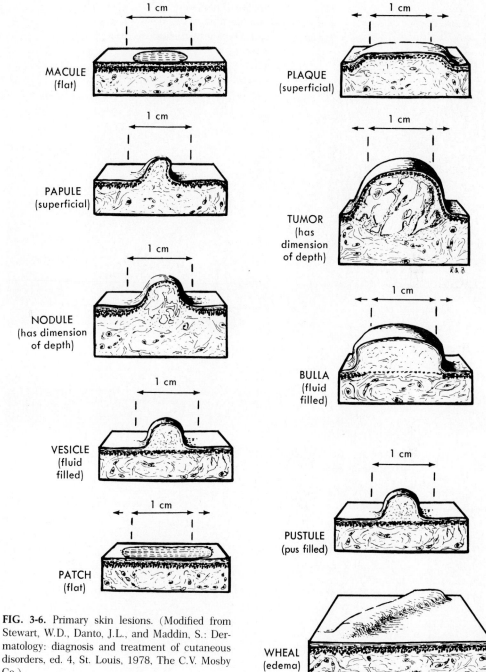

1 cm

MACULE (flat)

1 cm

PLAQUE (superficial)

1 cm

PAPULE (superficial)

1 cm

TUMOR (has dimension of depth)

1 cm

NODULE (has dimension of depth)

1 cm

BULLA (fluid filled)

1 cm

VESICLE (fluid filled)

1 cm

PUSTULE (pus filled)

1 cm

PATCH (flat)

WHEAL (edema)

**FIG. 3-6.** Primary skin lesions. (Modified from Stewart, W.D., Danto, J.L., and Maddin, S.: Dermatology: diagnosis and treatment of cutaneous disorders, ed. 4, St. Louis, 1978, The C.V. Mosby Co.)

## Clinical guidelines—cont'd

| THE STUDENT WILL: | TO IDENTIFY: | |
| --- | --- | --- |
| | **NORMAL** | **DEVIATIONS FROM NORMAL** |
| | Freckles (prominent in sun-exposed areas) Some birthmarks Some flat and raised nevi (in various shades of brown, tan, or near skin color) Patchy depigmented areas (vitiligo unassociated with inflammation, scaling, or scarring) (Fig. 3-7) | Increased vascularity Mixed lesions |

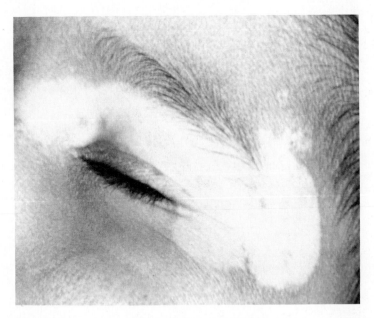

**FIG. 3-7.** Vitiligo. (From Stewart, W., Danto, J., and Maddin, S.: Dermatology: diagnosis and treatment of cutaneous disorders, ed. 4, St. Louis, 1978, The C.V. Mosby Co.)

| THE STUDENT WILL: | NORMAL | DEVIATIONS FROM NORMAL |
| --- | --- | --- |
| **i.** Trauma-induced surface alterations | | Bruises, scabs Lacerations Needle marks |
| **3.** Identify and inspect all pressure-prone areas for immobilized, recumbent, or chair-bound client (Fig. 3-8) for: | | |
| **a.** Color | Initial pallor (if there has been sustained pressure) quickly becomes red; redness (reactive hyperemia) then returns to original skin color | Prolonged blanching (ischemia) or, most often, redness (reactive hyperemia) is marked and extends over a prolonged period of time (area is engorged with blood) |
| **b.** Surface temperature | Localized area is same temperature as surrounding skin | Localized area is warmer than surrounding tissue |

TO IDENTIFY:

| THE STUDENT WILL: | NORMAL | DEVIATIONS FROM NORMAL |
|---|---|---|

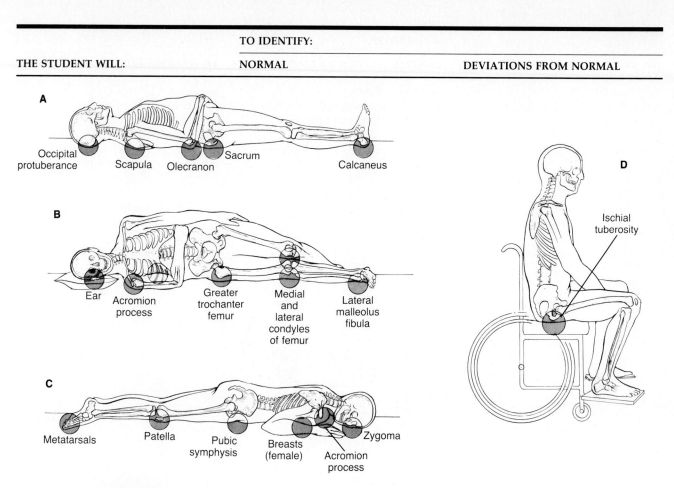

**FIG. 3-8.** Bony prominences vulnerable to pressure. **A,** Supine. **B,** Side lying. **C,** Prone. **D,** Sitting. (Modified from Forbes, E.J., and Fitzsimons, V.M.: The older adult: a process for wellness, St. Louis, 1981, The C.V. Mosby Co.)

| THE STUDENT WILL: | NORMAL | DEVIATIONS FROM NORMAL |
|---|---|---|
| **c.** Surface characteristics | Skin is intact | Cell and skin damage stages:<br>1. Prolonged redness with unbroken skin<br>2. Prolonged redness (that does not blanch) with excoriation<br>3. Full thickness of skin is lost Serosanguineous drainage<br>4. Invasion of deeper tissues (subcutaneous and/or muscle)<br>Open ulcer (may be necrotic, bone may be visible)<br>Purulent drainage (thick crust may be present) |
| **4.** Inspect and palpate the nails for:<br>  **a.** Configuration | Nail edges smooth and rounded<br>Nail base angle 160°<br>Nail surface flat or slightly curved | Edges bitten, ragged<br>Clubbing<br>Spooning, transverse depressions |
| **b.** Consistency | Smooth, hard surface<br>Uniform thickness | Excessive and/or irregular thickening; flaking |

## Clinical guidelines—cont'd

| THE STUDENT WILL: | TO IDENTIFY: | |
| --- | --- | --- |
| | NORMAL | DEVIATIONS FROM NORMAL |
| **c.** Color | Variations of pink<br>Dark-skinned individual may have pigment deposits in nail beds | Cyanotic<br>Very pale<br>Splinter hemorrhages<br>Redness at nail bed (paronychia) |
| **d.** Adherence to nail bed | Nail base feels firm when palpated | Nail base not firm<br>Nail base tender on palpation |
| **5.** Inspect and palpate scalp and hair for: | | |
| **a.** Surface characteristics | Scalp smooth<br>Hair shiny | Scalp flaky; scaling, reddened, or open lesions<br>Hair dull |
| **b.** Distribution and configuration | "Normal" varies with individuals; hair may be present on scalp, lower face, nares, ears, axillae, anterior chest around nipples, arms, legs, back of hands and feet, back, and buttocks | Sudden or marked increase or decrease in body hair |
| | Female pubic configuration forms inverted triangle (Fig. 3-9) (hairline may extend up linea alba)<br>Male configuration is upright triangle with hair extending up linea alba to umbilicus (Fig. 3-10) | Alteration of pubic configuration appropriate to male or female |
| **c.** Texture | Scalp hair may be fine or coarse<br>Fine hair over body<br>Coarse hair in pubic and axillary areas | Increased coarseness of body hair<br>Dryness, brittleness, or coarseness of scalp hair |
| **d.** Color | Wide variation from pale blond to black<br>Color may be masked or changed with rinses, dyes | |
| **6.** Inspect hair for: | | |
| **a.** Quantity | "Normal" varies according to individuals<br>Gradual symmetrical balding of scalp hair in some men | Excess body hair (hirsutism)<br>Female: hair growth intensified on upper lip, chin, cheeks, chest, and from pubic crest to umbilicus<br>Excessive loss of body hair<br>Scalp hair: asymmetrical or patchy balding (alopecia)<br>Marked hair loss |
| **b.** Parasites | | Body lice (especially in pubic and axillary areas)<br>Head lice and nits in scalp |

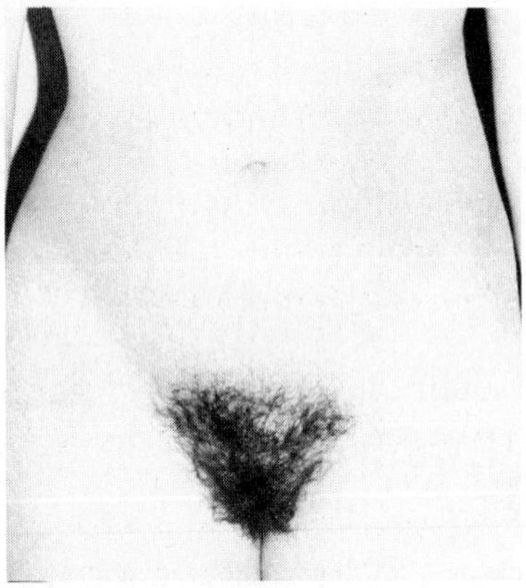

**FIG. 3-9.** Normal triangular configuration of female pubic hair.

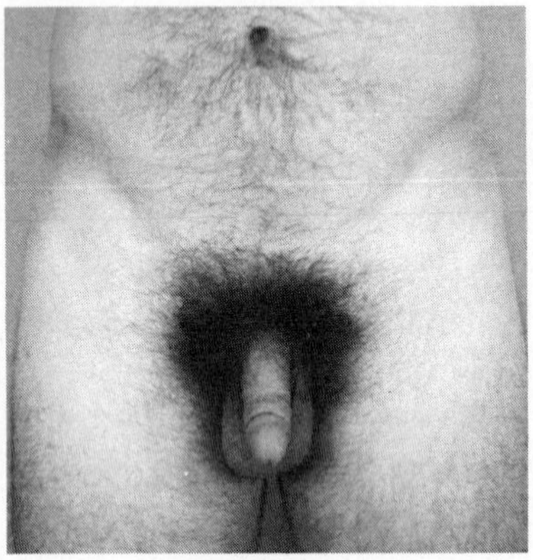

**FIG. 3-10.** Normal male pubic hair configuration.

## Clinical strategies

1. Be certain to have the client completely undressed for skin inspection. Examination of face and exposed extremities does not constitute a full assessment. Clients may be unaware of lesions or problems in areas that are inaccessible to them (e.g., the back, under skinfolds, bottom of feet).
2. Be certain to carefully inspect skinfolds (e.g., axillary, groin, area under pendulous breasts). These areas are usually warm and moist and may harbor bacteria, parasites (e.g., scabies), and fungi. Obese people have more skinfolds, so inspecting their skin will probably consume more time.
3. Be certain to remove shoes and socks or stockings to inspect *bottom of feet* and *between toes!* Elderly people and diabetics sometimes manifest decreased sensitivity to pain (especially in extremities). Open, infected, ulcerated lesions can be missed when direct inspection is neglected.
4. Long, jagged, thick toenails should be viewed as a problem. Inquire about the client's attempts to cut them. Sometimes elderly, obese, or disabled people cannot reach their feet to provide self-care.
5. Long toenails can interfere with shoe fit.
6. Skin lesions or surface alterations should be described in terms of the following:
   a. Distribution and location (e.g., confined to face, trunk, extremities, sun-exposed areas, or general distribution with no pattern; or placement on symmetrical body parts)
   b. Surface and color characteristics (e.g., confluent, macular)
   c. Lesion dimension: use metric system; do not compare tumors or nodules to fruits or vegetables
   d. Color and condition of surrounding tissue

---

### SAMPLE RECORDING

*Skin:* Pink, moist, soft, warm, and elastic. No lesions, discolorations, excess thickening, trauma, odor, or edema.
*Nails:* Pink, smooth, and hard. No clubbing, biting, or thickening or tenderness on palpation.
*Body hair:* Moderate, uniform distribution. Male pubic configuration.
*Scalp and hair:* Moderately thick, evenly distributed brown hair. Scalp clean. No flaking, lesions, or tenderness.

---

7. Wearing gloves is appropriate when examining open lesions. Washing hands is a necessity after any inspection.
8. Beginning examiners often have a difficult time describing findings in a concise, accurate manner. The vocabulary section at the beginning of this chapter can be very useful. Many of the words are adjectives that convey an explicit lesion pattern or arrangement with brevity. For example, "confluent vesicles" is a very efficient way to state that small, fluid-filled lesions all run together. Become familiar with these terms.

## History and clinical strategies: the pediatric client

1. Although assessment of the skin is important at all stages of a child's development, findings can be assigned to one of four categories:
   a. Integumentary characteristics present at birth that are considered deviations within normal limits, including mongolian spots, hemangiomas, café au lait spots, and lanugo
   b. Integumentary characteristics present at birth or shortly thereafter that may indicate disease, including jaundice appearing within 24 hours of birth, cyanosis in the nonchilled infant, tufts of hair over the spine or sacrum, or dermatoglyphics of the palm
   c. Integumentary characteristics that change as the child develops, including appearance of pubic and axillary hair or acne
   d. Integumentary characteristics that occur as either primary or secondary lesions caused by local irritations, communicable diseases, or infectious processes, including the following*:
      (1) Primary lesions
         (a) Poor skin turgor resulting from dehydration
         (b) *Macules* seen in scarlet fever, rubeola, and roseola infantum
         (c) *Papules* seen in ringworm, pityriasis rosea, psoriasis, or eczema
         (d) *Vesicles* (or blisters) seen in poison ivy, chickenpox (varicella), and herpes zoster (shingles)
         (e) *Bullae* seen in burns or on the palms and soles of children with scarlet fever
         (f) *Pustules* filled with pus and seen in impetigo, acne, and staphylococcal infections

---

*Modified from Alexander, M.M., and Brown, M.S.: Pediatric history taking and physical diagnosis for nurses, ed. 2, New York, 1979, McGraw-Hill Book Co., p. 51.

(g) *Wheals* usually associated with pruritus and seen in insect bites, hives, and urticaria

(h) *Petechiae* usually associated with systemic disease such as meningococcemia, bacterial endocarditis, or nonthrombocytopenic purpura. Needs immediate referral.

(2) Secondary lesions, which are alterations in the skin caused by another problem, such as trauma, unclean surface area, or continuous irritation:

(a) *Scales* seen in very dry skin or cradle cap

(b) *Crusts* (dried blood, scales, pus) from infected dermatitis, such as impetigo

(c) *Excoriation* seen in scrapes after falling

(d) *Erosions or ulcers* seen in infected, sloughing tissue or pressure sores

(e) *Scars* seen in healing tissue

(f) *Lichenification* seen over body areas where the child chronically rubs or scratches

2. The integumentary history of the pediatric client should include all the components of the adult history. In addition, the examiner should inquire about the following situations:

a. Specific exposure to communicable diseases.

b. Specific exposure to other children with environmentally caused skin problems, such as poison ivy or scabies.

c. If integumentary signs were present at birth or shortly thereafter, how have these signs changed or progressed since birth or the last visit?

d. If signs such as cyanosis, pallor, or jaundice are found, an expanded, detailed history should be collected.

e. Care and cleansing routines for children with conditions such as diaper rash, dry skin, or acne.

f. Environmental contacts for children with rashes; dry, patchy skin; or areas of irritation.

g. Young children with rashes or skin irritations should have a detailed history taken regarding skin care routines, soap or lotions used, new foods eaten, new detergents or fabrics exposed to, as well as parental treatment techniques.

3. The pediatric client must be completely undressed for the integumentary system to be adequately evaluated. The age and shyness of the child will determine examination techniques.

a. *Newborns* can be undressed easily for a comprehensive integumentary examination. The practitioner must carefully examine all the baby's cracks and crevices, observing skin characteristics, irritations, or rashes. The baby must not be allowed to chill.

b. *Older babies and toddlers* usually enjoy being undressed, which makes the integumentary examination easy. Special attention should be given to the fat creases, the diaper area, and the scalp.

c. Because of the acquired modesty of *preschoolers and school-age children,* the integumentary examination is more difficult. It may become necessary for the examiner to integrate this examination with other components of the physical assessment, for example, to provide integumentary assessment of the abdominal area while evaluating the abdomen. The hazard of this approach is that subtle skin problems or changes may be missed. At the completion of the examination the examiner must feel confident that total integumentary evaluation has been achieved. Again, this includes all the cracks and crevices.

d. Modesty is perhaps the biggest concern of *older school-age children and adolescents.* Examination criteria are the same as those for the adult client. Special attention should be paid to acne, complexion, and rashes that can develop around the genital area.

4. As the examiner evaluates the skin, signs of child abuse or neglect must not go unnoticed. Examples of problems include multiple bruises above the knees and elbows, multiple bruises at different stages of healing, bruises reflecting belt or electrical cord marks; cigarette burns or burns with even lines of demarcation that could indicate submersion, or any injury that does not coincide with the history. For example, the parent states that her 18-month-old child fell into hot bathtub water, but the clinical observation shows a submersion burn up to the waist with an even line of termination. There is no evidence of splash burns of the hands, face, or chest. A more subtle observation of child neglect involves the parents' nontreatment of obvious integumentary problems, for example, a diaper rash that has been allowed to progress to the point of blistering, infection, and bleeding. These situations require in-depth investigation and referral.

5. If a rash is identified, it is important for the examiner to determine the body surface involved, the rash migration and evolutionary pattern, and home care tried.

# Clinical variations: the pediatric client

| CHARACTERISTIC OR AREA EXAMINED | NORMAL | DEVIATIONS FROM NORMAL |
|---|---|---|
| **1.** Skin color | | |
| **a.** General tone | Newborn reddish during first 8 to 24 hours, then pale pink with transparent tone | Cyanosis |
| | | Pallor |
| | Slight jaundice starting second or third day of life; may last up to a month | Beefy red color that persists beyond 24 hours |
| | Mottled appearance of hands and feet in newborn; disappears with warming | Jaundice within first 24 hours of life |
| | | Mottled appearance not disappearing with rewarming |
| | Black newborns: melanotic pigmentation not intense, with exception of nail beds and scrotum | Half of newborn's body reddened and other half pale (harlequin sign) |
| | Older children: same as adult | |
| **b.** Uniformity (compare color of upper and lower extremities) | Similar color tones | Increased cyanosis of lower extremities may indicate aortic or congenital heart defect |
| **2.** Moisture | Perspiration present in all children over 1 month of age | Perspiration in infant less than 1 month of age |
| | | Excessive sweating, as seen in children with fever, hypoglycemia, hyperthyroidism, or heart disease |
| **3.** Texture | Smooth, soft, flexible | Dryness or flakiness in children over 1 month |
| | Dryness and flakiness of skin in infants less than 1 month of age (shedding of vernix caseosa); may appear as white cheesy skin | |
| | Presence of *milia*—small white papules over nose and cheeks, which are plugged sebaceous glands that may remain for 2 months | |
| | | Dryness or scaling between fingers or toes (may be from ringworm) |
| | | Scaling over knees, elbows, or behind ears (may be from eczema) |
| | | Scaliness of palms and soles (seen with scarlet fever) |
| | | Dermatoglyphics—straight single folds seen across the upper palm of hands at base of fingers in children with Down syndrome |
| | | Dryness or chafing of diaper area |
| **4.** Thickness | Varying degrees of adipose tissue, dimpling of skin over joint areas | Skin dimpling at areas other than over joints |

## Clinical variations: the pediatric client—cont'd

| CHARACTERISTIC OR AREA EXAMINED | NORMAL | DEVIATIONS FROM NORMAL |
|---|---|---|
| 5. Mobility and turgor<br> a. Pinch large area of skin over lower abdomen | Skin rises with pinch but falls quickly when released | Skin remains in pinched position (Fig. 3-11) |

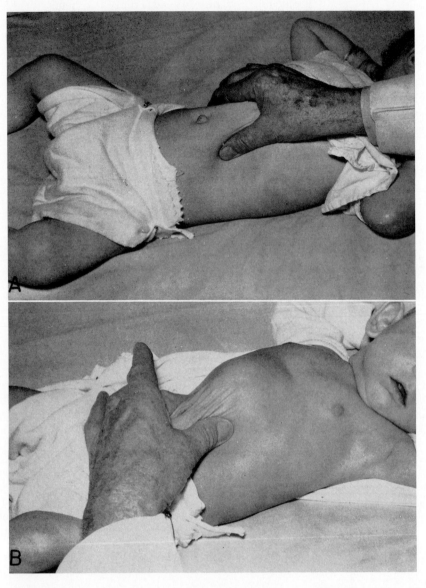

FIG. 3-11. **A,** Good tissue turgor. **B,** Poor tissue turgor. (From Prior, J.A., Silberstein, J.S., and Stang, J.M.: Physical diagnosis: the history and examination of the patient, ed. 6, St. Louis, 1981, The C.V. Mosby Co.)

| | | |
|---|---|---|
| b. Palpate the calf | Full, taut skin | Loose and "extra" skin<br>Edema |
| 6. Hygiene | Skin free from odor, clean | Dirty, crusted, or excoriated areas: skinfolds, diaper area, behind ears, neck region; dirty look |

| CHARACTERISTIC OR AREA EXAMINED | NORMAL | DEVIATIONS FROM NORMAL |
|---|---|---|
| **7.** Skin surface **a.** Alterations in pigmentation | *Mongolian spots*\*—irregularly shaped, darkened flat areas over sacral area and buttocks; usually seen in black or darkly pigmented children; may be gone by first or second year Note size and location | Vitiligo—absence of pigmentation in areas |
| | *Café au lait spots*\*—light, cream-colored spots found on darkened backgrounds Note size and location | Multiple areas of spots |
| | *Hemangiomas*\*—increase in pigmentation with crying I. *Flat capillary*    A. Storkbites: small red or pink spots often seen on back of neck, upper lip, or upper eyelid (Fig. 3-12); usually disappear by age 5 | |

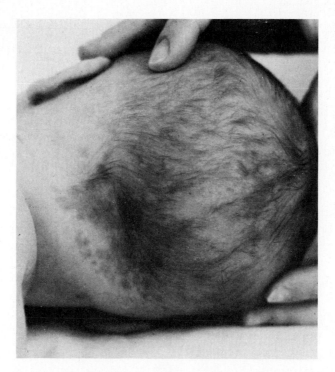

**FIG. 3-12.** Storkbite. (From Jensen, M., Benson, R., and Bobak, I.: Maternity care: the nurse and the family, ed. 2, St. Louis, 1981, The C.V. Mosby Co. Courtesy Mead Johnson & Co., Evansville, Ind.)

---

\*These lesions are commonly seen in the pediatric client. Many practitioners consider them a "normal" deviation. Beginners in assessment should consider all pigment alterations as problems until experience enables them to recognize common deviations within normal limits.

## Clinical variations: the pediatric client—cont'd

| CHARACTERISTIC OR AREA EXAMINED | NORMAL | DEVIATIONS FROM NORMAL |
| --- | --- | --- |
| | B. Port wine stain: large, flat, bluish purple capillary area; most frequently found on face along distribution of fifth cranial nerve (Fig. 3-13); usually does not disappear spontaneously | In children with port wine stains, screen for nervous system complications |
| | II. *Raised capillary:* strawberry mark, slightly raised, reddened area with sharp demarcation line; may be 2 to 3 cm in diameter; appears at birth or within first few months and usually gone by age 5 (Fig. 3-14) | |
| | Note size and location | |

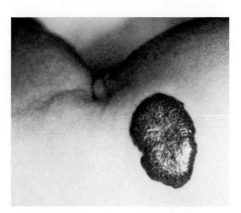

FIG. 3-14. Strawberry mark. (From Shirkey, H.: Pediatric therapy, ed. 5, St. Louis, 1975, The C.V. Mosby Co.)

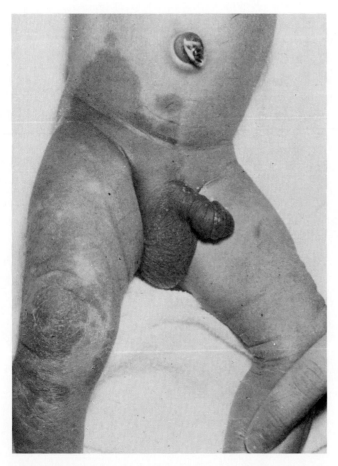

FIG. 3-13. Port wine stain. (From Jensen, M., Benson, R., and Bobak, I.: Maternity care: the nurse and the family, ed. 2, St. Louis, 1981, The C.V. Mosby Co. Courtesy Mead Johnson & Co., Evansville, Ind.)

| CHARACTERISTIC OR AREA EXAMINED | NORMAL | DEVIATIONS FROM NORMAL |
|---|---|---|
| | III. *Cavernous hemangioma:* reddish blue; round masses of blood vessels; may continue to grow until child is 10 to 15 months old<br>Note size and location<br>Child should be reevaluated frequently | Some may require surgical removal |
| | IV. *Nevus* (mole): may vary in size and number; brown in pigmentation<br>Note size, location and number<br>Those that are large or in irritating areas must be frequently evaluated for change | Large hairy nevi<br>Bathing trunk nevi |
| **b.** Common lesions | | *Macules,* as seen in measles, German measles, or drug rash ( Fig. 3-15)<br>*Papules,* as seen in tinea (ringworm) or psoriasis ( Fig. 3-16) |

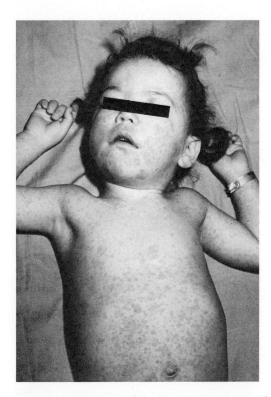

**FIG. 3-15.** Macule rash of measles. (From Krugman, S., and Katz, S.L.: Infectious diseases of children, ed. 7, St. Louis, 1981, The C.V. Mosby Co.)

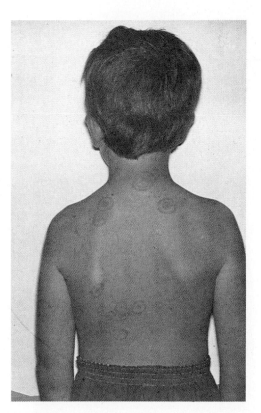

**FIG. 3-16.** Papules as seen in ringworm. (From Verbov, J., and Morley, N.: Color atlas of pediatric dermatology, Philadelphia, 1983, J.B. Lippincott Co.)

## Clinical variations: the pediatric client—cont'd

| CHARACTERISTIC OR AREA EXAMINED | NORMAL | DEVIATIONS FROM NORMAL |
|---|---|---|

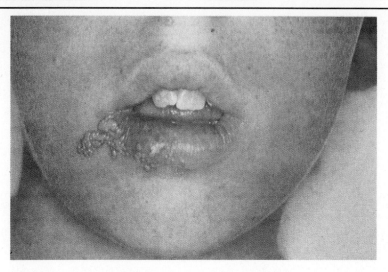

*Vesicles* (blebs), as seen in chickenpox, (herpes simplex), herpes zoster, or poison ivy (Fig. 3-17)

*Pustules*, as seen in impetigo or scabies (Fig. 3-18)

*Xanthomas*, small yellow plaques seen across nose of newborn

*Miliaria* (prickly heat), tiny red irritation (Fig. 3-19)

**FIG. 3-17.** Vesicles as seen in herpes simplex. (From Verbov, J., and Morley, N.: Color atlas of pediatric dermatology, Philadelphia, 1983, J.B. Lippincott Co.)

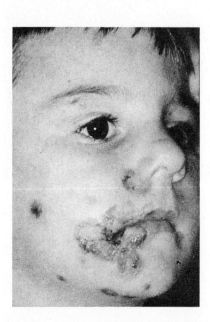

**FIG. 3-18.** Pustules as seen in impetigo. (From Verbov, J., and Morley, N.: Color atlas of pediatric dermatology, Philadelphia, 1983, J.B. Lippincott Co.)

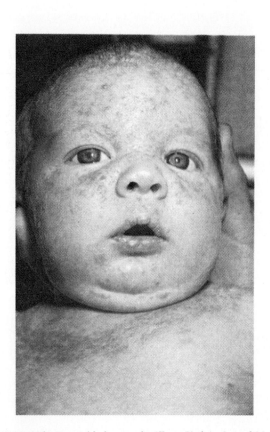

**FIG. 3-19.** Miliaria prickly heat rash. (From Verbov, J., and Morley, N.: Color atlas of pediatric dermatology, Philadelphia, 1983, J.B. Lippincott Co.)

| CHARACTERISTIC OR AREA EXAMINED | NORMAL | DEVIATIONS FROM NORMAL |
|---|---|---|

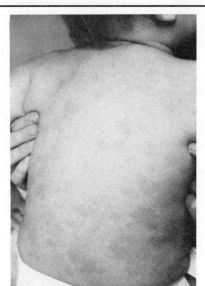

**FIG. 3-20.** Urticaria. (From Verbov, J., and Morley, N.: Color atlas of pediatric dermatology, Philadelphia, 1983, J.B. Lippincott Co.)

*Hives* (wheals or urticaria), as seen in allergic reactions (Fig. 3-20)
*Petechial rash,* or macular type of rash that does not blanch with palpation or pressure (may indicate meningococcemia, a medical emergency)
*Acne,* resulting in blackheads, papules, pustules, and cysts (Fig. 3-21)

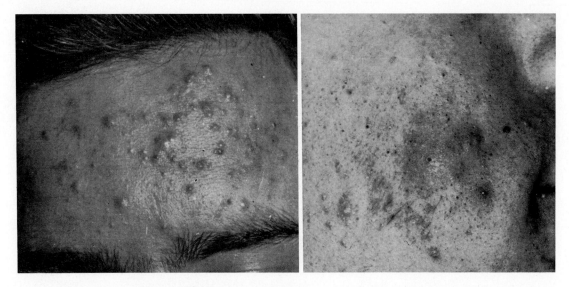

**FIG. 3-21.** Acne vulgaris. (From Stewart, W.D., Danto, J.L., and Maddin, S.: Dermatology: diagnosis and treatment of cutaneous disorders, ed. 4, St. Louis, 1978, The C.V. Mosby Co.)

| | | |
|---|---|---|
| | *Ecchymoses,* bruises commonly seen below knees and elbows | *Ecchymoses,* bruises seen elsewhere on body, or multiple bruises seen at different stages of healing |
| **8.** Nails | | |
| **a.** Configuration | Generally longer than wider | Nail beds wider than longer; may be seen in children with Down syndrome or other congenital malformations |

## Clinical variations: the pediatric client—cont'd

| CHARACTERISTIC OR AREA EXAMINED | NORMAL | DEVIATIONS FROM NORMAL |
|---|---|---|
| **b.** Consistency | Soft nails in infants and small children; become hardened with age<br>Vernix may be found under nails of newborns | Pitting of nails, as seen with fungal diseases |
| **c.** Color | Same as adult<br>Postmature infants may show yellow staining | |
| **d.** Adherence to nail bed | Same as adult | Paronychia, commonly seen infections around nail bed (Fig. 3-22) |

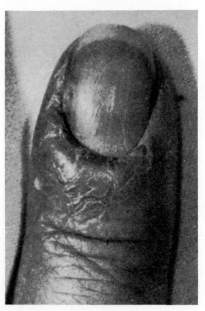

FIG. 3-22. Paronychia. (From Stewart, W.D., Danto, J.L., and Maddin, S.: Dermatology: diagnosis and treatment of cutaneous disorders, ed. 4, St. Louis, 1978, The C.V. Mosby Co.)

| | | |
|---|---|---|
| **9.** Scalp and hair | | |
| **a.** Scalp | Smooth, soft | Scaliness of scalp with crusting, seborrheic dermatitis (cradle cap) (Fig. 3-23)<br>Ringworm or eczema of scalp |

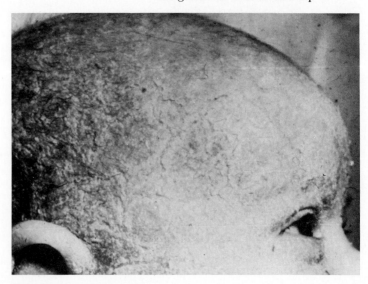

FIG. 3-23. Seborrheic dermatitis (cradle cap). (From Shirkey, H., Pediatric therapy, ed. 6, St. Louis, 1979, The C.V. Mosby Co.)

| CHARACTERISTIC OR AREA EXAMINED | NORMAL | DEVIATIONS FROM NORMAL |
|---|---|---|
| **b.** Scalp hair | Shiny, soft, fine texture; as child grows, hair takes on adult characteristics<br>Irregularity in pigmentation | Brittle hair may be seen in children with hypothyroidism, ringworm of scalp, or other conditions<br>Presence of nits |
| **c.** Distribution and configuration of body hair | Newborn displays lanugo, fine hair over body, mostly over shoulders and back; will disappear during first 3 months of life | Hairy trunk may be seen in children with Cushing syndrome<br>Tufts of hair seen anywhere over spine, especially over sacrum (may mark spot of spina bifida) |
| | Pubic hair begins to develop between 8 and 12 years; smooth hair at first, changing to coarse, curly hair; followed approximately 6 months later by axillary hair; followed approximately 6 months later by facial hair in boys | Absence of secondary hair characteristics |

## History and clinical strategies: the geriatric client

1. Differentiating normal from abnormal skin changes is very difficult when assessing elderly clients. A novice examiner should consult regularly with an experienced clinician.
2. "Normal" lesions must be considered a problem if they are causing client distress (e.g., cosmetic concern, clothing rubbing or irritating lesion).
3. Elderly clients sometimes exhibit a more intense response to skin irritations. The client may feel more pain or more severe itching. Lesions or dermatitis problems may respond more slowly to treatment.
4. Elderly clients may manifest a *reduced* pain response to lesions (especially in extremities): (a) they may be unable to feel pain; (b) they may accept chronic discomfort as part of aging and fail to report it.
5. If a client complains of itching and scratching (a fairly common complaint among elderly clients), assess the fingernails. Dirty, jagged fingernails often contribute to the problem.
6. The integumentary system reflects an individual's relationship to the outer as well as the inner environment. Some of the variables affecting the skin, hair, and nails follow:
   a. Outer environment
      (1) Cold weather conditions: increased sensitivity to cold.
      (2) Humidity and moisture: low humidity (especially in winter) will irritate dry skin; individuals who habitually soak in warm water (to relieve arthritic pain) may develop dry skin.
      (3) Sun: chronic exposure (especially with light-skinned individuals) results in a higher incidence of precancerous and cancerous growths. Sun sensitivity may develop; certain drugs and chemicals contribute to phototoxic reactions: sulfonamides, thiazide diuretics, antibacterial soaps.
      (4) Skin irritants: soaps, detergents, lotions with high alcohol content, disinfectants, and woolen clothing may aggravate dry skin.
      (5) Allergic reactions: occur fairly often; jewelry, dark blue or black dyes in clothing or shoes, chemicals in crease-resistant clothing, and linens or clothing containing residual soap or detergent are some of the more common causative factors.
      (6) Decreased activity (pressure friction) will stress the system.
   b. Internal environment
      (1) Medications (often numerous with the elderly) may create problems (rash, itching).
      (2) Systemic/chronic disease (itching).
      (3) Nutritional deficiencies (e.g., vitamin A deficiency may result in rough, dry skin).
      (4) Decreased circulation lowers skin resistance to infection.

## Clinical variations: the geriatric client

| CHARACTERISTIC OR AREA EXAMINED | NORMAL | DEVIATIONS FROM NORMAL |
|---|---|---|
| 1. Skin color | | |
| a. General tone | Caucasian skin appears white | Pallor associated with anemia |
| b. Uniformity | More freckles, uneven tanning, or pigment deposits in sun-exposed areas (more evident on fair skin) (Fig. 3-24) | Hypersensitivity to sun (marked reddening, eczematous changes) |
| | Hypopigmented patches | |

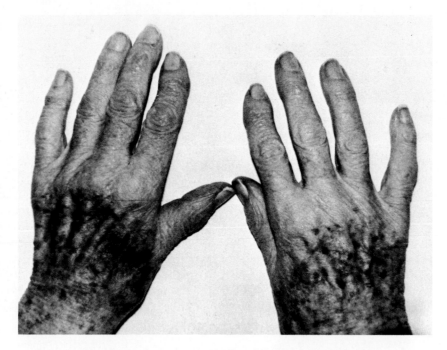

FIG. 3-24. Marked pigmentation deposits associated with aging.

| | | |
|---|---|---|
| 2. Moisture | Increased dryness (especially extremities) | Marked flaking |
| | Decreased perspiration | |
| 3. Texture | Flaking, scaling (associated with dry skin, especially over lower extremities | Scaling associated with dryness, itching, and scratching (erythema, excoriation may be present) |
| 4. Thickness | Thinner skin (especially over dorsal surface of hands and feet, forearms, lower legs, bony prominences such as scapula, trochanter, knees) | |
| | Other skin areas may be thicker (abdomen, torso) | Torso obesity distribution associated with disease |
| 5. Mobility and turgor | General loss of elasticity; appears lax | |

| CHARACTERISTIC OR AREA EXAMINED | NORMAL | DEVIATIONS FROM NORMAL |
|---|---|---|
| | Increased wrinkle pattern (more marked in sun-exposed areas, in fair skin, in expressive areas of face) (Fig. 3-25) | Marked wrinkling or sagging associated with weight loss (Fig. 3-26)<br>Perlèche—deep wrinkling, fissures or maceration at corners of mouth; monilial infection often develops in this moist area (associated with overclosure of mouth because of ill-fitting dentures or edentulous state) (Fig. 3-27) |
| | Pendulous parts sag or droop (skin under chin, earlobes, breasts, scrotum) | Pendulous scrotal tissue may become excoriated or damaged because of client sliding or sitting on it |

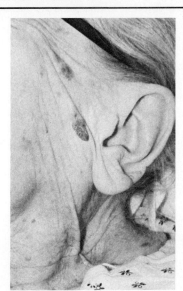

FIG. 3-25. Increased wrinkling and skinfolds associated with aging.

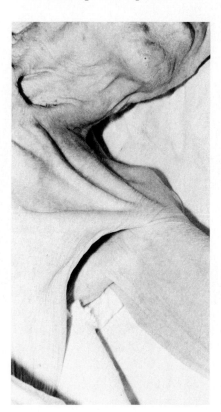

FIG. 3-26. Marked weight loss. Note bony prominences and sagging skinfolds.

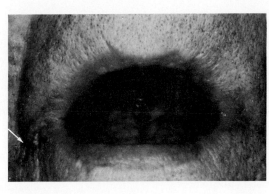

FIG. 3-27. Perlèche. (Courtesy Dr. George Blozis, The Ohio State University College of Dentistry.)

| | | |
|---|---|---|
| **6.** Hygiene | | Hard-to-reach areas may be less clean (e.g., feet, axillary area, buttocks, or inguinal skinfolds) |
| **7.** Skin surface<br>  **a.** Alterations or lesions | Nevi (common moles) often become lighter in color or disappear | Evaluated in same manner as with adult client |

## Clinical variations: the geriatric client—cont'd

| CHARACTERISTIC OR AREA EXAMINED | NORMAL | DEVIATIONS FROM NORMAL |
|---|---|---|
| 1. Seborrheic keratosis* | | *Seborrheic dermatitis†* |
| a. Location | Temples, neck, back, under pendulous breasts | Face, scalp, upper chest (oil-rich areas of body) |
| b. Size | 2 to 3 cm in diameter | Wide variation |
| c. Color | Light tan to black | Reddish or yellowish scaling |
| d. Surface characteristics | Appears "stuck on"; lobulated or warty, scaly, thickened | Demarcated scaling, redness, and itching; may erupt into red-brown papules with yellowish scaling |
| e. Distribution | Often multiple (Fig. 3-28) | Singular or multiple (often associated with illness, confinement, and inability to maintain good hygiene) (Fig. 3-29) |

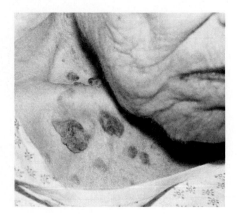

**FIG. 3-28.** Seborrheic keratosis.

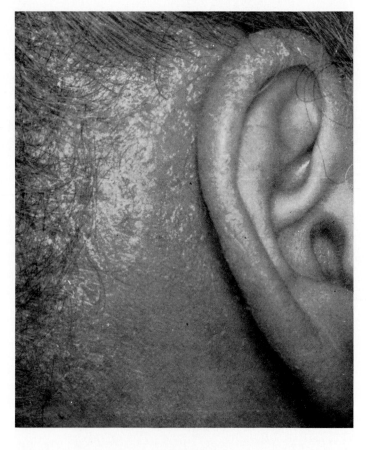

**FIG. 3-29.** Seborrheic dermatitis of postauricular area. (From Stewart, W.D., Danto, J.L., and Maddin, S.: Dermatology: diagnosis and treatment of cutaneous disorders, ed. 4, St. Louis, 1978, The C.V. Mosby Co.)

| CHARACTERISTIC OR AREA EXAMINED | NORMAL | DEVIATIONS FROM NORMAL |
|---|---|---|
| 2. Skin tags (acrochordons)* | | *Herpes zoster†* |
| a. Location | Side of neck, face, axillary folds | Can be anywhere on body: thorax, abdomen (most common), forehead and temple, neck and shoulders |
| b. Size | 1 mm to 1 cm | Under 1 cm (multiple vesicles) |
| c. Color | Pinkish tan to light brown | Red |

*These lesions commonly occur in elderly adults. They are described by some authors as "normal," in that the chief concern for the client is cosmetic. Beginners in assessment should consider all lesions as problems until experience enables them to recognize common deviations within normal limits.

†These lesions are fairly common in elderly adults. They are all considered "abnormal" and should be treated.

| CHARACTERISTIC OR AREA EXAMINED | NORMAL | DEVIATIONS FROM NORMAL |
|---|---|---|
| d. Surface | Soft, pedunculated | Multiple, confluent vesicles preceded by pain and burning and followed by weeping, crusting, and healing; postzoster neuralgia (severe pain) may persist for weeks or months |
| e. Distribution | Often multiple, may be singular (Fig. 3-30) | Over a segmented sensory nerve area (Fig. 3-31) |

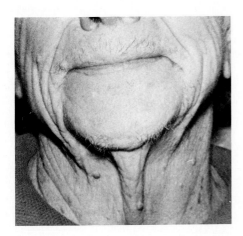

**FIG. 3-30.** Skin tags in the neck and bristly facial hair.

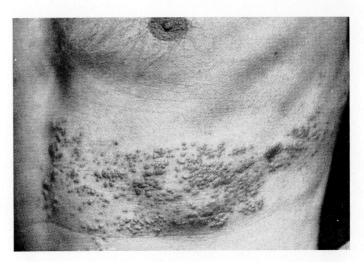

**FIG. 3-31.** Herpes zoster. (From Stewart, W.D., Danto, J.L., and Maddin, S.: Dermatology: diagnosis and treatment of cutaneous disorders, ed. 4, St. Louis, 1978, The C.V. Mosby Co.)

| | | |
|---|---|---|
| 3. Senile angiomas* | | *Dry skin dermatitis†* |
|    a. Location | Trunk, proximal extremities, scrotum | Lower legs (most common), arms, hands, trunk |
|    b. Size | 1 to 5 mm diameter | Wide variation |
|    c. Color | Purplish or red | Whitish flakes, redness with inflammation |
|    d. Surface | Smooth, soft, dome-shaped May bleed if traumatized | Flaking, redness, fissures, itching |
|    e. Distribution | Singular or multiple | Multiple |
| 4. Sebaceous hyperplasia* (more common in males) | | *Actinic keratosis†* |
|    a. Location | Forehead, nose, cheeks | Dorsum of hands, forehead, ears, face, neck |
|    b. Size | 2 to 3 mm diameter | Varies |
|    c. Color | Yellow | Whitish scales, mild erythema |
|    d. Surface | Papular, flat, may be umbilicated or lobular | Small, macular with scales and varying degree of mild erythema (premalignant, slow growing) |

## Clinical variations: the geriatric client—cont'd

| CHARACTERISTIC OR AREA EXAMINED | NORMAL | DEVIATIONS FROM NORMAL |
|---|---|---|
| e. Distribution | Singular or multiple (Fig. 3-32) | May be singular or may erupt in multiple spots over sun-exposed areas<br>*Basal cell carcinoma†*<br>Location: lower lip, face (especially on eyelid, nose, earlobe); can occur anywhere<br>Size: small; varies, but usually 0.5 to 1 cm<br>Color: varies<br>Surface: Varies; usually begins as small, pearly-translucent papule that breaks down into an ulcer with bleeding and crusting; border of crater is elevated and pearly in appearance; painless<br>Distribution: Usually singular (see Fig. 5-28)<br>*Squamous cell carcinoma†*<br>Location: most often on lip, cheek, ear, temple, neck; can occur anywhere<br>Size: varies, usually 1 cm<br>Color: varies<br>Surface: variety of forms; usually begins as red-brown nodule that breaks down into a necrotic ulcer (develops more rapidly than basal cell); may begin as a persistent scale that eventually ulcerates<br>Distribution: usually singular, may be multiple<br>Use extra caution in assessing lesions or changes in (1) sun-exposed areas, (2) moist folds (monilial infections frequently erupt in genital or inframammary areas), or (3) lower extremities (look for reddening, flaking, dusky appearance, blanching, mottling) |
| | | |
| b. Skin alterations: trauma induced | Bruises, lacerations, excoriations may heal more slowly | Large number of bruises<br>Tearing of thin skin<br>Reddened areas from pressure (bony prominences)<br>Fissures or hyperkeratosis associated with friction (heels, toes, side of foot rubbing against shoe)<br>Evaluated in same manner as with adult client |

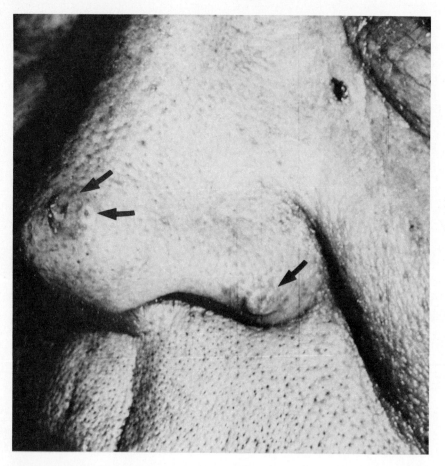

**FIG. 3-32.** Sebaceous hyperplasia. (From Steinberg, F.U., editor: Care of the geriatric patient, ed. 6, St. Louis, 1983, The C.V. Mosby Co.)

†These lesions are fairly common in elderly adults. They are all considered "abnormal" and should be treated.

| CHARACTERISTIC OR AREA EXAMINED | NORMAL | DEVIATIONS FROM NORMAL |
|---|---|---|
| 8. Nails<br>  **a.** Configuration | Toenails may be thickened, distorted (toenails treated for fungal infection may not return to normal configuration) (Fig. 3-33) | Toenail thickening associated with fungal infection (yellowish discoloration, granular surface)<br>Uncut toenails curled over foot |

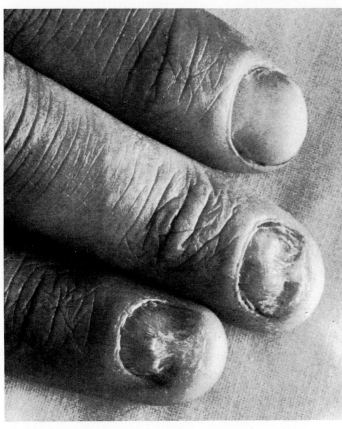

FIG. 3-33. Fungal infection of nails. (From Stewart, W.D., Danto, J.L., and Maddin, S.: Dermatology: diagnosis and treatment of cutaneous disorders, ed. 4, St. Louis, 1978, The C.V. Mosby Co.)

| | | |
|---|---|---|
| **b.** Consistency | Fingernails may be more brittle, may peel | |
| **c.** Color | Toenails may lose translucency | |
| 9. Hair and scalp | | |
| **a.** Surface | Sebaceous hyperplasia may extend into scalp | Evaluated in same manner as with adult client |
| **b.** Distribution | Increased facial hair (especially women), bristly quality (Fig. 3-30) | |
| | Men may have coarse hair in ears, nose, eyebrows | |
| | Decreased scalp hair (scalp may be visible) | Sudden hair loss |
| | Symmetrical balding in men (most often frontal or occipital) | Patchy, asymmetrical hair loss |
| | Decreased pubic and axillary hair | |
| **c.** Texture | Facial hair coarse, body hair fine | Sudden change in texture |
| **d.** Color | Graying, whitening (hairs that do not lose pigment often become darker) | |
| **e.** Quantity | General decrease of body and scalp hair | |

**Cognitive self-assessment**

Following is a series of statements about integumentary function and formation. Mark each statement "T" or "F."

1. _____ Skin without epidermis is freely permeable.
2. _____ Corns and calluses are areas of hypertrophied horny epidermis.
3. _____ Eccrine sweat glands are widely distributed over the body and contribute to temperature regulation.
4. _____ Skin turgor (normal firmness) is determined by the amount of subcutaneous tissue available.
5. _____ Calluses may distort normal skin coloration.
6. _____ Effective resistance to skin injury is determined in part by adequate circulation.
7. _____ Effective resistance to skin injury is determined in part by the presence of sufficient subcutaneous tissue.
8. _____ Apocrine sweat glands are widely distributed over the body.
9. _____ The amount of skin moisture normally varies according to environmental conditions.
10. _____ Pallor, in dark skin, may be observable by noting the absence of underlying red tones.

For questions 11 through 17, all the statements but one are true. Pick the false one.

11. The stratum corneum:
    - ☐ a. is composed of keratin
    - ☐ b. is part of the epidermis
    - ☐ c. is composed of dead cells
    - ☐ d. absorbs water readily
    - ☐ e. lies under the subcutaneous layer

12. The epidermal layer:
    - ☐ a. is avascular
    - ☐ b. is uniformly paper thin
    - ☐ c. is a barrier to external substances
    - ☐ d. prevents excessive water loss
    - ☐ e. contains melanin

13. Keratin:
    - ☐ a. originates in the dermis
    - ☐ b. is the principal constituent of nails and hair
    - ☐ c. is a tough fibrous protein
    - ☐ d. originates in the epidermis

14. Melanin:
    - ☐ a. produces varying skin shades of yellow, brown, and black
    - ☐ b. is produced in some people in response to ultraviolet rays
    - ☐ c. deposits are usually heavier in the palms, soles, and nail beds
    - ☐ d. acts as a barrier to ultraviolet radiation
    - ☐ e. deposits may normally be patchy or uneven

15. The dermis:
    - ☐ a. is well supplied with blood and lymph vessels
    - ☐ b. contains the peripheral nervous system
    - ☐ c. is freely permeable
    - ☐ d. is nourished by the epidermis
    - ☐ e. contains sebaceous glands

16. Sebum:
    - ☐ a. is an oily secretion produced in the apocrine glands
    - ☐ b. glands are more numerous on the face and scalp

☐ c. production is increased at the time of puberty
☐ d. production is decreased when peripheral circulation is impaired
☐ e. accumulation on the skin can cause skin irritation

17. The subcutaneous layer:
    ☐ a. stores fat
    ☐ b. contributes to body heat conservation
    ☐ c. varies greatly in amounts among individuals
    ☐ d. supplies melanocytes for pigmentation
    ☐ e. acts as a cushion

18. Systematic integument evaluation is especially important when the client:
    ☐ a. is receiving treatments (e.g., topical medications, soaks) that involve the skin
    ☐ b. has impaired circulation
    ☐ c. depends on others for physical care or protection (e.g., infants, debilitated or immobilized individuals)
    ☐ d. has been living under unhygienic circumstances
    ☐ e. is known to have particularly sensitive or delicate skin.
    ☐ f. a, b, and c
    ☐ g. all the above
    ☐ h. all except d
    ☐ i. all except e

19. Which of the following statements are true?
    ☐ a. Prolonged anoxemia will result in clubbing of the nails.
    ☐ b. Spider angiomas can be associated with pregnancy.
    ☐ c. Hypothyroidism can cause scalp hair to be dry and coarse.
    ☐ d. Acne is likely to be more prominent on the face, scalp, chest, and back.
    ☐ e. Scabies is likely to be more prominent on the wrists, hands, axillae, and inguinal area.
    ☐ f. all except b
    ☐ g. a, d, and e
    ☐ h. all the above
    ☐ i. all except c

Match the definitions in column B with the terms in column A.

| Column A | Column B |
|---|---|
| 20. _____ Macule | a. Large, superficial, fluid-containing elevation greater than 0.5 cm |
| 21. _____ Papule | |
| 22. _____ Nodule | b. Loss of superficial epidermis, moist but not bleeding |
| 23. _____ Vesicle | |
| 24. _____ Bulla | c. Circumscribed, flat, change in skin color |
| 25. _____ Pustule | d. Thin flakes of exfoliated epidermis |
| 26. _____ Wheal | e. Deep linear crack in the skin |
| 27. _____ Scale | f. Solid elevated mass, usually less than 1.0 cm |
| 28. _____ Crust | g. Solid mass extending into subcutaneous or dermal tissue |
| 29. _____ Erosion | |
| 30. _____ Scar | h. Replacement of skin by fibrous tissue |
| 31. _____ Fissure | i. Elevation containing purulent exudate |
| | j. Small superficial elevation, less than 1.0 cm, containing serous fluid |
| | k. Dried residue of serum, pus, or blood |
| | l. Flat-topped, superficial, and well-circumscribed elevation |

PEDIATRIC QUESTIONS

32. All the following skin color characteristics are normal except one. Pick the statement that indicates an abnormal finding.
    - ☐ a. Beefy red color seen in a newborn less than 24 hours old
    - ☐ b. Jaundice appearing on the third day of life
    - ☐ c. Jaundice of the palms and soles of a toddler who loves carrots
    - ☐ d. Jaundice appearing within 24 hours of birth
    - ☐ e. Mottled appearance of the hands and feet of a newborn

33. A healthy newborn may show which of the following skin characteristics?
    - ☐ a. Flakiness of skin around wrists and ankles
    - ☐ b. Milia—small white papules over nose
    - ☐ c. Dermatoglyphics—straight lines across upper palms of hands
    - ☐ d. Mongolian spots
    - ☐ e. Hair over shoulders and upper back
    - ☐ f. all except d
    - ☐ g. a, b, and d
    - ☐ h. b and c
    - ☐ i. all except c
    - ☐ j. all the above

Mark each statement "T" or "F."

34. _____ A "strawberry mark" is a red, raised, and soft capillary hemangioma.

35. _____ Tufts of hair found over the spine are generally considered to be a sign of retardation.

36. _____ An example of a disease having papules is poison ivy.

GERIATRIC QUESTIONS

For questions 37 through 39, all the statements are true except one. Pick the false statement.

37. A number of epidermal and dermal changes occur with aging.
    - ☐ a. Outer skin moisture and suppleness often directly reflect the amount of moisture available in the environment.
    - ☐ b. Toenails may be thicker and somewhat disfigured.
    - ☐ c. The loss of melanocytes may contribute to a pale appearance in Caucasians.
    - ☐ d. Precancerous lesions are a noted hazard for brown- and yellow-skinned people.
    - ☐ e. Pigment deposits (lentigines) may be more numerous in sun-exposed skin areas.

38. Subcutaneous fat decreases with aging.
    - ☐ a. Bony prominences emerge.
    - ☐ b. Sensitivity to cold weather increases.
    - ☐ c. Sensitivity to warm weather increases.
    - ☐ d. A folded, wrinkled, and lax appearance of the skin increases.
    - ☐ e. The abdomen may remain obese in spite of fat loss over arms and legs.

39. A healthy elderly person might manifest the following integumentary changes.
    - ☐ a. Hyperkeratosis
    - ☐ b. Vitiligo
    - ☐ c. Increased coarsening of facial hair
    - ☐ d. Decrease and thinning of body hair
    - ☐ e. Patchy balding (men)

## SUGGESTED READINGS
### General

Bates, B.: A guide to physical examination, ed. 3, Philadelphia, 1983, J.B. Lippincott Co., pp. 43-53.

Capell, P.T., and Case, D.B.: Ambulatory care manual for nurse practitioners, Philadelphia, 1976, J.B. Lippincott Co., pp. 283-313.

Davis, M.: Getting to the root of the problem: hair grooming techniques for black patients, Nursing '77 **7**(4):60-65, 1977.

Forbes, E.J., and Fitzsimons, V.M.: The older adult: a process for wellness, St. Louis, 1981, The C.V. Mosby Co., pp. 203-207.

Malasanos, L., and others: Health assessment, ed. 2, St. Louis, 1981, The C.V. Mosby Co., pp. 180-204.

Nordmark, M.T., and Rohweder, A.W.: Scientific foundations of nursing, ed. 3, Philadelphia, 1975, J.B. Lippincott Co., pp. 221-238.

Prior, J.A., Silberstein, J.S., and Stang, J.M.: Physical diagnosis: the history and examination of the patient, ed. 6, St. Louis, 1981, The C.V. Mosby Co., pp. 64-70.

Roach, L.B.: Color changes in dark skin, Nursing '77 **7**(1):48-51, 1977.

Shmunes, E.: The importance of pre-employment examinations in the prevention and control of occupational skin disease, J. Occup. Med. **22**(6):407-409, 1980.

Wasson, J., and others: The common symptom guide, New York, 1975, McGraw-Hill Book Co., pp. 270-271, 280-284.

### Pediatric

Alexander, M., and Brown, M.S.: Pediatric history taking and physical diagnosis for nurses, ed. 2, New York, 1979, McGraw-Hill Book Co., pp. 42-54.

Barness, L.: Manual of pediatric physical diagnosis, ed. 5, Chicago, 1981, Year Book Medical Publishers, Inc., pp. 23-47.

Brown, M.S., and Murphy, M.A.: Physical examination. III. Examining the skin, Nursing '73 **3**(9):39-43, 1973.

Cohen, S.: Skin rashes in infants and children, Programmed instruction, Am. J. Nurs. **78**(6):1041-1072, 1978.

DeAngelis, C.: Basic pediatrics for the primary health care provider, Boston, 1975, Little, Brown & Co., pp. 38-42, 249-264.

Verbov, J., and Morley, N.: Color atlas of pediatric dermatology, Philadelphia, 1983, J.B. Lippincott Co.

Whaley, L.F., and Wong, D.L.: Nursing care of infants and children, ed. 2, St. Louis, 1983, The C.V. Mosby Co., pp. 118-121.

### Geriatric

Burnside, I.M. editor: Nursing and the aged, ed. 2, New York, 1981, McGraw-Hill Book Co., pp. 32-34, 414.

DeVillez, R.L.: Externally and internally caused skin problems of aging, Geriatrics **38**(1):71-78, 1983.

Malasanos, L., and others: Health assessment, ed. 2, St. Louis, 1981, The C.V. Mosby Co., pp. 630-631.

Palmore, E., editor: Normal aging II: reports from the Duke Longitudinal Studies, Durham, N.C., 1974, Duke University Press, pp. 18-23.

Shelley, W.B., and Shelley, E.D.: The ten major problems of aging skin, Geriatrics **37**(9):107-113, 1982.

Steinberg, F.U., editor: Care of the geriatric patient, St. Louis, 1983, The C.V. Mosby Co., pp. 199-215.

Uhler, D.: Common skin changes in the elderly, Am. J. Nurs. **78**(8):1342-1344, 1978.

Wells, T.J.: In geriatric patients: that "minor" skin problem could be trouble, R.N. **41**(7):41-46, 1978.

Wright, E.T.: Identifying and treating common benign skin tumors, Geriatrics **33**(6):37-44, 1978.

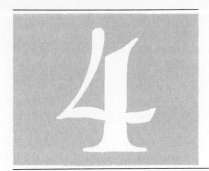

# Head and neck

## VOCABULARY

**alopecia** Absence or loss of hair.

**anterior triangle (of neck)** Landmark area for palpating the submaxillary, submental, and anterior cervical lymph nodes; sectioned by the anterior surface of the sternocleidomastoid muscle, the mandible, and an imagined line running from the chin to the sternal notch.

**cricoid cartilage** Lowermost cartilage of the larynx.

**fontanel** Unossified space or soft spot lying between the cranial bones of an infant.

**frontal bone** Forehead bone.

**goiter** Hypertrophy of the thyroid gland, usually evident as a pronounced swelling in the neck.

**hirsutism** Excessive body hair, usually in a masculine distribution, owing to heredity, hormonal dysfunction, porphyria, or medication.

**hyoid** Single bone suspended from the styloid process of the temporal bone.

**isthmus (glandulae thyroideae)** Narrow portion of the thyroid gland connecting the left and right lobes.

**lymphadenitis** Inflammation of the lymph nodes.

**lymphoma** General term for growth of new tissue in the lymphatic area; ordinarily a malignant growth.

**manubrium** Uppermost of the three bones of the sternum.

**mastoid process** Conical projection of the temporal bone extending downward and forward behind the external auditory meatus.

**occipital bone** Bone in the lower back part of the skull between the parietal and temporal bones.

**parietal bone** One of the pair of bones that forms the sides of the cranium.

**posterior triangle (of neck)** Landmark area for palpating the posterior cervical chain, the supraclavicular chain, and the occipital lymph chain; sectioned along the anterior border by the sternocleidomastoid muscle, the posterior border by the trapezius muscle, and the bottom by the clavicle.

**"shotty" node** Lymph node that feels hard and nodular; generally moveable and nontender; may show evidence of having been infected many times in the past.

**sternocleidomastoid muscle** Major muscle that rotates and flexes the head; originates by two heads from the sternum and clavicle and inserts on the mastoid process and the occipital bone.

**trapezius muscle** Major muscle that rotates and extends the head; originates along the superior curved line of the occiput and the spinous processes of the seventh cervical and all thoracic vertebrae and inserts at the clavicle, acromion, and base of the scapula.

## Cognitive objectives

At the end of this chapter the learner will demonstrate knowledge of assessment of the head and neck by the ability to do the following:

1. Systematically list structures of the head and neck evaluated during the physical examination.
2. Describe the characteristics of a lymph node that must be evaluated.
3. Describe the lymphatic drainage of the head and neck.
4. Explain the significance of and methods for examining the thyroid gland and trachea.
5. Apply the terms in the vocabulary section.
6. Identify selected elements of the pediatric head and neck examination.
7. Identify selected elements of the geriatric head and neck examination.

## Clinical objectives

At the end of this chapter the learner will perform a systematic assessment of the head and neck, demonstrating the ability to do the following:

1. Obtain a pertinent health history from the client.
2. Demonstrate and describe the results of inspection and palpation of the following aspects of the head:
   a. Skull for contour and size
   b. Scalp for texture and color
   c. Hair for distribution, quality, and quantity
   d. Facies for symmetry, quality, color, expression, and movements
   e. Head movements
3. Demonstrate and describe the results of inspection and palpation of the neck and thyroid gland for:
   a. Symmetry
   b. Muscular development and movement
   c. Landmarks and location of the trachea
   d. Location, size, shape, delineation, mobility, consistency, and surface characteristics of the faciocervical lymph nodes
   e. Placement, symmetry, and characteristics of the thyroid gland
4. Summarize results of the assessment with a written description of findings.

## Health history additional to screening history

1. Head injury profile
   a. Events associated with the injury
      (1) Predisposing factors leading to injury, such as epilepsy or seizure disorder, blackout, poor vision, dizziness, light-headedness
      (2) Precipitating factors leading to injury, such as unsafe conditions, wet floors, getting up too fast
   b. If possible, describe the exact details of the injury
      (1) Specifically, what happened?
      (2) How did client appear immediately following injury (unconscious, dazed, crying, convulsive)?
      (3) How was client 5 minutes later (vomited, complained of headache, appeared fine, same as immediately following, or different)?
      (4) In general, has client gotten progressively worse or better or been unchanged since injury?
   c. Associated symptoms
      (1) State of consciousness: unconscious (momentary vs. prolonged—describe), dazed, sleepy
      (2) Neck or head pain (see headache profile that follows)
      (3) Visual problems: droopy eyes, blurred or double vision
      (4) Vomiting: number of times, associated distress, projectile in nature
      (5) Motor or sensory changes: staggered gait, tremors, numbness of limbs
      (6) Ear or nasal discharge: serous or bloody discharge from nose or ears
      (7) Loss of urine or bowel control since injury
      (8) Loss of memory: recent or long term
   d. Medications
      (1) Those routinely being taken
      (2) Any discontinued within 1 week before injury
2. Headache profile
   Because of the vast complexity of headaches, profile questioning will incorporate the symptom analysis format presented in Chapter 1.
   a. When was client last entirely well?
      (1) When did *this type* of headache start occurring?
      (2) How long has client been bothered with headaches in general?
   b. Date of current problem onset: If headache has been going on for some time, try to determine beginning date.
   c. Character
      (1) Constant bandlike pressure
      (2) Throbbing, pounding
      (3) Single area pressure
      (4) Single area pain (dull vs. sharp)
      (5) Shooting pains (dull vs. sharp)
      (6) Severity of headache
   d. Nature of problem onset
      (1) Slowly over several weeks, days, hours
      (2) Abrupt onset over several minutes

e. Client's hunch of precipitating factors
   (1) Stress
   (2) Sudden movement or exercise
   (3) Alcohol
   (4) Medication
f. Course of problem
   (1) Lasts for minutes, hours, days, weeks before disappearing; relieved by medication
   (2) Lasts for minutes, hours, days, weeks before disappearing; medication not necessary for relief
   (3) Appears in clusters (several over given time period), then disappears for extensive period before returning
g. Location of problem
   (1) Occipital region
   (2) Frontal region
   (3) Temporal region
   (4) Neck region
   (5) Maxillary sinus region
   (6) Behind eyes
   (7) Unilateral or bilateral
   (8) Generalized or specific
h. Relation to other entities
   (1) Visual changes (decreased acuity or blurring, tearing)
   (2) Nausea and vomiting (which came first: headache or nausea and vomiting?)
   (3) Nasal stuffiness and discharge
   (4) Muscle aches and pains
   (5) Cough, sore throat
   (6) Neck pain and/or stiffness
   (7) Fever

   (8) Change in level of consciousness as headache increases
   (9) Movement aggravates headache symptoms
i. Patterns
   (1) Timing
      (a) Worse in AM or PM
      (b) Occurs only during sleep
      (c) Worse or better as day progresses
   (2) Duration
      (a) Episodes getting closer together and worse
      (b) Getting worse but no closer together
      (c) Lasting longer
j. Efforts to treat
   (1) Physician help sought for headache
   (2) Current medications taken, prescription and over the counter
   (3) Body positions that help headache
   (4) Other remedies that help headache
k. How do headaches interfere with client's activities of daily living?
3. Complaints of neck pain
   a. Head or neck injury or strain
   b. Swelling of neck
   c. Limitations of neck movement (continuous vs. sporadic)
   d. Does neck movement aggravate or alleviate neck pain?
   e. Radiation patterns to arms, shoulders, hands, down back
4. If the client complains of dizziness, it is important to determine exactly what is meant. The term *dizziness* means the inability to maintain equilibrium. In the objective type the room spins; in the subjective type the client is moving.

## Clinical guidelines

|  | TO IDENTIFY: | |
|---|---|---|
| **THE STUDENT WILL:** | **NORMAL** | **DEVIATIONS FROM NORMAL** |

**1.** Ask client to sit and remove wigs or hairpieces

**2.** Inspect and palpate:

   **a.** Skull (Fig. 4-1)

|  |  |  |
|---|---|---|
|     1. Contour | Rounded and symmetrical with frontal, parietal, and bilateral occipital prominences | Lumps, marked protrusions, depressions |
|     2. Size | Wide variety of sizes | Greatly enlarged<br>Abnormally small<br>Protruding mandible |

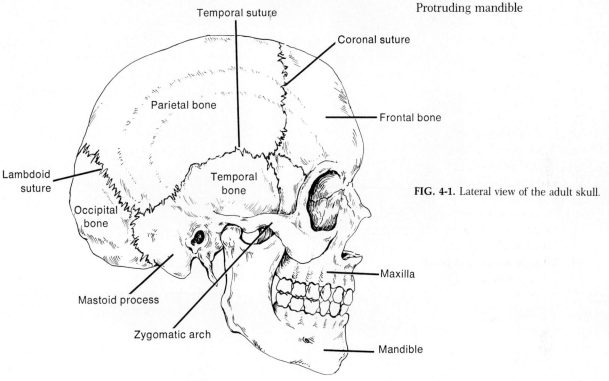

FIG. 4-1. Lateral view of the adult skull.

   **b.** Scalp (Fig. 4-2)

|  |  |  |
|---|---|---|
|     1. Texture | Skin intact | Lesions, scabs<br>Tenderness<br>Scaliness<br>Superficial nodules |

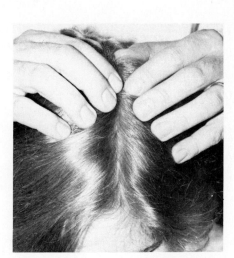

FIG. 4-2. Scalp palpation.

## Clinical guidelines—cont'd

| THE STUDENT WILL: | TO IDENTIFY: | |
|---|---|---|
| | NORMAL | DEVIATIONS FROM NORMAL |
| | Smooth and even skin | Thickening of skin, which becomes coarse, leathery, oily and develops thick folds |
| | | Skin and bone changes also seen in jaw and facial bones, hands, feet (acromegaly) (Fig. 4-3) |

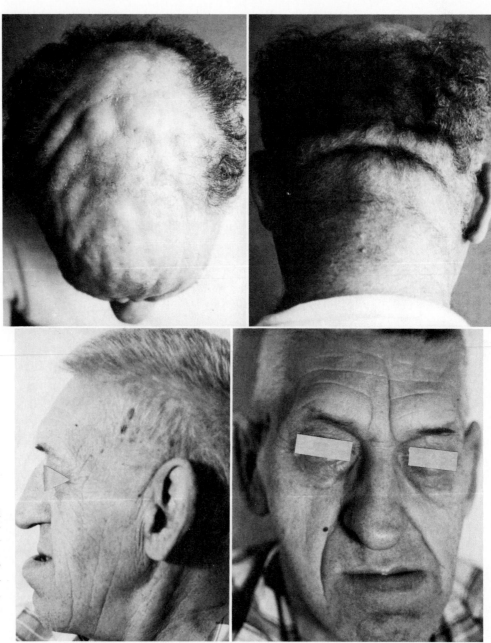

FIG. 4-3. Scalp and facial changes noted with acromegaly. (From Prior, J.A., Silberstein, J.S., and Stang, J.M.: Physical diagnosis: the history and examination of the patient, ed. 6, St. Louis, 1981, The C.V. Mosby Co.)

| | | |
|---|---|---|
| 2. Color | Pigmentation will vary depending on race | Reddened areas |
| | | Areas of increased or decreased pigmentation |
| c. Hair | | |
| 1. Foreign bodies | | Flaking |
| | | Nits |

| THE STUDENT WILL: | TO IDENTIFY: | |
| --- | --- | --- |
| | NORMAL | DEVIATIONS FROM NORMAL |
| 2. Distribution | Even<br>Bilateral, symmetrical balding (Fig. 4-4, *A*) | Patchy, asymmetrical alopecia (Fig. 4-4, *B*) |

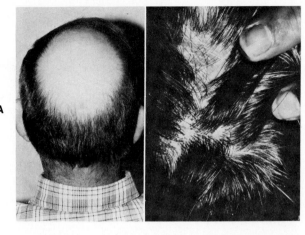

A          B

FIG. 4-4. **A,** Normal balding pattern. **B,** Abnormal balding pattern. (From Stewart, W.D., Danto, J.L., and Maddin, S.: Dermatology: diagnosis and treatment of cutaneous disorders, ed. 4, St. Louis, 1978, The C.V. Mosby Co.)

| | | |
| --- | --- | --- |
| 3. Quantity | Thick, thin, sparse | Excessive loss |
| 4. Quality | Shiny, smooth | Dull, brittle<br>Excessive coarseness or dryness |
| 5. Hygiene | Clean | Odor; matted, dirty |
| **d.** Face | | |
| 1. Symmetry | Symmetrical placement and shape of eyes, ears, mouth, eyebrows, nasolabial folds | Marked asymmetry |
| 2. Quality | Facial qualities vary according to race and body build<br>(Note slight facial asymmetry in photograph below.) (Fig. 4-6, *A*) | Edema (especially of eyelids) (Fig 4-5)<br>Exceptionally coarse features<br>Puffiness<br>Excessive perspiration<br>Waxy pallor<br>Lesions<br>Lip lesions, fissures, swelling<br>Acne, scarring |

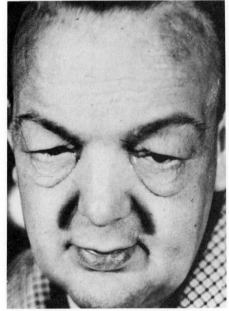

FIG. 4-5. Periorbital edema and facial puffiness as seen in myxedema. (From Prior, J.A., Silberstein, J.S., and Stang, J.M.: Physical diagnosis: the history and examination of the patient, ed. 6, St. Louis, 1981, The C.V. Mosby Co.)

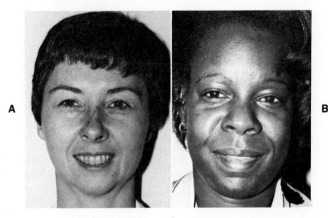

A          B

FIG. 4-6. Variations of facial structures.

## Clinical guidelines—cont'd

| THE STUDENT WILL: | TO IDENTIFY: | |
| --- | --- | --- |
| | NORMAL | DEVIATIONS FROM NORMAL |
| 3. Color | Pigmentation varies with race | Jaundice |
| | | Cyanosis (especially around lips) |
| | | Pigmentation variations |
| 4. Expression | Alert; response appropriate to conversation | No responsiveness |
| | | Tense, drawn muscles |
| | | Inappropriate expression |
| 5. Movements | Controlled, smooth | Involuntary |
| **3.** Evaluate head and neck movements | | |
|   **a.** Instruct client to: | | |
|     1. Move chin to chest | Controlled and smooth throughout series of movements | Rachety movement |
|     2. Move head back so that chin is pointing toward ceiling | Movement of neck from neutral upright position | Bounding (up and down), synchronizes with pulse |
|     3. Move head so that ear is moved toward shoulder (do not allow client to move shoulder up to ear) |   Chin toward chest, 45° flexion<br>  Chin upward toward ceiling, 55° extension<br>  Lateral bending, 40° each way<br>  Rotation 70° for both right and left directions | Rhythmic movement or tremor |
|     4. Move head and neck in lateral rotation so that while head is upward and pointed forward the client's chin is placed on first one shoulder and then the other | No discomfort or limitation of movement (Fig. 4-7) | Pain throughout movement |
| | | Pain at particular points during movement |
| | | Spasms or tics |
| | | Limited range of motion |
| | | Unable to touch points (as indicated) |

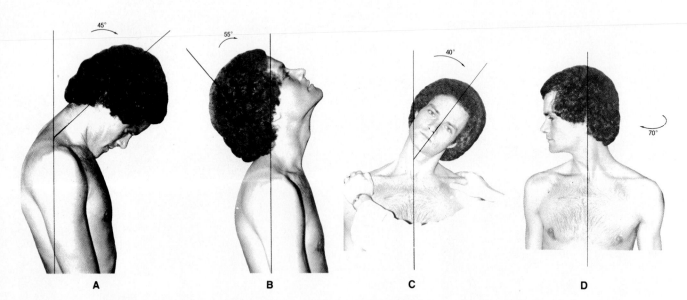

**FIG. 4-7.** Normal range of motion of the neck. **A,** Flexion. **B,** Extension. **C,** Lateral bending. **D,** Rotation.

| THE STUDENT WILL: | TO IDENTIFY: | |
| --- | --- | --- |
| | NORMAL | DEVIATIONS FROM NORMAL |
| **b.** Neck range of motion may be evaluated by a single rotary movement incorporating the four touch points | | |
| **c.** Neck symmetry (Fig. 4-8) | Head position centered<br>Bilateral symmetry of trapezius and sternocleidomastoid muscles | Head tilted<br>Muscle shortening, wasting<br>Tenderness on palpation<br>Masses, scars |

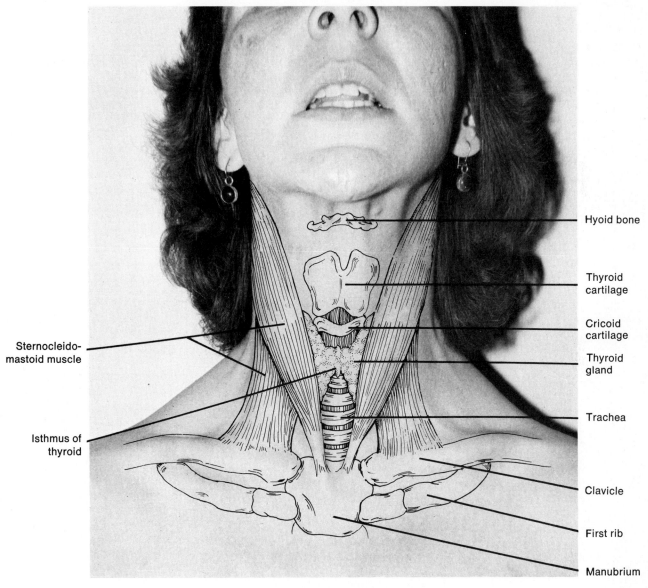

**FIG. 4-8.** Anatomical structure of the neck.

## Clinical guidelines—cont'd

| THE STUDENT WILL: | TO IDENTIFY: NORMAL | DEVIATIONS FROM NORMAL |
|---|---|---|
| **4.** Palpate trachea (easiest just above suprasternal notch) | | |
|    **a.** Location | Central placement | Lateral displacement<br>Tenderness on palpation |
|    **b.** Landmarks | Tracheal rings<br>Cricoid cartilage<br>Thyroid cartilage | |
| **5.** Inspect thyroid | | |
|    **a.** Instruct client to: | | |
|      1. Put chin up as if drinking from glass | | |
|      2. Swallow | | |
|    **b.** Note symmetry and placement | Gland usually not visible | Unilateral or bilateral lobe enlargement* (Fig. 4-9) |
|    **c.** Palpate thyroid | | |
|      1. Stand behind client | | |
|      2. Instruct client to flex head slightly | | |
|      3. Tilt chin slightly toward side you are examining | | |
|      4. Place your fingers anteriorly with finger pads over client's trachea | | |

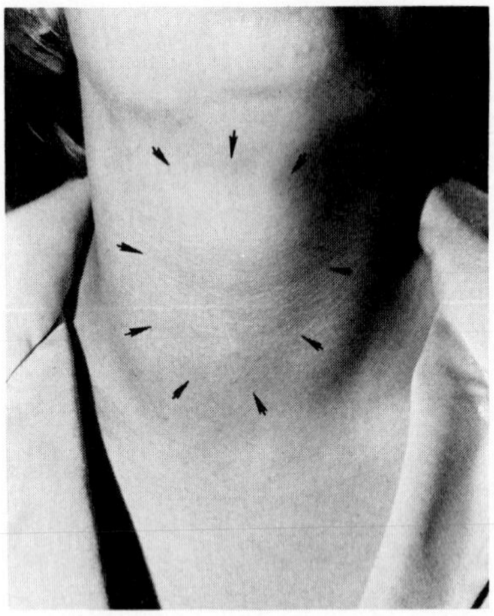

**FIG. 4-9.** Minimal thyroid enlargement encroaching on the sternocleidomastoid muscle. Note full appearance of the neck.

| | | |
|---|---|---|
|      5. Instruct client to swallow periodically so that you can locate identifying landmarks, including: | | |
|        a. Thyroid cartilage | Smooth<br>Centrally located | |
|        b. Cricoid cartilage | Smooth ringlike structure | |
|        c. Isthmus | Smooth tissue found approximately 1 cm below cricoid cartilage<br>May not be felt<br>With swallowing may feel smooth tissue slide under skin | |

*Auscultate the thyroid gland if enlargement is found (use bell of stethoscope). Evidence of abnormality is systolic bruit or continuous venous hum in supraclavicular areas.

| THE STUDENT WILL: | TO IDENTIFY: | |
| --- | --- | --- |
| | NORMAL | DEVIATIONS FROM NORMAL |
| d. Thyroid lobes on lateral border of gland | | |
| (1) Right lobe felt with chin slightly to right | Lobes may not be felt<br>If lobes felt, they are small, smooth, nontender, and rise freely with swallowing | Enlarged lobes<br>Palpated easily without swallowing<br>Nodular or irregular lobe consistency<br>Tender to palpation<br>Gland not freely moving with swallowing |
| (2) Place right fingertips directly behind sternocleidomastoid muscle | | |
| (3) Fingertips of left hand slightly displace trachea to right | | |
| (4) Instruct patient to swallow (Fig. 4-10) | Right lobe larger than left | |
| e. Main body of gland | | |
| (1) Right lobe felt with chin slightly to right | | |
| (2) Place right fingertips directly in front of sternocleidomastoid muscle | | |
| (3) Fingertips of left hand slightly displace trachea to right | | |
| (4) Instruct patient to swallow (Fig. 4-11) | | |
| f. Reverse procedure for left lobe evaluations | | |

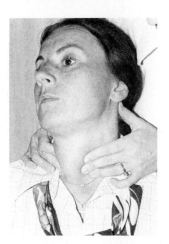

**FIG. 4-10.** Palpating the thyroid behind the client. Displace the trachea with the left hand. Palpate the thyroid lobe with the right hand behind the sternocleidomastoid muscle.

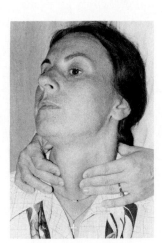

**FIG. 4-11.** Palpating the thyroid behind the client. Displace the trachea with the left hand. Palpate the thyroid lobe with the right hand in front of the sternocleidomastoid muscle.

## Clinical guidelines—cont'd

| THE STUDENT WILL: | TO IDENTIFY: | |
| --- | --- | --- |
| | NORMAL | DEVIATIONS FROM NORMAL |

**6.** Lymphatic nodes
    **a.** Inspect lateral neck (Fig. 4-12)

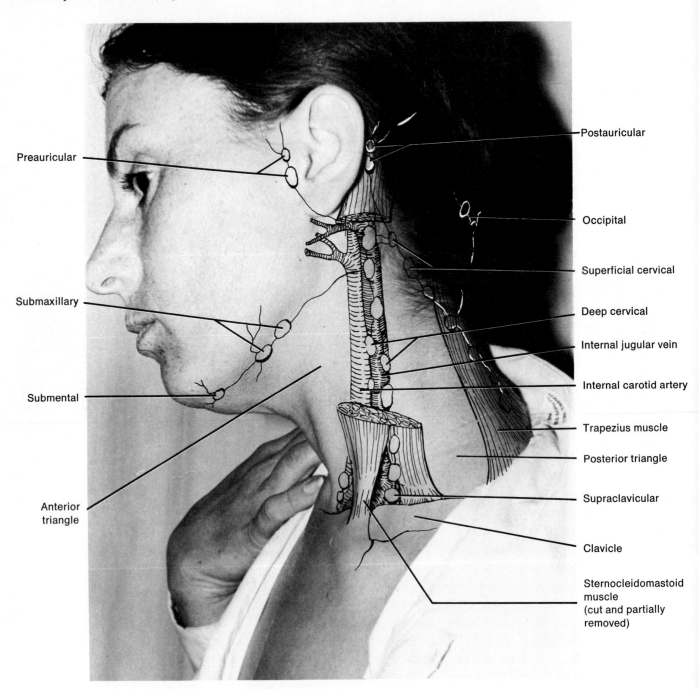

Preauricular

Submaxillary

Submental

Anterior
triangle

Postauricular

Occipital

Superficial cervical

Deep cervical

Internal jugular vein

Internal carotid artery

Trapezius muscle

Posterior triangle

Supraclavicular

Clavicle

Sternocleidomastoid
muscle
(cut and partially
removed)

**FIG. 4-12.** Lateral view of anatomical lymph structures of the neck with nodes.

| THE STUDENT WILL: | TO IDENTIFY: | |
| --- | --- | --- |
| | **NORMAL** | **DEVIATIONS FROM NORMAL** |

**b.** Palpate the following nodes:
1. Preauricular (Fig. 4-13)
2. Postauricular and occipital (Fig. 4-14)
3. Tonsillar, submaxillary, and submental (Fig. 4-15)
4. Superficial and deep cervical (Fig. 4-16)
5. Posterior cervical (Fig. 4-17)
6. Supraclavicular (Fig. 4-18)

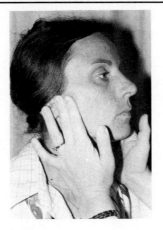

**FIG. 4-13.** Palpating preauricular lymph nodes.

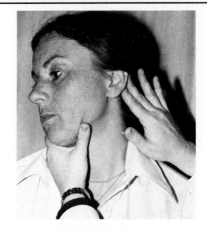

**FIG. 4-14.** Palpating posterior auricular chain of lymph nodes.

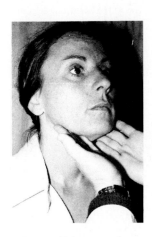

**FIG. 4-15.** Palpating submaxillary lymph nodes.

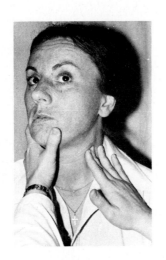

**FIG. 4-16.** Palpating deep cervical chain of lymph nodes.

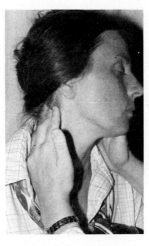

**FIG. 4-17.** Palpating posterior cervical chain of lymph nodes.

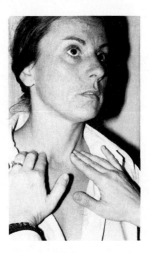

**FIG. 4-18.** Palpating supraclavicular chain of lymph nodes.

| | | |
| --- | --- | --- |
| **c.** Size (cm) and shape | Nodes usually not palpable<br>If palpable, small, mobile, discrete, nontender | Palpable nodes<br>Large, round, cylindrical, irregular |
| **d.** Delimitation | | Multiple discrete or matted nodes |
| **e.** Mobility | | Fixed to underlying tissue<br>Fixed to overlying tissue<br>Induration |
| **f.** Consistency | | Hard, firm; soft, spongy |
| **g.** Surface characteristics | | Smooth, nodular |
| **h.** Tenderness | | Tender on palpation |
| **i.** Heat | | Present |
| **j.** Erythema | | Present |

*Note:* Inspection and palpation of the jugular vein and carotid arteries and auscultation of the carotid arteries are described in Chapter 9.

## Clinical strategies

1. Abnormal hair or scalp texture or quantity should be carefully explored with the client. Most clients are aware of recent or marked changes in texture. Thinning hair, loss of elasticity, or changing pigmentation may be part of the normal aging process. Change in hair care habits can contribute to hair texture changes.

2. Nits can be confused with dandruff. Nits are creamy, yellowish, ovoid, and smooth. They cling to a strand of hair. Dandruff flakes will shake away from scalp or hair and are irregularly shaped.

3. When palpating the skull/scalp, use the palmar surface of finger pads. Some beginning examiners tend to use the distal tips of the fingers instead of the finger pads. The finger pads are much more sensitive to subtle changes.

4. Have the client flex the neck slightly forward for thyroid and trachea palpation. This permits muscle relaxation in this area so that the examiner's fingers can probe more effectively.

5. When palpating the neck and thyroid, have the client comfortably seated so that the neck is relaxed. Some examiners actually encourage the client to rest the back of the head against the examiner's chest.

6. Some textbooks present both anterior and posterior thyroid palpation. Posterior position thyroid palpation is presented here because it is the easiest technique for the beginner to master.

7. There are many teaching techniques for cervical lymph node palpation. Each text the beginning student reads may give slightly different locations for the nodes and use slightly different names. The important points for the student to remember follow:
   a. Find the text you believe best describes node locations and stick to that text for memorization and practice.
   b. Although general anatomical node positions are described in texts, individual locations vary.
   c. When palpating for lymph nodes, the examiner must screen the *entire area* of the anticipated nodes before summarizing clinical findings.
   d. *Light* palpation is necessary to pick up smaller, more superficial nodes.
   e. At times it is helpful for the examiner to place one hand on the client's head and to palpate with the other. In this way the client's head can be moved into any desired position.

8. If you find identifiable lymph nodes, note the following:

   a. Node size, shape, perimeters, mobility, consistency, and tenderness.
   b. Systemic symptoms that may be related to node enlargement. Table 4-1 is helpful in evaluations of this type. It describes node locations and the areas of the body drained by them.

## History and clinical strategies: the pediatric client

1. The head and neck examination of a child is easy to do because it is not considered an intrusive procedure; it is difficult, however, because the size of the examiner's hands may be too large to accurately assess the tiny structures of a child's head and neck.

   a. The fontanels usually present no difficulty in palpation. The examiner must remember that even though babies are born with six fontanels, generally only the frontal and occipital fontanels are palpated. The examiner must have a firm understanding of normal findings so that there can be early identification of deviations.

   b. Head circumference should be evaluated for every child during each visit until the age of 2 years. Because cloth tape measures can stretch, the examiner should use either a metal or paper tape measure. The tape measure should be placed in front at midforehead level and in the back at the level of the occipital protuberance.

   c. For successful evaluation of the child's cervical lymph nodes, the neck muscles must be relaxed. We have found it most helpful to palpate both sides of the child's neck at the same time.

---

**SAMPLE RECORDING**

*Skull:* Normocephalic. No tenderness, lesions, or masses.

*Hair:* Normal female hair distribution. Dark-brown natural color with beginning graying. No nits or flaking noted.

*Face:* Symmetrical. Skin smooth and moist. No involuntary movements noted.

*Neck:* Symmetrical and supple. Trachea midline; thyroid not palpable. No palpable nodes or masses. Full and strong range of motion without discomfort.

**TABLE 4-1.** Lymphatic drainage pattern for cervical lymph nodes

| NODE | LOCATION | RECEIVES DRAINAGE FROM |
|---|---|---|
| Preauricular | In front of tragus of external ear | Scalp, external auditory canal, forehead or upper facial structures, lateral portion of eyelids |
| Postauricular | Behind ear on mastoid process | Parietal region of scalp, external auditory canal |
| Occipital | Midway between external occipital protuberance and mastoid process | Parietal region of scalp |
| Tonsillar | At angle of mandible | Tonsils, posterior palate, thyroid, floor of mouth |
| Submaxillary | Halfway between angle and tip of mandible | Tongue, submaxillary glands, mucosa of lips and mouth |
| Submental | In midline behind tip of mandible | Tongue, mucosa of lips and mouth, floor of mouth |
| Superficial cervical chain | Superficial to sternocleidomastoid muscle | Skin of neck, ear |
| Posterior cervical chain | Along anterior edge of trapezius muscle | Posterior scalp, thyroid, posterior skin of neck |
| Deep cervical chain | Under sternocleidomastoid muscle; includes four separate chains extending over larynx, thyroid gland, and trachea | Larynx, thyroid, trachea, ear, and upper part of esophagus |
| Supraclavicular | Deep in angle formed by sternocleidomastoid muscle and clavicle | Upper abdomen, lungs, breast, arm |

This permits comparison of unilateral or bilateral findings.

   d. The techniques for evaluating the thyroid are the same as those for the adult. The examiner should use only two fingers of each hand as the tracheal stabilizer and lobe palpator, as opposed to all four fingers with an adult client.

   e. Because of the lack of neck muscle stability in the infant, the examiner may elect to evaluate the thyroid from an anterior position with the infant supine.

2. Lymph node presence in children seems to be the norm rather than the exception. The important point is to draw a relationship between the presence of lymph nodes and the general wellness or illness of the child. Barness states: "Shotty, discrete, movable, cool, nontender nodes up to 1 cm in the cervical region are normal when found in the child under 12 years of age."*

3. When examining the child's head and neck, evaluate also the range of motion of the neck. Although an older child is instructed to perform this maneu-ver, younger children and infants should be passively moved through the ranges of neck motion.

4. Before remarking on the "funny looking" facial characteristics of a child, be sure to take a good look at the parents.

5. Risk factors for the pediatric client follow:

   a. Child whose fontanels close earlier than scheduled or remain open longer than scheduled

   b. Fontanels with diameters larger than 4 or 5 cm

   c. Child with overriding suture lines or prolonged, separated suture lines

   d. Child whose head and chest circumferences are disproportionate before age 2

   e. Any bulge areas noted on the scalp or skull

   f. Child with multiple lymph nodes palpated (unexplained presence)

   g. Child with any supraclavicular nodes palpated

   h. Child whose neck does not seem to be growing in proportion to the body

   i. Any neck stiffness or crying with range of motion exercise

   j. Child who maintains a tonic neck reflex beyond 3 to 5 months

   k. Infant unable to hold head up by 2 months

   l. Infant, when in sitting position, unable to hold head steady by 4 months

*From Barness, L.: Manual of pediatric physical diagnosis, ed. 5, Chicago, 1981, Year Book Medical Publishers, Inc., p. 55.

## Clinical variations: the pediatric client

| CHARACTERISTIC OR AREA EXAMINED | NORMAL | DEVIATIONS FROM NORMAL |
|---|---|---|
| **1.** Head | | |
| **a.** Contour | Symmetry noted with frontal, parietal, and bilateral occipital prominences<br>Long heads in Nordic children<br>Broad heads in Oriental children | Asymmetry, marked depressions or protrusions<br>Flattening of part of head<br>Odd-shaped heads that do not follow racial heritage<br>Frontal bulging |
| **b.** Size (Measure during every visit until age 2 years.) | At birth the head measures between 32 and 38 cm; head is normally about 2 cm larger than the chest; by age 2 years both chest and head circumferences are same size; during childhood chest becomes 5 to 7 cm larger than head (Table 4-2) | Any sudden increase in head size<br>Failure of head to grow |

**TABLE 4-2.** Head circumference norms for young children*

| AGE | BOYS (by percentile) | | | GIRLS (by percentile) | | |
|---|---|---|---|---|---|---|
| | 10 | 50 | 90 | 10 | 50 | 90 |
| Birth | 33.5† | 35.3 | 37.0 | 33.4 | 34.7 | 36.0 |
| 3 mo | 39.2 | 40.9 | 42.1 | 38.5 | 40.0 | 41.7 |
| 6 mo | 42.7 | 43.9 | 45.4 | 41.3 | 42.8 | 44.5 |
| 9 mo | 44.5 | 46.0 | 47.1 | 43.1 | 44.6 | 46.3 |
| 12 mo | 45.5 | 47.3 | 48.4 | 44.3 | 45.8 | 47.7 |
| 15 mo | 46.3 | 48.0 | 49.2 | 44.9 | 46.3 | 48.4 |
| 18 mo | 47.0 | 48.7 | 49.9 | 45.4 | 47.1 | 49.0 |
| 2 yr | 48.0 | 49.7 | 51.0 | 46.4 | 48.1 | 50.1 |
| 2.5 yr | 48.5 | 50.2 | 51.6 | 47.0 | 48.8 | 50.8 |
| 3 yr | 48.9 | 50.4 | 51.9 | 47.5 | 49.3 | 51.1 |

Data from Waring, W.W., and Jeansonne, L.O., III: Practical manual of pediatrics: a pocket reference for those who treat children, ed. 2, St. Louis, 1982, The C.V. Mosby Co.
*Head circumference growth rates:
    Full-term newborn-3 mo    2 cm/mo
    3 mo-6 mo    1 cm/mo
    6 mo-1 yr    0.5 cm/mo
†Measurements are given in cm.

| CHARACTERISTIC OR AREA EXAMINED | NORMAL | DEVIATIONS FROM NORMAL |
|---|---|---|
| **2.** Sutures and fontanels (Fig. 4-19) | Suture ridges may be palpated until approximately 6 months<br>Anterior fontanel: small or absent at birth, then enlarges to average 2.5 × 2.5 cm; normally closes between 9 months and 2 years<br>Posterior fontanel: may or may not be able to palpate at birth; usually closes between 1 and 2 months | Sutures that are overriding or remain open beyond 6 months<br>Late closure of fontanel (beyond 2 years) |

| CHARACTERISTIC OR AREA EXAMINED | NORMAL | DEVIATIONS FROM NORMAL |
|---|---|---|

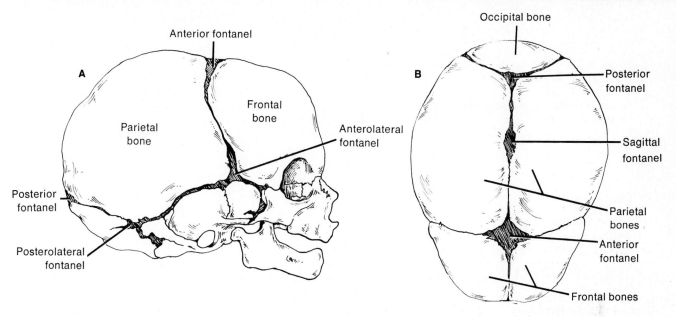

**FIG. 4-19.** Anatomical structures of an infant's skull. **A,** Lateral view. **B,** Superior view.

| CHARACTERISTIC OR AREA EXAMINED | NORMAL | DEVIATIONS FROM NORMAL |
|---|---|---|
| **a.** Palpate fontanel for quality (Infant should be sitting and *not* crying; lying or crying may give fontanel a full or bulging appearance.) | No bulging<br>Slight depression normal<br>Slight palpitations | Bulging or significant depression<br>Bounding palpitations |
| **3.** Scalp texture | Skin intact | Crusting<br>Lesions, scabs<br>Tenderness<br>Scaliness<br>Ringworm patches<br>Superficial nodules |
| **4.** Hair | | White streaks from forehead toward crown (Waardenburg syndrome symptom)<br>Lack of hair pigment<br>Flaking |
| **a.** Foreign bodies | None present | Nits |
| **b.** Distribution | Even | Patchy, asymmetrical alopecia |
| **c.** Quantity | Thick, thin, sparse | Excessive loss |
| **d.** Quality | Shiny, smooth | Dull, brittle<br>Excessive coarseness or dryness |
| **e.** Hygiene | Clean | Odor; matted, dirty |
| **5.** Face | | |
| **a.** Symmetry | Eyes same level<br>Symmetrical placement and shape of eyes, ears, mouth, eyebrows, nasolabial folds | Wide-set or close-set eyes<br>Marked asymmetry<br>Wide bulge at base of nose |

## Clinical variations: the pediatric client—cont'd

| CHARACTERISTIC OR AREA EXAMINED | NORMAL | DEVIATIONS FROM NORMAL |
|---|---|---|
| **b.** Quality | | Edema (especially of eyelids) |
| | | Markedly coarse features |
| | | Puffiness |
| | | Excessive perspiration |
| | | Waxy pallor |
| | | Lesions |
| | | Lip lesions, fissures, swelling |
| | | Acne, scarring |
| **c.** Color | Pigmentation will vary with race | Jaundice |
| | | Cyanosis (especially around lips) |
| | | Pigmentation variations |
| **d.** Expression | Alert; response appropriate to conversation | No responsiveness |
| | | Tense, drawn muscles |
| | | Inappropriate expression |
| **e.** Movements | Controlled, smooth | Involuntary |
| **6.** Head and neck movements | | |
| **a.** Passive range of motion with infants | Able to hold head up by 2 months from prone position | Unable to hold head up by 2 months |
| | Infants younger than 3 months have head lag when pulled into sitting position | Head lag present beyond 3 months |
| | Tonic neck reflex up to 5 months | Tonic neck beyond 5 months |
| | Infant in sitting position able to hold head steady by 4 months | Unable to hold head steady by 4 months |
| **b.** Active range of motion with older children | Controlled and smooth throughout series of movement | Ratchety movement |
| | | Bounding (up and down), synchronizes with pulse |
| | No discomfort or limitations of movement | Pain throughout movement |
| | | Pain of particular points during movement |
| | | Spasms or tics |
| | | Limited range of motion |
| | | Unable to touch points |
| **7.** Neck | | |
| **a.** Symmetry | Head position centered | Head tilted |
| | Bilateral symmetry of trapezius and sternocleidomastoid muscles | Muscle shortening, wasting |
| | | Masses, scars |
| | | Webbing (seen as extra folds of skin) |
| **b.** Palpate (Slightly extend chin upward to expose as much anterior neck as possible.) | | |
| 1. Location | Central placement | Lateral displacement |
| | | Tenderness on palpation |
| 2. Landmarks | Tracheal rings | |
| | Cricoid cartilage | |
| | Thyroid cartilage | |

| CHARACTERISTIC OR AREA EXAMINED | NORMAL | DEVIATIONS FROM NORMAL |
|---|---|---|
| **8.** Thyroid (Palpation should be done using two or three fingers; evaluation will depend on cooperation of child.) | | |
|    **a.** Thyroid cartilage | Smooth<br>Centrally located | |
|    **b.** Cricoid cartilage | Smooth ringlike structure | |
|    **c.** Isthmus | Smooth tissue found below cricoid cartilage<br>May not be felt<br>With swallowing may feel smooth tissue slide under skin | |
|    **d.** Thyroid lobes | Lobes may not be felt<br>If lobes are felt, they are small, smooth, nontender, and rise freely with swallowing | Enlarged lobes<br>Palpated easily without swallowing<br>Nodular or irregular lobe consistency<br>Tender on palpation<br>Gland not freely moving with swallowing |
| **9.** Lymphatic nodes | | |
|    **a.** Palpate the following nodes:<br>     1. Preauricular<br>     2. Postauricular<br>     3. Occipital<br>     4. Tonsillar<br>     5. Submaxillary<br>     6. Submental<br>     7. Superficial cervical<br>     8. Posterior cervical<br>     9. Deep cervical<br>    10. Supraclavicular | | |
|    **b.** Size and shape | Usually not palpable<br>or<br>Small, mobile, discrete, nontender nodes<br>Single nodes up to 1 cm; may appear as shotty, discrete, movable, cool, and nontender | Palpable<br>Large, round, cylindrical, irregular<br>Multiple discrete or matted nodes<br>Similar findings in children over 12 years of age |
|    **c.** Mobility | | Fixed to underlying or overlying tissue<br>Induration |
|    **d.** Consistency | | Hard, firm, soft, spongy |
|    **e.** Surface characteristics | | Smooth, nodular |
|    **f.** Tenderness | | Tender on palpation |
|    **g.** Heat | | Present |
|    **h.** Erythema | | Present |

## History and clinical strategies: the geriatric client

1. Mild tremors (rhythmic) of the head are reported by some authors as normal for some elderly people. However, beginning examiners should report any finding of this nature on the problem list.
2. Head and neck range of motion should be assessed slowly and carefully. The single rotary movement recommended in the adult section for this assessment should not be performed with elderly individuals. Each movement should be evaluated separately for the following symptoms:
   a. Pain on movement
   b. Limited movement
   c. Jerky or "cogwheel" motion
   d. Dizziness accompanying or resulting from movement
   e. Crepitation
   f. Tension of muscles in neck during movement
3. If neck pain and/or limitation of movement is a complaint, be certain to get full information about the following:
   a. Duration of problem
   b. Association of problem with trauma (e.g., from lifting, falling)
   c. Any additional discomfort or sensation (e.g., pain radiating to shoulders, arms, chest, or numbness in fingers or hands)
   d. Aggravating factors (e.g., necessity for stooping, lifting at home or work)
   e. Interference with activities of daily living (e.g., housework, driving automobile, discomfort during sleep, inability to look down while climbing or descending stairs)
4. Complaints of dizziness associated with head and neck movement can pose a serious safety problem for the client. Inquire about client's ability to drive an automobile and to move about in the home and community safely.
5. In palpating for nodes or swellings under the mandible, the examiner is usually able to palpate the submandibular parotid glands. These glands are rather large, soft, and symmetrical and lie approximately midway between the chin and the mandible angles on either side.
6. Occasionally a client may complain of sudden (i.e., within 10 to 30 minutes) swelling under the mandible (usually just anterior to the ear). This may be associated with parotid gland response to obstruction of a duct, duct spasm, or a stone in the duct. Be certain to clarify the timing of onset of swelling, duration (swelling may subside within 30 to 60 minutes), and whether swelling is associated with eating (during or immediately following). The gland may remain enlarged or may swell periodically. This should be considered a problem for referral, but the preceding information assists with final differential diagnosis.
7. Refer to the adult section for additional history and clinical strategy considerations.

# Clinical variations: the geriatric client

| CHARACTERISTIC OR AREA EXAMINED | NORMAL | DEVIATIONS FROM NORMAL |
| --- | --- | --- |
| **1.** Skull | | |
|   **a.** Contour | Rounded and symmetrical with frontal, parietal, and bilateral occipital prominences | Lumps, marked protrusions, depressions |
|   **b.** Size | "Normal" encompasses a wide variety of sizes | Lateral expansion of skull <br> Noticeably enlarged <br> Abnormally small <br> Protruding mandible |
| **2.** Scalp | | |
|   **a.** Surface characteristics | Skin intact and smooth | Lesions, scabs <br> Tenderness <br> Scaliness <br> Superficial nodules |
|   **b.** Color | Pigmentation varies with race | Reddened areas <br> Areas of increased or decreased pigmentation |
| **3.** Hair | | |
|   **a.** Foreign bodies | None present | Flaking <br> Nits, pediculi |
|   **b.** Distribution | Even <br> Bilateral, symmetrical balding <br> Women may exhibit increased facial hair over upper lip or on chin | Patchy, asymmetrical alopecia |
|   **c.** Quantity | Often less hair; appears thin or sparse | Sudden or excessive loss |
|   **d.** Quality | Smooth; may have less luster than younger adult | Brittle <br> Excessive coarseness or dryness |
|   **e.** Hygiene | Clean | Odor; matted, dirty |
| **4.** Face | | |
|   **a.** Symmetry | Usually symmetrical; however, dentures or loss of some teeth may alter facial arrangement | Marked asymmetry (especially eyelids, nasolabial folds, smile pattern) |
|   **b.** Quality | Expression is alert, responsive <br> Wrinkling of skin, especially at forehead, mouth, eyes | Flat or expressionless (limited eye blinking) <br> Edema (especially of eyelids) <br> Markedly coarse features <br> Puffiness <br> Excessive perspiration <br> Waxy pallor <br> Lesions <br> Lip lesions, fissures <br> Swelling <br> Cachectic <br> Acne, scarring |
|   **c.** Color | Pigmentation varies with race <br> Color evenly distributed | Jaundice <br> Cyanosis (especially around lips) <br> Pigmentation variations |
|   **d.** Expression | Alert; eye contact in response to conversation | Tense, drawn muscles <br> Inappropriate expression |
|   **e.** Movements | Controlled, smooth | Tremors, twitches, tics, involuntary movements (e.g., grinding motion of jaws, tremors either localized to lips or eyes or over entire head) |

## Clinical variations: the geriatric client—cont'd

| CHARACTERISTIC OR AREA EXAMINED | NORMAL | DEVIATIONS FROM NORMAL |
|---|---|---|
| **5.** Head and neck position | | |
| **a.** Observe head and neck while client is relaxed and looking straight ahead | Head, neck, and lower jaw may be thrust slightly forward (particularly if client manifests a kyphotic stance) | Head and neck held rigidly (diminished or absent cervical concavity); inability to thrust head forward normally |
| | Females may show a "dowager's hump," an accumulation of posterior fat over the cervical vertebrae | |
| **b.** Involuntary movements | None present | Tremors (coarse or fine) |
| | | Bounding (up and down) |
| | | Synchronizes with pulse |
| **c.** Instruct client to: | | |
| 1. Move chin to chest (Examiner places one hand over back of neck.) | Many elderly clients with cervical arthritis cannot touch chin to chest | Pain with movement (*Note:* Pain may be referred to the ear.) |
| | No discomfort or marked limitation | Crepitation (felt by examiner) |
| | | Gross limitation of movement or jerky motion |
| 2. Move chin toward right shoulder | Movement smooth and easily controlled | Client experiences pain, dizziness with side movements |
| 3. Move chin to left shoulder (Do not permit client to shrug or elevate shoulders.) | Smooth, easy motion | Crepitation or limitation |
| | No gross limitation (movement approximately 70° from straight-ahead gaze in both directions) | |
| 4. Move head toward right shoulder (so that client's ear is directed toward shoulder) | Client should be able to move head 40° from midline in either direction | Pain, grossly limited movement |
| | | Crepitation |
| 5. Move head toward left shoulder | | |
| 6. Move head back so chin points toward ceiling | 30° back from straight-up position | Pain, grossly limited movement |
| | | Crepitation |
| **6.** Neck | | |
| **a.** Symmetry | Head position centered | Head tilted |
| | Bilateral symmetry of trapezius and sternocleidomastoid muscles | Muscle asymmetry or shortening |
| **b.** Surface | Neck veins prominent; loss of subcutaneous fat | Marked muscle wasting or tension |
| | Overlying skin is thin | |
| | Smooth, symmetrical, and nontender on palpation | Tenderness, masses |
| **7.** Trachea | | |
| **a.** Location | Central placement | Lateral displacement |
| | | Tenderness on palpation |
| **b.** Landmarks | Tracheal rings | |
| | Cricoid cartilage | |
| | Thyroid cartilage | |
| **8.** Thyroid | | |
| **a.** Symmetry | Gland usually not visible | Unilateral or bilateral lobe enlargement |
| **b.** Palpate along trachea for: | Smooth | |
| 1. Thyroid cartilage | Centrally located | |
| 2. Cricoid cartilage | Smooth ringlike structure | |
| 3. Isthmus | Smooth tissue found approximately 1 cm below cricoid cartilage | |
| | May not be felt | |
| | With swallowing may feel smooth tissue slide under skin | |

| CHARACTERISTIC OR AREA EXAMINED | NORMAL | DEVIATIONS FROM NORMAL |
|---|---|---|
| 4. Thyroid lobes | Lobes may not be felt<br>If lobes are felt, they are small, smooth, rise freely with swallowing<br>Nontender | Enlarged lobes<br>Palpated easily without swallowing<br>Nodular or irregular lobe consistency<br>Tender to palpation<br>Gland not freely moving with swallowing |
| **9.** Lymphatic nodes<br>  **a.** Inspect and palpate the following nodes:<br>    1. Preauricular<br>    2. Postauricular<br>    3. Occipital<br>    4. Tonsillar<br>    5. Submaxillary<br>    6. Submental<br>    7. Superficial cervical<br>    8. Posterior cervical<br>    9. Deep cervical<br>    10. Supraclavicular | | |
|   **b.** Size and shape | Usually not palpable | Palpable |
|   **c.** Delimitation | | Large, round, cylindrical, irregular<br>Multiple discrete, or matted nodes |
|   **d.** Mobility | | Fixed to underlying or overlying tissue<br>Induration |
|   **e.** Consistency | | Hard, firm, soft, spongy |
|   **f.** Surface characteristics | | Smooth, nodular |
|   **g.** Tenderness | | Tender on palpation |
|   **h.** Heat | | Present |
|   **i.** Erythema | | Present |

## Cognitive self-assessment

1. Which *one* of the following statements about cervical lymph nodes is *not* true?
   - ☐ a. The deep cervical chain is largely obscured by the sternocleidomastoid muscle.
   - ☐ b. Normally, fasciocervical lymph nodes are not palpable in an adult.
   - ☐ c. Lymphatics from the thorax drain up to the supraclavicular nodes.
   - ☐ d. Deep, firm palpation is necessary to effectively reach the tonsillar nodes.
   - ☐ e. Nodes enlarged as a consequence of prior inflammation are frequently palpable.
2. An ear infection might involve all the following lymph nodes except one. Identify the *one not involved.*
   - ☐ a. Preauricular
   - ☐ b. Superficial cervical
   - ☐ c. Posterior cervical chain
   - ☐ d. Deep cervical chain
   - ☐ e. Postauricular

3. An infected tooth might involve all the following lymph nodes except one. Identify the *one not involved.*
   - ☐ a. Posterior cervical
   - ☐ b. Submental
   - ☐ c. Submaxillary
   - ☐ d. Tonsillar
   - ☐ e. Deep cervical
4. The anterior triangle of the neck includes all but one of the following structures. Identify the *one not included.*
   - ☐ a. Thyroid gland
   - ☐ b. Anterior cervical nodes
   - ☐ c. Trachea
   - ☐ d. Carotid artery
   - ☐ e. Omohyoid muscle
5. The largest endocrine gland in the body is the:
   - ☐ a. adrenal gland
   - ☐ b. parotid gland
   - ☐ c. thyroid gland
   - ☐ d. ovary
   - ☐ e. submaxillary gland
6. Swallowing causes the lateral parts of the thyroid tissue to __ against the examiner's fingers.
   - ☐ a. fall
   - ☐ b. rise
   - ☐ c. bulge
   - ☐ d. remain stationary
7. The thyroid isthmus is most easily palpated:
   - ☐ a. just above the cricoid cartilage
   - ☐ b. just below the cricoid cartilage
   - ☐ c. just below the thyroid cartilage
   - ☐ d. just above the thyroid cartilage
   - ☐ e. just below the hyoid bone

Identify the lymph nodes in the illustration on the opposite page.
   8. _____ Preauricular
   9. _____ Occipital
   10. _____ Tonsillar
   11. _____ Postauricular
   12. _____ Submental
   13. _____ Submaxillary
   14. _____ Superficial cervical
   15. _____ Deep cervical
   16. _____ Posterior cervical
   17. _____ Supraclavicular

**PEDIATRIC QUESTIONS**

18. When palpating the skull of a 4-month-old child, the examiner would *expect* the following *normal findings*.
    □ a. Skull size 36 cm
    □ b. Sagittal suture palpated
    □ c. Coronal suture palpated
    □ d. Anterior fontanel approximately 2 cm × 2 cm; soft, not full
    □ e. Posterior fontanel approximately 1 cm × 1 cm; soft, not full
    □ f. All except b
    □ g. All except c
    □ h. All except a
    □ i. All except e
    □ j. All the above

19. All the following statements about lymph node palpation in the child are true except *one*. Identify the false statement.
    □ a. Multiple palpable lymph nodes less than 1 cm in diameter may be normal.
    □ b. Single palpable lymph nodes less than 3 mm in diameter may be normal.
    □ c. Palpable supraclavicular nodes are considered abnormal regardless of size.
    □ d. Shotty nodes are considered "red flags" for possible systemic infections.
    □ e. Because of a child's fat or short neck, it may be impossible to palpate any cervical lymph nodes.

**GERIATRIC QUESTIONS**

20. When assessing an elderly client for head and neck range of motion:
    - ☐ a. a single rotary motion is a good screening mechanism
    - ☐ b. assess for dizziness associated with movement
    - ☐ c. crepitation may be felt by the examiner
    - ☐ d. assess for jerky motions
    - ☐ e. ask client to shrug shoulders to complete full range of motion testing
    - ☐ f. all the above
    - ☐ g. b, c, and d
    - ☐ h. a, c, and e
    - ☐ i. all except b

21. Painful limited head and neck motion:
    - ☐ a. can be accompanied by pain radiating to shoulders and arms
    - ☐ b. can impose safety risks on client
    - ☐ c. can always be resolved with proper exercises and rest
    - ☐ d. all the above
    - ☐ e. a and b

## SUGGESTED READINGS
### General

Bates, B.: A guide to physical examination, ed. 3, Philadelphia, 1983, J.B. Lippincott Co., pp. 54-124.

Examination of the head and neck, Am. J. Nurs. **75**(5):1-24, 1975.

Malasanos, L., and others: Health assessment, ed. 2, St. Louis, 1981, The C.V. Mosby Co., pp. 246-255, 260-266.

Prior, J.A., Silberstein, J.S., and Stang, J.M.: Physical diagnosis: the history and examination of the patient, ed. 6, St. Louis, 1981, The C.V. Mosby Co., pp. 71-98.

Werner, S.C., and Ingbar, S.H.: The thyroid: a fundamental and clinical text, ed. 4, New York, 1978, Harper & Row, Publishers, Inc.

### Pediatric

Barness, L.: Manual of pediatric physical diagnosis, ed. 5, Chicago, 1981, Year Book Medical Publishers, Inc., pp. 48-109.

Brown, M.S., and Alexander, M.: Physical examination. IV. The lymph system, Nursing '73 **3**(10):49-52, 1973.

Brown, M.S., and Alexander, M.: Physical examination. VI. The head, face, and neck, Nursing '74 **4**(1):47-50, 1974.

### Geriatric

Caird, F.I., and Judge, T.G.: Assessment of the elderly patient, London, 1977, Pitman Medical Publishing Co., Ltd., pp. 53-55, 59-61.

Carotenuto, R., and Bullock, J.: Physical assessment of the gerontologic client, Philadelphia, 1980, F.A. Davis Co., pp. 63-68.

# Nose, paranasal sinuses, mouth, and oropharynx

## VOCABULARY

**alveolar ridge** Bony prominences of the maxilla and mandible that support the teeth; in edentulous clients these structures support dentures.

**aphthous ulcer (canker sore)** A painful ulcer on the mucous membrane of the mouth.

**attrition of teeth** Wearing away of the occlusal surfaces of the teeth from many years of chewing or excessive grinding.

**bruxism** Grinding of the teeth; usually an unconscious act occurring during sleep.

**buccal** Pertaining to the inside of the cheek.

**epistaxis** Bleeding from the nose.

**epulis** Any growth on the gum.

**Fordyce spots** Small yellowish spots on the buccal membrane that are visible sebaceous glands; a normal phenomenon seen in many adults, but sometimes mistaken for abnormal lesions; also called *Fordyce granules.*

**frenulum (lingual)** Band of tissue that attaches the ventral surface of the tongue to the floor of the mouth.

**gingiva** Pertaining to the gum.

**glossitis** An inflammation of the tongue.

**leukoplakia** Well-circumscribed, thickened, white patch that can appear on any mucous membrane; sometimes precancerous; often a response to chronic irritation, such as pipe smoking.

**nares (singular: naris)** Nostrils; the anterior openings of the nose.

**papilla** General term for a small projection; dorsal surface of the tongue is composed of a variety of forms of papillae that contain openings to the taste buds.

**periodontitis (pyorrhea)** Inflammation and deterioration of the gums and supporting alveolar bone; occurs in varying degrees of severity; if neglected, this condition will result in loss of teeth.

**perlèche (cheilosis, cheilitis)** Fissures at the corners of the mouth that become inflamed; causes are overclosure of the mouth in an edentulous client, marked loss of alveolar ridge, or riboflavin deficiency; saliva irritates the area, and moniliasis is a common complication.

**plaque** Film that accumulates on the surface of teeth; made up of mucin and colloidal material from saliva, plaque is subject to bacterial invasion.

**ptyalism** Excessive salivation.

**rhino-** Combining form pertaining to the nose. EXAMPLE: *Rhinitis* is an inflammation of the mucous membrane of the nose.

**stoma** General term that means opening or mouth. EXAMPLE: *Stomatitis* refers to a general inflammation of the oral cavity.

**torus palatinus** Exostosis, or benign outgrowth of bone, located on the midline of the hard palate; a fairly common finding that appears in a variety of shapes and sizes.

**turbinates** Extensions of the ethmoid bone located along the lateral wall of the nose; these fingerlike projections are covered with erectile mucosal membranes that become swollen or inflamed in response to allergy or viral invasion.

**vermilion border** A demarcation point between the mucosal membrane of the lips and the skin of the face; common site for recurrent infections, such as herpes infections, and carcinoma; blurring of this border may be an early sign of lesion development.

**xerostomia** Dryness of the mouth.

## Cognitive objectives

At the end of this chapter the learner will demonstrate knowledge of assessment of the nose, paranasal sinuses, mouth, and oropharynx by the ability to do the following:

1. List inspection criteria and processes for evaluating the external and internal nose, including nasal structure, turbinates, meatuses, and septum.
2. List inspection and palpation criteria for evaluating the maxillary and frontal sinuses.
3. Discuss a systematic method to test intactness of the olfactory nerve (CN I).
4. Identify the anterior and posterior boundaries of the mouth.
5. Describe characteristics of the lips, gums, tongue, teeth, and buccal mucosa that are relevant to assessment.
6. Point out characteristics of the oropharynx that are relevant to assessment.
7. Identify selected common physical variations with pediatric and geriatric clients.
8. Apply the terms in the vocabulary section.

## Clinical objectives

At the end of this chapter the learner will perform a systematic assessment of the nose, paranasal sinuses, mouth, and oropharynx by demonstrating the ability to do the following:

1. Obtain a pertinent health history from a client.
2. Demonstrate and describe results of inspection and palpation of the following:
   a. External and internal nose for structure, septum position, patency, turbinates, and meatuses
   b. Frontal and maxillary sinuses
   c. Temporomandibular joint for mobility, tenderness, crepitus, referred pain, and occlusion
   d. Lips for color, symmetry, moisture, and surface characteristics
   e. Gingivobuccal fornices and buccal mucosa for color, landmarks, and surface characteristics
   f. Gums for color and surface characteristics
   g. Teeth for number, color, form, surface characteristics, and insertion
   h. Tongue for symmetry, movement, color, surface characteristics, and texture
   i. Floor of mouth for color and surface
   j. Hard and soft palates for color and surface
3. Demonstrate and describe results of inspection and observation of mouth odor and the oropharynx for landmarks, color, and surface.
4. Summarize results of the assessment with a written description of the findings.

## Health history additional to screening history

1. If client states that the nose is "stopped up" or obstructed, ask the following questions:
   a. History of nasal surgery?
   b. History of blow or injury to nose?
   c. Are both nares usually obstructed, or just right or left naris?
   d. Often necessary to breathe through the mouth (especially at night)?
   e. History of discharge followed by crusting and localized pain? Is nose picking or scratching contributing to the problem?
   f. Nose drops or nasal spray used? Clarify type, amount, frequency, and how long client has used medication.
2. If client has a history of nosebleeds, ask the following questions:
   a. Bleeding usually from both nostrils, or just right or left naris?
   b. Is bleeding aggravated by crusting? Is pain followed by picking or scratching?
   c. Do full symptom analysis with this complaint.
3. History of repeated sinusitis? General treatment?
4. History of chronic postnasal drip? Is it associated with seasons or weather changes?
5. If mouth or dental problems are observed, the following inquiries are appropriate:
   a. Do you experience pain? If so, how severe and how often? Do you treat the pain? What medications? How often? Do you apply anything locally to teeth or gums? What and how often?
   b. Do your mouth problems interfere with or alter food intake? Describe foods that you can no longer eat.
   c. Are other members of the family having dental or mouth problems?
6. If lesions are observed on mouth or lips, inquire about:
   a. Efforts to treat (medications or local applications).
   b. Whether lesions disappear and reappear. Identify pattern, if possible, associated with foods, stress, seasons, fatigue.
   c. Whether others close to client have lesions.
   d. Whether client smokes a pipe.
7. If client wears dentures, inquire about their effectiveness. Are they worn all the time? Just for meals? Do they permit the eating and chewing of all foods? Are they loose or wobbly? Do they click or whistle or interfere with talking? Does client use any adhesive to retain dentures in place? Ask about den-

ture cleaning habits. Are gums or palate ever irritated or tender? Does client feel that the dentures are cosmetically satisfactory?

8. If client complains of, or offers a history of, sore throat, ask the following questions:
   a. Are others in your home ill at present time, or do others close to you often have colds or sore throats?
   b. Do you have to inhale dust or fumes at work?
   c. Does it feel as though you have a lump in your throat?
   d. Does it hurt to swallow?
   e. Is the sore throat associated with fever, cough, headache, decreased appetite?
   f. Is your nose obstructed ("stopped up"); do you have to breathe through your mouth?
   g. Is your throat more tender in the morning? Evening?
   h. Is your home dry (humidity level)?
   i. Is sore throat associated with hoarseness?
   j. Treatment (medications, gargling)?
9. If client complains of a hoarse voice (either acute, intermittent, or chronic), ask:
   a. Do you use your voice a lot?
   b. Is hoarseness associated with fever, sore throat, or cold symptoms?
   c. Does the weather affect your voice?
   d. In addition to hoarseness, has your voice changed (e.g., weak, husky, higher or lower pitch)?
   e. Do you have a constant urge to clear your throat?

## Clinical guidelines

| THE STUDENT WILL: | TO IDENTIFY: | |
| --- | --- | --- |
| | NORMAL | DEVIATIONS FROM NORMAL |
| 1. Assemble necessary equipment:<br>   a. Penlight<br>   b. Otoscope with broad-tipped nasal speculum or nasal speculum | | |
| 2. Inspect general appearance of nose | | |
|    a. Surface/skin | Smooth, intact<br>Skin color same as face | Lesions, warty appearance<br>Redness, discoloration<br>Vascularization |
|    b. Contour | External alignment symmetrical (or nearly symmetrical) | Marked asymmetry<br>Swelling or hypertrophy (bulbous appearance) |
|    c. Nares | Symmetrical<br>Dry, no crusting<br>No flaring or narrowing associated with breathing | Marked asymmetry<br>Discharge present, crusting<br>Narrowing on inspiration (associated with chronic obstruction and mouth breathing) |
| 3. Press finger on side of client's nose to occlude one naris, and ask client to close mouth and breathe through opposite side to test for patency; repeat with other naris | Noiseless, free exchange of air through each naris | Breathing noisy or obstructed |
| 4. Palpate external nose for:<br>   a. Stability<br>   b. Tenderness | Firm<br>Nontender | Unstable<br>Tender on palpation; masses |
| 5. Evaluate olfactory nerve (CN I): ask client to close eyes and mouth; occlude one naris at a time and hold aromatic substance (lemon extract, coffee) under each nostril for odor identification | Client able to identify odor | Incorrect identification of odor |

## Clinical guidelines—cont'd

| THE STUDENT WILL: | TO IDENTIFY: | |
| --- | --- | --- |
| | NORMAL | DEVIATIONS FROM NORMAL |

**6.** Inspect internal nasal cavity using nasal speculum: hold speculum in left hand and stabilize with index finger against side of nose; insert approximately 1 cm and dilate outer naris as much as possible (Fig. 5-1); use right hand to adjust client's head and to hold penlight, or use otoscope with nasal speculum attached; observe naris:

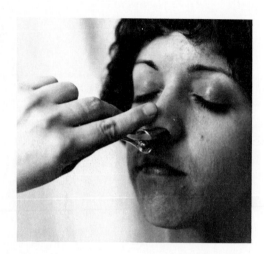

**FIG. 5-1.** Nasal speculum insertion.

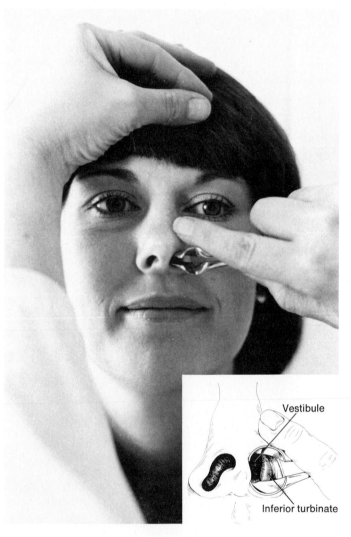

Vestibule

Inferior turbinate

**FIG. 5-2.** Nasal speculum inserted; view of naris with head in upright position.

| | | |
| --- | --- | --- |
| **a.** With client's head erect (Fig. 5-2) | Floor of nose (vestibule)<br>Inferior turbinate<br>Nasal hairs present<br>Mucosa slightly darker (redder) than oral mucosa | Furuncle (most often present in vestibule)<br>Tenderness<br>Marked redness<br>Crusting, discharge<br>Lesions or masses |

|  | TO IDENTIFY: | |
| THE STUDENT WILL: | NORMAL | DEVIATIONS FROM NORMAL |
| **b.** With client's head back ( Fig. 5-3) | Middle meatus<br>Middle turbinate<br>Turbinates same color as surrounding nasal mucosa | Sinus drainage<br>Polyps, masses<br>Turbinates appear pale, swollen (allergic responses)<br>Mucosa markedly red with copious discharge |
| **c.** With client's head to side ( Fig. 5-4); repeat with opposite naris | Film of clear discharge (small amount)<br>Lower third is vascular area (Kiesselbach area)<br>Septum midline and straight<br>(*Note:* Many normal individuals show a slight deviation of the septum without symptoms of occlusion.) | Yellow, thick, green discharge<br>Bleeding, crusting<br>Tenderness<br>Lesions<br>Marked deviation of septum |

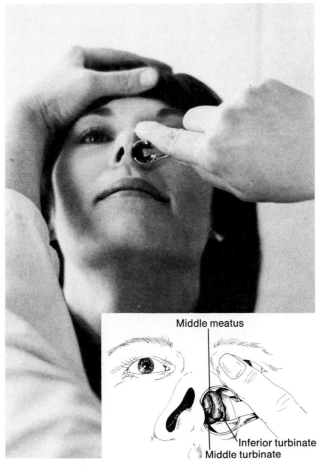

Middle meatus

Inferior turbinate
Middle turbinate

**FIG. 5-3.** Nasal speculum inserted; view of naris with head tilted back.

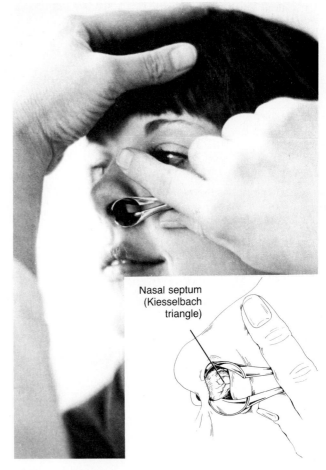

Nasal septum
(Kiesselbach triangle)

**FIG. 5-4.** Nasal speculum inserted; view of naris with head turned to side.

## Clinical guidelines—cont'd

| THE STUDENT WILL: | TO IDENTIFY: | |
| --- | --- | --- |
| | NORMAL | DEVIATIONS FROM NORMAL |
| **d.** Inspect and palpate paranasal sinuses for tenderness and swelling<br>1. Frontal (Fig. 5-5)<br>2. Maxillary (Fig. 5-6) | Nontender<br>No swelling | Tender on palpation<br>Swelling of soft tissue over sinus area |
| **7.** Assemble equipment for examination of mouth and pharynx:<br>**a.** Penlight<br>**b.** Two tongue blades<br>**c.** Two 4 × 4-inch gauze sponges<br>**d.** Gloves or finger cots | | |
| **8.** Inspect, palpate, and maneuver temporomandibular joint: place fingers in front of each ear and ask client to open and close mouth slowly (Fig. 5-7) | | |

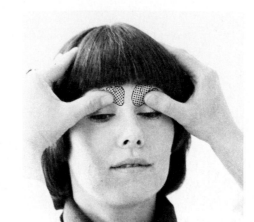

FIG. 5-5. Palpating frontal sinuses.

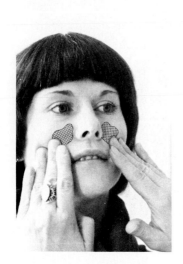

FIG. 5-6. Palpating maxillary sinuses.

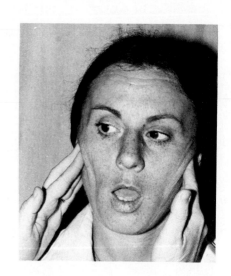

FIG. 5-7. Palpating the temporomandibular joint.

| | | |
| --- | --- | --- |
| **a.** Mobility | Smooth jaw excursion, 3.5 to 4.5 cm (1⅓ to 1¾ inches) | Limited excursion |
| **b.** Tenderness | Absent on palpation | Present on palpation |
| **c.** Crepitus | Absent | Present |
| **d.** Referred pain | Absent | Present (especially on closure of jaw) |

|  | TO IDENTIFY: | |
| --- | --- | --- |
| **THE STUDENT WILL:** | **NORMAL** | **DEVIATIONS FROM NORMAL** |
| **9.** Inspect closed mouth: ask client to clench teeth and smile <br> **a.** Occlusion | Top back teeth rest directly on lower teeth; upper incisors slightly override lowers (Fig. 5-8) | Protrusion of upper incisors <br> Protrusion of lower incisors <br> Upper incisors do not overlap lowers on closure (Fig. 5-9) <br> Lateral displacement of teeth; back teeth do not occlude <br> Separation or malalignment of individual teeth |

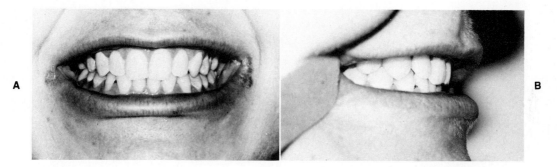

**FIG. 5-8.** Normal occlusion. **A,** Front view. Note vesicular and ulceration patterns at the corners of the mouth. **B,** Lateral view.

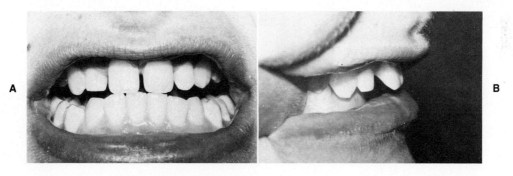

**FIG. 5-9.** Example of malocclusion. **A,** Front view. **B,** Profile.

| | | |
| --- | --- | --- |
| **10.** Inspect and palpate lips for: <br> **a.** Color | Pink | Pale, cyanotic, reddened |
| **b.** Symmetry | Vertical and lateral symmetry at rest or on movement | Swelling (general or localized), induration |
| **c.** Moisture | Smooth and moist | Dry, flaking, cracked |

## Clinical guidelines—cont'd

| | TO IDENTIFY: | |
| --- | --- | --- |
| **THE STUDENT WILL:** | **NORMAL** | **DEVIATIONS FROM NORMAL** |
| **d.** Surface characteristics | Slight vertical linear markings | Lesions: plaques, vesicles (Fig. 5-10), nodules, ulcerations<br>Inflamed fissures at corners |

**11.** Ask client to remove any dental appliances and to open mouth partially; inspect and palpate inner lips and upper and lower gingivobuccal fornices; ask client to open wide to inspect buccal mucosa; use tongue blade and penlight

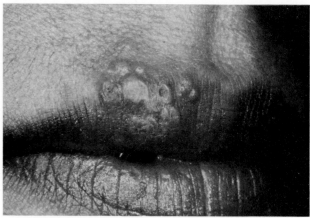

**FIG. 5-10.** Herpes simplex I. (Courtesy Dr. George Blozis, The Ohio State University College of Dentistry.)

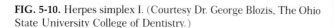

| | | |
| --- | --- | --- |
| **a.** Color | Pale coral, pink<br>Increased pigmentation (general or localized) with dark-skinned individuals | Pale, cyanotic, reddened<br>Local deposits of brown pigmentation |
| **b.** Landmarks | Parotid duct (pinpoint red marking); may be slightly elevated (Fig. 5-11) | |

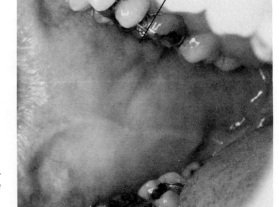

Parotid duct

**FIG. 5-11.** Occlusion line on buccal membrane. Note parotid (Stensen) duct. (Courtesy Dr. George Blozis, The Ohio State University College of Dentistry.)

| THE STUDENT WILL: | TO IDENTIFY: | |
| --- | --- | --- |
| | NORMAL | DEVIATIONS FROM NORMAL |
| **c.** Surface characteristics | Smooth<br>Where teeth meet, occlusion line may appear on adjacent mucosa (Fig. 5-11)<br>Clear saliva over surface | Ulcers<br>White patches<br>White plaques<br>Swelling (local/general)<br>Bleeding<br>Excessively dry mouth<br>Excessive salivation |
| **12.** Inspect and palpate gums for:<br>  **a.** Color<br>  **b.** Surface characteristics | Pink, coral<br>Slightly stippled (Fig. 5-12)<br>Clearly defined, tight margin at tooth<br>Patchy brown pigmentation (usually with dark-skinned individuals) | Reddened, pale<br>Swelling (stippling disappears)<br>Bleeding with slight pressure<br>Enlarged crevice between teeth and gums<br>Pockets containing debris at tooth margin (Fig. 5-13)<br>Gingivitis and edema can develop into advanced pyorrhea with erosion of gum tissue, destruction of underlying bone, and loosening of teeth (Fig. 5-14) |

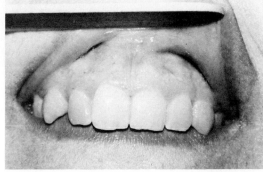

**FIG. 5-12.** Slightly stippled gum surface is a normal characteristic.

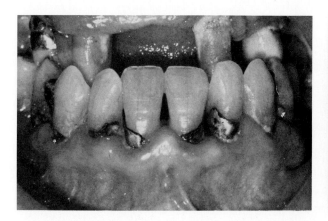

**FIG. 5-13.** Pockets containing debris at tooth margin.

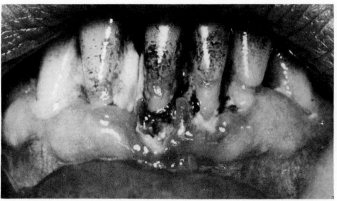

**FIG. 5-14.** Advanced pyorrhea. (From DeWeese, D.D., and Saunders, W.H.: Textbook of otolaryngology, ed. 6, St. Louis, 1982, The C.V. Mosby Co.)

## Clinical guidelines—cont'd

| THE STUDENT WILL: | TO IDENTIFY: | |
|---|---|---|
| | NORMAL | DEVIATIONS FROM NORMAL |
| | Hypertrophy may appear at puberty or during pregnancy (Fig. 5-15)<br>If inflammation (gingivitis) appears, client should be referred for appraisal by dentist | Ulcers, epulis<br>Blue-black line at gum margin<br>Marked enlargement (Fig. 5-16)<br>Tenderness on palpation<br>White patches (especially with edentulous clients) |

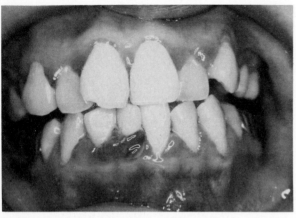

**FIG. 5-15.** Pregnancy gingivitis with hypertrophy. (Courtesy Dr. George Blozis, The Ohio State University College of Dentistry.)

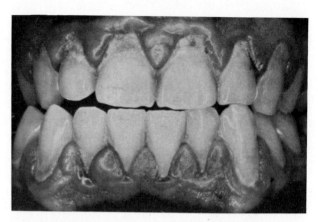

**FIG. 5-16.** Marked enlargement of gums. (Courtesy Dr. Leonard K. Ebel, The Ohio State University College of Dentistry.)

| | | |
|---|---|---|
| **13.** Inspect teeth for: | | |
|    **a.** Number | Thirty-two (full adult)<br>Upper and/or lower third molars sometimes congenitally absent | Missing teeth |
|    **b.** Color | White, yellowish, or grayish hues | Darkened, stained (individual teeth or all) |
|    **c.** Form | Smooth edges | Central incisor notching<br>Irregular notching<br>Broken<br>Peglike |
|    **d.** Surface characteristics | Smooth<br>Dental restorations present | Debris present (especially at gum line)<br>Caries (Fig. 5-17)<br>Much tooth neck exposed, with receding gums |

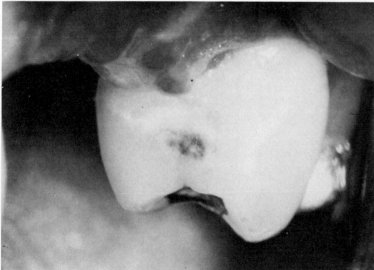

**FIG. 5-17.** Early tooth decay with surface intact. (Courtesy Dr. George Blozis, The Ohio State University College of Dentistry.)

| THE STUDENT WILL: | TO IDENTIFY: | |
| --- | --- | --- |
| | NORMAL | DEVIATIONS FROM NORMAL |
| **14.** Maneuver teeth for tightness | No movement or slight movement | Marked movement (generalized or localized) |
| **15.** Inspect and palpate tongue: ask client to protrude tongue | | |
| **a.** Symmetry and movement | Forward thrust smooth and symmetrical | Unilateral atrophy |
| | Appearance of tongue symmetrical | Lateral movement |
| | | Fasciculation |
| **b.** Color | Pink | Red |
| **c.** Surface characteristics | Dorsal and lateral: | |
| | Moist, glistening coating | Papillae absent |
| | | Lesions |
| | Papillae present | |
| | Elongated vallate papillae | |
| | Fissures present (Fig. 5-18) | |

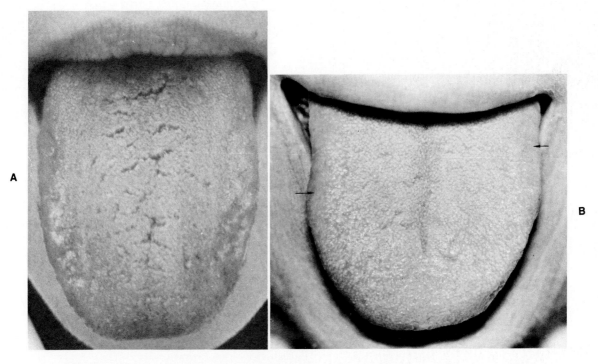

**FIG. 5-18. A,** Normal dorsal surface of tongue. Note papillae, small fissures, and scalloped effect along left lateral border, a normal deviation caused by adjacent teeth. **B,** Dorsal surface on elderly individual's tongue. Arrows indicate smoothness (papillary atrophy) on lateral borders.

| | | |
| --- | --- | --- |
| **16.** Grasp tongue with 4 × 4-inch gauze pad and palpate all sides for texture | Smooth, even tissue | Lumps, nodules |
| | | Induration |

## Clinical guidelines—cont'd

|  | TO IDENTIFY: | |
| --- | --- | --- |
| THE STUDENT WILL: | NORMAL | DEVIATIONS FROM NORMAL |
| **17.** Ask client to put tongue to roof of mouth; inspect and palpate ventral surface and floor of mouth for: | Pink and smooth, with large veins (Fig. 5-19) | Lesions, patches |
| **a.** Color | Pale, coral, pink | Pallor; redness |
| **b.** Surface characteristics | Frenulum (centered) Submaxillary duct opening | Lesions, lumps |

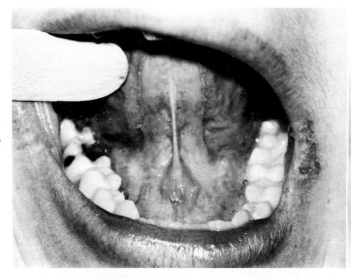 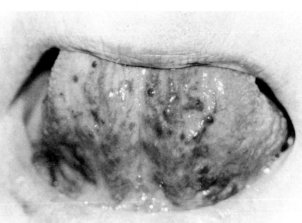

**FIG. 5-19. A,** Normal ventral surface of tongue showing vessels, septum, and floor of mouth. **B,** Ventral surface of elderly individual's tongue. Note engorged and nodular vessels.

|  | | |
| --- | --- | --- |
| **18.** Inspect and palpate hard and soft palates for: | | |
| **a.** Color | Hard palate: pale | Reddened |
| | Soft palate: pink | Pallor; redness |
| | (*Note:* Heavy smokers may show small red dots on surface of hard palate as shown in Fig. 5-20.) | |

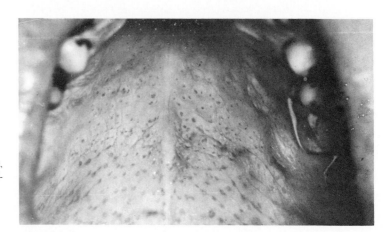

**FIG. 5-20.** Nicotine stomatitis. (From DeWeese, D.D., and Saunders, W.H.: Textbook of otolaryngology, ed. 6, St. Louis, 1982, The C.V. Mosby Co.)

| THE STUDENT WILL: | TO IDENTIFY: | |
| --- | --- | --- |
| | NORMAL | DEVIATIONS FROM NORMAL |
| **b.** Surface characteristics | Hard palate immovable, with irregular transverse rugae | Patches, lesions |
| | | Petechiae |
| | Midline exostosis (torus palatinus) may be present (Fig. 5-21) | |
| | Soft palate movable | Lesions |
| | Symmetrical elevation | |
| | Smooth | |

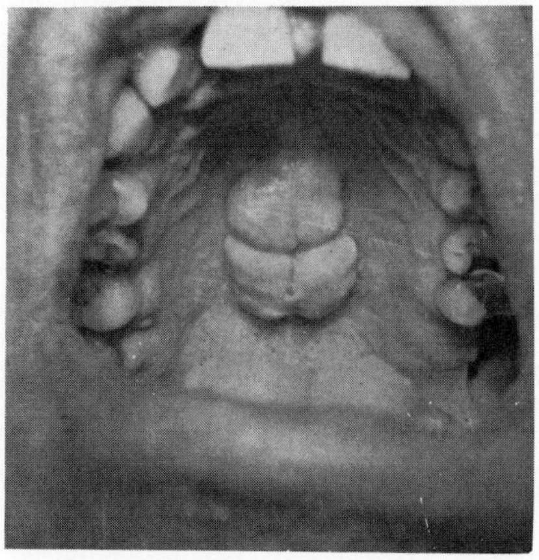

**FIG. 5-21.** Torus palatinus. (From DeWeese, D.D., and Saunders, W.H.: Textbook of otolaryngology, ed. 6, St. Louis, 1982, The C.V. Mosby Co.)

| | | |
| --- | --- | --- |
| **19.** Observe for mouth odor | Absent or sweet | Fetid, musty, or acetonic |
| **20.** Inspect oropharynx for: | | |
|    **a.** Landmarks | Anterior and posterior pillars symmetrical | |
| | Uvula midline | Pulled laterally |
| | Tonsils (may be partially or totally absent); may also be called *tonsil tag* (Fig. 5-22) | Hypertrophied (adult) |
|    **b.** Color | Posterior wall pink | Reddened |
|    **c.** Surface characteristics | Smooth | Lesions, plaques |
| | Tonsils may be cryptic (Fig. 5-22) | Increased vascularity |
| | Posterior wall: slight vascularity may be present | Crypts inflamed or filled with debris or exudate |
| | | Vertical reddened lines or general redness |
| | | Swelling, exudate |
| | | Grayish membrane |

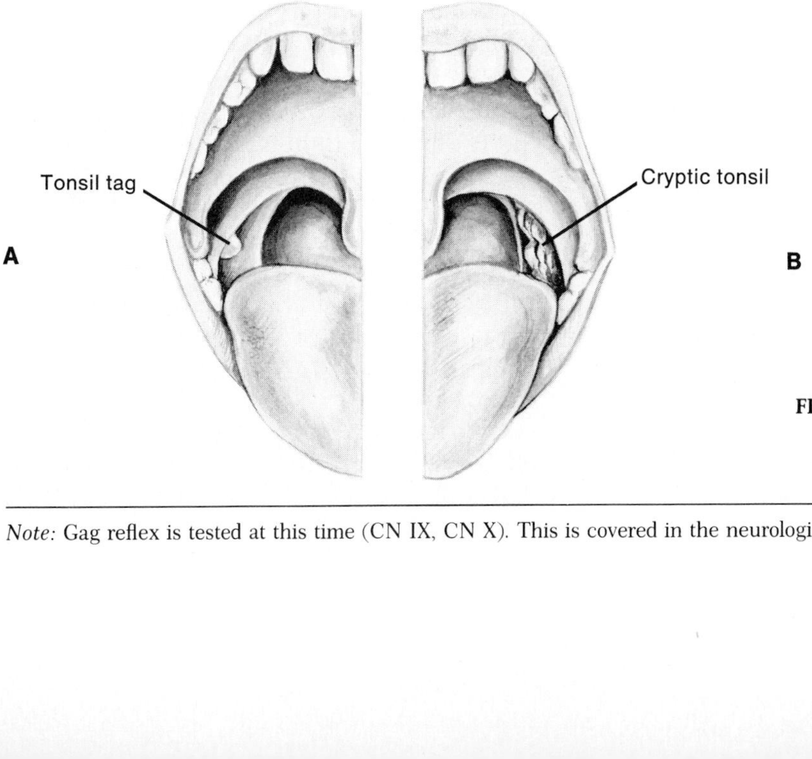

Tonsil tag

Cryptic tonsil

A

B

**FIG. 5-22. A,** Tonsil tag. **B,** Cryptic tonsil.

*Note:* Gag reflex is tested at this time (CN IX, CN X). This is covered in the neurological assessment (Chapter 15).

## Clinical strategies

1. A prolonged examination of the nose or mouth should be carried out with client comfort in mind. The head needs to be supported. Having the client lie down may be easiest for both of you. (Remember that the head must be tilted at various angles for viewing the nose.)

2. To visualize the lower and middle turbinates, the examiner must insert the nasal speculum at least 1.3 cm (½ inch) into the nares.

3. Stabilize the nasal speculum with the index finger against the side of the patient's nose to avoid jiggling the speculum unnecessarily while it is in the naris.

4. The nasal speculum (if otoscope not in use) is to be inserted with the blades up and down to avoid pressure of the speculum blades against the septum, which can cause much discomfort. Open the blades as wide as possible for optimum viewing.

5. Watch out for hair in the nose. Be careful not to pinch hair as you remove the speculum.

6. For oral examination some practitioners use angled mouth mirrors. They are helpful for viewing posterior angles.

7. Early dental caries cannot be recognized without the use of radiography. An examination of teeth with the use of a penlight, mirror, and tongue blade does not constitute adequate screening for dental caries.

8. Open, crusted lesions on the lips or in the mouth should be palpated with a gloved hand.

9. The tongue blade on the posterior dorsal surface of the tongue will usually cause a gag reflex. For most of the examination the tongue blade, when used, should rest lightly on the anterior part of the tongue.

10. Many clients can elevate their soft palate and depress their own tongue for viewing of the pharyngeal wall, so that the examiner does not have to use a tongue depressor.

11. Explain your procedure to the client *before* beginning (especially when grasping the tongue).

## History and clinical strategies: the pediatric client

1. It is important to assess individually the nose, mouth, teeth, and oropharynx of all children. The frontal and maxillary sinuses are routinely palpated in children over 8 years of age.

2. Because of the intrusive nature of these examinations, the examiner should delay assessment until the end of the entire examination.

3. Although it is desirable to assess the nose, mouth, and throat while the child is sitting, a young or uncooperative child will need to be firmly restrained. Following are examination strategies:

   a. Infants to 1 year are usually restrained in a supine position with the child's arms extended over the head and secured in position by a parent or helper.

   b. Toddlers may be restrained in either a supine position as just described or when sitting on the parent's lap. If the second method is used, the child's legs are trapped between the parent's knees, and the arms and chest are restrained with one of the parent's arms while the other hand is used to restrain the child's head firmly against the chest (Fig. 5-23).

   c. For preschoolers, spend time getting to know the child; allow him to play with the tongue blade during the examination, and play smiling and "aah" games as a buildup to the actual mouth and throat examination. Although these techniques may work for some children, others will need to be restrained with one of the techniques just described. Regardless of the technique used for the throat examination, we have discovered that it may be helpful to divide the examination of the mouth and throat into two phases and evaluate each at different times during the total assessment. The mouth eval-

---

### SAMPLE RECORDING

*Nose:* Appears straight and symmetrical with nostrils patent. Odors properly identified. Nasal mucosa pink, moist, with no discharge or lesions. Sinuses nontender on palpation.

*Mouth and pharynx:*
Temporomandibular joint fully mobile, without tenderness or crepitus.
Lips pink, moist, without lesions.
Buccal mucosa, gingivae and hard and soft palates pink, with no lesions, inflammation, patches, or swelling.
Teeth: 28 (all third molars absent). Firmly seated, with five gold restorations. No debris, staining, obvious caries. No inflammation at gingivae.
Tongue: midline, symmetrical. No lesions or fasciculations.
Floor of mouth without lesions.
Uvula midline, tonsils absent. Pharyngeal wall pink with no lesions, exudate, or swelling. Mouth odor faintly sweet.

uation is easily done early in the examination process. If the examiner simply approaches the sitting child with a flashlight and asks the child to show lips, teeth, and tongue, an initial assessment can be made. A more thorough evaluation of unexposed spots and the throat should be postponed until the end of the examination (Fig. 5-24).

    d. School-age children are usually cooperative and willing to show off their new teeth or the absence of their teeth. The mouth and throat are easiest to evaluate if the child is sitting upright on the cart.

4. It is a universal problem to attempt to open the mouth of an uncooperative child whose teeth are clenched tight. Although not every technique will work on every child, the following might be helpful. Slowly advance the tongue blade along the lips to the posterior teeth. Carefully ease the blade between the teeth toward the pharynx. If possible, maintain a downward motion on the tongue blade so that the tongue is pushed forward and the base of the tongue is pressed downward. The child will suddenly gag, and the mouth will open wide. During what appears to be a split second of visibility the examiner must view all the structures therein. Repeated practice is necessary to develop the inclusive scanning view required during mouth and throat evaluation.

5. Several techniques can be used to facilitate the posterior pharynx viewing while avoiding the gag reflex. A common one is to instruct the child to pant like a puppy while sticking the tongue far forward. This technique lowers the posterior tongue and raises the uvula. The second technique requires placing the tongue blade along the lateral aspect of the tongue instead of down the middle.

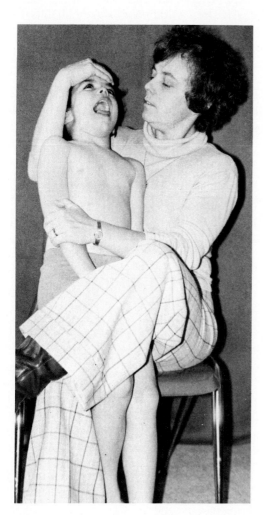

**FIG. 5-23.** Technique to restrain child for mouth examination.

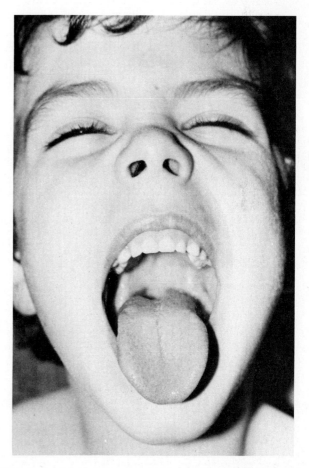

**FIG. 5-24.** Cooperative preschooler participating in mouth examination.

6. Whenever the nose is inspected or whenever there is a history of unilateral nasal drainage or a "strange" odor about the child's head or mouth, a foreign body in the nose must be considered.

7. Bruising or lacerations about the lips, gums, frenulum, or buccal mucosa of an infant or young child must be further evaluated as a possible sign of child abuse. Forced feedings by either a bottle or spoon may cause such bruising.

8. It is important to inquire about tooth brushing from the time the first tooth appears. Brushing habits as well as who brushes the child's teeth are important.

9. In young children with extensive caries of the central upper teeth, the examiner should inquire about the child's continuing use of a bottle, especially as a nighttime routine.

10. When inspecting the child's occlusion, instruct the child to bite down as if chewing food. If the examiner instructs the child to show his teeth, a purposeful malocclusion might be noted.

11. The clinical evaluation of the pediatric client's sinuses differs from that of the adult. Because of the difficulty and reliability of clinical assessment, the frontal and maxillary sinuses are not normally evaluated until about age 8. From that age on the technique of evaluation is the same as for the adult client, testing for disorders such as puffiness or tenderness to palpation.

12. Because of the smallness of the subject and the difficulty in adult technique instrumentation, the nasal evaluation may best be done using the otoscope with the nasal speculum.

13. In trying to evaluate the patency or possibility of a naris obstruction, the examiner may either listen for patency by using a stethoscope at the naris opening or by using a small mirror to detect spot fogging during exhalation.

14. Risk factors of the pediatric client include the following:
   a. History of recurrent nosebleeds
   b. Obvious nasal septal deviation following trauma
   c. Obvious malocclusion
   d. History of thumbing sucking, especially as secondary teeth erupt
   e. "Bottle babies," those who routinely have access to a bottle especially after teeth erupt; continue to evaluate for caries.
   f. Children with poor hygiene habits or those who do not routinely seek preventive dental care
   g. Recurrent mouth infections, thrush, gingivostomatitis, or canker sores
   h. Recurrent tonsil infections
   i. Noted bruising to the gums, lips, or hard palate
   j. No teeth by age 12 months

## Clinical variations: the pediatric client

| CHARACTERISTIC OR AREA EXAMINED | NORMAL | DEVIATIONS FROM NORMAL |
|---|---|---|
| **1.** Nose | | |
| **a.** Outer surface | Smooth, intact | Lesions |
| | Skin color same as face | Eczema |
| | Newborns may show milia | Acne |
| | May have some redness around nares openings if child has a cold | |
| **b.** Contour | External alignment symmetrical or nearly symmetrical | |
| **c.** Form | Some children with allergies may show transverse ridge from chronic upward wiping of nares (called the *allergic salute*) | Flaring with inhalation |
| **d.** Patency of nares | Noiseless, free exchange of air through each naris | Breathing noisy or obstructed Unilateral patency (evaluate for foreign body or polyps) |
| **e.** Evaluation of olfactory nerve (CN I) not normally conducted in the pediatric client | | |

| CHARACTERISTIC OR AREA EXAMINED | NORMAL | DEVIATIONS FROM NORMAL |
|---|---|---|
| **2.** Internal nasal cavity—observe nares: | | |
| **a.** With client's head erect | Floor of nose (vestibule) | Septal deviation |
| | Inferior turbinate | Septal perforation (noted by viewing spot of light in other naris) |
| | Nasal hairs present | Furuncle (most often present in vestibule) |
| | Mucosa slightly darker (redder) than oral mucosa | Tenderness |
| | | Marked redness |
| | | Crusting, discharge |
| | | Lesions or masses |
| **b.** With client's head back | Middle meatus | Sinus drainage |
| | Middle turbinate | Polyps, masses |
| | Turbinates same color as surrounding nasal mucosa | Turbinates appear pale, swollen (allergic responses) |
| | | Mucosa markedly red with copious discharge present |
| | Film of clear discharge (small amount) | Yellow, thick, green discharge |
| **c.** With client's head to side | Septum | Bleeding, crusting |
| | Lower third is vascular area (Kiesselbach area) | Tenderness |
| | | Lesions |
| | Septum midline and straight | Marked deviation of septum |
| **3.** Frontal and maxillary sinuses (See clinical strategy no. 11.) | Nontender | Tender on palpation |
| | No swelling | Swelling of soft tissue over sinus area |
| **4.** Temporomandibular joint (to be evaluated if the child is cooperative) | | |
| **a.** Mobility | Smooth jaw excursion | Limited excursion |
| **b.** Tenderness | Absent on palpation | Present on palpation |
| **c.** Crepitus | Absent | Present (especially on closure of jaw) |
| **d.** Referred pain | Absent | Present (especially on closure of jaw) |
| **5.** Occlusion | Top back teeth rest directly atop lower teeth; upper incisors slightly override lowers | Protrusion of upper incisors |
| | | Protrusion of lower incisors |
| | | Upper incisors do not overlap lowers on closure |
| | | Lateral displacement of teeth |
| **6.** Jaw size | Appears appropriate for face size | Very *small* or *large* mandible, seen in numerous congenital diseases |
| **7.** Lips | | |
| **a.** Color | Pink | Pale, cyanotic |
| | | Cherry pink |
| | | Marked circumoral pallor |
| **b.** Symmetry | Vertical and lateral symmetry at rest or on movement | Swelling (general or localized), induration, twisting, drooping clefts |
| **c.** Moisture | Smooth and moist | Dry, flaking, cracking, corners are especially common (evaluate for impetigo) |
| **d.** Surface characteristics | Slight vertical linear markings | Fissures |
| | Breast- or bottle-fed babies may develop a sucking tubercle in the middle of the upper lip | Lesions: plaques, vesicles, nodules, ulcerations |
| **8.** Inner lips and buccal mucosa | | |
| **a.** Color | Pale coral, pink | Pale, cyanotic, reddened |
| | Increased pigmentation (general or localized) with dark-skinned individuals | Local deposits of brown pigmentation |
| | | Blackish, blue areas |

## Clinical variations: the pediatric client—cont'd

| CHARACTERISTIC OR AREA EXAMINED | NORMAL | DEVIATIONS FROM NORMAL |
|---|---|---|
| **b.** Landmarks | Parotid duct (pinpoint red marking) may be slightly elevated | Puffy, reddened area |
| **c.** Surface characteristics | Smooth<br>Fine grayish ridge<br>Where teeth meet, occlusion line may appear<br>Salivation in children between 3 months and 2 years may be normal<br>If child also appears ill, salivation should be considered abnormal until proved otherwise | Ulcers<br>White patches (*Candida albicans*, or thrush) where scraped-off patches are reddened and tend to bleed<br>White plaques<br>Swelling<br>Bleeding<br>Excessively dry mouth (observe for other signs of dehydration, fever, or possible atropine ingestion)<br>Excessive salivation may be seen in gingivostomatitis (child appears ill and usually drools) or in child with multiple caries |
| **9.** Gums<br>  **a.** Color<br>  **b.** Surface characteristics | Pink, coral<br>Slightly stippled<br>Sharp margin at tooth<br>Patchy brown pigmentation (usually with dark-skinned individuals)<br>Hypertrophy may appear at puberty<br>May see downward extension of alveolar frenulum as child's central incisors separate; should self-correct<br>Small pearly white cysts (Epstein pearls) may be seen along gums of infants; usually disappear by age 2 or 3 months; called *Bohn nodules* when on midpalate | Reddened, pale<br>Swelling (stippling disappears)<br>Bleeding (with slight pressure)<br>Enlarged crevice between teeth and gums<br>Pockets containing debris at tooth margin<br>Ulcers, epulis<br>Blue-black line at gum margin<br>Marked hypertrophy<br>Tenderness on palpation<br>Hypertrophy of gum tissue may be indicative of mouth breathers, vitamin deficiency, or phenytoin (Dilantin) ingestion |
| **10.** Teeth<br>  **a.** Number: note eruption timing, sequence of eruption, and positioning of teeth<br>  **b.** Color | See Fig. 5-25 for normal number of teeth at given age<br><br>White, yellowish, or grayish hues | No teeth by age 1 year<br>Missing teeth inappropriate for age<br><br>Darkened teeth<br>Brownish teeth (may indicate decay)<br>Mottled or pitted permanent teeth (may indicate decreased fluoride or tetracycline ingestion)<br>Green or black teeth (iron ingestion; will go away on withdrawal) |
|   **c.** Surface characteristics | Smooth, regularly formed teeth | Excessive smoothness (may indicate grinding of teeth)<br>Debris present, especially at gum line<br>Caries |

| CHARACTERISTIC OR AREA EXAMINED | NORMAL | DEVIATIONS FROM NORMAL |
|---|---|---|

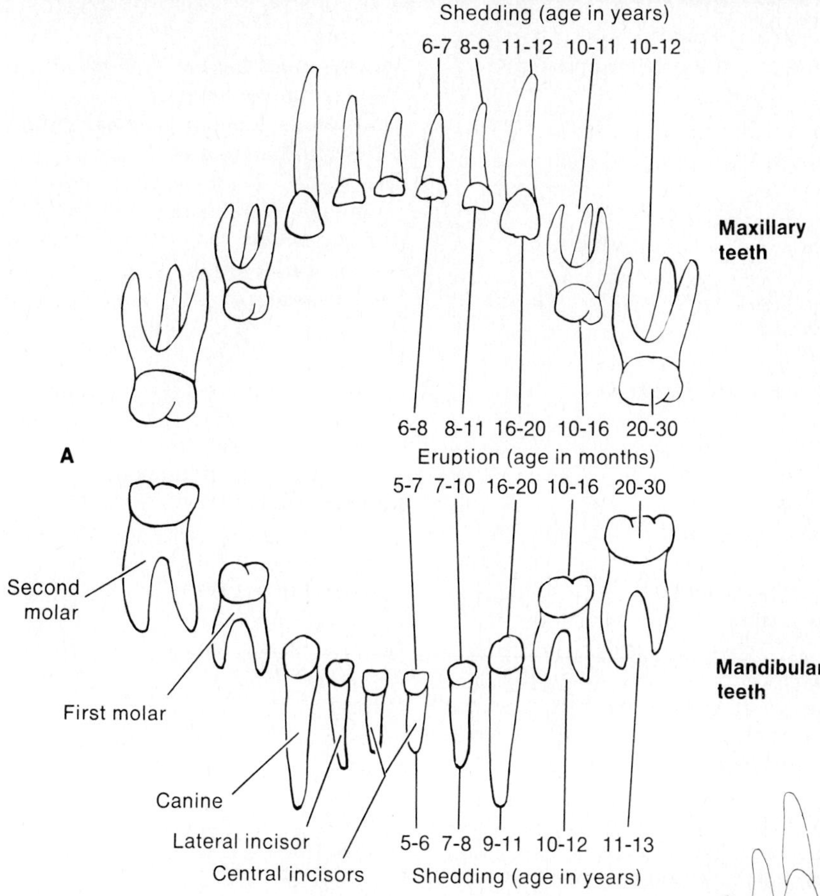

**A**

Shedding (age in years)

6-7 8-9 11-12 10-11 10-12

**Maxillary teeth**

6-8 8-11 16-20 10-16 20-30
Eruption (age in months)

5-7 7-10 16-20 10-16 20-30

Second molar

First molar

Canine

Lateral incisor

Central incisors

**Mandibular teeth**

5-6 7-8 9-11 10-12 11-13
Shedding (age in years)

**FIG. 5-25. A,** Average age of eruption and shedding of deciduous teeth. **B,** Average age of eruption of permanent teeth.

**B**

**Maxillary teeth**

7-8 8-9 11-12 10-11 10-12 6-7 12-13
Eruption of permanent teeth (age in years)

6-7 7-8 9-11 10-12 11-13 6-7 12-13

Second molar

First molar

Second premolar

First premolar

Canine

Lateral incisor

Central incisor

**Mandibular teeth**

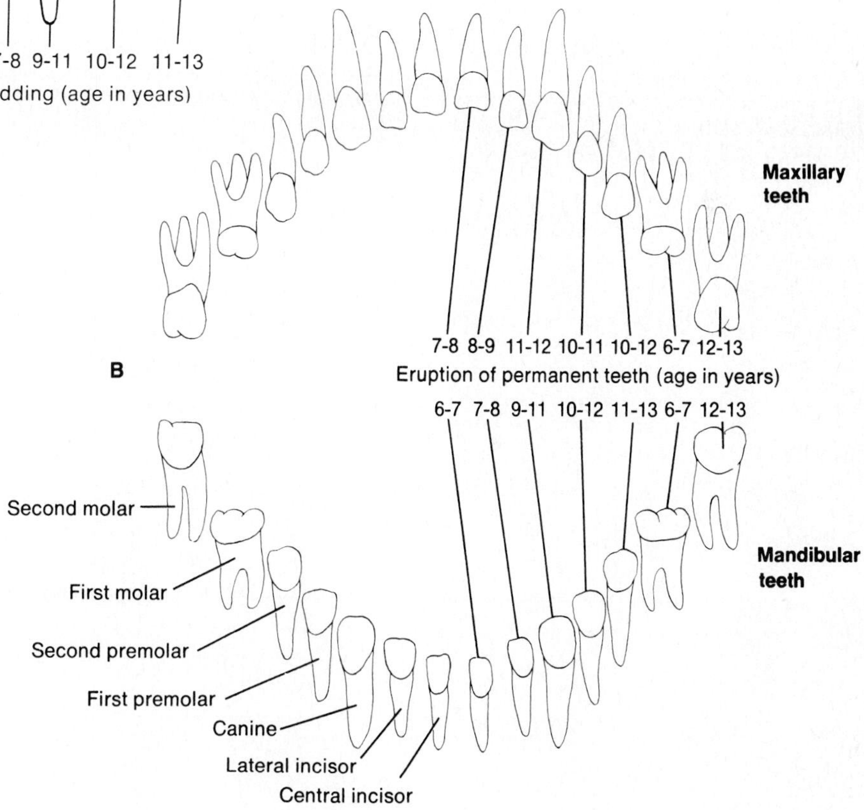

## Clinical variations: the pediatric client—cont'd

| CHARACTERISTIC OR AREA EXAMINED | NORMAL | DEVIATIONS FROM NORMAL |
|---|---|---|
| **11.** Tongue | | |
| **a.** Symmetry and movement | Smooth and even tissue | Fissures |
| | Able to touch tongue to upper lips | Tongue appearing too large for mouth (protrusion of tongue) |
| | | Glossoptosis: tongue attached farther forward than usual |
| | | Tongue-tied: child unable to advance tongue forward to lips |
| **b.** Color | Pink | Red, strawberry tongue (may be seen with scarlet fever) |
| **c.** Surface characteristics | Dorsal and lateral: moist, glistening coating | Papillae absent |
| | Papillae present | Lesions |
| | Elongated vallate papillae | |
| | Fissures present | |
| | Texture smooth, even | Furrows in tongue |
| | Ventral: pink and smooth, with large veins | Lumps, nodules, induration |
| | | Lesions, patches |
| **12.** Floor of mouth | | |
| **a.** Color | Pale, coral, pink | Pallor, reddened |
| **b.** Surface characteristics | Frenulum (centered) | Lesions, lumps |
| | Submaxillary duct opening | |
| **13.** Hard palate | | |
| **a.** Color | Pale pink | Reddened |
| **b.** Surface characteristics | Immovable with irregular transverse rugae | Patches |
| | Bohn nodules in newborn (gone by 2 or 3 months) | Lesions |
| | | Petechiae |
| | Very high or narrow arch requires further evaluation; may be linked to multiple other syndromes | Clefts |
| | | Bruising |
| **14.** Soft palate | | |
| **a.** Color | Pink | Reddened |
| | | Pallor |
| **b.** Surface characteristics | Movable | Discharge |
| | Symmetrical elevation | Edema |
| | Smooth | Patches |
| | | Lesions |
| **15.** Mouth odor | Absent | Fetid, musty (further investigate poor hygiene, local or systemic infections, sinusitis, mouth breathers) |
| | | Foreign body in nose |
| | | Acetonic or very sweet smell |

| CHARACTERISTIC OR AREA EXAMINED | NORMAL | DEVIATIONS FROM NORMAL |
|---|---|---|
| **16.** Oropharynx<br>  **a.** Landmarks | Anterior and posterior pillars symmetrical<br>Uvula midline<br>Tonsils pink<br>Size may vary from barely visible to very large (Fig. 5-26)<br>Cryptic | Lateral deviation<br>Bifid uvula<br>Uvula with lateral deviation<br>Reddened; pus, coating, exudate present<br>Tonsils occluding swallowing or breathing<br>White or yellow follicles filling crypts<br>Ulcerative |

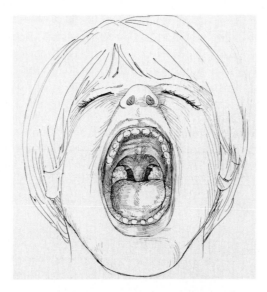

**FIG. 5-26.** Large tonsils in a child.

| | | |
|---|---|---|
|   **b.** Color<br>  **c.** Surface characteristics | Posterior wall pink<br>Posterior wall may show slight vascularity | Reddened<br>Vertical reddened lines or general redness<br>Swelling, exudate, grayish membrane |

## History and clinical strategies: the geriatric client

1. A number of variables contribute to mouth problems in elderly adults.
   a. Bone resorption is considered a normal aging process, but it can be escalated by systemic disease or local factors within the mouth.
   b. The diminished flow of saliva decreases the self-cleaning process within the mouth.
   c. Slower healing processes decrease the oral tissue's potential for repairing minor trauma from food, cold, or other assaults from the external environment.
   d. The presence of systemic disease (more common with geriatric clients) often manifests local changes or problems in the mouth.
   e. Physical disability (especially loss of manual dexterity or visual problems) decreases the individual's potential for a high level of self-care.
   f. Time itself has an effect: (1) old dental restorations deteriorate; (2) tooth enamel calcifies, erodes, and deteriorates from years of overly vigorous brushing; (3) gum tissue resorbs and exposes the neck of the tooth, which is vulnerable to decay; (4) attrition of the teeth (wearing down of the occlusal surface) occurs; and (5) gingival tissue becomes less elastic and more vulnerable to trauma.
   g. Other problems sometimes associated with aging interfere with mouth care: nutritional deficiency, emotional or mental changes, financial concerns.
2. The practitioner must take a careful history of self-care habits, frequency of visits to the dentist, and client's concerns about problems that interfere with self-care. (See history in adult section for specific questions related to nose, sinus, mouth, and throat assessment.)
3. Below is a list of risk factors that can serve as a "red flag" to examiners as they assess the oral cavities of elderly clients.
   a. Confused clients (even transient confusion or a shortened attention span can drastically alter self-care habits)
   b. Physically disabled clients (unable to provide adequate self-care)
   c. Poor eating habits: no intake of "cleaning" foods, high sugar content, limited intake of foods that require chewing
   d. Chronic mouth breathing (increases vulnerability of oral tissue to trauma, inflammatory response)
   e. History of chronic smoking (associated with higher incidence of oral cancer)
   f. History of chronic use of alcohol (higher associated incidence of cancer)
   g. Systemic diseases (only a sample of relevant diseases included)
      (1) Osteoporosis (associated with bone resorption)
      (2) Cirrhosis of liver (higher associated incidence of cancer of mouth)
      (3) Any disease disrupting protein metabolism
      (4) Anemia; blood dyscrasias
      (5) Diabetes mellitus
   h. Illness that creates general disability (e.g., fatigue, weakness) and thus interferes with self-care
   i. Local irritants chronically assaulting oral tissues (e.g., pipe smoking, chewing tobacco)
   j. History of poor dental care habits

## Clinical variations: the geriatric client

| CHARACTERISTIC OR AREA EXAMINED | NORMAL | DEVIATIONS FROM NORMAL |
|---|---|---|
| **1.** General appearance of nose | | |
| **a.** Surface/skin | Smooth, intact | Lesions, warty appearance |
| | Skin color same as face | Redness, discoloration |
| | | Vascularization |
| **b.** Contour | External alignment symmetrical (or nearly symmetrical) | Marked asymmetry |
| | | Swelling or hypertrophy (bulbous appearance) |
| **c.** Nares | Symmetrical | Marked asymmetry |
| | Dry, no crusting | Discharge present, crusting |
| | No flaring or narrowing associated with breathing | Narrowing on inspiration (associated with chronic obstruction and mouth breathing) |
| | Increase in bristly hairs (especially men) | |
| **d.** Patency | Noiseless, free exchange of air through each naris | Patency may be occluded because of nose drying out and crusting; associated with inflammatory response |
| | | Breathing noisy or obstructed |
| **e.** Stability | Firm | Unstable |
| **f.** Tenderness | Nontender | Tender on palpation; masses |
| **2.** Sense of smell and odor identification | Sense of smell somewhat decreased with aging, but client should be able to identify strong odor | Unable to identify strong odor |
| **3.** Internal nasal cavity—observe nares: | | |
| **a.** With client's head erect | Floor of nose (vestibule) | Furuncle (most often present in vestibule) |
| | Inferior turbinate | |
| | Nasal hairs present | Tenderness |
| | Mucosa slightly darker (redder) than oral mucosa | Marked redness |
| | | Crusting, discharge |
| | | Lesions or masses |
| **b.** With client's head back | Middle meatus | Sinus drainage |
| | Middle turbinate | Polyps, masses |
| | Turbinates same color as surrounding nasal mucosa | Turbinates appear pale, swollen (allergic responses) |
| | Mucosa tends to be dryer | Increased friability of tissues |
| | | Increased vulnerability to inflammatory response |
| | | Mucosa markedly red with copious discharge present |
| **c.** With client's head to side | Film of clear discharge (small amount) | Yellow, thick, green discharge |
| | Septum | Bleeding, crusting |
| | Lower third is vascular (Kiesselbach area) | Tenderness |
| | | Lesions |
| | Septum midline and straight | Marked deviation of septum |
| **4.** Sinuses (frontal and maxillary) | Nontender | Tender on palpation |
| | No swelling | Swelling of soft tissue over sinus area |
| **5.** Temporomandibular joint | | |
| **a.** Mobility | Smooth jaw excursion, 3.5 to 4.5 cm (1⅓ to 1¾ inches) | Joint may dislocate when mouth opened wide (associated with loss of elasticity of joint ligaments) |
| | | Limited excursion |
| **b.** Tenderness | Absent on palpation | Present on palpation |
| **c.** Crepitus | Absent | Present |
| **d.** Referred pain | Absent | Present (especially on closure of jaw) |

## Clinical variations: the geriatric client—cont'd

| CHARACTERISTIC OR AREA EXAMINED | NORMAL | DEVIATIONS FROM NORMAL |
|---|---|---|
| **6.** Occlusion | May be changed because of missing teeth<br>Marked overclosure of jaws may be associated with edentulous client<br>Individuals who stoop and thrust head forward tend to habitually protrude lower jaw | Protrusion of upper incisors<br>Protrusion of lower incisors<br>Upper incisors do not overlap lowers on closure<br>Lateral displacement of teeth; back teeth do not occlude |
| **7.** Lips | | |
| **a.** Color | Pink | Pale, cyanotic, reddened |
| **b.** Symmetry | Vertical and lateral symmetry at rest or on movement | Swelling (general or localized), induration |
| **c.** Moisture | Decreased supply of saliva may contribute to dryer lips | Dry, flaking, cracked |
| **d.** Surface | Increased vertical markings<br>"Purse-string" appearance associated with edentulism or overclosure of jaws | Marked, deep wrinkling and fissures at corner of mouth (perlèche) associated with inflammatory response to severe overclosure or vitamin deficiency)<br>Lesions at vermilion border (Figs. 5-27 and 5-28) or development of indistinct border<br>Fissures radiating across lip border<br>Lesions: plaques, vesicles, nodules, ulcerations<br>Inflamed fissures at corners |

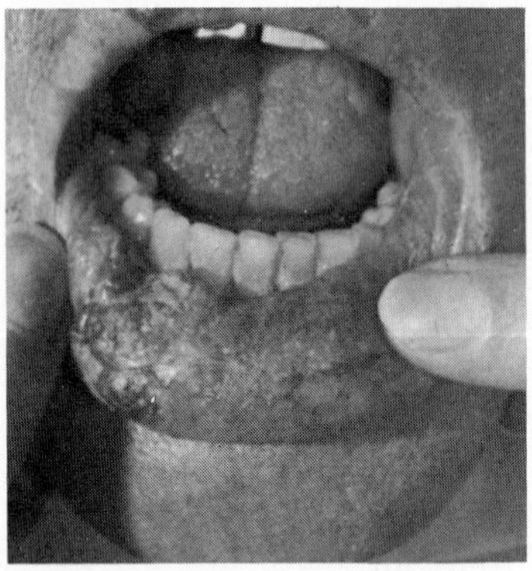

**FIG. 5-27.** Squamous cell carcinoma. (From Stewart, W.D., Danto, J.L., and Maddin, S.: Dermatology: diagnosis and treatment of cutaneous disorders, ed. 4, St. Louis, 1978, The C.V. Mosby Co.)

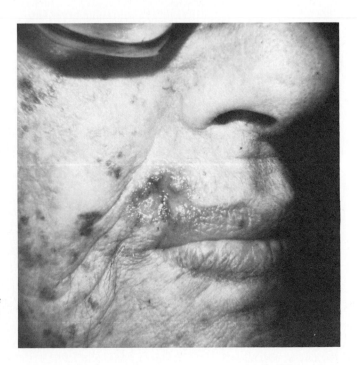

**FIG. 5-28.** Basal cell carcinoma. (From Steinberg, F.U., editor: Care of the geriatric patient, ed. 6, St. Louis, 1983, The C.V. Mosby Co.)

| CHARACTERISTIC OR AREA EXAMINED | NORMAL | DEVIATIONS FROM NORMAL |
|---|---|---|
| **8.** Ask client to remove any dental appliances; inner lips and buccal mucosa | | |
| **a.** Color | Pale coral, pink | Pale, cyanotic, reddened |
| | Increased pigmentation (general or localized) with dark-skinned individuals | Local deposits of brown pigmentation |
| **b.** Landmarks | Parotid duct (pinpoint red marking); may be slightly elevated | |
| **c.** Surface characteristics | Mucosa becomes thinner and less vascular; may appear shinier than in younger adult | White or gray patches (Fig. 5-30) |
| | | Monilial patches fairly common problem |
| | Fordyce granules common (Fig. 5-29) | Hyperkeratotic response (whitish areas, may be raised, rough); might be normal response to trauma but should be referred for validation |
| | | Petechiae |
| | | Swelling (local/general) |
| | | Bleeding |
| | | Ulcers |
| | | Excessively dry mouth |
| | | Excessive salivation |

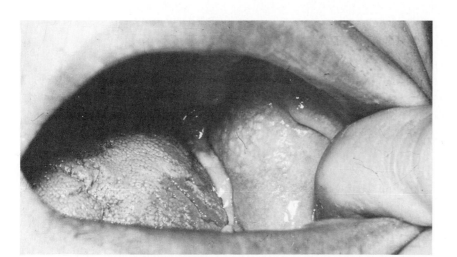

**FIG. 5-29.** Fordyce granules on buccal mucosa. (From DeWeese, D.D., and Saunders, W.H.: Textbook of otolaryngology, ed. 6, St. Louis, 1982, The C.V. Mosby Co.)

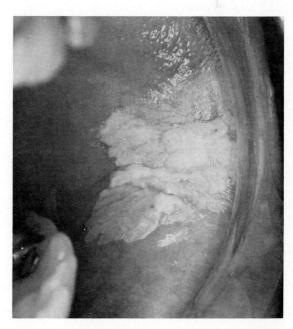

**FIG. 5-30.** Leukoplakia. (Courtesy Dr. George Blozis, The Ohio State University College of Dentistry.)

## Clinical variations: the geriatric client—cont'd

| CHARACTERISTIC OR AREA EXAMINED | NORMAL | DEVIATIONS FROM NORMAL |
|---|---|---|
| **9.** Gums | | |
|   **a.** Color | May appear slightly paler | Reddened, excessively pale |
|   **b.** Surface characteristics | Stippling may be somewhat decreased | Increased friability of gums; bleeding with slight pressure |
| | | Lesions, redness, uneven ridges, spurs, white patches, or tenderness of edentulous gums |
| | | Marked pallor (fibrotic changes) of gums |
| | Clearly defined, tight margin at tooth | Enlarged crevices between teeth and gums |
| | Patchy brown pigmentation (usually with dark-skinned individuals) | Pockets containing debris at tooth margin |
| **10.** Teeth | | |
|   **a.** Number | Thirty-two (full adult) | Missing teeth |
| | Third molars, upper and/or lower, sometimes congenitally absent | |
|   **b.** Color | May appear more yellowish or slightly darker (uniformly) | Darkened, stained (individual teeth or all) |
|   **c.** Form and surface characteristics | Teeth may appear elongated (increased root surface or neck of tooth exposure associated with resorption of supporting bone) (Fig. 5-13) | Enamel of old teeth may display cracks with stains (Fig. 5-13) |
| | | Old dental restorations may be deteriorated (especially at the margins) |
| | | Dentin surface may appear abraded |
| | | Occlusal surfaces markedly worn down (leaving hollow surface appearance) |
| | | Cusps of teeth may break off |
|   **d.** Maneuverability | No movement or slight movement | Loosening of teeth a special hazard, associated with periodontal disease, bone resorption |
| **11.** Tongue | | |
|   **a.** Symmetry and movement | Forward thrust smooth and symmetrical | Unilateral atrophy |
| | | Lateral movement |
| | | Fasciculation |
| | Appearance of tongue is symmetrical | Tongue lies limp on floor of mouth |
|   **b.** Color | Pink | Red |
|   **c.** Surface characteristics | Dorsal and lateral: | Papillae absent |
| | Moist, glistening coating | Lesions |
| | Papillae may appear slightly smoother, shinier (Fig. 5-18, *B*) | Very smooth tongue (associated with vitamin deficiency) |
| | Fissures present | |
|   **d.** Texture | Smooth, even tissue | Lumps, nodules |
| | | Induration |
| | Ventral: | Lesions, patches |
| | Epithelium thin and loosely attached | |
| | Veins often varicosed (Fig. 5-19, *B*)* | |
| **12.** Floor of mouth | | |
|   **a.** Color and surface | Pale coral, pink | Pallor, redness |
| | Frenulum (centered) | Lesions, lumps |
| | Submaxillary duct opening | Watch for retention cysts at salivary duct opening |

---

*Varicosities should be considered a problem for consultation by the beginning examiner.
*Note:* Gag reflex is tested at this time (CN IX, CN X). This is covered in the neurological assessment (Chapter 15).

| CHARACTERISTIC OR AREA EXAMINED | NORMAL | DEVIATIONS FROM NORMAL |
|---|---|---|
| **13.** Hard and soft palates | | |
|    **a.** Color | Hard palate pale | Reddened |
| | Soft palate pink | Pallor, redness |
|    **b.** Surface characteristics | Hard palate immovable, with irregular transverse rugae | Patches, lesions |
| | Midline exostosis (torus palatinus) may be present | Petechiae<br>Watch for injuries, lesions related to denture trauma |
| | Soft palate movable | Mucosal glands may become inflamed in heavy smokers |
| | Symmetrical elevation | |
| | Smooth | |
| **14.** Mouth odor | Absent or sweet | Fetid, musty, or acetonic |
| **15.** Oropharynx | | |
|    **a.** Landmarks | Anterior and posterior pillars symmetrical | |
| | Uvula midline | Pulled laterally |
| | Tonsils may be partially or totally absent; may also be called *tonsil tag* | Hypertrophied (adult) |
|    **b.** Color | Posterior wall pink | Reddened |
|    **c.** Surface characteristics | Smooth | Lesions, plaques |
| | Tonsils may be cryptic (Fig. 5-22, *B*) | Increased vascularity |
| | Slight vascularity may be present on posterior wall | Crypts inflamed or filled with debris or exudate |
| | | Vertical reddened lines or general redness |
| | | Swelling, exudate |
| | | Grayish membrane |

# Cognitive self-assessment

1. The function of the nasal turbinates is to:
   - ☐ a. warm the air
   - ☐ b. detect odors
   - ☐ c. provide humidity
   - ☐ d. stimulate tear formation
   - ☐ e. all the above
   - ☐ f. b, c, and d
   - ☐ g. b and d
   - ☐ h. a, c, and d
   - ☐ i. a and c
2. With a nasal speculum and penlight, an examiner is able to view:
   - ☐ a. vestibule
   - ☐ b. anterior septum
   - ☐ c. inferior turbinate
   - ☐ d. middle turbinate
   - ☐ e. a and c
   - ☐ f. b, c, and d
   - ☐ g. a, b, and d
   - ☐ h. all the above

3. A nasal speculum is inserted:
   - ☐ a. 0.5 cm ($^1/_5$ inch)
   - ☐ b. 1 cm ($^1/_3$ inch)
   - ☐ c. 2 cm ($^3/_4$ inch)

4. It is then opened:
   - ☐ a. transversely
   - ☐ b. vertically
   - ☐ c. transversely, initially; then vertically

5. The _____ of the nose is bone.
   - ☐ a. upper third
   - ☐ b. upper two thirds
   - ☐ c. lower half
   - ☐ d. entire middle partition

6. The paranasal sinuses directly evaluated are:
   - ☐ a. sphenoid
   - ☐ b. frontal
   - ☐ c. splanchnic
   - ☐ d. ethmoid
   - ☐ e. maxillary
   - ☐ f. a, c, and d
   - ☐ g. c and e
   - ☐ h. b and c
   - ☐ i. b and e
   - ☐ j. b, c, and d

7. About 90% of all nosebleeds originate from the:
   - ☐ a. inferior turbinate
   - ☐ b. middle concha
   - ☐ c. dorsum nasi point
   - ☐ d. Kiesselbach area

8. One sign by which allergies may be distinguished from a common cold is that in allergies:
   - ☐ a. the nasal mucosa is red, inflamed, and swollen
   - ☐ b. the nasal mucosa is comparatively pale
   - ☐ c. the discharge is clear and watery at the beginning
   - ☐ d. the presence of nasal congestion is prominent

9. The paranasal sinuses drain into:
   - ☐ a. the superior turbinate
   - ☐ b. the middle turbinate
   - ☐ c. the middle meatus
   - ☐ d. the vestibule

10. The anterior and posterior boundaries of the mouth are:
    - ☐ a. the gingivobuccal fornices and the posterior pharyngeal wall
    - ☐ b. the lips and the soft palate and uvula
    - ☐ c. the teeth and the laryngopharynx
    - ☐ d. none of the above

11. Which statement(s) is/are true about the lips?
    - ☐ a. Overclosure of the mouth can cause fissuring at the mouth angles.
    - ☐ b. A chancre on the lip might resemble a carcinoma or a cold sore.
    - ☐ c. There is a rich blood and lymphatic supply to the lips.
    - ☐ d. Aging tends to diminish the pattern on the vermilion surface.
    - ☐ e. Herpetic vesicles of the lip are common.
    - ☐ f. All the above
    - ☐ g. All except d

    ☐ h.  b, c, and e

    ☐ i.  All except b

12.  Which statement(s) is/are true about the gums?

    ☐ a.  The gums are composed of fibrous tissue covered with mucous membrane.

    ☐ b.  The most common irritant to gums are calculus deposits around the necks of teeth.

    ☐ c.  Stippling of gums is an early indicator of periodontal disease.

    ☐ d.  *Interdental papillae* is a term describing the gums between the teeth.

    ☐ e.  Gingival enlargement (hypertrophy) can occur in healthy as well as disease states.

    ☐ f.  All except e

    ☐ g.  b, c, and d

    ☐ h.  a, b, and e

    ☐ i.  All except c

    ☐ j.  a and b

13.  Which statement(s) is/are true about the buccal mucosa?

    ☐ a.  Fordyce spots are an early indicator of rubeola.

    ☐ b.  Aphthous ulcers are painless and might be precancerous lesions.

    ☐ c.  Leukoplakia may be a precancerous lesion.

    ☐ d.  The Wharton duct opens into the buccal membrane opposite the second molar.

    ☐ e.  Cheek biting can result in a hyperkeratotic reaction.

    ☐ f.  c and e

    ☐ g.  b, d, and e

    ☐ h.  All except b

    ☐ i.  None of the above

    ☐ j.  a, b, and d

14.  Which statement(s) is/are true about the tongue?

    ☐ a.  A whitish coating of the tongue is associated with vitamin B deficiency.

    ☐ b.  Carcinoma of the tongue first appears on the posterior dorsal surface.

    ☐ c.  Tongue fissures may appear with aging.

    ☐ d.  Tongue functions include speech, mastication, taste, and swallowing.

    ☐ e.  The lingual frenulum attaches the ventral surface of the tongue to the mandibular gingivae.

    ☐ f.  All the above

    ☐ g.  d only

    ☐ h.  c, d, and e

    ☐ i.  a, b, and d

    ☐ j.  All except e

15.  Which statement(s) is/are true about the teeth?

    ☐ a.  The crowns of teeth may become reduced in length by attrition.

    ☐ b.  Teeth are firmly anchored in the gingivae except during pregnancy or puberty.

    ☐ c.  The biting surface of incisors may become abraded by opening bobby pins.

    ☐ d.  Radiography is necessary for early detection of caries.

    ☐ e.  Teeth can darken because of some systemic medications, local exposure (e.g., smoking), or trauma.

    ☐ f.  All except a

    ☐ g.  All the above

☐ h.  b, c, and d
☐ i.  All except b

16. Which statement(s) is/are true about the oropharynx?
☐ a.  Smoking may result in a generalized redness of the oropharynx.
☐ b.  Malignant tumors may arise from the tonsils.
☐ c.  Benign tumors may arise from the tonsils.
☐ d.  Tonsils may be enlarged without being infected.
☐ e.  Streptococcal pharyngeal infection produces classic signs and is easily diagnosed.
☐ f.  All except b
☐ g.  a, b, and d
☐ h.  All except e
☐ i.  a and d
☐ j.  None of the above

**PEDIATRIC QUESTIONS**

17. Transverse creasing across the bridge of a child's nose is most often indicative of:
☐ a.  chromosomal abnormality
☐ b.  an allergic child
☐ c.  child with Down syndrome
☐ d.  trauma to the nose
☐ e.  a birth defect

18. Normally, salivation in the child is noted about age:
☐ a.  birth
☐ b.  1 month
☐ c.  3 months
☐ d.  5 months
☐ e.  none of the above

19. Which of the following findings indicates an abnormality requiring additional assessment and referral?
☐ a.  Pink tonsils extending almost to midline of throat; no difficulty swallowing or breathing
☐ b.  Cryptic tonsils
☐ c.  Transverse tongue fissures
☐ d.  Epstein pearls
☐ e.  None of the above

20. Any child with a strange mouth odor must be evaluated for:
☐ a.  possible ingestion
☐ b.  poor hygiene habits
☐ c.  certain diseases including diphtheria and diabetes
☐ d.  foreign object in nose
☐ e.  multiple caries
☐ f.  a, b, and e
☐ g.  b, c, and d
☐ h.  all but c
☐ i.  all the above
☐ j.  none of the above

21. Which of the following is not routinely evaluated in the pediatric client?
☐ a.  Tongue
☐ b.  Nares
☐ c.  Olfactory nerve
☐ d.  Gums
☐ e.  Hard palate

**GERIATRIC QUESTIONS**

22. Some studies show that the most common reason for loss of teeth with elderly clients is:
    - ☐ a. dental caries
    - ☐ b. root canal problems
    - ☐ c. soft enamel
    - ☐ d. periodontal disease

23. Lesions commonly found in the mouth of geriatric clients are:
    - ☐ a. Fordyce granules
    - ☐ b. hyperkeratosis
    - ☐ c. petechiae
    - ☐ d. purpura
    - ☐ e. all except d
    - ☐ f. a and b
    - ☐ g. a and c
    - ☐ h. all except c

24. Xerostomia:
    - ☐ a. is caused by bone resorption
    - ☐ b. is rare and occurs in people over 80 years of age
    - ☐ c. interferes with self-cleaning of the mouth
    - ☐ d. only occurs following poor oral self-care habits

25. Some of the risk factors that could alert a practitioner to potential mouth or dental problems are:
    - ☐ a. cirrhosis of the liver
    - ☐ b. use of chewing tobacco
    - ☐ c. severe arthritis of the hands
    - ☐ d. osteoporosis
    - ☐ e. chronic heavy smoking
    - ☐ f. all the above
    - ☐ g. all except d
    - ☐ h. a, b, and e
    - ☐ i. b and e

**SUGGESTED READINGS**
**General**

Bates, B.: A guide to physical examination, ed. 3, Philadelphia, 1983, J.B. Lippincott Co., pp. 62-65, 85-91, 116-122.

DeGowin, E., and DeGowin, R.: Bedside diagnostic examination, ed. 3, New York, 1976, Macmillan Publishing Co., Inc., pp. 126-139.

Judge, R.D., and Zuidema, G., editors: Methods of clinical examination: a physiologic approach, Boston, 1974, Little, Brown & Co., pp. 81-91.

Keough, G., and Niebel, H.N.: Oral cancer detection, Am. J. Nurs. 73(4):684-686, 1973.

Malasanos, L., and others: Health assessment, ed. 2, St. Louis, 1981, The C.V. Mosby Co., pp. 213-222.

Patient assessment: examination of the head and neck, Programmed instruction, Am. J. Nurs. 75:5, 1975.

Prior, J.A., Silberstein, J.S., and Stang, J.M.: Physical diagnosis: the history and examination of the patient, ed. 6, St. Louis, 1981, The C.V. Mosby Co., pp. 166-188.

Sana, J., and Judge, R.D.: Physical appraisal methods in nursing, Boston, 1975, Little, Brown & Co., pp. 97-98, 100-101, 136-141.

**Pediatric**

Barness, L.: Manual of pediatric physical diagnosis, ed. 5, Chicago, 1981, Year Book Medical Publishers, Inc., pp. 48-109.

Brown, M.S., and Alexander, M.: Physical examination. IX. Examining the nose, Nursing '74 4(7):35-38, 1974.

Brown, M.S., and Alexander, M.: Physical examination. X. Mouth and throat, Nursing '74 4(7):57-61, 1974.

DeAngelis, C.: Basic pediatrics for the primary health care provider, Boston, 1975, Little, Brown & Co., pp. 46-50.

**Geriatric**

Carotenuto, R., and Bullock, J.: Physical assessment of the gerontologic client, Philadelphia, 1980, F.A. Davis Co., pp. 51-58.

Langer, A.: Oral signs of aging and their clinical significance, Geriatrics 31(12):63-69, 1976.

Steinburg, Franz U., editor: Care of the geriatric patient, ed. 6, St. Louis, 1983, The C.V. Mosby Co., pp. 388-405.

# Ears and auditory system

## VOCABULARY

**anulus** The dense fibrous ring surrounding the tympanic membrane.

**auricle** Flap of the external ear; also called the *pinna*.

**cerumen** Waxy secretion of the glands of the external acoustic meatus; earwax.

**cochlea** Conical bony structure of the inner ear; perforated by numerous apertures for passage of the cochlear division of the acoustic nerve.

**darwinian tubercle** Blunt point projecting up from the upper part of the helix of the ear.

**dizziness** Disturbed sense of relationship to space.

**eustachian tube** Tube, lined with mucous membrane, that joins the nasopharynx and the tympanic cavity, allowing equalization of air pressure with atmospheric pressure.

**helix** Margin of the external ear.

**incus** One of three ossicles in the middle ear; Resembling an anvil, it communicates sound vibrations from the malleus to the stapes.

**injection** Redness or congestion of the tympanic membrane caused by dilatation of blood vessels secondary to an inflammatory or infectious process.

**labyrinth** Complex structure of the inner ear that communicates directly with the acoustic nerve, transmitting sound vibrations from the middle ear through the fluid-filled network of three semicircular canals that join at a vestibule connected to the cochlea.

**light reflex** A triangular landmark area on the tympanic membrane that most brightly reflects the examiner's light source.

**malleus** Innermost ossicle of the middle ear; resembling a hammer, it is connected to the tympanic membrane and transmits sound vibrations to the incus, which communicates with the stapes.

**mastoid process** Conical projection of the caudal posterior portion of the temporal bone.

**nystagmus** Involuntary rhythmical movement of the eyes; oscillations may be horizontal, vertical, rotary, or mixed.

**otalgia** Pain in the ear.

**otitis** Inflammation or infection of the ear.

**otitis externa** Inflammation or infection of the external canal or auricle of the external ear.

**otitis media** Inflammation or infection of the middle ear.

**pars flaccida** The small portion of the tympanic membrane between the mallear folds.

**pars tensa** The larger portion of the tympanic membrane.

**pinna** Auricle or projected part of the external ear.

**presbycusis** Impairment of hearing in old age.

**stapes** One of three ossicles in the middle ear; it resembles a tiny stirrup and transmits sound vibrations from the incus to the internal ear.

**tinnitus** Tinkling or ringing sound heard in one or both ears.

**tophi** Calculus, containing sodium urate deposits, that develops in periarticular fibrous tissue.

**tragus** Cartilaginous projection in front of the exterior meatus of the ear.

**umbo** Central depressed portion of the concavity on lateral surface of the tympanic membrane; marks the spot where the malleus is attached to the inner surface.

**vertigo** Sensation of a whirling motion, involving either oneself or external objects.

**vestibule** Middle part of the inner ear, located behind the cochlea and in front of the semicircular canals.

## Cognitive objectives

At the end of this chapter the learner will demonstrate knowledge of assessment of the ear and auditory system by the ability to do the following:

1. Systematically list examination criteria for evaluating the external ear, including:
   a. Anatomical positioning
   b. Surface characteristics of the external ear and ear canal
   c. Tympanic membrane (TM)
2. Describe the technique of manipulating the external ear and canal for otoscopic examination of the adult and the child.
3. List six methods to screen for hearing problems, three for the adult client and three for the pediatric client.
4. Identify selected common variations for pediatric and geriatric clients.
5. Differentiate testing methods for evaluating conductive and perceptive hearing loss. Describe the Rinne and Weber tests and discuss normal and abnormal findings for each.
6. List descriptors for evaluating the TM. Describe normal findings and the suggested significance of deviations from normal.
7. Use the terms in the vocabulary list.

## Clinical objectives

At the end of this chapter the learner will perform a systematic assessment of the ear and auditory system, demonstrating the ability to do the following:

1. Obtain a pertinent health history from a client.
2. Demonstrate inspection of the external ear and relate findings concerning:
   a. Ear position, size, and symmetry
   b. Skin color, intactness, deformities, and lesions
   c. Patency of external canal
3. Do palpation of the external ear and mastoid process and relate findings relevant to skin texture, tenderness, nodules, and swelling.
4. Demonstrate inspection of the external canal and TM and relate findings concerning:
   a. Color of canal tissue, evidence of tissue intactness, discharge, deformities, masses or lesions, cerumen presence, and characteristics
   b. Landmark identification, including umbo, malleus, light reflex, pars tensa, pars flaccida, anulus
   c. Color of the TM
   d. Tension of the TM
   e. Intactness, scars, or deformities of the TM

5. Evaluate the client's auditory system by using screening techniques, including the Rinne and Weber tests, and interpret findings.
6. Summarize results of the assessment with a written description.

## Health history additional to screening history

1. Is there a family history of hearing problems or hearing loss?
2. Is there history of frequent ear problems or infections during childhood? Describe typical treatment techniques and course of the problem.
3. Is there history of any ear injury or hearing problems related to trauma?
4. If the client complains of painful ears, the examiner should collect descriptive data using the analysis of a symptom format. In addition, the possibility of trauma to the ears, either by foreign body, harsh cleaning, or environmental noise, must be investigated; and related complaints, including recent problems with mouth, teeth, paranasal sinuses, or throat, must be inquired about.
5. If itching of the ears is a complaint, ask the client about where the sensation is felt, the duration of the sensation, and what he has done to correct the problem. In addition, inquire about swimming, showering, and ear cleansing techniques.
6. Medication history is especially important if the client has any complaints of tinnitus or extra noise in the ears. Special emphasis should be to collect information about ototoxic drugs, including acetylsalicylic acid, quinine, streptomycin, neomycin, gentamicin, or nitrofurantoin.
7. If the client complains of dizziness or vertigo, the examiner must collect detailed information to describe the exact nature of the problem.
   a. Vertigo is the sensation of whirling motion: with eyes open, the client states that the surroundings are moving; with eyes closed, the client feels himself in motion. Dizziness is the disturbed sense of relationship to space.
   b. How does the sensation change with the client's change in position (e.g., lying down, bending, standing)?
   c. Is the client taking medications, or is there a systemic disease?
   d. Does the symptom (e.g., falling, losing balance) interfere with the client's activities of daily living?
8. If the client complains of a hearing loss, the examiner should inquire about the following:

a. Sudden or slow onset of hearing problem
b. Environmental factors such as factory noise
c. Specific types of sounds or tones that the client has difficulty hearing, such as conversation or a telephone ringing
d. To what degree the hearing problem interferes with the client's activities of daily living; wheth-er it causes a problem on the job, in television viewing, phone conversations, etc.
e. What types of corrective devices the client has tried; where and from whom they were obtained

9. If environmental or employment noise is a problem, what precautions, if any, are taken? Head sets or ear plugs? What is the extent of the environmental exposure?

## Clinical guidelines

| THE STUDENT WILL: | TO IDENTIFY: | |
| | NORMAL | DEVIATIONS FROM NORMAL |
| --- | --- | --- |
| 1. Collect equipment:<br>    **a.** Otoscope with bright light, several sizes of ear specula, pneumatic bulb<br>    **b.** Tuning fork (500 to 1000 cps)<br>2. Perform physical assessment of the ear<br>    **a.** Inspect both ears for alignment and configuration | Ears of equal height and size<br>Located so that pinna is on line with corner of eye (Fig. 6-1)<br>Ear within 10° angle of vertical position | Abnormal configuration<br>Low-set or unequal positioning (Fig. 6-1) |

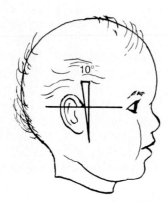 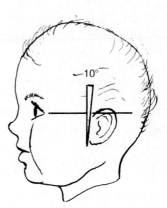

**FIG. 6-1.** Ear alignment.

| THE STUDENT WILL: | TO IDENTIFY: | |
| | NORMAL | DEVIATIONS FROM NORMAL |
| --- | --- | --- |
| **b.** Inspect external ear (anterior and posterior bilateral and mastoid areas) (Fig. 6-2) | Skin color pink, uniform<br>Skin intact | Redness<br>Swelling<br>Deformities, lesions, nodules such as darwinian tubercle (Figs. 6-3 and 6-4)<br>Tophi (Fig. 6-3)<br>Cauliflower ear (Fig. 6-4)<br>Furuncles |

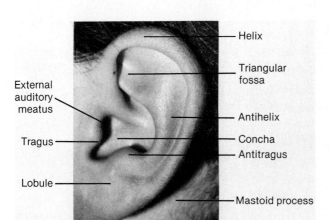

FIG. 6-2. Landmarks of ear.

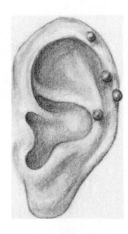

FIG. 6-3. Tophi.

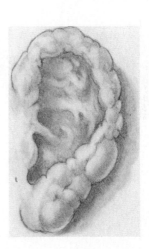

FIG. 6-4. Cauliflower ear.

| | | |
| --- | --- | --- |
| **c.** Palpate external ear (auricles and mastoid areas) | Intact<br>Smooth, nontender | Tenderness<br>Pain<br>Swelling<br>Nodules |

## Clinical guidelines—cont'd

| THE STUDENT WILL: | TO IDENTIFY: | |
| --- | --- | --- |
| | NORMAL | DEVIATIONS FROM NORMAL |
| **d.** Use otoscope to examine:<br>  1. External auditory canal (see clinical strategies for technique and Fig. 6-5 for structures) | Cerumen present; note color (may vary: black, brown, dark red, creamy, brown-gray); texture (may vary from moist waxy to dry flaky or hard texture); no odor<br>Caucasians and blacks: generally have wet cerumen that is tan or brown<br>Asians and American Indians: generally have dry cerumen that is light to brown-gray<br>Hair present (Fig. 6-6)<br>Canal skin intact<br>Uniform pink color<br>Tenderness with deep speculum insertion | Cerumen impacting ear canal; unable to visualize canal or TM (Fig. 6-7)<br>Lesions, bleeding, discharge (note appearance and odor), foreign bodies (Fig. 6-8), inflammation, growths (Fig. 6-9), pain, tenderness, swelling, infection<br>Partial occlusion of auditory canal caused by improper retraction of auricle; can usually be remedied by correct traction (Fig. 6-10) |

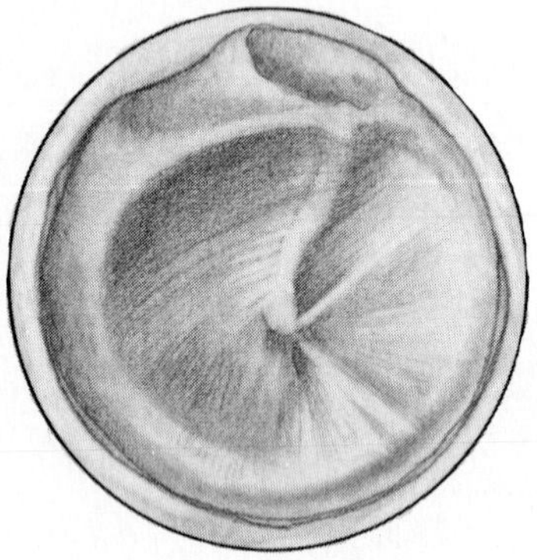

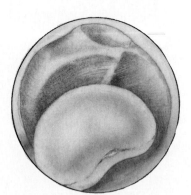

**FIG. 6-5.** Structures of ear.

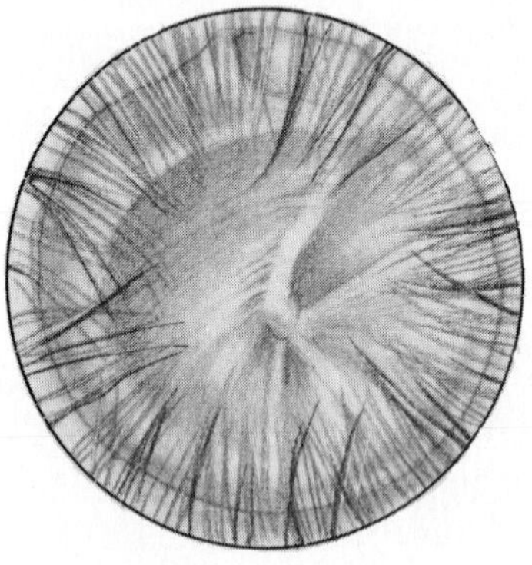

**FIG. 6-6.** Hairy ear canal.

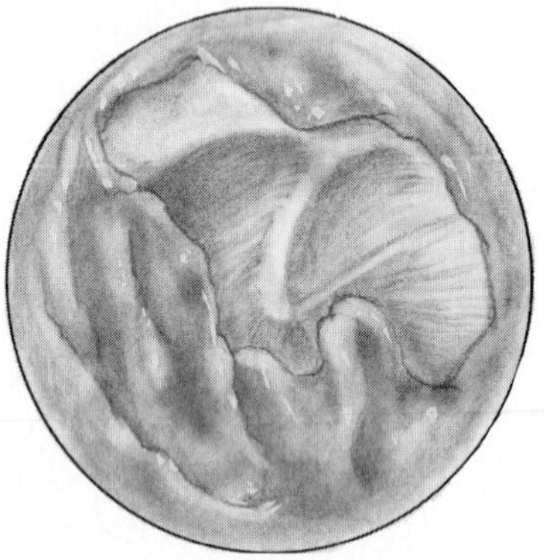

**FIG. 6-7.** Cerumen in ear canal.

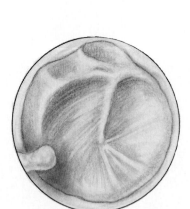

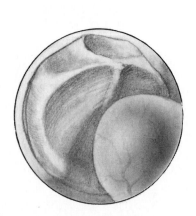

**FIG. 6-8.** Foreign object in ear canal.

**FIG. 6-9.** Polyp in external ear canal.

**FIG. 6-10.** Wall of ear canal obstructing view.

| THE STUDENT WILL: | TO IDENTIFY: | |
| --- | --- | --- |
| | NORMAL | DEVIATIONS FROM NORMAL |

2. Tympanic membrane (TM) (Fig. 6-11)

   a. Characteristics

Drum intact

Slight fluctuation present when swallowing

Membrane not intact (Fig. 6-12) or showing scarring (Fig. 6-13)

Membrane fixed and nonfluctuating or jerky fluctuation present

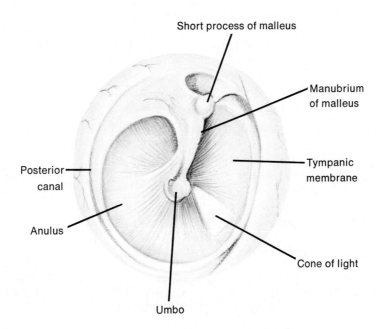

FIG. 6-11. Tympanic membrane landmarks.

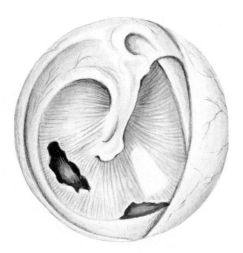

FIG. 6-12. Perforated membrane.

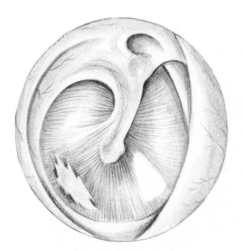

FIG. 6-13. Scarring of membrane.

## Clinical guidelines—cont'd

| THE STUDENT WILL: | TO IDENTIFY: | |
| --- | --- | --- |
| | NORMAL | DEVIATIONS FROM NORMAL |
| b. Color | Shiny, pearly gray, translucent appearance | Other TM colors indicating abnormality:<br>Serum—yellow-amber<br>Blood—blue or deep red<br>Pus—chalky white<br>Infection—red or pink<br>Fibrosis—dull surface<br>Diffuse or spotty light<br>Obliteration of some or all landmarks<br>Increased vascularization (injection) |
| c. Landmarks: follow anulus around periphery of pars tensa | Cone of light (pars tensa)<br>Umbo<br>Handle of malleus<br>Short process of malleus<br>Malleolar folds<br>Pars flaccida | Accentuated landmarks (indicating negative pressure behind TM)<br>Bulging membrane (indicating buildup of pressure behind TM) |
| **3.** Perform screening evaluation of auditory function | | |
| **a.** Whispered voice: stand 30 to 60 cm (1 to 2 feet) from client, mask client's opposite ear, exhale, then whisper in very low voice; increase intensity until client responds correctly at least 50% of time; use both monosyllabic and bisyllabic words; repeat other side | Able to hear softly whispered words at distance of 30 to 60 cm (1 to 2 feet)<br>Bilaterally equal response | Unilateral response or bilaterally unequal response<br>Unable to repeat words until whispered voice is louder |
| **b.** Watch tick: place ticking watch 2 to 5 cm (1 to 2 inches) from ear; mask opposite ear; repeat other side | Able to hear ticking watch at distance of 2 to 5 cm (1 to 2 inches) | Clients with high-frequency hearing loss unable to hear ticking |
| **c.** Tuning fork | | |
| 1. Rinne test (compares air conduction to bone conduction): softly strike tuning fork and place on client's mastoid process; when client is no longer able to hear tone, remove tuning fork and place it in front of same ear; tone should be heard approximately twice as long in this position (Fig. 6-14) | Air-conducted sound heard twice as long as bone-conducted sound (AC > BC); called *positive result* | Bone-conducted sound heard as long as or longer than air-conducted sound (BC ≥ AC); called *negative result;* a sign of conductive loss |

| THE STUDENT WILL: | TO IDENTIFY: | |
| --- | --- | --- |
| | NORMAL | DEVIATIONS FROM NORMAL |

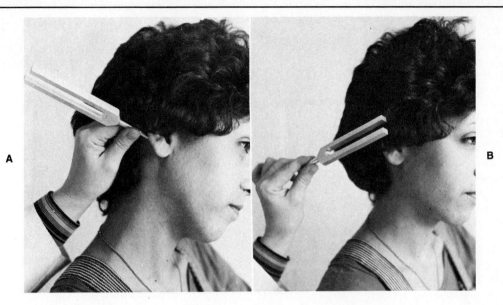

**FIG. 6-14.** Rinne test. **A,** Behind ear, on mastoid process. **B,** In front of ear.

| | | |
| --- | --- | --- |
| 2. Weber test (assesses bone conduction by testing lateralization of sounds): softly strike tuning fork and place on midline of forehead (Fig. 6-15) | Bilaterally equal sound | If client has conductive loss, sound lateralizes to poorer ear<br>If client has sensorineural loss, sound lateralizes to good ear |

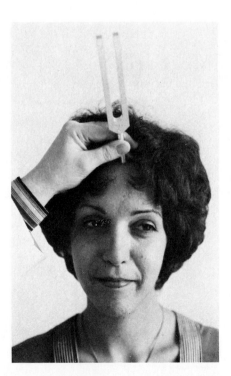

**FIG. 6-15.** Weber test. Tuning fork is placed on forehead.

## Clinical guidelines—cont'd

| THE STUDENT WILL: | TO IDENTIFY: | |
|---|---|---|
| | NORMAL | DEVIATIONS FROM NORMAL |

**4.** Evaluate vestibular portion of auditory nerve (CN VIII)

   **a.** Test for nystagmus using cold caloric test (procedure is not normally done during screening examination and should not be performed if client is thought to have acute middle ear infection or perforated eardrum): client sits with head tilted 60° in extension (backward) position; irrigate against eardrum with 10 ml of ice water (32°-50° F) over 20-second period; test one ear at a time and note response

*NORMAL:* Nausea, dizziness, and nystagmus, appearing in about 30 seconds and lasting approximately 1½ minutes (Fig. 6-16)

*DEVIATIONS FROM NORMAL:* Bilaterally unequal response
Unduly prolonged unilateral nystagmus

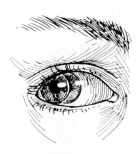

**FIG. 6-16.** Nystagmus associated with CN VIII vestibular malfunction.

   **b.** Nylen-Bárány test (for positional nystagmus): Client lies supine with head hanging 45° backward over end of table and turned to one side; make observation; then instruct client to turn head to other direction

*NORMAL:* No nystagmus noted

*DEVIATIONS FROM NORMAL:* Nystagmus noted; observe duration and direction

   **c.** Test for falling (Romberg sign): client stands with feet together, eyes closed, arms to side; watch for steadiness of stance (stand close by in case client loses balance) (Fig. 6-17)

*NORMAL:* Swaying but able to maintain body and feet positioning

*DEVIATIONS FROM NORMAL:* Unable to maintain positioning
Need to widen base support
Unable to keep from falling

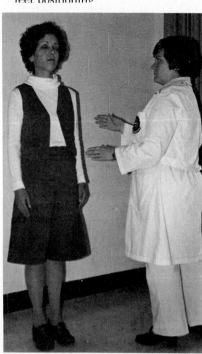

**FIG. 6-17.** Romberg test.

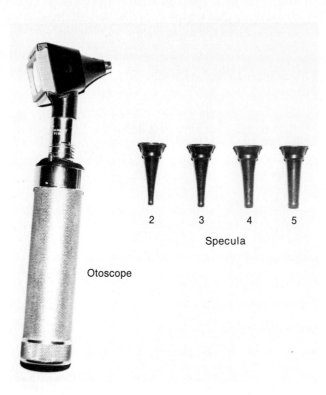

**FIG. 6-18.** Ostoscope with all sizes of available specula.

Specula

2   3   4   5

Otoscope

## Clinical strategies

1. Hearing evaluation should begin from the moment you meet the client. Note how the individual responds to your speaking; note *posturing of head* or types of words that need repeating.
2. When using the otoscope, consider the following guidelines:
   a. Use the largest speculum that will fit into the ear canal comfortably (Fig. 6-18).
   b. The otoscope must have good batteries or adequate illumination of the landmarks of the ear will be impossible. (Batteries should give off white, *not* yellow, light.)
   c. The adult client should be sitting with the head tilted toward the opposite shoulder.
   d. Hold the otoscope between the palm and the first two fingers of one hand. The handle may be positioned either downward (Fig. 6-19) or upward (Fig. 6-24). The examiner must determine which position provides better immobility between the otoscope and the client's head.
   e. With the other hand, grasp the pinna with the thumb and fingers and pull out, up, and back to straighten the canal (Fig. 6-19).
   f. Remember, the inner two thirds of the external ear canal are bony. It will *hurt* if the speculum

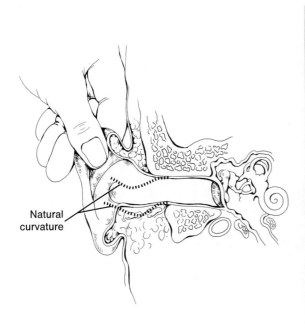

Natural curvature

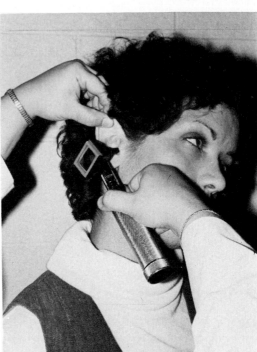

**FIG. 6-19.** Straighten external canal of adult ear by pulling helix up and out.

is pressed against either side (Fig. 6-20). If the examiner is having difficulty seeing the TM, a combination of repositioning the head, pulling the auricle in a slightly different position, and reangling the otoscope should be attempted.

   g. When placing the speculum in the client's ear, make sure to steady your hand against the client's head by extending one or two fingers from the hand holding the otoscope.

3. A cerumen spoon or irrigation may be used to remove cerumen from the external ear canal. If the cerumen is wet and waxy, a cerumen spoon works best; if it is dry, irrigation is preferable. The examiner must see the TM in any client with a history suggestive of hearing or ear problems.

4. If, because of bone structure or excessive hair in the ear canal, only about half of the TM is visualized, and if that half appears healthy and without disease, it can be assumed that the other half is also healthy.

5. When striking a tuning fork, be careful not to make the tone too loud. If this happens, it will take so long to quiet the tone enough for auditory testing that the client may become tired. It is usually sufficient to tap the fork gently on the knuckle or stroke the fork between the thumb and the index finger (Fig. 6-21).

6. During the whisper test, make sure to position yourself so that the client cannot read your lips.

7. The technique of masking is very important. The examiner should simply instruct the client to insert a finger into the ear that is not being tested and then wiggle it back and forth slightly to occlude hearing in that ear by masking it with noise. The technique is reversed during examination of the opposite ear.

## History and clinical strategies: the pediatric client

1. The basic evaluation of a child's ear is exactly like that of an adult's ear. For screening purposes the vestibular component is not evaluated.

2. The examiner must evaluate the same anatomical structures in both an adult's and a child's ears. It is important for the examiner to scale down expectations to maintain a gentle approach (Fig. 6-22). Consequently, insert the speculum into the canal between 0.6 and 1.2 cm ($\frac{1}{4}$ and $\frac{1}{2}$ inch).

3. One difference in examining a child's ear is the curvature of the external canal (Fig. 6-23). Because of the upward curvature of the canal in the infant and small child, the examiner must grasp the lower portion of the auricle and retract the ear downward and backward to straighten the canal. By age 3, the child's canal has changed to assume more of an adult position. Therefore with the child who is 3 years and older the pinna should be pulled up and back to straighten the canal.

4. Because young children can be "squirmy," we have found it best to examine the child's ear canal and TM in the following manner:

   a. Place the child in either a prone position with head to the side and arms downward (Fig. 6-24), or

---

**SAMPLE RECORDING**

*Ear:* Positioning bilaterally symmetrical; smooth auricles without lesions or discharge.
   External canal, small amount of dark cerumen noted.
   Tympanic membrane intact; all landmarks clearly identified.
*Auditory:* Can hear low whisper at 60 cm (2 feet).
   Rinne: AC > BC.
   Weber: equal lateralization.
*Vestibular:* CN VIII intact.

---

**FIG. 6-20.** Relationship of speculum insertion and bony prominence.

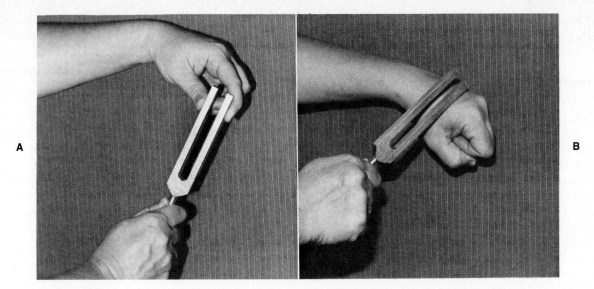

**FIG. 6-21.** Activating the tuning fork. Hearing is tested at *near-threshold* levels; therefore the fork should be made to ring softly. **A,** Stroking the fork. **B,** Tapping the fork gently on the knuckle.

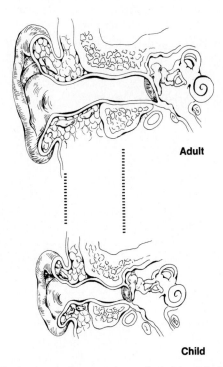

**FIG. 6-22.** Anatomical comparison of adult's and child's ear.

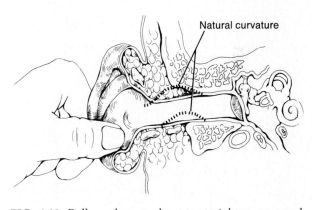

**FIG. 6-23.** Pull ear down and out to straighten ear canal.

b. Place the child in a supine position on the cart with arms extended overhead and secured by the parent (Fig. 6-25).

c. Hold the otoscope like a pencil, with the handle extending upward toward the top of the child's head. Brace the otoscope and your hand against the child's head by extending one or two fingers as securing forces (Fig. 6-24). This will allow your hand and the instrument to go along with any sudden movements.

d. The child *must* be securely immobilized during the ear examination.

5. Because of the sensitive nature of the ear examination, it is best left until the last part of the physical examination. Should the child become upset, this will permit immediate return to the parent for cuddling.

6. During the TM evaluation the examiner may decide to evaluate the fluctuating capacity of the TM by injecting small puffs of air against the membrane. This is especially important if the child is thought to have fluid or pressure buildup behind the TM. Slight fluctuation of the membrane is a normal response; no movement or jerky movement is abnormal. There are several instruments and procedures to perform this assessment (Fig. 6-26). The examiner must choose the largest speculum that will fit into the child's ear canal; the secure, tight fit will allow air pressure to move the TM.

7. Every child should have an ear evaluation. If the

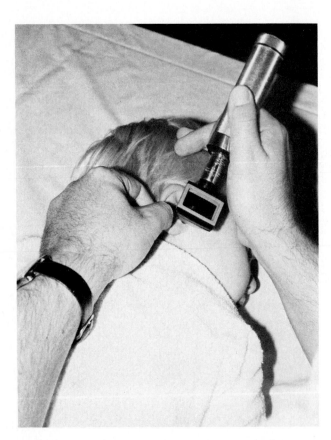

**FIG. 6-24.** Examination of child in prone position with arms to side.

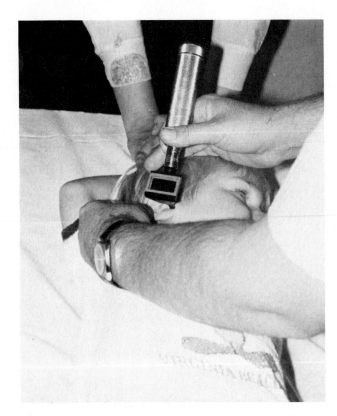

**FIG. 6-25.** Examination of child in supine position with arms overhead.

ear canal is occluded with wax, the examiner must use one of the common techniques to remove it. If the child is ill or running a fever, examination of the TM is an *absolute must*.

8. History questions specifically related to the pediatric client include the following:

   a. Recurrent infections of the throat or ears? Number during past 6 months? Usual treatment?
   b. Are ear problems becoming more frequent and/or severe?
   c. History of ear surgery? If so, what and when?
   d. Does child play with his ears frequently or have tendency toward putting objects in his ears?
   e. History of foreign body in ears?
   f. How does the parent clean the child's ears?
   g. Has child ever had his ears tested? If so, by whom and where?
   h. If the child has low-set ears, question extensively about kidney or other congenital problems.
   i. If a child has symptoms of ear or auditory dysfunction, it is specifically important to inquire about any past disease or drug usage that is considered potentially ototoxic. High-risk children are those who have had measles, mumps, otitis media, any disease with high fever, or drugs including streptomycin, kanamycin, and neomycin.

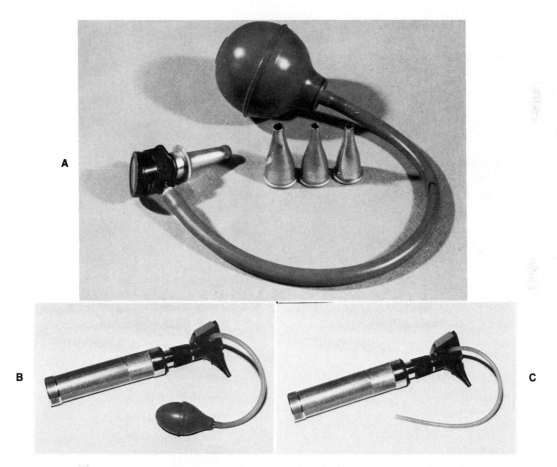

FIG. 6-26. **A,** Pneumatic otoscope. **B,** Regular otoscope with pneumatic bulb. **C,** Regular otoscope with pneumatic tube. End of the tubing is placed in the examiner's mouth, where small puffs of air are expelled against the child's tympanic membrane. (**A** from Prior, J.A., Silberstein, J.S., and Stang, J.M.: Physical diagnosis: the history and examination of the patient, ed. 6, St. Louis, 1981, The C.V. Mosby Co.)

## Clinical variations: the pediatric client

| CHARACTERISTIC OR AREA EXAMINED | NORMAL | DEVIATIONS FROM NORMAL |
|---|---|---|
| **1.** External ear | | |
| **a.** Alignment | Ears of equal height and size | Low-set or unequal positioning |
| | Located so that pinna is on line with corner of eye | |
| | Ear within 10° angle of vertical position | |
| **b.** Configuration | | Abnormal configuration |
| | | Deformities, lesions, nodules such as darwinian tubercle |
| | | Tophi |
| | | Cauliflower ear |
| | | Furuncles |
| **2.** External canal | | |
| **a.** Color and surface | Skin color pink, uniform | Redness |
| | Skin intact | Swelling |
| | Hair present | Lesions, bleeding, discharge (note appearance and odor), foreign bodies, inflammation, growths, pain, tenderness, swelling, infection |
| | Canal skin intact | |
| | Tenderness with deep speculum insertion | |
| | | Partial occlusion of auditory canal caused by improper retraction of auricle; can usually be corrected with traction |
| | Smooth, nontender | Tenderness |
| | | Pain |
| | | Swelling |
| | | Nodules |
| **b.** Cerumen | Cerumen present; note color (may vary: black to brown to creamy pink), texture (may vary from moist waxy to dry flaky or hard texture); no odor | Cerumen impacting ear canal; unable to visualize canal or TM |
| **3.** Tympanic membrane | | |
| **a.** Characteristics | Drum intact | Membrane not intact or showing scarring |
| | Presence of myringotomy tube (Fig. 6-27) in selected clients | |

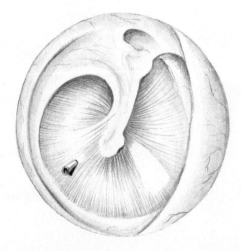

**FIG. 6-27.** Drainage tube inserted following myringotomy.

| CHARACTERISTIC OR AREA EXAMINED | NORMAL | DEVIATIONS FROM NORMAL |
|---|---|---|
| **b.** Tension: use pneumatic or squeeze bulb to evaluate TM fluctuation | Slight fluctuation of drum with air puffs | Fixed, nonfluctuating or jerky fluctuation |
| **c.** Color | Shiny, pearly gray, translucent appearance | Other TM colors indicating abnormality: <br> Serum: yellow-amber <br> Blood: blue or deep red <br> Pus: chalky white <br> Infection: red or pink <br> Fibrosis: dull surface |
| **d.** Landmarks | Cone of light (pars tensa) <br> Umbo <br> Handle of malleus <br> Short process of malleus <br> Malleolar folds <br> Pars flaccida | Diffuse or spotty light <br> Obliteration of some or all landmarks <br> Increased vascularization (injection) <br> Accentuated landmarks (indicating negative pressure behind TM) <br> Bulging membrane (indicating buildup of pressure behind TM) |
| **4.** Auditory function | | |
| **a.** Newborn: at distance of approximately 30.5 cm (12 inches), and so that infant does not see, snap fingers loudly or ring bell (may need to repeat several times) | Startle reflex or eye blink | No response |
| **b.** 2 to 3 months: at distance of approximately 30.5 cm (12 inches), and so that infant does not see, snap fingers loudly or ring bell | Eye blink, or stopping movement to listen for sound | No response |
| **c.** 3 months and older: at distance of approximately 30.5 cm (12 inches), and so that infant does not see, snap fingers loudly or ring bell | Turns head toward noise | No response |
| **d.** Older infants and toddlers: have child sit on parent's lap; stand behind parent; at first on one side and then the other, either ring bell, whisper "s" or "sh" words, or call child's name | Turns head toward noise | No response |
| **e.** Preschool and school age: should receive audiometric testing; for preschool and school-age client, if audiometry unavailable, use same screening as for adult client: | Able to hear 1000, 2000, 4000, and 6000 cps at 25 db | Unable to hear recommended levels |
| 1. Whispered voice | Able to hear whispered voice at 30 to 60 cm (1 to 2 feet) | Unilateral or unequal response <br> Unable to repeat words until whispered voice is louder |
| 2. Watch ticking | Able to hear ticking watch at distance of 2 to 5 cm (1 to 2 inches) | Unable to hear ticking |
| 3. Tuning fork: <br> Rinne test <br> Weber test | <br> AC > BC <br> Bilaterally equal sound | <br> AC = BC <br> Lateralization of sound |

## History and clinical strategies: the geriatric client

1. Formal hearing screening should be delayed until near the end of the assessment. Client anxiety or insecurity about ability to perform may exist at the beginning of the examination and may interfere with accurate assessment.

2. Informal hearing screening should occur at the beginning and throughout the assessment. Noting whether the client is able to respond appropriately to questions or conversation, with and/or without direct eye contact, is an important clue for assessment of hearing acuity.

3. Other clues or "red flags" indicating possible hearing difficulty follow:
   a. Client watches examiner's face and mouth movements closely.
   b. Client's speech volume control is erratic or constantly pronounced.
   c. Client's tone of voice is monotonous, unvaried.
   d. Client's speech is distorted (especially with use or omission of vowel sounds).

4. Fairly extensive hearing loss can occur before the client complains about it or reports it as a problem.

5. If hearing loss is offered as a complaint, the following questions should be asked:
   a. Is the loss in both ears or one ear?
   b. Was the onset sudden or gradual? (*Note:* A sudden onset is a "red flag" for immediate referral to a physician.) "Sudden" should be clarified in terms of instant loss (may be indicative of vascular disruption) versus a loss that occurred over a few hours or days (may indicate a viral disorder).
   c. Is all hearing diminished or just certain types of sounds (e.g., does conversation sound garbled, can you hear the telephone)?
   d. Do outside or environmental noises interfere with or distort your hearing (e.g., is it more difficult to understand conversation if a lot of people are talking at once)?
   e. Do you have a history of exposure to loud or continuous noises (e.g., the whine of machinery on the job)?
   f. Have you ever had any auditory training?
   g. Does your hearing loss interfere with your daily life (e.g., responses of family or friends to loss, general social or family relationships, ability to function at work or at home)?
   h. Have you ever used or do you now use a hearing aid?

6. Obtain a drug history. Salicylates, aminoglycosides (e.g., gentamicin, streptomycin), furosemide, quinine, and ethacrynic acid are commonly used drugs that diminish hearing.

7. If a hearing aid is used, the following questions should be asked:
   a. Do you feel it is effective? (*Note:* Adjustment to a new hearing aid may take 2 to 6 months.)
   b. How often do you wear it (all the time, on social occasions, rarely, never)?
   c. Do you have any difficulty operating it or using it (e.g., pushing small switches or buttons, inserting batteries, fastening aid to clothing, inserting earmold, untangling wires)?
   d. Do you have difficulty keeping it in good repair, or are you concerned about expenses related to repair?
   e. Do you have difficulty cleaning it? (*Note:* Cerumen or other debris can plug the tiny hole that carries sound through the earmolds.)
   f. When was it purchased? Who prescribed it?

8. Tinnitus may be interpreted by the client as a ringing, cracking, whistling, or buzzing sound. In addition to a full symptom analysis, be certain to clarify the quality of the sound.
   a. Tinnitis may be a pulsatile sensation (possibly associated with carotid bruits), a steady noise, or a transient complaint.
   b. Chronic tinnitis (6 months or more) should be differentiated from a similar complaint of short duration and/or sudden onset.

9. Vertigo must be differentiated from unsteadiness, which is fairly common with elderly people. If vertigo is established as a complaint, ask if it is associated with head or neck movement (in addition to doing a full symptom analysis).

10. Ear pain or a feeling of "fullness" may reflect a problem related to temporomandibular joint movement, cervical arthritis, or dental disease.

11. Following is a list of risk factors that can alert the examiner to possible hearing deficiency:
    a. History of long exposure to loud or continuous noise
    b. History of chronic nasal allergy
    c. Systemic disease (some of the more commonly associated diseases: cardiovascular disease, diabetes mellitus, nephritis)
    d. Sensitivity to some medications (see list in adult history section of this chapter)
    e. Chronic cigarette smoking
    f. General physical or emotional disability (some authors state there is a correlation between impaired physical and/or emotional well-being and diminished hearing acuity)
    g. Family history of deafness

12. See adult history in this chapter for further questions.

# Clinical variations: the geriatric client

| CHARACTERISTIC OR AREA EXAMINED | NORMAL | DEVIATIONS FROM NORMAL |
|---|---|---|
| **1.** External ear | | |
| **a.** Alignment | Ears of equal height and size<br>Located so that pinna is on line with corner of eye<br>Ear within 10° angle of vertical position | Low-set or unequal positioning |
| **b.** Configuration | Earlobes may appear pendulous | Abnormal configuration |
| **c.** Surface characteristics | Skin color pink, uniform<br>Skin intact | Redness<br>Swelling<br>Deformities, lesions, nodules such as darwinian tubercle<br>Tophi<br>Cauliflower ear<br>Furuncles |
| | Smooth, nontender | Tenderness<br>Pain<br>Swelling<br>Nodules |
| **2.** External canal | | |
| **a.** Color, surface characteristics, discharge | Canal skin intact<br>Uniform pink color<br>Tenderness with deep speculum insertion<br>Cerumen present; note color (may vary from black to brown to creamy pink) and texture (may vary from moist waxy to dry flaky or hard texture)<br>Impacted cerumen usually contains more keratin and may be more difficult to remove<br>Hair present | Cerumen impacting ear canal (*Note:* In older adults cerumen can become very dry and totally obstruct canal; canal can also be obstructed with impacted skin and hair [keratoses].)<br>Lesions, bleeding, discharge (note appearance and odor), foreign bodies (Fig. 6-8), inflammation, growths (Fig. 6-9), pain, tenderness, swelling, infection<br>Be alert for sebaceous cysts, furuncles, dermatosis, or increase in granulation tissue (*Note:* Earmolds—part of hearing aids—may cause irritation of canal, especially if they do not fit well.) |
| **3.** Tympanic membrane | | |
| **a.** Characteristics | Drum intact<br><br>Slight fluctuation present with swallowing | Membrane not intact (Fig. 6-12) or showing scarring (Fig. 6-13)<br>Fixed, nonfluctuating or jerky fluctuation |
| **b.** Color | Shiny, pearly gray, translucent appearance | Other TM colors indicating abnormality:<br>Serum: yellow-amber<br>Blood: blue or deep red<br>Pus: chalky white<br>Infection: red or pink<br>Fibrosis: dull surface |
| **c.** Landmarks: follow anulus around periphery of pars tensa | Cone of light (pars tensa)<br>Umbo<br>Handle of malleus<br>Short process of malleus<br>Malleolar folds<br>Pars flaccida<br>Landmarks may appear slightly more pronounced with atrophic or sclerotic tympanic changes | Diffuse or spotty light<br>Obliteration of some or all landmarks<br>Increased vascularization (injection)<br>Accentuated landmarks (indicating negative pressure behind TM)<br>Bulging membrane (indicating buildup of pressure behind TM) |

## Clinical variations: the geriatric client—cont'd

| CHARACTERISTIC OR AREA EXAMINED | NORMAL | DEVIATIONS FROM NORMAL |
| --- | --- | --- |
| **4.** Screening evaluation of auditory function | | |
| **a.** Whispered voice | Able to hear softly whispered words at distance of 30 to 60 cm (1 to 2 feet) Bilaterally equal response | Unilateral response or bilaterally unequal response Unable to repeat words until whispered voice is louder |
| **b.** Watch tick | Able to hear ticking watch at distance of 2 to 5 cm (1 to 2 inches) | Clients with high-frequency hearing loss unable to hear ticking |
| **c.** Tuning fork | | |
| 1. Rinne test | Air-conduction sound heard twice as long as bone conduction (AC > BC); called a *positive result* | Bone-conduction sound heard as long as or longer than air-conduction sound (*Note:* Air-conduction hearing time will exceed bone-conduction time with sensorineural loss but will be accompanied by unequal lateralization in Weber test.) |
| 2. Weber test | Bilaterally equal sound | If client has conductive loss, sound will lateralize to poorer ear If client has sensorineural loss, sound will lateralize to better ear |
| **5.** Vestibular portion of auditory (CN VIII) (evaluates labyrinth system) | | |
| **a.** Test for nystagmus | Slow movement of eyes in one lateral direction until they reach their limit; steady gaze in that position | Rapid compensatory rhythmic movement in eyes in opposite direction (Fig. 6-16) |
| **b.** Test for falling (Romberg sign): client stands with feet together, eyes closed, arms to side; watch for steadiness of stance; stand close by in case client loses balance | Swaying but able to maintain body and feet positioning | Unable to maintain positioning Need to widen base support Unable to keep from falling |

## Cognitive self-assessment

1. The eardrum divides the:
   - ☐ a. external ear from the inner ear
   - ☐ b. middle ear from the inner ear
   - ☐ c. external ear from the middle ear
2. When looking at the right tympanic membrane, the quadrant farthest away from the examiner is the:
   - ☐ a. anteroinferior
   - ☐ b. posteroinferior
   - ☐ c. anterosuperior
   - ☐ d. posterosuperior
3. One of the most likely spots to find perforations of the eardrum is:
   - ☐ a. along the malleus
   - ☐ b. at the light reflex
   - ☐ c. along the anulus
   - ☐ d. at the pars flaccida

4. When choosing a tuning fork for testing auditory function, pick one with frequencies between:
   - ☐ a.  200 and 500 cps
   - ☐ b.  400 and 800 cps
   - ☐ c.  500 and 1000 cps
   - ☐ d.  1000 and 2000 cps

5. Functions of the middle ear are to:
   - ☐ a.  transmit sounds across the ossicle chain to the inner ear
   - ☐ b.  transmit stimuli to the cochlear branch of the auditory nerve
   - ☐ c.  maintain balance
   - ☐ d.  protect the auditory apparatus from intense vibrations
   - ☐ e.  equalize air pressure
   - ☐ f.  a, c, and e
   - ☐ g.  b, d, and e
   - ☐ h.  a, c, d, and e
   - ☐ i.  a, d, and e
   - ☐ j.  all the above

6. The cochlear branch of the auditory nerve responsible for hearing is:
   - ☐ a.  CN II
   - ☐ b.  CN IV
   - ☐ c.  CN VIII
   - ☐ d.  CN IX
   - ☐ e.  none of the above

7. Which statements are true concerning the Rinne test?
   - ☐ a.  It is a test of bone conduction only.
   - ☐ b.  It is a test of bone conduction and air conduction.
   - ☐ c.  The sound is referred to the better ear because the cochlea or auditory nerve is functioning more effectively.
   - ☐ d.  A normal response would be that if the tuning fork were placed on the mastoid process until it were no longer heard and then placed in front of the auditory meatus, the sound would continue to be heard.
   - ☐ e.  A normal response would be that if the fork were placed in the middle of the forehead, the sound would radiate bilaterally and equally.
   - ☐ f.  a and d
   - ☐ g.  b, c, and d
   - ☐ h.  a, c, and e
   - ☐ i.  b and d
   - ☐ j.  none of the above

8. The structures of the inner ear include:
   - ☐ a.  stapes
   - ☐ b.  anulus
   - ☐ c.  vestibule
   - ☐ d.  organ of Corti
   - ☐ e.  ecderon
   - ☐ f.  a, b, and e
   - ☐ g.  b, c, and e
   - ☐ h.  b and d
   - ☐ i.  c, d, and e
   - ☐ j.  c and d

9. When examining the adult client's ear, the examiner should:
   - ☐ a. instruct the client to sit with head erect
   - ☐ b. instruct the client to sit with head tilted toward the opposite shoulder
   - ☐ c. pull the auricle out
   - ☐ d. pull the auricle out and down
   - ☐ e. pull the auricle out and up
   - ☐ f. a and c
   - ☐ g. a and e
   - ☐ h. a and d
   - ☐ i. b and d
   - ☐ j. b and e

**PEDIATRIC QUESTIONS**

10. The external ear of the child is:
    - ☐ a. normally at a position lower than the corner of the eye, but by the child's first birthday it is at its normal adult position
    - ☐ b. slanted backward at about a 10° angle
    - ☐ c. normally above the position of the corner of the eye, but by the child's first birthday it is at its normal adult position
    - ☐ d. directly vertical to the position of the head
    - ☐ e. normally at the same level as the corner of the eye
    - ☐ f. a and b
    - ☐ g. b and c
    - ☐ h. b and e
    - ☐ i. c and d
    - ☐ j. d and e

11. A child considered at high risk for auditory dysfunction is one who has:
    - ☐ a. had measles
    - ☐ b. had chickenpox
    - ☐ c. had mumps
    - ☐ d. been taking streptomycin
    - ☐ e. been taking kanamycin
    - ☐ f. all but e
    - ☐ g. all but c
    - ☐ h. all but b
    - ☐ i. all but a
    - ☐ j. all the above

Mark each statement "T" or "F."

12. \_\_\_\_ The best time to examine the child's ear is at the beginning of the examination to "get it over with."

13. \_\_\_\_ While looking at the TM, the examiner sees a dull, nonglistening spot. This is most likely a scar.

14. \_\_\_\_ The best method to remove dry, hard wax is with a cerumen spoon.

15. \_\_\_\_ The normal curvature of an infant's ear canal is downward.

16. \_\_\_\_ A child who received audiometry scoring at 1000, 2000, 4000, and 6000 at 60 db has normal hearing.

**GERIATRIC QUESTIONS**

17. Pick the false statement. Presbycusis:
    - ☐ a. is a progressive, bilaterally symmetrical hearing loss
    - ☐ b. can often be relieved with surgical repair
    - ☐ c. often involves auditory loss of high tones initially
    - ☐ d. when advanced may cause speech to sound garbled or distorted
    - ☐ e. can exist to a fairly advanced degree before a client will report it as a symptom

18. Pick the false statement. Tinnitus:
    - ☐ a. might be caused by cerumen impaction
    - ☐ b. can be associated with temporomandibular joint malfunction
    - ☐ c. can be associated with chronic emotional upset
    - ☐ d. is an early symptom of presbycusis
    - ☐ e. might occur with an arthritis client who is taking regular doses of an analgesic

Mark each statement "T" or "F."

19. _____ Speech can eventually become distorted with a client who has a prolonged severe hearing loss.

20. _____ A sudden hearing loss in an elderly client usually indicates mechanical obstruction and subsides quickly (within 3 days).

21. _____ Loss of general physical well-being may affect the client's auditory effectiveness.

22. _____ Earmolds (part of hearing aids) should fit very loosely when inserted into the canal to avoid friction or pressure irritation.

## SUGGESTED READINGS

### General

Bates, B.: A guide to physical examination, ed. 3, Philadelphia, 1983, J.B. Lippincott Co., pp. 60-62, 83-85.

DeGowin, E., and DeGowin, R.: Bedside diagnostic examination, ed. 3, New York, 1976, Macmillan Publishing Co., Inc., pp. 178-193.

DeWeese, D.D., and Saunders, W.H.: Textbook of otolaryngology, ed. 6, St. Louis, 1982, The C.V. Mosby Co.

Malasanos, L., and others: Health assessment, ed. 2, St. Louis, 1981, The C.V. Mosby Co.

Patient assessment: examination of the ear, Programmed instruction, Am. J. Nurs. **75**(3), 1975.

Prior, J.A., Silberstein, J.S., and Stang, J.M.: Physical diagnosis: the history and examination of the patient, ed. 6, St. Louis, 1981, The C.V. Mosby Co.

Sana, J., and Judge, R.D.: Physical appraisal methods in nursing, Boston, 1975, Little, Brown & Co., pp. 121-132.

### Pediatric

Alexander, M., and Brown, M.S.: Pediatric physical diagnosis for nurses, New York, 1974, McGraw-Hill Book Co., pp. 71-85.

Barness, L.: Manual of pediatric physical diagnosis, ed. 5, Chicago, 1981, Year Book Medical Publishers, Inc., pp. 48-109.

Bates, B.: A guide to physical examination, ed. 3, Philadelphia, 1983, J.B. Lippincott Co., pp. 478-481.

Brown, M.S., and Alexander, M.: Physical examination. VII. Examining the ear, Nursing '74 **4**(2):48-51, 1974.

Brown, M.S., and Alexander, M.: Physical examination. VIII. Hearing acuity, Nursing '74 **4**(4):61-65, 1974.

DeAngelis, C.: Basic pediatrics for the primary health care provider, Boston, 1975, Little, Brown & Co., pp. 79-82, 185-190.

### Geriatric

Holder, L.: Hearing aids: handle with care, Nursing '82, **12**:64-67, 1982.

Palmore, E., editor: Normal aging II: reports from the Duke Longitudinal Studies, Durham, N.C., 1974, Duke University Press, pp. 32-41.

Pearson, L.J., and Kotthoff, M.E.: Geriatric clinical protocols, Philadelphia, 1979, J.B. Lippincott Co., pp. 95-191.

Turner, J.S.: Treatment of hearing loss, ear pain, and tinnitis in older patients, Geriatrics **37**(8):107-118, 1982.

ASSESSMENT OF THE

# Eyes and visual system

## VOCABULARY

**accommodation** Process of visual focusing from far to near; accomplished by contraction of the ciliary muscle, which thickens and increases the convexity of the crystalline lens.

**amblyopia** Reduced vision that occurs after deprivation of visual stimulation during visual maturation (birth to 2 years); eye appears normal on examination; also called *suppression amblyopia*.

**ametropia** General term denoting a condition involving a refractive error. EXAMPLES: myopia, hyperopia.

**aphakia** Absence of the crystalline lens of the eye.

**arcus senilis** Gray ring composed of lipids deposited in the peripheral cornea; commonly seen in older adults; also called *arcus cornealis*.

**asthenopia** General eye discomfort or fatigue resulting from use of the eyes.

**astigmatism** Visual distortion resulting from an irregular corneal curvature that prevents light rays from being focused clearly on the retina.

**blepharitis** Inflammation of the eyelid.

**bulbar conjunctiva** Thin, transparent mucous membrane that covers the sclera and adjoins the palpebral conjunctiva, which lines the inner eyelid.

**canthus** Outer or inner angle between the upper and lower eyelids.

**cataract** Opacity of the crystalline lens of the eye.

**chalazion** Small localized swelling of the eyelid caused by obstruction and dilation of a meibomian gland.

**cycloplegia** Paralysis of the ciliary muscle resulting in loss of accommodation and a dilated pupil; usually induced with medication to allow for examination or surgery of the eye.

**diplopia** Double vision; is usually caused by an extraocular muscle malfunction or a muscle innervation disorder.

**dyslexia** Impairment of the ability to read (with no impairment of mental or intellectual function); letters or words may appear reversed, or the reader may have difficulty distinguishing right from left.

**ectropion** Abnormal outward turning of the margin of the eyelid.

**enophthalmos** The abnormal backward placement of the eyeball.

**entropion** Abnormal inward turning of the margin of the eyelid.

**exophthalmos** Abnormal forward placement of the eyeball.

**glaucoma** Eye disease characterized by abnormally increased intraocular pressure caused by obstruction of the outflow of aqueous humor.

**hordeolum (sty)** Infection of a sebaceous gland at the margin of the eyelid.

**hyperopia (farsightedness)** A refractive error in which light rays focus behind the retina.

**miosis** Condition in which the pupil is constricted; usually drug induced (agent is called a *miotic*).

**mydriasis** Dilation of the pupil; usually drug induced (agent is known as a *mydriatic*).

**myopia (nearsightedness)** Refractive error in which light rays focus in front of the retina.

**nicking** Abnormal condition showing compression of a vein at an arteriovenous crossing; viewed through an ophthalmoscope during a retinal examination.

**O.D. (oculus dexter)** Right eye.

**O.S. (oculus sinister)** Left eye.

**O.U. (oculus uterque)** Both eyes.

**palpebral conjunctiva** A thin, transparent mucous membrane that lines the inner eyelid and adjoins the bulbar conjunctiva, which covers the sclera.

**palpebral fissure** The opening between the upper and lower eyelids.

**PERRLA** Stands for "pupils equal, round, react to light, and accommodation."

**photophobia** Ocular discomfort caused by exposure of the eyes to bright light.

**presbyopia** Loss of accommodation (ability to focus on near objects) associated with aging.

**ptosis** Drooping of the upper eyelid; can be unilateral or bilateral; usually results from innervation or lid muscle disorder.

**refraction** Deviation of light rays as they pass from one transparent medium into another of different density.

**scotoma** Defined area of blindness within the visual field; can involve one or both eyes.

**strabismus** Condition in which the eyes are not directed at the same object or point.

## Cognitive objectives

At the end of this chapter the learner will demonstrate knowledge of assessment of the eyes and visual system by the ability to do the following:

1. Identify the purposes for measuring distant and near visual acuity.
2. Appropriately interpret the readings reporting distant visual acuity measurement.
3. State the purposes for testing the corneal light reflex.
4. Identify potential abnormal results when using the confrontation method for testing vision fields.
5. Explain the purpose of the cover-uncover test.
6. Identify the cranial nerves responsible for eyeball movement in the six fields of gaze.
7. Point out the physiological events that occur with direct and consensual pupillary response.
8. Identify the characteristics of normal anatomical structures of the external eye, including:
   a. Eyelids and lashes
   b. Spherical body in position within the socket
   c. Lacrimal apparatus
   d. Conjunctiva
   e. Cornea
   f. Iris and pupil
   g. Anterior chamber
9. Describe the proper and effective techniques for handling the ophthalmoscope.
10. Identify the characteristics of normal anatomical structures of the internal eye, including:
    a. Layers covering the eyeball
    b. Red reflex
    c. Retinal structures
       (1) Disc and physiological cup
       (2) Vessels
       (3) Retina surface
       (4) Macula and fovea centralis
11. Identify selected common variations of pediatric and geriatric clients.
12. Use the terms in the vocabulary section.

## Clinical objectives

At the end of this chapter the learner will perform a systematic assessment of the eyes and visual system, demonstrating the ability to do the following:

1. Obtain a pertinent health history from the client.
2. Demonstrate the correct procedures for testing a client for the following:
   a. Distant-vision acuity
   b. Near-vision acuity
   c. Visual fields (confrontation method)
   d. Extraocular movement control and parallel eye positioning by means of:
      (1) Corneal light reflex
      (2) Six fields of gaze
      (3) Cover-uncover test
   e. Corneal reflex
   f. Direct and consensual pupillary response
3. Demonstrate and describe the results of inspection and palpation of the following:
   a. Eyebrows for hair quality and distribution, skin surface, and bilateral movement
   b. Eyelids and lashes for height and bilateral dimension of palpebral fissures, lash formation and distribution, lid closure, blinking, tenderness, and surface characteristics
   c. Eyeball position in bony socket
   d. Lacrimal apparatus for puncta appearance and response to pressure at inner canthus
   e. Conjunctiva for color, tenderness, discharge, and surface characteristics
   f. Cornea: transparency, surface characteristics
   g. Anterior chamber and iris for transparency, iris color, surface and shape, and clearance between iris and cornea
   h. Pupil for shape and bilateral size
4. Show proper use of the ophthalmoscope.
5. Demonstrate a systematic inspection of the internal eye, including the following:
   a. Red reflex for color and shape
   b. Clear media of eye for transparency

  c. Optic disc for margin, shape, size, color, and physiological cup

  d. Retinal vessels for artery size, color, caliber, and distribution; vein size, color, caliber, and distribution

  e. Retinal surface for color and surface characteristics or alterations

  f. Macula and fovea centralis for color and surface characteristics

6. Summarize results of the assessment with a written description.

## Health history additional to screening history

1. History of eye surgery, injury or trauma? Describe what and when.

2. Currently taking or using any medications for eye problems? If so, describe. (*Note:* Eyedrops or ointments may not be reported as part of list of medications taken in original data base.)

3. Is client subject to work or environmental conditions that could irritate or injure the eyes (e.g., irritating fumes, dust, smoke, flying sparks, or particles in air)? If so, does client wear goggles? If client rides a motorcycle, are goggles worn?

4. Does client engage in any contact sport that creates problems with wearing corrective lenses or increases risk for eye injury?

5. If client wears contact lenses, the following questions should be asked:

  a. When prescribed? By whom?

  b. Any difficulty with pain (mild, acute), burning, excessive tearing, photophobia (mild or severe), feeling of dryness, foreign body sensation, eye infections, swelling of eyelids or eyes (conjunctiva)?

  c. Does client wear soft, hard, or extended-wear lenses?

  d. How often are lenses checked by a physician?

  e. What are client's habits concerning the wearing of lenses?

    (1) Duration (in a given day)?

    (2) Ever sleep with lenses in place?

    (3) Worn every day or just for special occasions?

    (4) Lenses alternated with glasses?

    (5) Removed for special activities (e.g., contact sports, swimming)?

  f. Ask client to describe:

    (1) Insertion/removal procedure

    (2) Cleaning/storage procedure

  g. Following are risk factors for contact lens wearers (or candidates):

    (1) Disorganized life-style (difficulty storing, cleaning, wearing for appropriate periods)

    (2) Swimming, contact sports

    (3) Poor hygiene habits

    (4) Susceptibility to infections (especially eye infections)

    (5) Severe allergy (sneezing, eye watering)

    (6) Limited or reduced manual dexterity

    (7) Limited motivation to endure adjustment to new lenses or to tolerate foreign body in eye

    (8) History of seizures

    (9) Environment or work situation where fumes, smoke, or eye irritants exist

    (10) Traveling (lens care and transport habits need to be considered, especially for soft lenses)

  h. Does client have any special problems with lenses? Keeping surface clean, free of scratches, lenses popping out, etc.?

  i. *Note:* Soft and extended-wear lenses often present a different set of problems from hard lenses. The corneal surface is often more subject to edema resulting from deprivation of tears and oxygen. Symptoms of blurred vision, halos around lights, or slight redness may occur in the absence of pain. Corneal abrasion or breakdown will occur with prolonged or severe edema, and pain will accompany this sign. Palpebral conjunctivitis (of upper eyelid) is also a problem. The wearer may have great difficulty opening his eyes in the morning. Eventually redness, swelling, and discharge will appear. Soft lenses may also absorb fumes or dust and cause corneal irritation.

6. *Note:* If client complains of *sudden onset* of any eye or visual symptoms (e.g., pain, loss of peripheral vision, blind spot, floaters, or any visual change), consider this an emergency for referral.

7. If client complains of blurring:

  a. Does it involve one or both eyes?

  b. Is it constant or transient?

  c. Can it be cleared by blinking several times?

  d. Does client have sensation that something is obstructing vision (e.g., cloudy or foggy interference), or are images out of focus?

  e. Do images appear bent or warped?

  f. Does squinting or frowning help to reduce blur?

  g. Is blurring related to fatigue or eye strain?

8. If client complains of eye strain, ask for a definition in terms of pain (localized in one or both eyes), headache (do symptom analysis), visual changes, association with time of day, use of cor-

rective lenses, and reading or other vision use demands.

9. If client complains of floaters or moving spots:
    a. Is the onset sudden (recent), or is this a chronic problem?
    b. Are there large numbers, just a few, or do they occur singly?
    c. Are they seen in one or both eyes?
10. If client complains of redness, watering, or discharge around eyes:
    a. Is there a history of allergies? Is the problem seasonal, associated with sports activities, swimming?
    b. Does anyone else in family or others in close contact with client have similar problems?
    c. Any environmental factors that could serve as irritants?
11. If client complains of diplopia (double vision):
    a. Is the onset sudden or gradual?
    b. Is it present all the time?
    c. Does it occur with both eyes open? Right eye closed? Left eye closed?
12. If client complains of blind spot or peripheral vision loss:
    a. Is the onset sudden or gradual?
    b. Does blind spot move with eye movement (i.e., does it remain in a constant position in relation to direction of gaze)?
13. Does client have any unusual or different eye symptoms or sensations (e.g., flashes of light, distortion of color such as brownish green or yellowish hues, confusion about differentiating colors, halos around lights)?
14. If client has a vision problem, how does this interfere with activities of daily living (e.g., getting around the house or community, caring for self, family, belongings, ability to read, driving a car, difficulty visualizing steps and curbs, difficulty maintaining job)?

## Clinical guidelines

| THE STUDENT WILL: | TO IDENTIFY: | |
| | NORMAL | DEVIATIONS FROM NORMAL |
| --- | --- | --- |
| **1.** Gather equipment necessary to perform eye and vision assessment: <br> **a.** Snellen chart <br> **b.** Near-vision chart or newsprint for testing near vision (Fig. 7-1) <br> **c.** Cover card (opaque) <br> **d.** Penlight <br> **e.** Cotton wisp <br> **f.** Cotton-tipped applicator <br> **g.** Ophthalmoscope | | |

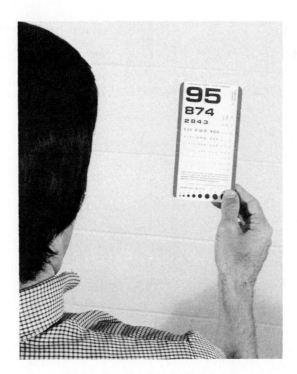

**FIG. 7-1.** Sample of a near-vision chart.

## Clinical guidelines—cont'd

|  | TO IDENTIFY: |  |
| --- | --- | --- |
| **THE STUDENT WILL:** | **NORMAL** | **DEVIATIONS FROM NORMAL** |

### Acuity and function

**1.** Perform measurement of distant vision (CN II)

   **a.** Stabilize Snellen chart on wall in well-lighted room (Fig. 7-2)

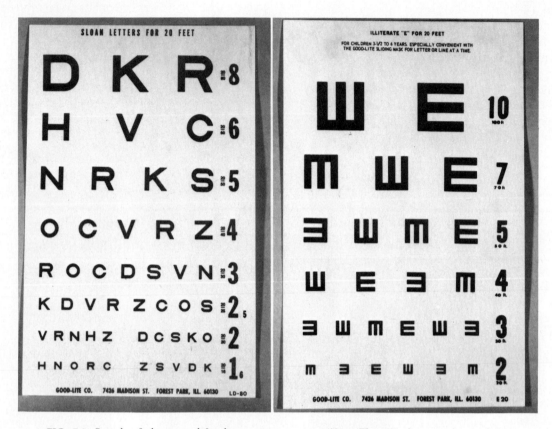

**FIG. 7-2.** Sample of charts used for distant-vision testing. (*Note:* The "E" chart can be used for illiterate clients.)

   **b.** Seat client comfortably 6 m (20 feet) from chart

   **c.** Ask client to cover one eye with cover card

   **d.** Ask client to repeat each letter as you point to it; begin pointing at letters in line where client is most comfortable reading—usually 20/30 or 20/20 line

   **e.** Urge client to read as many of smallest letters as possible, even if unable to complete a particular line

   **f.** Repeat procedure with other eye

| THE STUDENT WILL: | TO IDENTIFY: | |
| --- | --- | --- |
| | NORMAL | DEVIATIONS FROM NORMAL |
| **g.** Clients who wear corrective lenses for far vision should be tested first while wearing glasses and then without* | 20/20 O.D. and 20/20 O.S. | O.D. or O.S.: any letters missed in 20/20 line or above |
| **h.** Observe reading pattern and facial expression during acuity test | Reading pattern smooth, without hesitation<br>Eyes remain open without frowning or squinting | Behaviors indicating reading difficulty: frowning, squinting, "cheating," leaning forward, head tilting, hesitancy or difficulty naming letters |
| **2.** Perform measurement of near vision<br> **a.** Seat client comfortably<br> **b.** Ask client to hold near-vision chart or newsprint 35 cm (14 inches) from face | Near-vision chart:<br> 14/14 O.D.<br> 14/14 O.S.<br> Newsprint is read without hesitancy or attempt to position reading material closer or farther away | Unable to read letters at 35 cm (14 inch) distance<br>Pushes reading material farther away (*Note:* Myopic [nearsighted] individuals may be able to read at a normal distance [14 inches] if they remove their glasses. They will report this as a change in vision. Formerly, they would have been able to read while wearing glasses.) |
| **c.** Ask client to read aloud letters or words in sentence<br> **d.** If client wears corrective lenses for reading, perform test with glasses on | Eyes remain open without excessive blinking or facial distortions | Behaviors indicating difficulty: frowning, squinting, hesitancy, pulling reading material closer |
| **3.** Test for peripheral visual fields<br> **a.** Examiner and client sit directly facing each other at distance of 60 to 90 cm (2 to 3 feet)<br> **b.** Client covers one eye with cover card<br> **c.** Examiner covers own eye directly opposite client's covered eye<br> **d.** Client and examiner stare directly at each other's open eye<br> **e.** Examiner holds pencil or penlight in hand and extends it to farthest periphery (Fig. 7-3) temporally and gradually brings object closer to midline point (equal distance between client and examiner) | | |

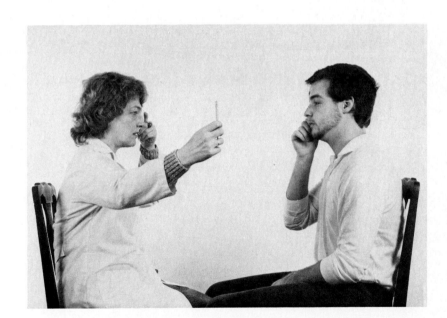

**FIG. 7-3.** Visual field testing; examiner holding object at midline.

---

*Note: Reading glasses should not be used for testing far vision.

## Clinical guidelines—cont'd

| THE STUDENT WILL: | TO IDENTIFY: | |
| --- | --- | --- |
| | NORMAL | DEVIATIONS FROM NORMAL |

| THE STUDENT WILL: | NORMAL | DEVIATIONS FROM NORMAL |
| --- | --- | --- |
| **f.** Ask client to report when object is first seen<br>**g.** Procedure is repeated upward, toward nose, and downward<br>**h.** Ask client to repeat entire procedure with other eye covered; examiner also covers other eye | Client and examiner report seeing object at approximately same time as it approaches from periphery; test assumes examiner has normal peripheral vision, described as:<br>Temporal peripheral—90°<br>Upward—50°<br>Toward nose—60°<br>Downward—70° | Client fails to report sighting object at same time as examiner in any one or in all directions (peripheral visual loss may involve both eyes or one eye)<br>(*Note:* Confrontation method is a crude measurement for peripheral vision loss. A "blind spot" can occur within the central visual field [within 30° of central vision] and not be detected with this method.) |
| **4.** Test for extraocular muscle function<br>  **a.** Assess corneal light reflex<br>    1. Ask client to stare straight ahead with both eyes open<br>    2. Shine penlight, held at midline and directed toward corneas<br>  **b.** Test movement of eyes in six cardinal fields of gaze (CN III, IV, VI) (Fig. 7-4)<br>    1. Client stabilizes head, looking directly ahead at examiner<br>    2. Client is asked to move *eyes only* to follow object in examiner's hand<br>    3. Examiner moves object from center position to upper and outer extreme (hold in position momentarily), back to center, and then to lower and inner extreme (Fig. 7-5)<br>    4. Examiner moves object to temporal-nasal extremes, holding object in extreme positions momentarily (Fig. 7-6) | Light reflections appear symmetrically in both pupils | Light reflections appear at different spots (asymmetrically) in each eye |

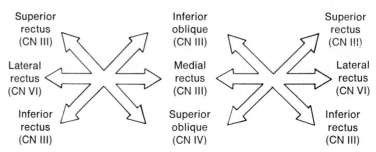

FIG. 7-4. Six cardinal fields of gaze.

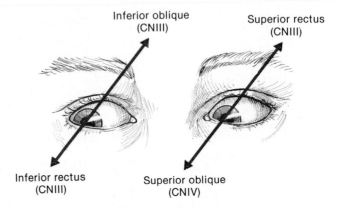

FIG. 7-5. Field testing position no. 1.

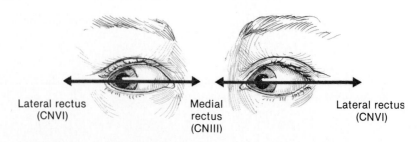

FIG. 7-6. Field testing position no. 2.

| THE STUDENT WILL: | TO IDENTIFY: | |
| --- | --- | --- |
| | NORMAL | DEVIATIONS FROM NORMAL |
| 5. Examiner moves object to opposite upper and outer extreme and back to opposite lower and inner extreme (Fig. 7-7) | Both eyes demonstrate coordinated, parallel movements in all directions<br><br>End-point nystagmus may occur if eye is held in extreme gaze (mild rhythmic twitching with quick movement in direction of gaze with slow drift in other direction) | Eye movements are not coordinated or parallel; one or both eyes fail to follow examiner's hand in any given direction<br><br>Sporadic or nonpurposeful eye movements<br><br>Pathological nystagmus (quick movement always in same direction regardless of direction of gaze) |

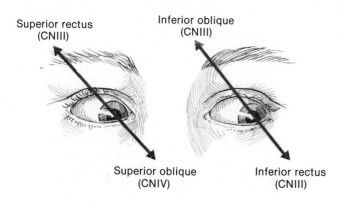

Superior rectus
(CNIII)

Inferior oblique
(CNIII)

Superior oblique
(CNIV)

Inferior rectus
(CNIII)

**FIG. 7-7.** Field testing position no. 3.

| | | |
| --- | --- | --- |
| **c.** Perform cover-uncover test<br>  1. Client is asked to stare straight ahead at fixed point<br>  2. Examiner covers one eye with cover card and observes uncovered eye for movement to focus on designated point | Uncovered eye does not move as examiner places card over other eye | Uncovered eye moves to focus on designated point (Fig. 7-8) |

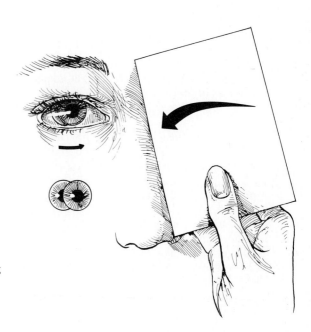

**FIG. 7-8.** Cover test for right eye demonstrating abnormal shift from lateral to central gaze.

# Clinical guidelines—cont'd

| THE STUDENT WILL: | TO IDENTIFY: NORMAL | DEVIATIONS FROM NORMAL |
|---|---|---|
| 3. Examiner removes card from same eye and observes newly uncovered eye for movement to focus | Newly uncovered eye does not move | Newly uncovered eye moves to focus on designated point (Fig. 7-9) |
|    4. Repeat steps 2 and 3 with other eye | | |
| 5. Test corneal reflex (CN V) | | |
|    a. Ask client to keep both eyes open and to look up | | |
|    b. Examiner approaches from side with wisp of cotton | | |
|    c. Examiner lightly touches cornea (not conjunctiva) with cotton | | |

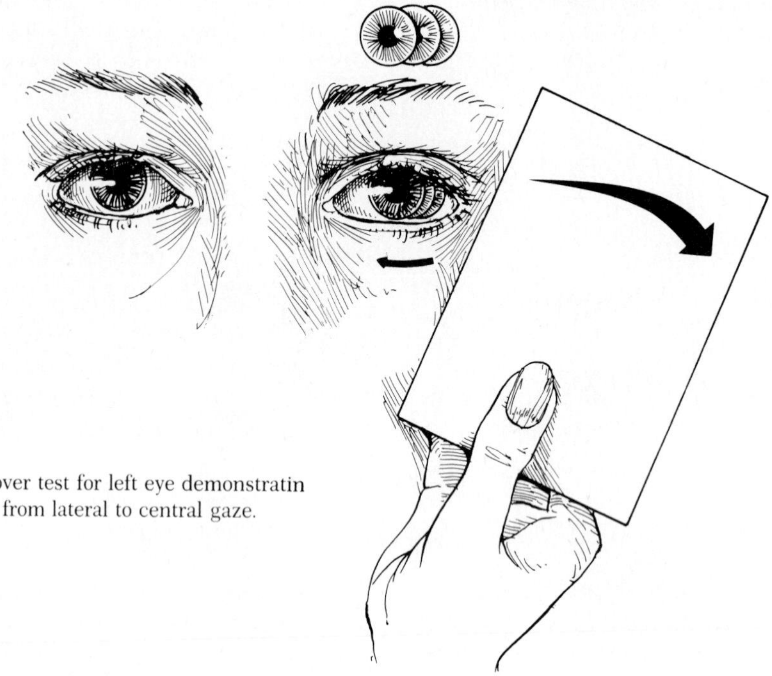

FIG. 7-9. Uncover test for left eye demonstratin abnormal shift from lateral to central gaze.

| THE STUDENT WILL: | NORMAL | DEVIATIONS FROM NORMAL |
|---|---|---|
|    d. Repeat procedure with other eye | Lids of both eyes close when either cornea is touched* | Lids of one or both eyes fail to respond |
| 6. Evaluate pupillary response (CN II, III) | | |
|    a. Evaluate direct and consensual reactions to light | | |
|      1. Room should be partially darkened | | |
|      2. Client holds both eyes open and fixes gaze straight ahead | | |
|      3. Examiner approaches with penlight beam from side and shines light on pupil | Illuminated pupil constricts (direct response) | Unequal (in size or speed) reflex responses or absent response |
|      4. Repeat procedure with other eye | Other eye (pupil) constricts simultaneously (consensual response) Speed of constrictive response (bilateral) may vary among clients | |
|    b. Test for accommodation | | |
|      1. Client fixes gaze at object directly ahead at distant point | | |
|      2. Examiner holds up object about 10 to 12 cm (4 or 5 inches) from client's nose | | |

*Note: Contact lenses will interfere with results.

| THE STUDENT WILL: | TO IDENTIFY: | |
| --- | --- | --- |
| | NORMAL | DEVIATIONS FROM NORMAL |
| 3. Ask client to adjust focus of gaze from distant object to object in front of nose | Pupils converge and constrict as eyes focus on near object<br>Symmetrical response (Fig. 7-10)<br>Client reports object in focus | Pupils fail to constrict or converge<br><br>Asymmetrical response |

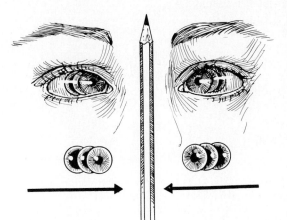

**FIG. 7-10.** Test for accommodation, with convergence of eyes and pupil constriction.

**External ocular structures**

| | | |
| --- | --- | --- |
| 1. Have client seated at eye level | | |
| 2. Inspect eyebrows, noting hair quality and distribution, skin quality, movement | Skin intact, without hair loss<br>Equal alignment and movement | Flakiness, loss of hair, scaling<br>Unequal alignment or movement |
| 3. Inspect eyelids and lashes, noting the following: | | |
|   **a.** Height of palpebral fissures | Bilaterally equal in position | Asymmetrical positioning |
|   **b.** Lid positioning | With eyes opened, lid margins overlie cornea at both superior and inferior borders | Sclera visible between upper lid(s); covers part of pupil |
|   **c.** Lid closure | Complete, with smooth, easy motion | Incomplete, or closure with difficulty or pain |
|   **d.** Blinking | Frequent involuntary, bilateral movements (average 15 to 20 blinks/min) | Rapid blinking<br>  Monocular blinking<br>  Absent or infrequent blinking |
|   **e.** Surface characteristics | Skin intact, without discharge<br>Lid margins flush against eyeball surface<br>Lashes equally distributed and curled slightly outward | Lesions, nodules, redness, flaking, crusting, excessive tearing, discharge<br>Creamy or yellowish plaques (xanthelasma) (Fig. 7-11) |

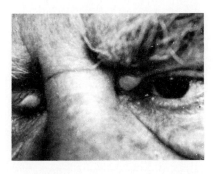

**FIG. 7-11.** Xanthelasma. (From Stewart, W., Danto, J., and Maddin, S.: Dermatology: diagnosis and treatment of cutaneous disorders, ed. 4, St. Louis, 1978, The C.V. Mosby Co.)

## Clinical guidelines—cont'd

| THE STUDENT WILL: | TO IDENTIFY: NORMAL | DEVIATIONS FROM NORMAL |
|---|---|---|
| | | Lid edema |
| | | Lid deformity |
| | | Lower lid pulled away, or drooping, from eyeball (Fig. 7-12) |
| | | Lower lid turned inward (Fig. 7-13) |
| | | Lashes absent |
| | | Lashes turned inward |

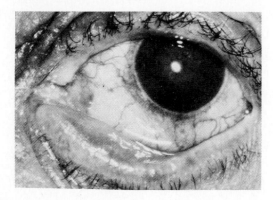

FIG. 7-12. Ectropion: atonic lower lid with excessive tearing and exposed conjunctiva. (From Newell, F.W.: Ophthalmology: principles and concept, ed. 5, St. Louis, 1982, The C.V. Mosby Co.)

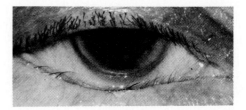

FIG. 7-13. Entropion: lower lid is turned inward (spastic) resulting in irritation of the eye. (From Newell, F.W.: Ophthalmology: principles and concepts, ed. 5, St. Louis, 1982, The C.V. Mosby Co.)

| THE STUDENT WILL: | TO IDENTIFY: NORMAL | DEVIATIONS FROM NORMAL |
|---|---|---|
| 4. Observe position of globe in bony socket | Caucasians: eyeball does not protrude beyond supraorbital ridge of frontal bone | Asymmetrical placement |
| | | Forward placement (exophthalmos) |
| | Negroes: eyeball may protrude slightly beyond supraorbital ridge | Backward placement (enophthalmos) |
| 5. Inspect and palpate lacrimal apparatus (puncta) and eyelids | | |
| a. Examiner presses index finger against lower orbital rim near inner canthus (Fig. 7-14); pressure slightly everts lower lid | Puncta seen on tiny elevations on nasal side of upper and lower lid margins | Puncta red, swollen, with response of tenderness to pressure |
| | Mucosa pink and intact with no response to pressure | Fluid or purulent material discharged from puncta in response to pressure |

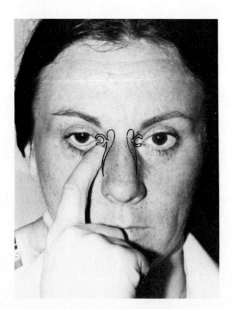

FIG. 7-14. Palpating the lacrimal puncta.

| THE STUDENT WILL: | TO IDENTIFY: | |
| --- | --- | --- |
| | **NORMAL** | **DEVIATIONS FROM NORMAL** |

| THE STUDENT WILL: | NORMAL | DEVIATIONS FROM NORMAL |
| --- | --- | --- |
| **b.** Gently palpate upper and lower lids for tenderness and nodules<br>Exert minimal pressure over eyeball with examining finger* | No tenderness or nodules | Tenderness, nodules, or irregularities |
| **6.** Inspect bulbar conjunctiva and sclera and palpebral conjunctiva<br>**a.** Separate lids widely with thumb and index finger, exerting pressure over bony orbit surrounding eye; ask client to look up, down, and to both sides<br><br>**b.** Pull down and evert lower lid, and ask client to look up<br>**c.** Eversion of upper lid is not ordinarily performed in screening examination; if indicated, the following steps should be performed†: | Bulbar conjunctiva clear; tiny red vessels may be visible<br>Sclera appears white<br>Tiny black dots (pigmentation) may appear near limbus (in dark-skinned individuals)<br>Slight yellowish cast (in dark-skinned individuals)<br>Palpebral conjunctiva pink, intact, without discharge<br>No tenderness or itching | Blood vessels dilated<br>Conjunctiva reddened<br>Lesions or nodules<br>Sclera yellow (jaundice) or significantly bluish<br>Foreign body<br>Tenderness (especially on eye movement)<br>Redness, lesions, nodules, discharge, tenderness, crusting |

1. Explain entire procedure to the client before beginning
2. Ask the client to look down but to keep his eyes slightly open. This relaxes the levator muscle, whereas closing the eyes contracts the orbicularis muscle, preventing lid eversion.
3. Gently grasp the upper eyelashes and pull gently downward. Do not pull the lashes outward or upward; this, too, causes muscle contraction (Fig. 7-15, *A*).
4. Place a cotton-tipped applicator about 1 cm above the lid margin on the upper tarsal border and push gently downward with the applicator while still holding the lashes. This everts the lid (Fig. 7-15, *B*).
5. Hold the lashes of the everted lid against the upper ridge of the bony orbit, just beneath the eyebrow, never pushing against the eyeball (Fig. 7-15, *C*).
6. Examine the lid for swelling, infection, a foreign object, and so on.

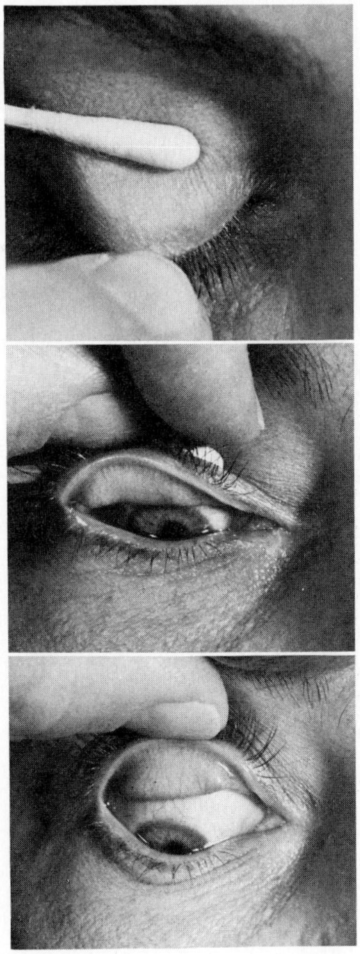

**FIG. 7-15.** Eversion of the upper eyelid. **A,** Lashes pulled gently downward and applicator positioned. **B,** Lid everts over applicator. **C,** Everted lid lashes stabilized against bony ridge. (From Newell, F.W.: Ophthalmology: principles and concepts, ed. 5, St. Louis, 1982, The C.V. Mosby Co.)

*If client complains of scratching or localized tenderness of eye, do not palpate over lid.
†Points 2 through 7 from Malasanos, L.: Health assessment, ed. 2, St. Louis, 1981, The C.V. Mosby Co., p. 234.

## Clinical guidelines—cont'd

| | TO IDENTIFY: | |
|---|---|---|
| **THE STUDENT WILL:** | **NORMAL** | **DEVIATIONS FROM NORMAL** |
| 7. To return the lid to its normal position, move the lashes slightly forward and ask the client to look up and then to blink. The lid returns easily to a normal position. | | |
| 7. Inspect cornea, using oblique lighting; slowly move light reflection over corneal surface and check for: | | |
|   **a.** Transparency | Transparent | Opacities |
|   **b.** Surface characteristics | Smooth<br>Clear, shiny | Irregularities appearing in light reflections on surface<br>Lesions, abrasions<br>Foreign body<br>Arcus senilis: whitish, opaque ring that encircles the limbus: may be abnormal in younger (under age 40) clients; often an insignificant sign with older clients<br>Tissue growth from periphery toward corneal center (pterygium) |
| 8. Inspect anterior chamber using oblique lighting for: | | |
|   **a.** Transparency | Transparent | Cloudiness or any visible material, blood |
|   **b.** Iris surface | Iris flat | Iris bulging toward cornea (crescent-shaped shadow may appear on far side of iris) |
|   **c.** Chamber depth | Adequate (approximately 3.3 mm) clearance between cornea and iris | Chamber appears shallow |
| 9. Inspect iris for: | | |
|   **a.** Shape | Round | Irregular shape |
|   **b.** Color and consistency | Consistent coloration | Inconsistent coloration in one eye or between two eyes |
| 10. Inspect pupil for: | | |
|   **a.** Shape | Round | Other than round |
|   **b.** Bilateral size | Equal in size | Unequal in size |

### Internal eye

| | | |
|---|---|---|
| 1. Use ophthalmoscope (see *Clinical strategies* for technique) to observe: | | |
|   **a.** Red reflex from about 30 cm (1 foot) away, at 0 setting | Bright, round, red-orange glow seen through pupil | Decreased redness or roundness of reflex |
|   **b.** Retinal structures (lens wheel usually remains at 0; it may need to be adjusted to allow for refractive errors: focus on a vessel and adjust lens until borders of image appear sharp and clear) (Fig. 7-16) | | Dark spots or any opacities |

| THE STUDENT WILL: | TO IDENTIFY: | |
|---|---|---|
| | **NORMAL** | **DEVIATIONS FROM NORMAL** |

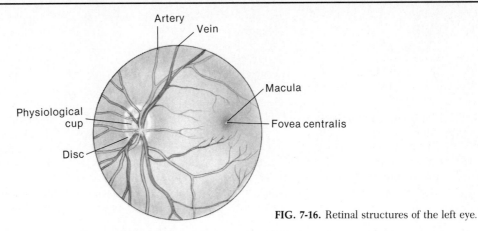

Artery
Vein
Macula
Physiological cup
Fovea centralis
Disc

**FIG. 7-16.** Retinal structures of the left eye.

| | | |
|---|---|---|
| 1. Optic disc margin | Regular, distinct<br>Sharp outline<br>Scattered or dense pigment deposits may be visualized at border<br>Grayish crescent may appear at temporal border | Margin blurred |
|   a. Shape | Round or slightly vertically oval | Irregular |
|   b. Size | Approximately 1.5 mm diameter (appears magnified 15 times to examiner)<br>Marked myoptic refractive errors may make disc appear larger<br>Hyperopic errors may make it appear smaller | Shape and size of discs not equal in both eyes |
|   c. Color | Creamy pink<br>Lighter than retina<br>Tiny vessels may be visible on disc surface | Diffuse pallor or pallor of section of disc, which always extends from center of disc to border<br>Hyperemic disc with engorged, tortuous vessels on surface |
|   d. Physiological cup | Small depression just temporal of center of disc, does *not* extend to disc border<br>Usually appears paler than disc, sometimes grayish<br>Usually occupies four tenths to five tenths of diameter of disc<br>Vessels entering disc may drop abruptly into cup or may appear to fade gradually<br>(Discs are more pronounced in some clients than others) | Cup extends to border of disc<br><br><br>Cup occupies more than five tenths of diameter of disc<br>Cup size or placement not equal in both eyes |
| 2. Retinal vessels: follow from disc to periphery, dividing retina into four quadrants | | |
|   a. Arteries | Usually about 25% narrower than veins (⅔ or ⅘ ratio; size varies with number of branches) | Arteries become narrow (¾ or ⅗ ratio or less) |

## Clinical guidelines—cont'd

| THE STUDENT WILL: | TO IDENTIFY: | |
| --- | --- | --- |
| | NORMAL | DEVIATIONS FROM NORMAL |
|     b. Veins | Narrow band of light may appear at center<br>Light red<br>Larger than arteries<br>No light reflection<br>Darker in color<br>Venous pulsations may be visible | Width of light reflex increases to cover over one third of artery<br>Opaque or pale<br>Veins become larger |
|     c. Distribution and pattern (*Note:* Vessel abnormalities are not evenly distributed; scan all quadrants in orderly fashion for observation.) | Vessel caliber should be regular and uniformly decreasing in size as it branches and moves toward periphery<br>Artery/vein crossings should not alter (or pinch) caliber of underlying vessel | Irregularities of caliber; dilation or constriction<br>Neovascularization (appears as compact patches of tortuous, narrow vessels)<br>Indentations or nicks of vessels at artery/vein crossing |
| 3. Retinal background: scan the four quadrants in orderly fashion | | |
|     a. Color and surface characteristics | Fine granular texture<br>Pink, usually uniform throughout<br>Negroid fundi are often heavily pigmented and uniformly dark<br>Choroidal vessels may be visible through retinal layer (appear as linear, light orange streaks)<br>Movable light reflections may appear on retinal surface (more prominent in young persons) | Pallor of fundus (general or localized)<br>Hemorrhage (may be linear, flame-shaped, round, dark or red, large or small)<br>Microaneurysms (appear as discrete, tiny red dots)<br>Soft or hard exudates (fuzzy or well-defined white patches) |
| 4. Macula and fovea centralis (located 2 DD [disc diameters] temporal to disc) | | |
|     a. Color and surface | Appears slightly darker than remainder of retina<br>Fovea may appear as tiny bright light in center of macula<br>Tiny vessels may appear on surface<br>Fine pigmentation and granular appearance may be visible | Any abnormalities or lesions described for remainder of retinal surface |
| **c.** Observe vitreous body (slowly move lens wheel into the positive numbers, from 0 to 15) | Clear<br>Transparent | Floating particles<br>Cloudiness |
| **d.** Observe cornea, anterior chambers, and lens (+15 to +20 setting) | Clear | Cloudiness or any visible material, blood |

## Clinical strategies

1. When testing with the Snellen chart, remember the following:
   a. Always use an opaque card for covering the client's eyes (in lieu of client's hand).
   b. Client "cheating" may not be deliberate; it may be an unconscious attempt to resolve the frustration of not being able to perform the test.
   c. Be certain that the client can read or identify the letters. An illiterate client may simply indicate an inability to see the letters.
   d. Proceed slowly enough to permit the client sufficient time to follow directions.
   e. Far-vision errors should be recorded in the following manner. If the client misses two letters in the 20/20 line with the left eye: O.S. 20/20−2; if the client reads only one letter correctly in the 20/20 line with the right eye: O.D. 20/25+1.

2. When testing by confrontation for visual fields, hold the object in the *midline* between you and the client. Beginning students often extend the object too far toward the client (this enables the examiner to spot the object first); or they hold the object too far back (Fig. 7-17). This gives the client the advantage in spotting the object.

3. When using the ophthalmoscope, the following procedures are helpful:
   a. Turn the diaphragm dial so that the small, round white light can be used. Turn on light to maximum brightness (old or defective batteries will reduce lighting).
   b. Client should be comfortably seated. Either stand or be seated facing the client.
   c. Client and examiner remove glasses. Removal of client's contact lenses is optional. It might help to reduce light reflection.
   d. The room should be darkened.

---

### SAMPLE RECORDING

Distant vision: 20/20 O.U.; near vision: 14/14 O.U., no glasses.
Visual fields intact (by confrontation).
Parallel corneal light reflex, EOM intact, no nystagmus.
Eyes symmetrical without deviation of gaze with cover test.
Brows, lids, and lashes intact without deformity, ptosis, or lesions.
Conjunctiva/sclera clear; puncta patent; no discharge.
Cornea smooth and clear.
Iris flat, round, PERRLA.
Ophthalmoscopy
  Full bilateral red reflex, discs round, cream color, well-defined margins.
  Vessels—2:3 (A/V ratio); arteries light red with narrow light reflex and even caliber.
  Retina uniform red-orange without exudates or lesions.
  Maculae 2 DD from discs; no lesions.

---

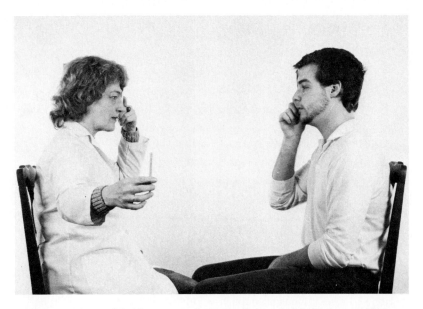

**FIG. 7-17.** Visual field testing; examiner fails to hold object at midline.

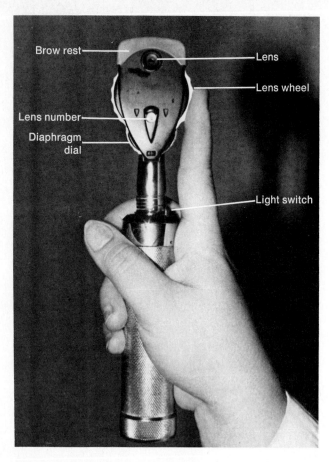

**FIG. 7-18.** Ophthalmoscope. Index finger is on lens wheel.

e.   Ask the client to hold both eyes open and to direct gaze slightly upward and straight ahead. Gaze should be fixed on some distant object and maintained even if the examiner's head gets in the way

f.   For examination of the client's right eye, hold the ophthalmoscope in your right hand, over your right eye. Stand slightly to the right, at about a 15° angle (temporally) from the client.

g.   The ophthalmoscope is held with the index finger on the lens wheel. Rotate the lens wheel to 0 diopter setting (a lens that neither converges nor diverges light rays) (Fig. 7-18).

h.   Place left hand over the client's right eye, with thumb on upper brow.

i.   Hold the ophthalmoscope firmly against your head and approach to within 30 cm (12 inches) of the client (Fig. 7-19). Direct ophthalmoscope light into the pupil. Continue approach, and red reflex will appear. Try to keep both eyes open.

j.   Continue the approach until 3 to 5 cm (1 to 2 inches) from client's eye (Fig. 7-20). Retinal structures should come into view. Clear focus can be established by looking closely at a vessel to see if the borders are sharp. Wheel adjustments need to be made for refractive errors. The myopic client's eyeball may be longer than normal, requiring rotation of the lens wheel into the red (minus) numbers for clarity. The hy-

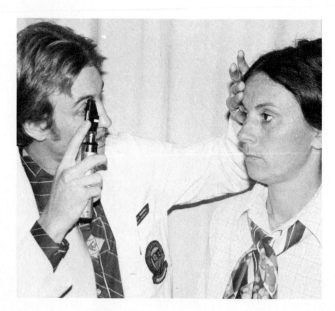

**FIG. 7-19.** Distance: 30.5 cm (12 inches); focus on pupil; red reflex visualized.

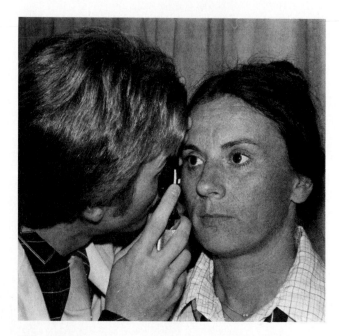

**FIG. 7-20.** Distance: 3 to 5 cm; lens wheel setting moves from +20 to 0; focuses from cornea to retina.

peropic or aphakic client will require lens wheel movement into the black (plus) numbers for clarity.

k. The examiner may not initially focus on the disc. It is helpful to follow vessel bifurcations that lead toward the disc.

l. After inspection of the disc, follow the vessels peripherally in each of four directions. Light must always be shown *through* the pupil as the examiner inspects in different directions. Beginning examiners often lose their view as they begin to scan the fundus. The client's pupil serves as a stable fulcrum while the examiner and ophthalmoscope move *as a unit* in viewing the retinal periphery (Fig. 7-21).

m. Inspect the retinal background and the macula (2 DD temporal to the disc).

n. After retinal inspection is completed, rotate the lens wheel slowly into the black numbers (0, +5, +10, +15, +20). As the numbers become larger, the anterior surfaces (vitreous, lens) come into view (Fig. 7-22).

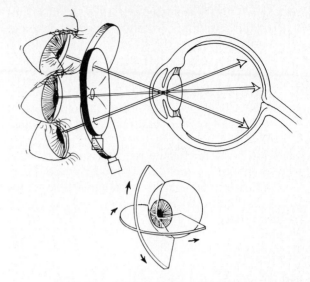

**FIG. 7-21.** Examiner directs ophthalmoscope light through client's pupil onto the retina. Ophthalmoscope must be stabilized against examiner's own eye as he or she moves to view different retinal surfaces. (*Note:* Examiner moves in two dimensions—not just up and down.)

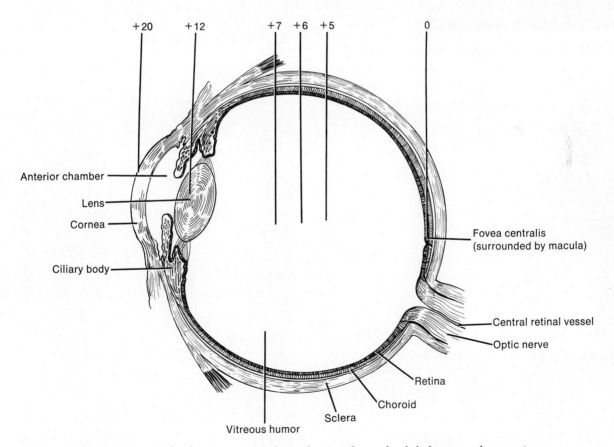

**FIG. 7-22.** Longitudinal cross section of eye showing focused ophthalmoscope lens setting.

o. Slowly rotate the lens wheel up to +20. This should bring the cornea and anterior chamber into focus.

p. Now change to the left eye. Start at client's left, holding the ophthalmoscope with the left hand and over the left eye.

q. *Note:* Clients who talk during the examination often tend to blink and move their eyes more often.

r. *Note:* Absence of the red reflex may indicate an abnormal eye, an improperly positioned ophthalmoscope, or that the client moved his eyes. If the red reflex is lost, back away and start over.

s. *Note:* It is extremely important that you consider your head and the ophthalmoscope as a unit. Be certain that the instrument is stabilized against your brow and cheek.

## History and clinical strategies: the pediatric client

1. When examining a newborn who was vaginally delivered, the practitioner should carefully inquire about vaginal infections the mother may have had before delivery. This is of particular importance if the baby shows conjunctival irritation, pus, redness, or granular development.

2. The practitioner should inquire about the devel-

**TABLE 7-1.** Sequence of visual development

| AGE | CHARACTERISTICS OF DEVELOPMENT |
|---|---|
| Birth | Pupils react to light <br> Moderate photophobia <br> Eyes usually kept closed <br> Blink reflex in response to light stimulus <br> Corneal reflex in response to touch <br> Retinoscopy indicates 1 to 3 diopters of hyperopia <br> Nystagmus may be present <br> Rudimentary fixation on objects with ability to follow to midline <br> Visual acuity approximately 20/300 |
| 2 to 4 weeks | Fixation ability advances; stares at light source <br> Follows to midline more readily <br> Tear glands begin to function |
| 4 to 12 weeks | Infant becoming alert to moving objects but convergence and following are jerky and inexact <br> Fascination for light objects and bright colors <br> Tear glands begin to display response to emotion <br> Binocular fixation established <br> Follows moving object with head and eyes through 180° |
| 12 to 20 weeks | Infant inspects hands <br> One-inch colored cubes stimulate immediate fixation within 60 cm (2 feet) of eyes <br> Accomodative convergence reflexes organizing <br> Able to fixate on objects more than 90 cm (3 feet) distant <br> Foveal pit becomes distinguishable as macula development proceeds <br> Pigmentation of fundus not developed; appearance of fundus pale <br> Visual acuity 20/200 |
| 20 to 28 weeks | Color preference for bright reds and yellows develops <br> Ciliary muscle function begins and accomodation convergence reflexes start to organize <br> Coordination between hand and eye developing <br> True blinking appears <br> Binocular fixation clearly established <br> Ultimate color of iris can now be determined <br> Able to rescue dropped block |

Based on Chinn, P., and Leitch, C.: Child health maintenance: a guide to clinical assessment, ed. 2, St. Louis, 1979, The C.V. Mosby Co., p. 75.

opmental maturation of the child's visual system. Table 7-1 indicates developmental milestones. Numerous studies have shown that mothers are *most commonly* the ones who identify vision problems in their children.

3. There is much controversy regarding novice practitioners using the ophthalmoscope with small children. We encourage the beginning examiner to attempt its use with all children. Although the findings may not equal the effort, repeated practice will increase the examiner's skill so that when there is a child who needs an ophthalmoscopic examination, the likelihood of seeing the internal structures will be increased. Following is a list of

suggested techniques for infants and small children:

a. Babies up to about 18 months should be lying on their backs on the examining table. The overhead examination room lights should be off, but some type of side-room lighting should be on.

b. Hold a penlight or lighted object at arm's length (using left hand) above the baby's head to attract his focus while using the right hand on the ophthalmoscope to perform the internal eye examination. Assistance will be necessary to immobilize baby's head or to hold light.

c. Do not attempt to pry the child's eye open. If

**TABLE 7-1.** Sequence of visual development—cont'd

| AGE | CHARACTERISTICS OF DEVELOPMENT |
|---|---|
| 28 to 44 weeks | About 36 weeks, depth perception begins development<br>Very interested in small objects, can accurately pick up 7 mm pellet<br>Follows in both vertical and horizontal planes<br>Tilts head backward to see upward<br>Visual acuity exceeds 20/200 |
| 44 weeks to 12 months | Central acuity approaches 20/100<br>Readily discriminates simple geometrical forms and gazes intently at facial expressions<br>Transverse diameter of cornea is 12 mm, the adult size<br>Full binocular vision developed<br>Amblyopia may develop with lack of binocularity |
| 12 to 15 months | Keen interest in pictures<br>Can identify forms and associate simple visual experience<br>Associates with visual experiences<br>Able to scribble on paper<br>Convergence becomes well established<br>Depth perception remains crude |
| 18 months to 2 years | Depth perception still immature<br>Accomodation well developed<br>Visual acuity 20/40 |
| 2 to 3 years | Convergence smooth<br>Fixation on small objects or pictures should approach 50 seconds<br>Able to recall visual images<br>Visual acuity 20/30 |
| 3 to 5 years | Acuity appears well established, but amblyopia can occur from disuse<br>Able to copy geometrical figures<br>Reading readiness may be present |
| 5 years | Only small potential for reduction of acuity from disuse (amblyopia development unlikely)<br>Color recognition well established |
| 6 years | Central acuity unconditionally established<br>Physiological hyperopia decreases<br>Visual acuity approaches 20/20<br>Gross attention span lengthened to 20 minutes, and detailed attention will last about 2 minutes<br>Color shading can be differentiated<br>Depth perception fully developed |

this technique is necessary, the child will not cooperate by focusing during the funduscopy examination.

d. Older children are likely to assist in the funduscopy examination if the examiner offers proper instructions and actually involves the child in the examination. This may include:

(1) Letting the child know in advance that the room lights will be turned out but that some small light will be left on

(2) Informing the child during the time the light is out that the examiner will be using a small flashlight to look into the child's eyes

(3) Reassuring him that the procedure will not hurt

(4) Instructing the child to look at a particular picture on the wall, or providing the child with a penlight to shine onto a picture on the wall and then look at the "lighted picture"

(5) Remembering that older children prefer to sit

e. The findings of the ophthalmoscopic examination for a child are very similar to those for an adult. The primary difference is the length of time the examiner has to survey the internal structures. The comparison is several seconds for the adult to split seconds for the child. During this time the examiner should at least attempt to do the following:

(1) Focus on the retina (most likely for children under 6 years old the lens wheel will be between 0 and −5).

(2) Observe disc and note flatness and sharpness of disc edges.

(3) Note color and gross characteristics of the retina.

4. Vision screening begins informally with the newborn examination as the examiner notes the child's following and fixation capabilities. This should continue during each physical assessment period. Although there is some disagreement about the exact age children should receive formalized vision screening, Table 7-2 serves as a guide.

5. Although it is impossible to perform an accurate vision screening on a newborn, the examiner must perform some method of visual screening to rule out gross vision problems. For example, use a penlight at a distance of about 25 cm (10 inches), blink it on and off several times, and then move it around slightly. The infant should indicate recognition of the light and should follow it momentarily. No recognition or following requires further vision evaluation.

6. When using either the Snellen "E" chart or the Snellen alphabet chart with children, it is necessary to have two examiners, one to show the various lines of the chart and to point to the desired item, and the other to assist the child to stand or sit in the correct spot and correctly cover the eye not being tested.

7. The alphabet chart is by far the more accurate, and whenever possible it should be used. Directions for using the Snellen chart have been previously discussed.

8. The mechanics of the "E" chart are generally the

**TABLE 7-2.** Vision screening schedule

| AGE | SCREENING | ANTICIPATED RESULTS | REFERRAL CRITERIA |
|---|---|---|---|
| Newborn | General vision ability | Should follow short distance | No recognition or blink |
| 3 mo | Strabismus screen | May be positive | |
| 6 mo-1 yr | Strabismus screen | Should be negative | Positive screen |
| 3 yr | "E" test | 20/30 to 20/40 | Grossly abnormal results |
| 4 yr | Color vision screening for boys (Ishihara test if possible) | Normal color identification | Abnormal color identification |
| | Visual field-confrontation screening | Sees objects at same time as examiner | Grossly abnormal results |
| 5-8 yr (test each year) | "E" test or Snellen test | 20/30 to 20/40 | 20/40 results after two screening periods Unequal results (e.g., 20/20 O.D., 20/40 O.S.) |
| 9-11 yr (test each year) | Snellen test | 20/20 to 20/30 | >20/30 results after two screening periods Unequal results |

same as with the alphabet chart. The child is instructed to point with his finger and entire arm to the direction which the "legs of the table" are pointing. This evaluates not only the ability to see the letter but also the ability to comprehend the idea of direction.

9. If the child wears glasses, vision screening should be done with glasses both on and off.
10. Problems with strabismus or heterophoria should be carefully evaluated in every child over the age of 6 months. Babies under 6 months may have intermittent eye crossing, which can be normal. Such a finding in any child over the age of 6 months is considered abnormal, and the client should be referred. The two techniques for evaluating the situation in which the child's eyes do not focus to transmit good coordinated binocular vision are the cover test and the corneal light reflex test. Both have been previously described; they should be evaluated at near-point (35 cm [14 inches]) and far-point (6 m [20 feet]) distances. The age and cooperation of the child will determine the success of the evaluation.
11. The importance of color vision screening is disputed among authorities. We believe it can be eas-

ily incorporated into a well-child examination and should therefore be done. Because color blindness is extremely rare among girls, only the boys need to be tested. Before beginning the evaluation, the examiner must first evaluate the child's knowledge and correct recognition of colors. Color testing needs to be done only once.
12. The eyesight of a child is so precious that the examiner should refer any questionable finding to a physician for further evaluation.

## Clinical variations: the pediatric client

The overall success of this evaluation depends on the cooperation of the child. It is desirable to evaluate each component during every well-child visit. If the child is uncooperative, the examiner must decide whether to postpone the component being evaluated until later during the examination or to wait until the child's next visit.

There are five components of the pediatric vision screening examination that are most important, including visual acuity, testing for farsightedness, strabismus screening, color vision screening, and visual field evaluation. These five components are incorporated into the following clinical guidelines.

| CHARACTERISTIC OR AREA EXAMINED | NORMAL | DEVIATIONS FROM NORMAL |
|---|---|---|
| **Acuity and function** | | |
| **1.** Distant vision (CN II) in children over age 3 years | 3 years: 20/20 to 20/40 | |
| | 5 to 8 years: 20/30 to 20/40 | >20/40 results after two screening periods or unequal results in either eye (5 to 8 years) |
| | 9 to 11 years: >20/20 to 20/30 | >20/30 results after two screening periods or unequal results in either eye (9 to 11 years) |
| **2.** Near vision: not routinely used until *older school-age evaluation;* when used, directions are same as for adult | Near-vision chart: 14/14 O.D. 14/14 O.S. | Client unable to read letters at 35 cm (14 inch) distance |
| | Newsprint is read without hesitancy or attempt to pull it closer or push it farther away | Note any other behaviors indicating difficulty (frowning, squinting, hesitancy, pulling reading material closer) |
| | Eyes remain open without excessive blinking or facial distortions | |
| **3.** Peripheral visual fields: should be evaluated from age 3 years on or as soon as child is able to cooperate by maintaining *his position* throughout procedure | Client and examiner report seeing object at approximately same time as it approaches from periphery; this test assumes that the examiner has normal peripheral vision | Client fails to report sighting object at same time as examiner, in any one direction or in all directions (peripheral visual loss may involve both eyes or one eye) |

## Clinical variations: the pediatric client—cont'd

| CHARACTERISTIC OR AREA EXAMINED | NORMAL | DEVIATIONS FROM NORMAL |
|---|---|---|
| | Another affirmative response is noting exact moment child changes head position to gaze toward object, indicating that child did see object coming into view (Examiner must be alert to judge if this is same instance that examiner saw object.)<br>Temporal peripheral vision: 90°<br>Upward: 50°<br>Toward nose: 60°<br>Downward: 70° | |
| **4.** Extraocular muscle function (also a test for strabismus); eye muscle coordination is not fully mature until 1 year; at this time it shows mature adult function | | |
|   **a.** Corneal light reflex<br><br>    Because infants are unable to cooperate, examiner must use penlight to attract infant's attention; while infant focuses on light, examiner must evaluate light reflection position | Light reflections appear symmetrically in pupils<br>If child is under 6 months of age, asymmetry of image may be normal | Light reflections appear at different spots (asymmetrically) in each eye<br>Refer for further evaluation if child is over 6 months |
|   **b.** Movement of eyes in six cardinal fields of gaze: test in children over 2 years of age; examiner may need to stabilize child's chin with hand to prevent entire head movement | Both eyes demonstrate coordinated, parallel movements in all directions<br>End-point nystagmus may occur if eye is held in extreme gaze (mild rhythmic twitching with quick movement in direction of gaze with slow drift in other direction) | Eye movements not coordinated or parallel (Fig. 7-23)<br>One or both eyes fail to follow examiner's hand in any given direction<br>Sporadic or nonpurposeful eye movements<br>Pathological nystagmus (quick movement always in same direction regardless of direction of gaze) |

A 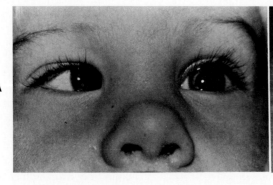 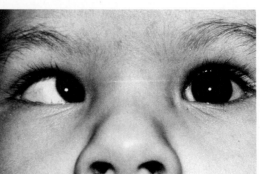 B

**FIG. 7-23.** Abnormal alignment of eyes. (From Helveston, E.M., and Ellis, F.D.: Pediatric ophthalmology practice, St. Louis, 1980, The C.V. Mosby Co.)

| CHARACTERISTIC OR AREA EXAMINED | NORMAL | DEVIATIONS FROM NORMAL |
|---|---|---|
| **c.** Cover-uncover test: performed on all children 3 months and older until school age; test should be done with child looking at object about 35 cm (14 inches) away and then repeated as he viewed object approximately 6 m (20 feet) away | Uncovered eye does not move as examiner places card over other eye<br>Newly uncovered eye does not move | Uncovered eye moves to focus on designated point<br>Newly uncovered eye moves to focus on designated point<br>Refer if child is over 6 months of age |
| **5.** Corneal reflex (CN V): not routinely tested in preschool children; when tested, technique is same as for adult | Lids of both eyes close when either cornea is touched | Lid(s) of one or both eyes fails to respond |
| **6.** Pupillary response: direct and consensual reaction to light | Pupil with light shining on it constricts (direct response)<br>Other eye (pupil) constricts simultaneously (consensual response)<br>Pupils converge and constrict as eyes focus on near object<br>Response symmetrical | Unequal (in size or speed) reflex responses or absent response<br><br>Pupils fail to constrict or converge<br><br>Asymmetrical response |
| **7.** Color vision: use Ishihara test if possible; single line testing for preschool boys | Able to correctly differentiate colors | Unable to correctly differentiate colors |

## External ocular structures

| | | |
|---|---|---|
| **1.** Have client seated at eye level. Note the following: | | |
| **a.** Position and alignment of eyes on face | Outer canthus of eye aligns with pinna of ear | Outer canthus does not align with pinna of ear; may be higher or lower than pinna |
| **b.** Symmetry | See Fig. 7-24 for measurement criteria | Large spacing between eyes (hypertelorism) is frequent sign of mental retardation (*Note:* Even though large spacing may be normal, examiner should refer child to specialist for verification.) |

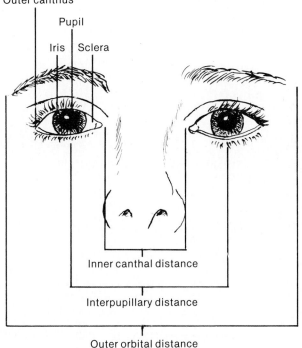

Outer canthus

Pupil

Iris  Sclera

Inner canthal distance

Interpupillary distance

Outer orbital distance

**FIG. 7-24.** Anatomical landmarks for distance measurements.

## Clinical variations: the pediatric client—cont'd

| CHARACTERISTIC OR AREA EXAMINED | NORMAL | DEVIATIONS FROM NORMAL |
|---|---|---|

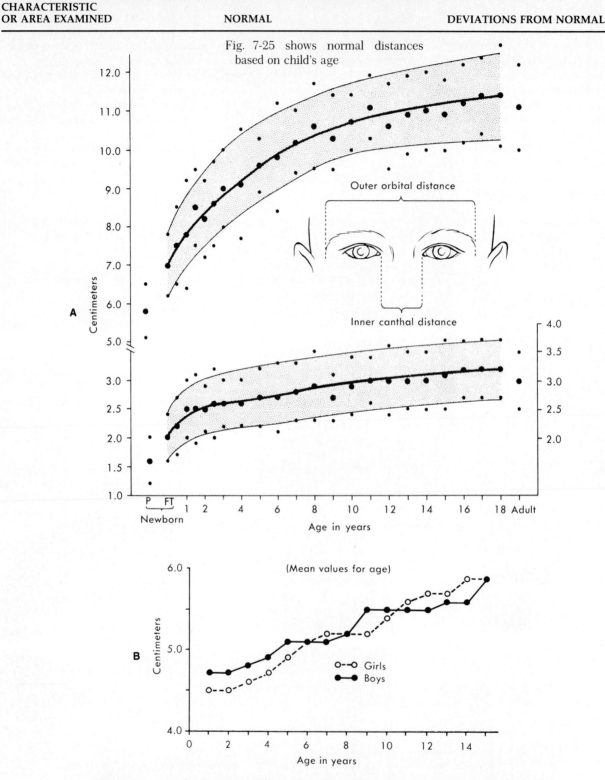

Fig. 7-25 shows normal distances based on child's age

**FIG. 7-25. A,** Graph of inner canthal and outer orbital distances. Large points represent mean value for each age group; smaller points represent two standard deviations from the mean. Heavy line approximates fiftieth percentile, and shaded area roughly encompasses range from third to ninety-seventh percentile. *P* = premature; *FT* = full term. Note that 70% of an adult's inner canthal distance is achieved by 2 years of age. **B,** Graph of interpupillary distance measurements (mean values for age) from 5570 normal white children. (From Laestadius, N.D., Aase, J.M., and Smith, D.W.: J. Pediatr. **74:**465-468, 1969.)

| CHARACTERISTIC OR AREA EXAMINED | NORMAL | DEVIATIONS FROM NORMAL |
|---|---|---|
| **2.** Eyebrows | | |
|    **a.** Hair quality/distribution and skin quality | Skin intact, without hair loss | Flakiness, loss of hair, scaling |
|    **b.** Movement | Equal alignment and movement | Unequal alignment or movement |
| **3.** Eyelids and eyelashes | | |
|    **a.** General slant of palpebral fissures: draw imaginary line through two points of medial canthus and across outer orbit of eyes with each eye on the line (Fig. 7-26) | Horizontal<br>Oriental children may have slightly upward slant | Upward slant in non-Oriental children and children with Down syndrome (Fig. 7-27) |

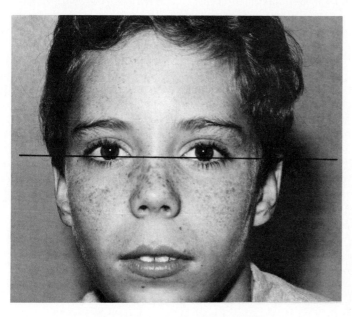

**FIG. 7-26.** Normal alignment of eyes.

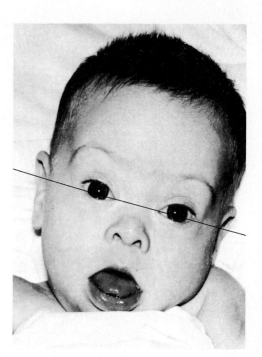

**FIG. 7-27.** Abnormal slanting seen in eyes of child with Down syndrome. (Modified from Reisman, L.E., and Matheny, A.P.: Genetics and counseling in medical practice, St. Louis, 1969, The C.V. Mosby Co.)

## Clinical variations: the pediatric client—cont'd

| CHARACTERISTIC OR AREA EXAMINED | NORMAL | DEVIATIONS FROM NORMAL |
|---|---|---|
| **b.** Lid positioning | With eyes opened, lid margins overlie cornea at both superior and inferior borders | Sclera visible between upper lid(s) and part of iris |
| **c.** Lid closure | Complete with smooth, easy motion | Incomplete, or closure with difficulty or pain |
| **d.** Blinking | Frequent involuntary, bilateral movements (average 15 to 20 blinks/min) | Rapid blinking<br>Monocular blinking<br>Absent or infrequent blinking |
| **e.** Surface characteristics | Skin intact, without discharge<br>Lid margins flush against eyeball surface<br>Lashes equally distributed and curled slightly outward | Lesions, nodules, redness, flaking, crusting, excessive tearing, discharge<br>Creamy or yellowish plaques (xanthelasma)<br>Lid edema, lid deformity (pulled away from eyeball or turned inward)<br>Lashes absent<br>Lashes turned inward |
| | Epicanthal folds (vertical folds of skin covering inner canthus of eye): may be considered normal in Oriental children (Fig. 7-28); should decrease greatly by age 10; position and degree of folds must be evaluated (Fig. 7-29) | Large epicanthal folds in non-Oriental children, or folds that remain past age 10<br>Any sign of ptosis needs referral |

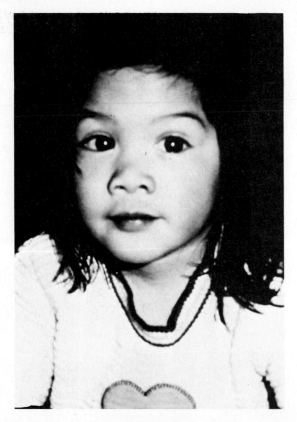

**FIG. 7-28.** Inner epicanthal folds may be normally seen in Oriental children. Note that this may give the appearance of pseudostrabismus. (From Whaley, L.F., and Wong, D.L.: Nursing care of infants and children, ed. 2, St. Louis, 1983, The C.V. Mosby Co.)

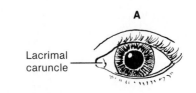
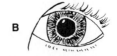

Lacrimal caruncle

**FIG. 7-29.** Position and degree of epicanthal folds. **A,** Normal eye without epicanthal fold. **B,** Partial epicanthal fold of eye. **C,** Epicanthal fold completely covering lacrimal caruncle.

| CHARACTERISTIC OR AREA EXAMINED | NORMAL | DEVIATIONS FROM NORMAL |
| --- | --- | --- |
| **4.** Position of globe in socket | Caucasians: eyeball does not protrude beyond supraorbital ridge of frontal bone<br>Blacks: may protrude slightly beyond supraorbital ridge | Forward displacement (exophthalmos)<br>Backward displacement (enophthalmos)<br>Sunken eyes may need further evaluation for dehydration or malnutrition |
| **5.** Lacrimal apparatus | No tearing during first month | Excessive tearing before third month<br>No tearing by second month |
| **a.** Examiner presses index finger against lower orbital rim near inner canthus; pressure slightly everts lower lid<br>**b.** Gently palpate upper and lower lids for tenderness and nodules; exert minimal pressure over eyeball with examining finger | Puncta seen on tiny elevations on nasal side of upper and lower lid margins<br>Mucosa pink and intact with no response to pressure<br>No tenderness or nodules | Puncta red, swollen, with tenderness on pressure<br>Fluid or purulent material discharged from puncta in response to pressure<br>Tenderness, nodules, or irregularities |
| **6.** Bulbar conjunctiva and sclera | Infant sclera may have blue tinge caused by thinness<br>Bulbar conjunctiva clear; tiny red vessels may be visible<br>Sclera appears white<br>Tiny black dots (pigmentation) may appear near limbus in dark-skinned persons<br>Some pigmented deposits may appear<br>Slight yellowish cast in dark-skinned persons | Darker blue sclera<br>Blood vessels dilated<br>Conjunctiva reddened<br>Lesions or nodules<br>Sclera yellow (jaundice)<br>Foreign body<br>Tenderness (especially on eye movements) |
| **a.** Lower lid eversion: not routinely performed in children unless examiner expects irritation, infection, or foreign body<br>**b.** Upper lid eversion: not ordinarily performed in screening examination unless examiner expects irritation, infection, or foreign body; when performed, techniques are same as for adult | Palpebral conjunctiva pink, intact, without discharge<br>No tenderness or itching | Redness, lesions, nodules, discharge, tenderness, crusting |
| **7.** Cornea (using oblique lighting)<br>**a.** Transparency<br>**b.** Surface characteristics | Transparent<br>Smooth<br>Clear, shiny | Opacities<br>Irregularities appearing in light reflections on surface<br>Lesions, abrasions<br>Foreign body<br>Arcus senilis<br>Tissue growth from periphery toward corneal center (pterygium)<br>Corneal ulcerations |
| **8.** Anterior chamber: child must be old enough to cooperate<br>**a.** Transparency<br>**b.** Iris surface | Transparent<br>Iris flat | Cloudiness or any visible material, blood<br>Iris bulging toward cornea (crescent-shaped shadow may appear on far side of iris) |

## Clinical variations: the pediatric client—cont'd

| CHARACTERISTIC OR AREA EXAMINED | NORMAL | DEVIATIONS FROM NORMAL |
| --- | --- | --- |
| c. Chamber depth | Adequate clearance between cornea and iris | Chamber appears shallow |
| 9. Iris | | |
| a. Shape | Round | Irregular shape |
| b. Color and consistency | Coloration from newborn to 6 months may be blue<br>Generally between 6 and 9 months permanent color is determined<br>By 1 year all children should have permanent iris color | Inconsistency of coloration (in one eye or between two eyes) |
| 10. Pupil | Round | Other than round |
| a. Shape | Equal in size | Unequal in size |
| b. Bilateral size | | |
| **Internal eye** | | |
| (See both adult and pediatric *Clinical strategies* for techniques) | | |
| 1. Red reflex | Bright, round, red-orange glow seen through pupil (even in infants) | Decreased redness or roundness of reflex<br>Dark spots or any opacities |
| 2. Retinal structures (lens wheel at −5 to 0) | | |
| a. Optic disc margin | Regular, distinct<br>Sharp outline scattered or dense pigment deposits may be visualized at border<br>Grayish crescent may appear at temporal border | Margin blurred |
| 1. Shape | Round or slightly vertically oval | Irregular |
| 2. Size | Approximately 1.5 mm diameter (appears magnified 15 times to examiner)<br>Marked myopic refractive errors may make disc appear larger<br>Hyperopic errors may make it appear smaller | Shape and size of discs not equal in both eyes |
| 3. Color | Creamy pink<br>Lighter than retina<br>Tiny vessels may be visible on disc surface | Diffuse pallor or pallor of section of disc, which always extends from center of disc to border<br>Hyperemic disc (with engorged, tortuous vessels on disc surface) |
| 4. Physiological cup | Small depression just temporal of center of disc; does *not* extend to disc border<br>Usually appears paler than disc, sometimes grayish<br>Usually occupies four tenths to five tenths of diameter of disc<br>Vessels entering disc may drop abruptly into cup or may appear to fade gradually<br>Discs are more pronounced in some people than others | Cup extends to border of disc<br><br><br>Cup occupies more than five tenths of diameter of disc<br>Cup size or placement not equal in both eyes |

| CHARACTERISTIC OR AREA EXAMINED | NORMAL | DEVIATIONS FROM NORMAL |
|---|---|---|
| **b.** Retinal vessels: follow from disc to periphery, dividing retina into four quadrants | | |
| 1. Arteries | Usually about 25% narrower than veins (2:3 or 4:5 ratio; size varies with number of branches) | Arteries become narrow (2:4 or 3:5 ratio or less) (hypertension) |
| | Narrow band of light may appear at center | Width of light reflex increases to cover over one third of artery |
| | Light red | Opaque or pale in color |
| 2. Veins | Larger than arteries | Veins become larger |
| | No light reflection | |
| | Darker in color | |
| | Venous pulsations may be visible | |
| 3. Distribution and pattern (*Note:* Vessel abnormalities are not evenly distributed; scan all quadrants in orderly fashion for observation.) | Vessel caliber should be regular and uniformly decreasing in size as it branches and moves toward periphery | Irregularities of caliber; dilation or constriction |
| | | Neovascularization (appears as compact patches of tortuous, narrow vessels) |
| | Artery/vein crossings should not alter (or pinch) caliber of underlying vessel | Indentations or nicks of vessels at artery/vein crossing |
| **c.** Retinal background: scan four quadrants in orderly fashion | | |
| 1. Color and surface characteristics | Pink, usually uniform throughout | Pallor of fundus (general or localized) |
| | Fundi of black clients often are heavily pigmented or uniformly dark | Hemorrhage (may be linear, flame-shaped, rounded, dark or red, large or small) |
| | Choroidal vessels may be visible through retinal layer (appear as linear, light orange streaks) | Microaneurysms (appear as discrete, tiny red dots) |
| | Movable light reflections may appear on retinal surface (more prominent in young persons) | Soft or hard exudates (fuzzy or well-defined white patches) |
| **d.** Macula and fovea centralis: not fully mature until end of first year | | |
| 1. Color and surface | Appears slightly darker than remainder of retina | Any abnormalities or lesions described for remainder of retinal surface |
| | Fovea may appear as tiny bright light in center of macula | |
| | Tiny vessels may appear on surface | |
| | Fine pigmentation and granular appearance may be visible | |
| **3.** Vitreous body (lens wheel from 0 to +15) | Clear | Floating particles |
| | Transparent | Cloudiness |
| **4.** Cornea, anterior chamber, and lens (lens wheel from +15 to +20) | Clear | Cloudiness |
| | | Blood |

## History and clinical strategies: the geriatric client

1. Glaucoma symptoms and information follow:
   a. Open-angle, or chronic simple, glaucoma is the most common type of glaucoma in elderly clients.
   b. Early symptoms are absent or subtle:
      (1) Vague loss of peripheral vision (which client may not notice or just attribute to aging)
      (2) Aching or discomfort around eyes
      (3) Difficulty adjusting to darkness (a common complaint *not* associated with glaucoma, caused by normal pupillary decrease in size)
   c. May be familial (tonometry screening should be performed with other family members)
   d. Usually bilateral
   e. Noncompliancy with treatment prescribed for glaucoma may be a problem because:
      (1) The disease itself is often asymptomatic, and the miotic drops create difficulty in adjusting to darkness.
      (2) Clients may have difficulty administering medication.
   f. Clients with acute closed-angle glaucoma have acute symptoms, and it is regarded as an emergency medical problem. The symptoms are:
      (1) Severe eyeball pain and headache
      (2) Colored halos around lights
      (3) Sudden decrease in visual acuity
      (4) Nausea, vomiting
   g. Clients with closed-angle (or narrow-angle) glaucoma can also have acute intermittent attacks alternating with remissions.
2. Cataract symptoms and information follow:
   a. The extent of client visual loss or blurring may not correlate with the extent of opacity viewed by the examiner.
   b. Opacities may be nuclear (central)—which tend to interfere with central vision—peripheral, or scattered.
   c. Lens opacities increase glare (e.g., lights at night, bright sunlight, highly polished floors).
   d. Cataracts are usually bilateral; however, they can progress at different rates in each eye.
   e. Common symptoms accompanying cataracts are:
      (1) General darkening of images
      (2) Glare
      (3) Sense of dimness
      (4) Image distortion
   f. If the cataracts have been removed and corrective lenses are worn, the client may have good central vision, but images appear closer and larger than they really are. Peripheral vision will be diminished. Safety concerns such as using stairs, learning to turn head to side to view peripheral images, maneuvering in traffic, and adjusting to visual change should be covered.
   g. Corneal contact lenses can be prescribed for individuals who have had cataracts removed. Peripheral vision is more accurate with these lenses. However, adjustment to wearing lenses is difficult (see adult history section for some details).
   h. Intraocular lens implantation is being performed increasingly for clients who have had cataracts removed. The implantation offers more normal central and peripheral vision. Miotic eyedrops are prescribed to ensure that the lens remains in place.
3. The examiner will probably be working with clients who are chronically visually handicapped. Some common problems follow:
   a. Blurred or diminished vision acuity
   b. Decreased ability to perceive depth
   c. Difficulty adjusting to darkness; light, in general, appears dimmer
   d. Increased glare
   e. Diminished peripheral vision
   f. Loss of color perception acuity (lens becomes more yellowish with aging, and objects appear more yellow; difficulty differentiating blue/green hues)
4. The problems just mentioned may be perceived by the client as mild inconveniences or as major problems. The practitioner must take an adequate history to cover safety concerns and successful and satisfactory performance of activities of daily living (see original data base screening, pp. 26, 32, for details). Particular safety and convenience concerns to inquire about follow:
   a. Sufficient lighting available in home (dark hallways, stairways, night light)
   b. Sufficient lighting for close work (reading, sewing, writing)
   c. Safety concerns at night or in the dark (driving, walking on irregular surfaces)
   d. Reduction of glare and excess lighting ("cool" lighting contributes to glare), windows without curtains, highly polished floors
   e. If depth perception is altered, concerns about using stairs, stepping off curbs
   f. If necessary, client access to special materials available for visually handicapped (e.g., large-print books, magazines, and calendars, special dials for telephone)
   g. Resources available for help (e.g., relatives, neighbors, local community agencies)

h. Difficulty with administration of medication
i. Adequacy of *total* sensory input with visually handicapped clients (e.g., is client alone for long periods; able to use television or radio as a means of receiving information?)
5. When interviewing visually handicapped clients, the following behaviors are helpful:
   a. Remember that this individual is probably in a strange environment and is receiving a multitude of sensory stimuli. New sounds, odors, environmental temperatures, and a busy, crowded environment may overload a client whose vision is diminished to the extent that he cannot ac-

commodate. Privacy, a quiet area, and the use of touch to communicate is helpful.
   b. Questions should be worded distinctly and slowly, allowing client sufficient time to respond.
   c. The examiner must explain every activity *before* it happens.
6. Review *Health history* and *Clinical strategies* in the adult section of this chapter for additional information related to eye and visual examination.
7. *Note:* Testing for intraocular pressure with a tonometer has not been covered in this chapter. It is considered a necessary component of regular eye/vision screening for adults over 40 years of age.

## Clinical variations: the geriatric client

| CHARACTERISTIC OR AREA EXAMINED | NORMAL | DEVIATIONS FROM NORMAL |
|---|---|---|
| **Visual acuity and function** | | |
| 1. Distant-vision measurement (CN II) | 20/20 to 20/30 O.D., O.S. (with corrective lenses) | O.D. or O.S.: any letters missed in 20/20 to 20/30 line or above* |
| a. Reading patterns | Smooth, without hesitation. Eyes remain open without frowning or squinting | Behaviors indicating difficulty reading (frowning, squinting, "cheating," leaning forward, head tilting, hesitancy or difficulty naming letters) |
| 2. Near-vision measurement | One author states that average individual over age 60 cannot focus more closely than 3 feet without corrective lenses. With corrective lenses: 14/14 O.D. 14/14 O.S. | Inability to read newsprint or near-vision chart at 35 cm (14 inches) with corrective lenses. Tendency to push reading material farther away. (*Note:* Myopic (nearsighted) individuals may be able to read at normal (14-inch) distance if they *remove* their glasses. They will report this as a change in vision. Formerly, they should have been able to read while wearing glasses. *Older adults* may report sudden improvement in near vision. This may result from cataract formation, which causes lens contraction and increases lens curvature. Such a change should be referred.) |
| a. Reading patterns | Newsprint or chart is read without hesitancy or attempt to pull it closer or push it farther away. Eyes remain open without excessive blinking or facial distortions | Note any other behaviors indicating difficulty (frowning, squinting, hesitancy, pulling reading material closer) |

*Several authors state that distant visual acuity begins to decrease in the sixth decade, and that only about 15% of the individuals over 80 years measure at 20/20. However, for screening purposes any measurement less than 20/20 to 20/30 is considered a problem for referral regardless of client age.

## Clinical variations: the geriatric client—cont'd

| CHARACTERISTIC OR AREA EXAMINED | NORMAL | DEVIATIONS FROM NORMAL |
|---|---|---|
| 3. Peripheral visual fields (confrontation method) | Client and examiner report seeing object at approximately same time as it approaches from periphery; this test assumes that examiner has normal peripheral vision<br>Normal described as:<br>Temporal peripheral vision: 90°<br>Upward: 50°<br>Toward nose: 60°<br>Downward: 70° | Client fails to report sighting object at same time as examiner in any one direction or in all directions (peripheral visual loss may involve both eyes or one eye)<br>(*Note:* Confrontation method is a crude measurement for peripheral visual loss. Central visual losses [e.g., blind spots or scotomas] will not be detected with this method.) |
| 4. Extraocular muscle function<br>a. Corneal light reflex | Light reflection appears symmetrically in the two pupils | Light reflection appears at different spots (asymmetrically) in each eye |
| b. Movement of eyes in six cardinal fields of gaze (CN III, IV, VI) | Both eyes demonstrate coordinated, parallel movements in all directions<br>End-point nystagmus may occur if eye is held in extreme gaze (mild rhythmic twitching with quick movement in direction of gaze with slow drift in other direction) | Eye movements not coordinated or parallel<br>One or both eyes fail to follow examiner's hand in any given direction<br>Sporadic or nonpurposeful eye movements<br>Pathological nystagmus (quick movement always in same direction regardless of direction of gaze)<br>*Note:* Clients with Parkinson disease tend to manifest restriction of conjugate upward gaze |
| c. Cover-uncover test | Uncovered eye does not move as examiner places card over other eye<br>Newly uncovered eye does not move | Uncovered eye moves to focus on designated point<br>Newly uncovered eye moves to focus on designated point |
| 5. Corneal reflex (CN V) | Lids of both eyes close when either cornea is touched | Lid(s) of one or both eyes fails to respond |
| 6. Pupillary response (CN II, III)<br>a. Direct and consensual reaction to light | Constriction response (bilateral) somewhat delayed: pupil with light shining on it constricts (direct response); other pupil constricts simultaneously (consensual response) | Unequal (in size or speed) reflex response or absent response |
| b. Accommodation | Pupil constriction remains intact in response to accommodation<br>Client will probably report that near object is out of focus (near-vision reading test measures client's ability to focus on near objects) | Pupils fail to constrict<br>Asymmetrical response |

### External ocular structures

| | | |
|---|---|---|
| 1. Eyebrows<br>a. Hair quality and distribution, skin quality | Skin intact, without marked or patchy hair loss<br>Moderate thinning of brows (especially at temporal side)<br>Brows in equal alignment | Flaking, scaling, lesions<br>Marked or patchy hair loss<br><br>Unequal alignment |
| b. Movement | Equal (bilateral) | Asymmetrical |
| 2. Eyelids/lashes<br>a. Height of palpebral fissures | Bilaterally equal in position | Asymmetrical positioning |
| b. Lid positioning | Upper lids may droop to greater extent than in young adult (lids overlie cornea at both superior and inferior borders) | Lids droop to extent of interfering with vision<br>Sclera visible between upper and/or lower lid margins and iris |

| CHARACTERISTIC OR AREA EXAMINED | NORMAL | DEVIATIONS FROM NORMAL |
|---|---|---|
| **c.** Lid closure | Complete with smooth, easy motion | Incomplete, or closure with difficulty or pain |
| **d.** Blinking | Frequent involuntary, bilateral movements (average 15 to 20 blinks/min) | Rapid blinking<br>Monocular blinking<br>Absent or infrequent blinking |
| **e.** Surface characteristics | Numerous wrinkles, thin skinfolds<br>Skin intact, without discharge<br>Lower lid margins may droop slightly away from eyeball surface | Flaking, crusting<br>Lesions (basal cell carcinoma most commonly found in this area) (Fig. 7-30) |

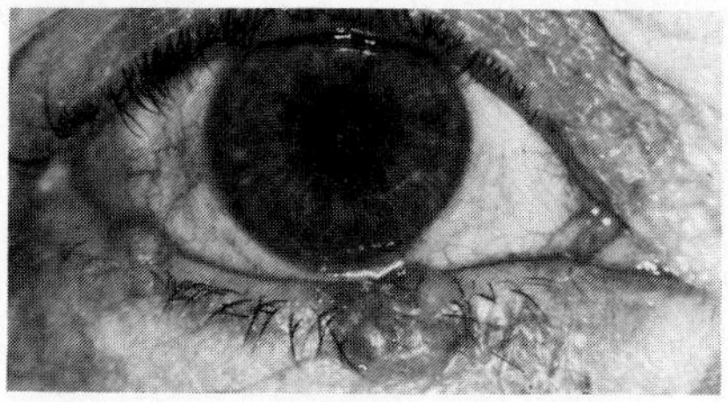

FIG. 7-30. Basal cell carcinoma of the lower lid. (From Newell, F.W.: Ophthalmology: principles and concepts, ed. 5, St. Louis, 1982, The C.V. Mosby Co.)

| | | |
|---|---|---|
| | Lashes curled outward (lashes may be sparse)<br>Creamy yellowish plaques, sometimes raised, may appear (especially near inner canthus) (xanthelasma, Fig. 7-11) | Ectropion, with tearing (Fig. 7-12) (may become infected)<br>Entropion (may become infected), lashes curled inward or absent (Fig. 7-13) |
| **3.** Position of globe in socket | Globe sinks deeper into socket (loss of fat cushion) | Forward displacement (exophthalmos)<br>Marked backward displacement (enophthalmos)<br>Asymmetrical placement |
| **4.** Lacrimal apparatus<br>  **a.** Puncta and eyelids (on palpation) | Puncta seen on tiny elevations on nasal side of upper and lower lid margins<br>Mucosa pink and intact with no response to pressure<br>Occasionally lacrimal gland can be viewed if upper eyelid is raised or everted (loss of circumorbital fat) | Puncta red, swollen with tenderness on pressure<br>Fluid or purulent material discharged from puncta in response to pressure |
|   **b.** Upper and lower lids | No tenderness or nodules | Tenderness, nodules, or irregularities |
| **5.** Bulbar conjunctiva, sclera, palpebral conjunctiva | Bulbar conjunctiva may appear somewhat dry, lacking luster of younger adult<br>Bulbar conjunctiva clear; tiny red vessels may be visible<br>Sclera appears white<br>Tiny black dots (pigmentation) may appear near limbus in dark-complexioned persons<br>Some pigmented deposits may appear<br>Slight yellowish cast in dark-complexioned persons<br>Palpebral conjunctiva pink, intact, without discharge<br>No tenderness or itching | Profuse tearing<br>Blood vessels dilated<br>Conjunctiva reddened<br>Lesions or nodules<br>Sclera yellow (jaundice) or significantly bluish<br>Foreign bodies<br>Tenderness (especially on eye movement)<br>Redness, lesions, nodules, discharge, tenderness, crusting |

## Clinical variations: the geriatric client—cont'd

| CHARACTERISTIC OR AREA EXAMINED | NORMAL | DEVIATIONS FROM NORMAL |
|---|---|---|
| **6.** Cornea (use oblique lighting) | | |
|   **a.** Transparency | Transparent | Opacities |
|   **b.** Surface characteristics | Smooth | Irregularities appearing in light reflections on surface |
| | Clear, shiny | |
| | Arcus senilis (deposit of white-yellow material around periphery of cornea; may be slightly elevated) (Fig. 7-31) | Lesions, abrasions, foreign body |
| | | Tissue growth from periphery toward corneal center (pterygium) |

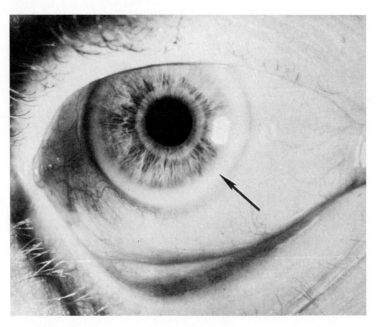

**FIG. 7-31.** Arcus senilis. (From Steinberg, F.U., editor: Care of the geriatric patient, ed. 6, St. Louis, 1983, The C.V. Mosby Co.)

| | | |
|---|---|---|
| **7.** Anterior chamber (use oblique lighting) | | |
|   **a.** Transparency | Transparent | Cloudiness or any visible material, blood |
|   **b.** Iris surface | Iris flat | Iris bulging toward cornea (crescent-shaped shadow may appear on far side of iris) |
|   **c.** Chamber depth | Chamber becomes shallower with aging; however, clearance between cornea and iris is maintained | Marked shallowness |
| **8.** Iris | | |
|   **a.** Shape | Round (wedge or portion of iris may be absent in clients who have had cataract removal) | Irregular |
|   **b.** Color and consistency | May be some irregularity of density of pigmentation (bilateral) | Inconsistency of coloration between eyes |
| | Normal pigment replaced by pale brownish coloration | |
| **9.** Pupil | | |
|   **a.** Shape and size | Round (shape may appear somewhat irregular or square with intraocular lens implant following cataract surgery) | Irregular shape |

| CHARACTERISTIC OR AREA EXAMINED | NORMAL | DEVIATIONS FROM NORMAL |
|---|---|---|
| | Aged pupils often smaller in size (sometimes markedly so) | |
| | Elderly client receiving topical miotic agents (for glaucoma) will have constricted pupils | |
| **b.** Bilateral size | Equal | Unequal |
| **Internal eye** | | |
| **1.** Red reflex | Bright, round, red-orange flow seen through pupil | Opacities or decreased redness or roundness of reflex |
| | Increasing opacities of lens viewed as part of normal aging; examiner may commonly see various patterns of dark spots or clouds (either central, peripheral, or scattered) in aged client's reflex | |
| | For screening purposes all opacities should be viewed as problem for referral | |
| **2.** Cornea, anterior chamber, lens | Clear | Cloudy or any visible materials, blood |
| **3.** Vitreous body | Clear | Cloudy |
| | Transparent | Floating particles |
| **4.** Retinal structures | | |
| **a.** Optic disc margin | Regular, distinct | Margin blurred |
| | Sharp outline scattered or dense pigment deposits may be visualized at border | |
| | Grayish crescent may appear at temporal border | |
| 1. Shape | Round or slightly vertically oval | Irregular |
| 2. Size | Approximately 1.5 mm diameter (appears magnified 15 times to examiner) | Shape and size of discs not equal in both eyes |
| | Marked myopic refractive errors may make disc appear larger | |
| | After cataract extraction, disc appears very small | |
| | Hyperopic errors may make it appear smaller | |
| 3. Color | Creamy pink | Diffuse pallor or pallor of section of disc, which always extends from center of disc to border |
| | Lighter than retina | |
| | Tiny vessels may be visible on disc surface | Hyperemic disc (with engorged, tortuous vessels on disc surface) |
| 4. Physiological cup | Small depression just temporal of center of disc; does *not* extend to disc border | Cup extends to border of disc |
| | Usually appears paler than disc, sometimes grayish | |
| | Usually occupies four tenths to five tenths of diameter of disc | Cup occupies more than five tenths of diameter of disc |
| | Vessels entering disc may drop abruptly into cup or may appear to fade gradually | Cup size or placement not equal in both eyes |
| | Discs are more pronounced in some clients than others | |

## Clinical variations: the geriatric client—cont'd

| CHARACTERISTIC OR AREA EXAMINED | NORMAL | DEVIATIONS FROM NORMAL |
|---|---|---|
| **b.** Retinal vessels | | |
| 1. Arteries | Arteriolar reflex is slightly widened | Arteries become narrow (2:4 or 3:5 ratio or less) (hypertension) |
| | Arteriolar column may appear slightly narrower, straighter with slight irregularities in caliber (Fig. 7-32) | Width of light reflex increases to cover over one third of artery |
| | Arteries may appear more opaque, grayish | Opaque or pale in color |
| | Adult arteries usually about 25% narrower than veins (2:3 or 4:5 ratio; size varies with number of branches) | |
| | Narrow band of light may appear at center | |
| | Light red | |

FIG. 7-32. Retinal changes in the aging eye. Arteriolar columns are narrower, straighter with slight irregularities in caliber. Retina may appear paler and more transparent (showing choroidal vessels).

| CHARACTERISTIC OR AREA EXAMINED | NORMAL | DEVIATIONS FROM NORMAL |
|---|---|---|
| 2. Veins | Larger than arteries | Veins become engorged |
| | No light reflection | |
| | Darker in color | |
| 3. Distribution and pattern | Vessel caliber should be regular and uniformly decreasing in size as it branches and moves toward periphery | Irregularities of caliber; dilation or constriction |
| | | Neovascularization (appears as compact patches of tortuous, narrow vessels) |
| | Artery/vein crossings should not alter (or pinch) caliber of underlying vessel | Indentations or nicks of vessels at artery/vein crossing |
| **c.** Retinal background | | |
| 1. Color and surface characteristics | Fine granular surface | Pallor of fundus (general or localized) |
| | Pink, usually uniform throughout | White choroid and vessels clearly visible through thinned or absent retina |
| | Negroid fundi are often heavily pigmented and uniformly dark | Hemorrhage (may be linear, flame-shaped, rounded, dark or red, large or small) |
| | Choroidal vessels may be visible through retinal layer (appear as linear, light orange streaks) | Microaneurysms (appear as discrete, tiny red dots) |
| | Movable light reflections may appear on retinal surface (more prominent in young clients) | Drusen commonly seen (usually located symmetrically in both eyes) |
| | | Any fuzzy or well-defined white or yellow patches |
| **d.** Macula and fovea centralis | Appears slightly darker than rest of retina (slight dispersion of granular pigment) | Macular degeneration manifests small areas or clumps of black pigment in and around macula (degree of pigmentation does not always correlate with visual loss symptoms) |
| | Foveal (light) reflex may be less bright than in young adult | May be hemorrhage visible in area |
| | Tiny vessels may appear on surface | |

     ☐ h.  a, b, and d
     ☐ i.   all except b
     ☐ j.   all except c

11. The eyeball is a sphere suspended within a bony orbit by means of:
     ☐ a.  muscles
     ☐ b.  ligaments
     ☐ c.  fat cushion
     ☐ d.  scleral tissue
     ☐ e.  nasolacrimal ducts
     ☐ f.  all the above
     ☐ g.  a, b, and c
     ☐ h.  a, c, and d
     ☐ i.   b and e

12. When examining the lacriminal apparatus, only one portion is actually observed; this is the:
     ☐ a.  lacrimal gland
     ☐ b.  puncta
     ☐ c.  lacrimal sac
     ☐ d.  nasolacrimal duct

13. The conjunctiva:
     ☐ a.  is the transparent lining of the eyelids
     ☐ b.  is the transparent covering of the anterior portion of the eyeball
     ☐ c.  is the white, porcelain-like covering of the eyeball
     ☐ d.  normally contains a few visible vessels
     ☐ e.  surfaces are kept moist and clean by a film of tears
     ☐ f.  a and e
     ☐ g.  c and d
     ☐ h.  a, b, and e
     ☐ i.   all except b
     ☐ j.   all except c

14. The cornea:
     ☐ a.  is normally transparent
     ☐ b.  may normally show a somewhat irregular surface
     ☐ c.  covers the pupil and meets the conjunctival layer at the pupillary border
     ☐ d.  surface, when touched, transmits the sensation through CN V (trigeminal nerve)
     ☐ e.  abrasions can often be detected through oblique light reflections on its surface
     ☐ f.  all the above
     ☐ g.  a, b, and e
     ☐ h.  c and e
     ☐ i.   a, d, and e
     ☐ j.   all except b

15. You are holding the ophthalmoscope 4 cm from the client's eye. You want to examine the anterior chamber of the lens. You should set the lens wheel at _____ for the best focus.
     ☐ a.  −3
     ☐ b.  0
     ☐ c.  −10 to −15
     ☐ d.  +5 to +2
     ☐ e.  +15 to +20

16. When using the ophthalmoscope:
    - ☐ a. approach the client about 15° temporally
    - ☐ b. move the ophthalmoscope forward and backward in front of your eye until the red reflex comes into focus
    - ☐ c. stabilize the client's head with your free hand
    - ☐ d. ask the client to look at the ophthalmoscope light
    - ☐ e. keep the client talking to distract him from the examination
    - ☐ f. all the above
    - ☐ g. b, c, and d
    - ☐ h. a and c
    - ☐ i. a, d, and e
    - ☐ j. all except d

17. Three layers of tissue cover the eyeball. Which of the following statements are true?
    - ☐ a. The sclera is the external layer.
    - ☐ b. The choroid layer is vascular, and these vessels can sometimes be viewed through the retina.
    - ☐ c. The choroid contains many nerve cells that react to light.
    - ☐ d. The iris, part of the middle layer, is muscular in function.
    - ☐ e. The retina, the innermost layer, is visible to the examiner when using the ophthalmoscope.
    - ☐ f. all the above
    - ☐ g. b, c, and e
    - ☐ h. a and d
    - ☐ i. all except c
    - ☐ j. all except b

18. Absence or diminishment of the red reflex may be an indication of:
    - ☐ a. xanthelasma
    - ☐ b. opacity
    - ☐ c. CN III malfunction
    - ☐ d. glaucoma
    - ☐ e. hypertension

19. The normal color of the optic disc is:
    - ☐ a. creamy pink
    - ☐ b. pinkish red
    - ☐ c. pale gray
    - ☐ d. bluish gray

20. The physiological depression (cup) within the disc:
    - ☐ a. is just temporal of the center of the disc
    - ☐ b. may normally extend to the disc border with hyperopic clients
    - ☐ c. normally appears paler than the disc
    - ☐ d. usually occupies approximately half the diameter of the disc
    - ☐ e. may normally be more pronounced in one eye
    - ☐ f. all the above
    - ☐ g. a and d
    - ☐ h. b and e
    - ☐ i. all except e
    - ☐ j. a, c, and d

21. Normal retinal arteries visible to the examiner are:
    - ☐ a. about 25% narrower than the veins
    - ☐ b. darker in color than the veins
    - ☐ c. opaque in appearance
    - ☐ d. about 50% narrower than the veins
    - ☐ e. none of the above

22. Normal retinal veins visible to the examiner:
    - ☐ a. are about 25% narrower than the arteries
    - ☐ b. are lighter in color than the arteries
    - ☐ c. often manifest a band of light at the center of the vessel
    - ☐ d. are over twice as wide as the arteries
    - ☐ e. none of the above
23. The normal retinal surface visible to the examiner:
    - ☐ a. may show a fine granular texture
    - ☐ b. may show marked dark-pigmented spots
    - ☐ c. may show light orange streaks (choroidal vessels)
    - ☐ d. a and b
    - ☐ e. a and c
24. The macula:
    - ☐ a. is about 1 DD in size
    - ☐ b. is nourished by the choroid layer vessels
    - ☐ c. is 2 DD toward the nose
    - ☐ d. a and b
    - ☐ e. a and c

**PEDIATRIC QUESTIONS**

25. Which of the following findings alone indicate referral of the child for further physician evaluation?
    - ☐ a. Four-month-old child whose eyes periodically cross
    - ☐ b. Four-year-old child whose visual acuity was 20/40 both eyes
    - ☐ c. Six-year-old child whose visual acuity was 20/30 O.D., 20/40 O.S.
    - ☐ d. Ten-month-old child who demonstrates right eye drifting with cover test
    - ☐ e. Five-year-old boy who excessively blinks but shows no signs of corneal irritation or infection
    - ☐ f. all except b
    - ☐ g. b and c
    - ☐ h. a, d, and e
    - ☐ i. c and d
    - ☐ j. none of the above
26. All the following are true but one. Identify the *false* statement.
    When performing vision screening on kindergarten children using the Snellen "E" chart, the examiner should:
    - ☐ a. test each eye separately
    - ☐ b. test both eyes together
    - ☐ c. evaluate only those children who have never been tested before
    - ☐ d. place the child 20 feet from the chart
    - ☐ e. retest any child who scores over 20/40
27. If you were to develop a vision screening program for 4-year-olds, which of the following techniques would you include?
    - ☐ a. Peripheral visual field testing
    - ☐ b. Cover test
    - ☐ c. Near-vision screening
    - ☐ d. Snellen visual acuity testing using either alphabet or "E" chart
    - ☐ e. Color vision screening using Ishihara test; test boys only
    - ☐ f. all the above
    - ☐ g. a, c, and d
    - ☐ h. b, d, and e
    - ☐ i. all except c
    - ☐ j. all except e

**GERIATRIC QUESTIONS**

28. Cataracts
    - ☐ a. are inherited
    - ☐ b. are chiefly associated with diabetic clients
    - ☐ c. do not create any visual problems until they become "ripe"
    - ☐ d. all the above
    - ☐ e. none of the above

29. Glaucoma:
    - ☐ a. is readily recognized in elderly clients because of the associated acute symptoms
    - ☐ b. can be diagnosed in its early stages by careful examination of the optic disc
    - ☐ c. is usually bilateral
    - ☐ d. all the above
    - ☐ e. none of the above

30. Presbyopia:
    - ☐ a. is synonymous with hyperopia
    - ☐ b. affects most individuals over 60 years of age
    - ☐ c. does not occur if the individual is myopic
    - ☐ d. is rare
    - ☐ e. none of the above

31. If an elderly client complains of difficulty adjusting to darkness, this might mean:
    - ☐ a. that his pupil is smaller and admits less light to the retina
    - ☐ b. advanced macular degeneration
    - ☐ c. optic atrophy
    - ☐ d. retinal detachment

## SUGGESTED READINGS

### General

Bates, B.: A guide to physical examination, ed. 3, Philadelphia, 1983, J.B. Lippincott Co., pp. 55-59, 70-82, 96-111.

Binder, P.S.: The physiologic effects of extended wear soft contact lenses, Ophthalmology 87(8):745-749, 1980.

Boyd-Monk, H.: Taking a closer look at contact lenses, Nursing '78 8(10):38-43, 1978.

Houde, W.L., and Rubin, M.L.: Extended-wear lenses: an update, Surv. Ophthalmol. 26(2):103-105, 1981.

Judge, R.D., and Zuidema, G., editors: Methods of clinical examination: a physiologic approach, Boston, 1974, Little, Brown & Co., pp. 61-80.

Malasanos, L., and others: Health assessment, ed. 2, St. Louis, 1981, The C.V. Mosby Co., pp. 223-245.

Melamed, M.: Complications of contact lenses, Emergency Medicine, pp. 218-224, Feb. 28, 1982.

Nordmark, M.T., and Rohweder, A.W.: Scientific foundations of nursing, ed. 3, Philadelphia, 1975, J.B. Lippincott Co., pp. 261-264.

Patient assessment: examination of the eye, Part I, Programmed instruction, Am. J. Nurs. 74(11), 1974.

Patient assessment: examination of the eye, Part II, Programmed instruction, Am. J. Nurs. 75(1), 1975.

Prior, J.A., Silberstein, J.S., and Stang, J.M.: Physical diagnosis: the history and examination of the patient, ed. 6, St. Louis, 1981, The C.V. Mosby Co., pp. 99-148.

Sana, J., and Judge, R.C., editors: Physical appraisal methods in nursing, Boston, 1975, Little, Brown & Co., pp. 105-120.

### Pediatric

Alexander, M., and Brown, M.S.: Pediatric history taking and physical diagnosis for nurses, ed. 2, New York, 1979, McGraw-Hill Book Co., pp. 85-113.

Alexander, M., and Brown, M.S.: Physical examination. V. Examining the eye, Nursing '73 3(12):41-46, 1973.

Barness, L.: Manual of pediatric physical diagnosis, ed. 5, Chicago, 1972, Year Book Medical Publishers, Inc., pp. 48-92.

Chinn, P., and Leitch, C.: Child health maintenance: a guide to clinical assessment, ed. 2, St. Louis, 1979, The C.V. Mosby Co.

DeAngelis, C.: Basic pediatrics for the primary health care provider, Boston, 1975, Little, Brown & Co., pp. 44-45, 82-84, 191-196.

Helveston, E.M., and Ellis, F.D.: Pediatric ophthalmology practice, St. Louis, 1980, The C.V. Mosby Co.

Laestadius, N., Aase, J., and Smith, D.: Normal inner canthal and outer orbital dimensions, J. Pediatr. 74:465-468, 1969.

Powell, M.L.: Assessment and management of developmental changes and problems in children, ed. 2, St. Louis, 1981, The C.V. Mosby Co., pp. 37-40.

Whaley, L.F., and Wong, D.L.: Nursing care of infants and children, ed. 2, St. Louis, 1983, The C.V. Mosby Co., pp. 125-132.

### Geriatric

Burnside, I.M., editor: Nursing and the aged, ed. 2, New York, 1981, McGraw-Hill Book Co., pp. 498-500.

Caird, F.I., and Judge, T.G.: Assessment of the elderly patient, London, 1977, Pitman Medical Publishing Co., Ltd., pp. 56-59.

Carotenuto, R., and Bullock, J.: Physical assessment of the gerontologic client, Philadelphia, 1980, F.A. Davis Co., pp. 45-51.

Jones, D., Dunbar, C.F., and Jirovec, M.M.: Medical-surgical nursing: a conceptual approach, New York, 1978, McGraw-Hill Book Co., pp. 1257-1274.

Marmor, M.: The eye and vision in the elderly, Geriatrics 32(8):63-67, 1977.

Steinberg, F.U., editor: Care of the geriatric patient, ed. 6, St. Louis, 1983, The C.V. Mosby Co., pp. 450-461.

ASSESSMENT OF THE

# Thorax and lungs

## VOCABULARY

**adventitious sounds** Sounds that are not normal within the lungs.

**angle of Louis** Point of tracheal bifurcation.

**asthma** Paroxysmal dyspnea that is accompanied by wheezing and caused by spasm of the bronchial tubes or by swelling of their mucous membranes.

**Biot breathing** Breathing characterized by several short breaths followed by long, irregular periods of apnea.

**bradypnea** Breathing that is abnormally slow.

**bronchitis** Inflammation of the bronchi.

**bronchophony** Increased vocal resonance detected over a bronchus that is surrounded by consolidated lung tissue.

**bronchovesicular breathing** This refers to breath sounds at a pitch intermediate between bronchial or tracheal sounds and alveolar sounds.

**consolidation** Increasing density of lung tissue caused by pathological engorgement.

**costal angle** Costal margin angle formed on the anterior chest wall at the base of the xiphoid process, where the ribs separate.

**cyanosis** Bluish-gray discoloration of the skin resulting from the presence of, or abnormal amounts of, reduced hemoglobin in the blood.

**diaphragmatic excursion** The extent of movement of the lungs.

**dyspnea** Breathing that is labored or difficult

**egophony** Bleating nasal sound heard during auscultation of the chest when the client speaks in a normal tone.

**emphysema** A chronic pulmonary disease characterized by overdistended lung tissue.

**friction rub** Sound produced by the rubbing of the pleura of the lung.

**hemoptysis** The expectoration of blood from the lungs or bronchial tubes.

**hyperpnea** Respiration that is deeper and more rapid than that usually experienced during normal activity.

**hyperresonance** Sound elicited by percussion; its pitch lies between that of resonance and tympany.

**Kussmaul respiration** Deep, gasping type of respiration, often associated with diabetic acidosis.

**kyphosis** Exaggeration or angulation of the normal posterior curve of the spine.

**manubrium of sternum** Upper segment of the sternum that articulates with the clavicle and the first pair of costal cartilages.

**orthopnea** Difficulty in breathing in any position other than an upright one.

**pectus carinatum** Abnormal prominence of the sternum.

**pectus excavatum** Abnormal depression of the sternum.

**pleximeter** Finger placed on the skin surface to receive the blow from the percussion hammer or plexor.

**rale** Abnormal wet or dry respiratory sound heard during auscultation of the chest.

**rhonchus** Coarse, dry rale heard in the bronchial tubes.

**scoliosis** Lateral curvature of the spine.

**singultus** Hiccup.

**stridor** Shrill, harsh sound heard during inspiration and caused by laryngeal obstruction.

**tactile fremitus** Vibratory sensations of the spoken voice felt through the chest wall on palpation.

**tympany** Low-pitched note heard on percussion of the distended thorax.

**vesicular breathing** The normal breath sounds heard over most of the lungs.

**whispered pectoriloquy** Transmission of whispered words through the chest wall, heard during auscultation; indicates solidification of the lungs.

## Cognitive objectives

At the end of this chapter the learner will demonstrate knowledge of assessment of the respiratory system by the ability to do the following:

1. Systematically list the elements included in inspection of the respiratory system.
2. Correctly locate or diagram landmarks of the anterior thorax, including:
   a. Suprasternal notch
   b. Second rib
   c. Costochondral junctions
   d. Manubrium of sternum
   e. Costal angle
   f. Sternal angle
   g. Clavicle
   h. Midsternal line
   i. Midclavicular line
   j. Anterior axillary line
3. Correctly locate or diagram landmarks of the posterior thorax, including:
   a. C7
   b. T1
   c. Scapula
   d. Inferior angle of scapula T6 and seventh rib
   e. Vertebral line
   f. Midscapular line
   g. Posterior axillary line
4. Describe the qualities of the following breath sounds and indicate the location in which they are normally heard in adults and children.
   a. Bronchial
   b. Bronchovesicular
   c. Vesicular
5. Describe the significance of each of the sounds in no. 4 when heard in areas other than their normal locations.
6. Describe the normal respiratory rates for children and adults.
7. Describe the following respiratory patterns:
   a. Kussmaul respirations
   b. Cheyne-Stokes breathing
   c. Sighing respirations
   d. Biot breathing
   e. Tachypnea
   f. Bradypnea
   g. Air trapping
8. Systematically list the elements included in palpating the thorax.
9. Describe the techniques for palpating expansion of the thorax.
10. Identify the following:
    a. One condition that increases lung expansion
    b. Four conditions that limit lung expansion
    c. One condition that results in asymmetrical expansion
11. Describe identifying characteristics of the following adventitious sounds:
    a. Rales
    b. Rhonchi
    c. Wheeze
    d. Pleural friction rub
12. Define the significance of and describe the procedures for eliciting:
    a. Tactile fremitus
    b. Bronchophony
    c. Egophony
    d. Whispered pectoriloquy
    e. Diaphragmatic excursion
13. State a rationale for palpating for tenderness of the costovertebral angle.
14. Describe a systematic method for percussing the thorax.
15. Describe four percussion tones elicited throughout the body and state their normal locations.
16. Identify selected common variations with pediatric and geriatric clients.
17. Apply the terms in the vocabulary list.

## Clinical objectives

At the end of this chapter the learner will perform systematic assessment of the thorax and lungs by demonstrating the ability to do the following:

1. Obtain a pertinent health history from the client.
2. Demonstrate inspection of the thorax and relate findings relevant to:
   a. General body build
   b. Thorax configuration
   c. Skin, nail, and lip color
   d. Chest movement
   e. Pattern of respiration, including type of breathing, rate, and depth
3. Demonstrate palpation of the thorax and relate findings relevant to:
   a. Chest expansion
   b. Tenderness or pulsations
   c. Skin texture and lesions
   d. Subcutaneous structures or masses
   e. Tactile fremitus in symmetrical areas of the chest
   f. Position of the trachea
4. Demonstrate percussion of the thorax and relate findings relevant to:
   a. Characteristics of percussion tones heard in various areas of the thorax
   b. Intensity, pitch, quality, and duration of tones heard
   c. Diaphragmatic excursion

5. Demonstrate the ability to identify and differentiate lung sounds, including vesicular, bronchovesicular, and bronchial sounds, rales, rhonchi, and friction rub.
6. Demonstrate systematic auscultation of the lungs and relate findings relevant to:
   a. Characteristics of auscultatory sounds heard throughout the lungs
   b. Checking abnormal findings by using tests for bronchophony, egophony, and whispered pectoriloquy
7. Summarize findings of the assessment with a written description.

## Health history additional to screening history

1. Coughing is basically caused by either internal or external stimuli. Internal stimuli include allergic responses or response to an inflammatory process. External stimuli include irritants such as smoke, dust, or gas. When compiling history data from a client complaining of a cough, collect as much descriptive information as possible. The data should include the following:
   a. Duration of the coughing problem
   b. Frequency of the cough; whether it is related to time of day
   c. Type of cough: hacky, dry, bubbly, throaty, barky, hoarse, congested
   d. Sputum production versus nonproductive cough
   e. If sputum is produced, describe characteristics: mucoid versus purulent, color, odor, blood-tinged (note that some medications, such as those containing catecholamines, may cause pink-tinged sputum), amount
   f. Circumstances related to cough, such as activity, time of day, client position (lying vs. sitting), anxiety, talking
   g. Whether activity makes cough better or worse (sitting, walking, exercise)
   h. History of allergies in client or others in family (see data base allergy profile in Chapter 1)
   i. Is client's cough currently being treated? By whom? With what: over-the-counter medications, prescription medications, other techniques such as a vaporizer?
   j. Client's concern about cough
   k. Is cough tiring?
2. If the client complains of shortness of breath or dyspnea on exertion:
   a. Does cough or diaphoresis accompany dyspnea?
   b. Describe the onset of breathing problems (severity, duration, efforts to treat).
   c. Is breathing problem associated with pain or discomfort?
   d. How does different positioning affect the dyspnea (lying vs. sitting)?
   e. Time of day when dyspnea is likely to occur
   f. Does dyspnea interfere with, alter, or slow down any daily activities?
   g. How much walking creates shortness of breath (number of steps, flights of stairs, or blocks)?
   h. Are there stairs at home or work? How often must they be climbed each day? How does this affect breathing problem?
   i. How much walking or other types of exertion must the client do each day? How does this affect breathing problem?
3. If the client complains of difficulty breathing or breathlessness:
   a. History of asthma, bronchitis, emphysema, or tuberculosis? (Have client describe what these mean personally and to the family.)
   b. Does breathing problem cause lips or fingernails to become cyanotic?
   c. During a "breathing attack," what does the client do (positioning, breathing aids such as medications or oxygen)?
   d. How does the breathing problem interfere with the client's activities of daily living or work?
   e. Client's view of breathing problem
   f. Does the client think the overall breathing problem is getting worse or staying about the same?
4. Has the client had any previous respiratory illnesses, hospitalizations, or surgeries for lung or breathing problems? Describe what and when.
5. When was the client's last chest x-ray examination, tuberculosis test, or pulmonary function test? What were the results?
6. Is the client currently taking any medications for breathing or allergy problems? If so, describe.
7. Is the client subject to work or environmental conditions that could irritate the respiratory system (e.g., chemical plants, dry-cleaning fumes, coal mines)? If so, what does the client do for protection or monitoring the exposure conditions (e.g., masks, frequent pulmonary function tests or chest x-ray examinations, or ventilatory systems in factory with chemical exposure analysis)?
8. Certain "fumes" cause specific respiratory or systemic irritation. If the client reports a pollution exposure history as well as these symptoms, the examiner must be alert to their interrelationship:

a. Carbon monoxide may cause dizziness, headache, or fatigue.

b. Sulphur oxide may cause irritation to the respiratory tract, resulting in a cough or congestion.

c. Nitrogen oxides may irritate the mucous membranes, resulting in a cough or congestion.

9. If the client smokes:
   a. What does he smoke?
   b. How long has client smoked?
   c. How much each day does client smoke?
   d. Does client inhale?
   e. Does client have cough related to smoking?
   f. When did cough begin? Has cough gotten worse since that time?
   g. Does client desire to quit smoking?
   h. If so, what techniques has client used in an attempt to stop?
   i. If client has tried to quit but has failed, what does he see as the reason for failure?
10. If the client formerly smoked but has quit:

a. What had client been smoking?
b. How long did client smoke?
c. How much each day did client smoke?
d. Why did the client quit?

## Clinical guidelines

The following clinical guidelines have been developed to simulate the clinical setting. Total assessment of the thorax and lungs can be carried out with the client in a sitting position. The sequence of assessment techniques is inspection, palpation, percussion, and auscultation. A detailed discussion of the techniques of percussion and auscultation can be found in *Clinical strategies* in this chapter.

Inspection of the anterior and posterior chest should be carried out first. Following inspection the examiner should perform palpation, percussion, and auscultation of the posterior chest; then the examiner palpates, percusses, and auscultates the anterior chest. This places the examiner in front of the client, where he can proceed to cardiovascular assessment.

| THE STUDENT WILL: | TO IDENTIFY: | |
| --- | --- | --- |
| | NORMAL | DEVIATIONS FROM NORMAL |

1. Secure equipment needed for assessment of thorax and lungs, including:
   a. Stethoscope
   b. Ruler
   c. Marker
2. Instruct client to undress to waist so that thorax may be examined (Females will need anterior cover during posterior examination.)

**Inspection of anterior and posterior chest**

1. Instruct client to sit on edge of examination table for general inspection of anterior and posterior chest (Gown should be removed.) (Fig. 8-1)
2. Observe:

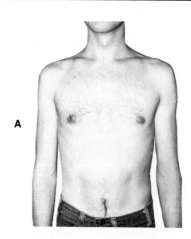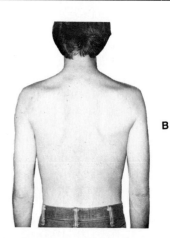

FIG. 8-1. **A,** Inspection of anterior chest. **B,** Inspection of posterior chest.

| | | |
| --- | --- | --- |
| a. Skin color of thorax and lips | Pink, well oxygenated | Cyanosis, pallor<br>Spider nevi |
| b. Nail beds and nail configuration | Smooth<br>Flat surface | Clubbing of nail and distal finger |

| THE STUDENT WILL: | TO IDENTIFY: | |
|---|---|---|
| | NORMAL | DEVIATIONS FROM NORMAL |
| **c.** General appearance | Relaxed posture | Apprehensive<br>Tense forward posture<br>Restless<br>Nostrils flaring<br>Supraclavicular retractions<br>Intercostal retractions<br>Intercostal bulging with expiration<br>Use of accessory muscles during breathing |
| **d.** Chest wall configuration<br>  1. Imagine topographical landmarks of thorax ( Fig. 8-2) | Symmetrical<br>Equal muscular development | |

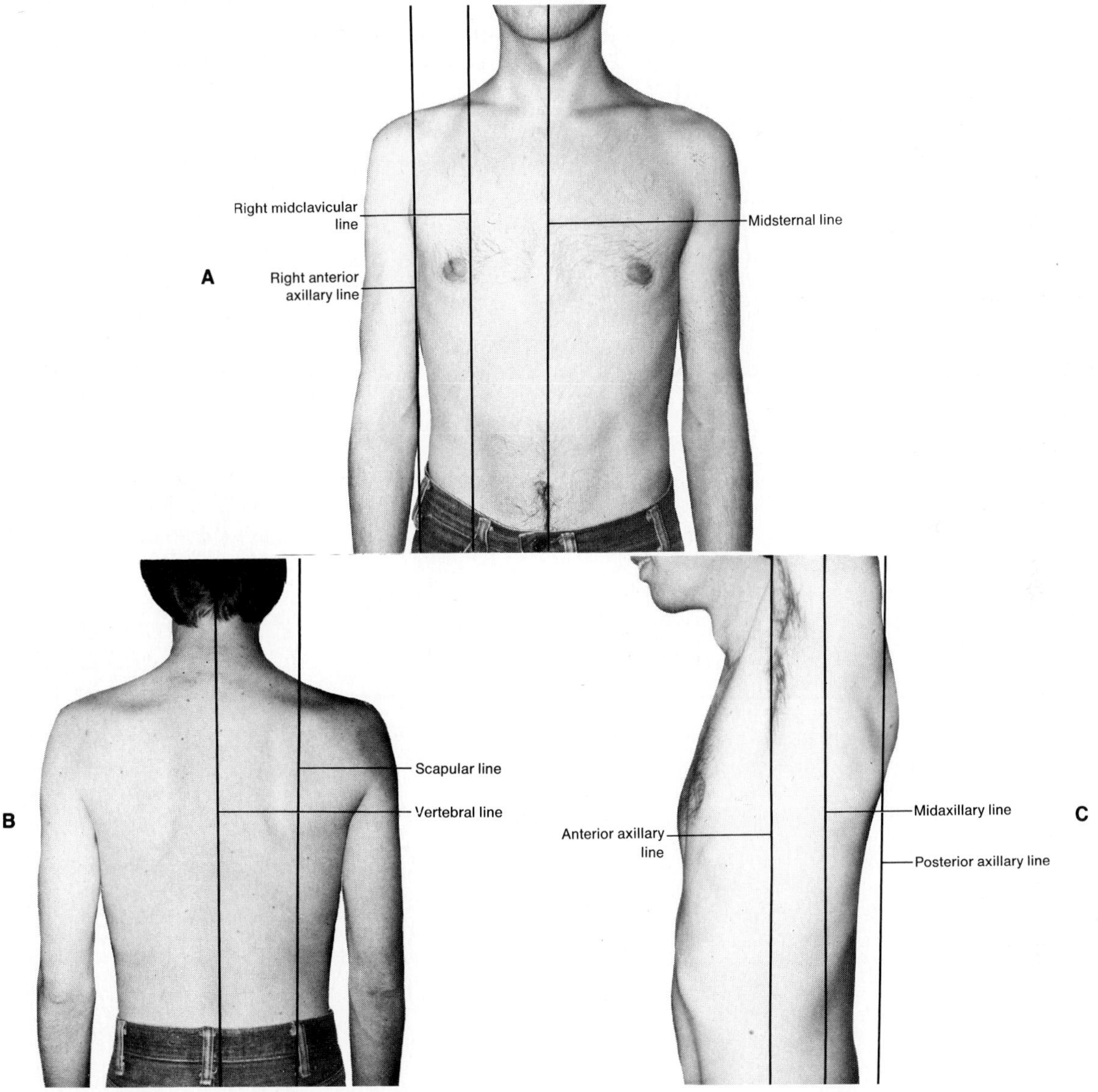

**FIG. 8-2. A,** Topographical landmarks of anterior thorax. **B,** Topographical landmarks of posterior thorax. **C,** Topographical landmarks of thorax (lateral view).

## Clinical guidelines—cont'd

|  | TO IDENTIFY: | |
|---|---|---|
| **THE STUDENT WILL:** | **NORMAL** | **DEVIATIONS FROM NORMAL** |
| 2. Imagine underlying structures of thorax (Fig. 8-3) | *Posterior*<br>  T4: angle of Louis<br>*Anterior*<br>  Second rib: angle of Louis, atria of heart | |

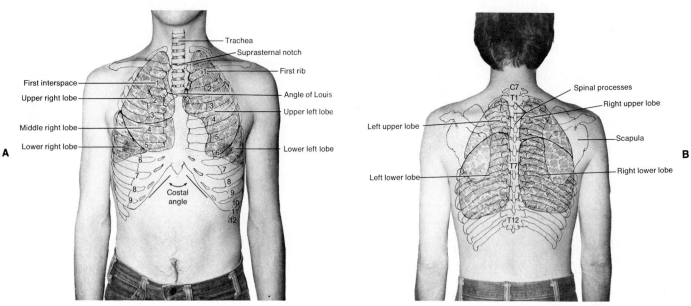

**FIG. 8-3. A,** Anterior view of anatomy of thorax. **B,** Posterior view of anatomy of thorax.

|  | | |
|---|---|---|
| 3. Anteroposterior (AP) diameter of chest | 1:2 to 5:7 (AP:transverse diameter) flat connections of rib cartilage with sternum | Barrel chest (Fig. 8-4)<br>Pectus carinatum<br>Pectus excavatum |

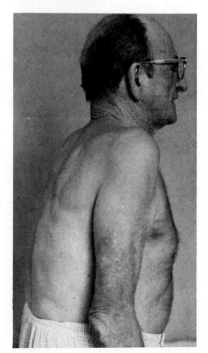

**FIG. 8-4.** Barrel chest. Note increased anteroposterior diameter.

| THE STUDENT WILL: | TO IDENTIFY: NORMAL | DEVIATIONS FROM NORMAL |
|---|---|---|
| **e.** Symmetry of chest | Bilaterally equal musculature (may be slightly more muscle development on client's dominant side)<br>Straight spinal processes (C7, T1 through T12)<br>Symmetrical scapular placement<br>Downward and equal slope of ribs<br>Costal angle 90° or less | Atrophy, tremors<br>Asymmetry<br>Loss of or accentuated spinal curvature, scoliosis, kyphosis, deformities<br>Asymmetrical scapular placement<br>Horizontal ribs<br>Costal angle greater than 90° |
| **f.** Breathing pattern | Diaphragmatic (male)<br>Thoracic (female)<br>Smooth, even breathing<br>Passive breathing 12 to 20 per minute; ratio of respiratory to pulse rate 1:4 | Abnormal, irregular breathing<br>Cheyne-Stokes |
| | Even pattern | Increase in rate and depth<br>Hyperpnea >20 per minute |
| | | Decrease in rate<br>Bradypnea <12 per minute |
| | Occasional sighing respirations | Increase in rate and depth >20 per minute<br>Kussmaul respirations |
| | During inspiration, chest expands, costal angle increases, and diaphragm descends and flattens | Many sighing respirations accompanied by other characteristics of anxiety<br>Biot breathing: shallow breathing followed by periods of apnea (may also be seen in some healthy persons) |
| | | Air-trapping breathing in clients with pulmonary disease: because of obstructive process, air becomes trapped in lungs |

## Clinical guidelines—cont'd

| THE STUDENT WILL: | TO IDENTIFY: | |
|---|---|---|
| | NORMAL | DEVIATIONS FROM NORMAL |

**Palpation of posterior chest**

1. Use one or two hands to palpate skin and thorax of posterior chest; examiner should use palmar surface of hand, including palmar base of fingers (Fig. 8-5)

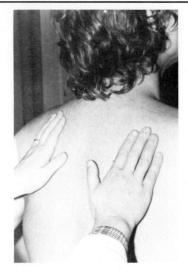

FIG. 8-5. Palpating posterior thorax.

| THE STUDENT WILL: | NORMAL | DEVIATIONS FROM NORMAL |
|---|---|---|
| 2. Evaluate and/or identify: | | |
| a. Skin texture and temperature, spinal process | Smooth, warm skin | Dry or moist skin<br>Poor skin turgor |
| b. C7, T1 | Straight spine, nontender | Crepitation<br>Curved spine<br>Scoliosis, kyphosis |
| c. Scapulae and surrounding musculature | Symmetrical location with developed musculature | Unequal musculature development |
| d. Chest wall | Stable ribs, nontender | Unstable chest wall<br>Masses<br>Tenderness<br>Subcutaneous emphysema |
| 3. Use palmar surface of one hand to assess vocal fremitus: examiner should place hand over equal positions of right and left lung fields and instruct client to repeat "one, two, three" or "how now brown cow" (Fig. 8-6); technique should be continued down posterior and posterolateral chest wall, comparing response of one side to other; do not test over bone areas | Varies from person to person because of intensity and pitch of voice<br>Bilaterally equal mild vibratory sensation<br>Most intense area to feel vibration is upper posterior chest wall medial to scapulae | *Increased fremitus* or increased vibratory sensation as seen in pneumonia or consolidation of lung<br>*Decreased fremitus* or decreased vibratory sensation seen when there is decreased production of sound (air blockage) or increase in space vibration must pass before it reaches skin surface; example is chronic obstructive pulmonary disease |

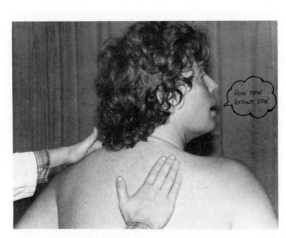

FIG. 8-6. Palpating for fremitus.

| THE STUDENT WILL: | TO IDENTIFY: | |
|---|---|---|
| | NORMAL | DEVIATIONS FROM NORMAL |

**4.** Palpate lateral chest wall excursion during deep respirations: examiner should place hands on lower posterior chest wall at about tenth rib level; examiner's thumbs should almost touch at spinal process; fingertips should wrap laterally around ribs (Fig. 8-7); instruct client to take several deep breaths; evaluate outward expansion

Bilaterally equal expansion of ribs during deep inspiration; thumbs move equally away from spine
Nonpainful breathing
No coughing

*Unequal fremitus*
Unequal excursion or pain with deep inspiration

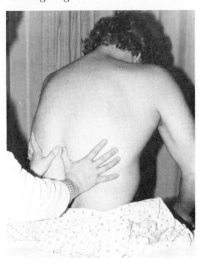

FIG. 8-7. Hand position for measuring respiratory excursion.

**5.** Percuss posterior chest: instruct client to sit and pull shoulders forward by crossing arms; this technique spreads scapulae and permits more lung area for evaluation (Fig. 8-8) (See *Clinical strategies* for percussion techniques.)

*Resonance* throughout lung fields
   Intensity: loud
   Pitch: low
   Duration: long
   Quality: hollow
   (Fig. 8-9)

*Hyperresonance* found over emphysematous lung
   Intensity: very loud
   Pitch: very low
   Duration: longer
   Quality: booming

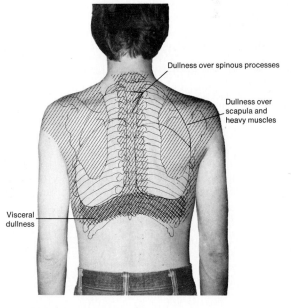

Dullness over spinous processes

Dullness over scapula and heavy muscles

Visceral dullness

FIG. 8-9. Percussion tones of the posterior chest.

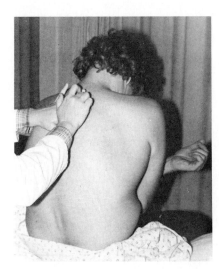

FIG. 8-8. Posture of posterior chest for percussion.

## Clinical guidelines—cont'd

| THE STUDENT WILL: | TO IDENTIFY: | |
|---|---|---|
| | NORMAL | DEVIATIONS FROM NORMAL |
| | *Flat sound* over bone or heavy muscle such as shoulder or scapula, spinal processes<br>Intensity: soft<br>Pitch: high<br>Duration: short<br>Quality: extreme dullness | *Dullness* over lung field occurs when fluid or solid tissue replaces normal lung tissue or fluid in pleural space<br>To identify consolidation, consolidated area must be at least 2 to 3 cm in diameter |
| 6. Percuss down posterior chest, comparing one side to other; avoid percussing over bone surface (Fig. 8-10)<br>　a. During percussion, listen and feel for intensity, pitch, duration, and quality of each percussed sound | *Dull sound* over viscera and liver border<br>Intensity: medium<br>Pitch: medium high<br>Duration: medium<br>Quality: thudlike<br>*Tympany sound* over stomach and gas bubble in intestine<br>Intensity: loud<br>Pitch: high<br>Duration: medium<br>Quality: drumlike | |

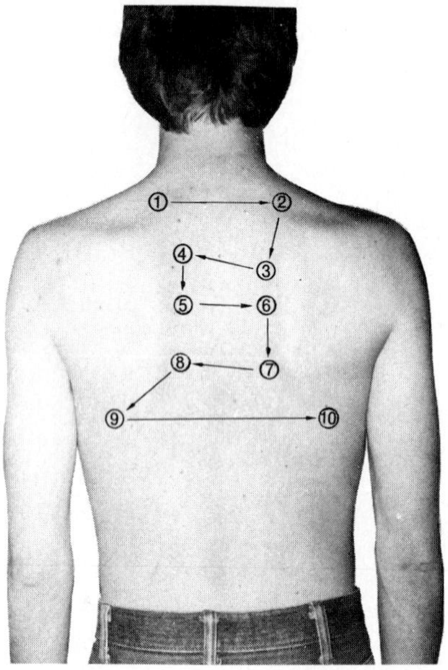

FIG. 8-10. Sequence for systematic percussion of the posterior thorax.

| | | |
|---|---|---|
| 7. Percuss diaphragmatic excursion of posterior lungs; client sits upright and breathes several times, then takes deep breath and holds it<br>　a. At this time percuss down posterior chest, starting at apex of scapulae<br>　b. Percussion continues downward until tone changes; mark that point with marker; then instruct client to breathe several times, exhale completely, and hold breath<br>　c. Again, percuss down line of apex of scapulae until tone changes; mark that point with marker<br>　d. Instruct client to breathe again | Resonance should be heard first; this tone becomes *dull* at bottom of lungs<br>Indicates level of diaphragm<br>Should occur around tenth rib<br><br>Higher diaphragm level may be present in pregnant women; may also have slightly narrower excursion volume | Unusually high level may accompany pleural effusion or atelectasis |
| 8. Repeat procedure on other side of posterior chest | Equal response on both sides | Unequal responses |

| THE STUDENT WILL: | TO IDENTIFY: | |
| --- | --- | --- |
| | NORMAL | DEVIATIONS FROM NORMAL |
| 9. With ruler, measure and record distance between two lines (Fig. 8-11)<br><br>(The purpose of this technique is to determine client's lung expansion capabilities.) | 4 to 6 cm (1½ to 2½ inches) downward excursion | Less than 4 cm (1½ inches) downward excursion |

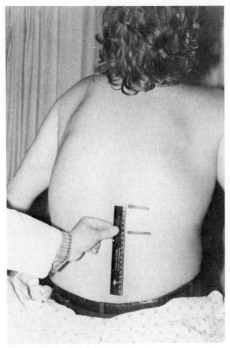

**FIG. 8-11.** Measurement of respiratory excursion.

### Auscultation of posterior chest

1. Auscultate posterior chest from apex to base; client should be seated; diaphragm of stethoscope should be used for breath sound auscultation (Fig. 8-12)

Vesicular breath sounds heard over almost all of posterior lung fields

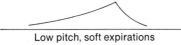

Low pitch, soft expirations

Bronchial breath sounds over peripheral lung

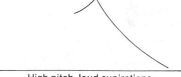

High pitch, loud expirations

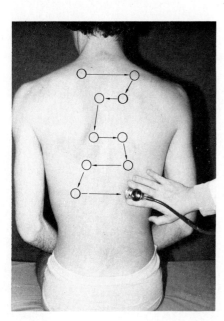

**FIG. 8-12.** Auscultatory pattern of posterior thorax with stethoscope.

## Clinical guidelines—cont'd

| THE STUDENT WILL: | TO IDENTIFY: | |
| --- | --- | --- |
| | NORMAL | DEVIATIONS FROM NORMAL |
| **2.** Instruct client to take slow, deep breaths in and out of mouth during auscultation; demonstrate breathing style for client | Bronchovesicular breath sounds over right upper posterior lung field | Bronchovesicular breath sounds over peripheral lung |
| | Medium pitch, medium expirations | |
| **3.** Slowly move stethoscope from one spot to next; compare sounds of one side of posterior chest to other; make sure to remain in one spot long enough to clearly analyze both inspiratory and expiratory sounds. (Fig. 8-13) | | Adventitious sounds, including rales and fine rales, high-pitched crackling sound, heard toward end of inspiration; indicates inflammation or congestion |

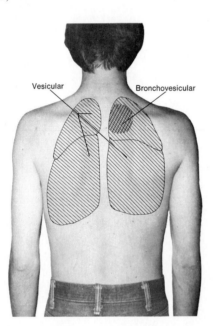

FIG. 8-13. Auscultatory sounds of the posterior chest.

| | | |
| --- | --- | --- |
| **a.** If abnormal sound is heard, instruct client to cough, then reexamine to evaluate if adventitious sound has changed or disappeared | | Medium rales: lower, more moist sound, heard about halfway through inspiration<br>Found in clients with pneumonia or pulmonary edema (not cleared by cough) |

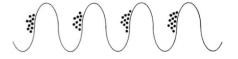

| THE STUDENT WILL: | TO IDENTIFY: | |
| --- | --- | --- |
| | NORMAL | DEVIATIONS FROM NORMAL |

| | | |
| --- | --- | --- |
| | | Coarse rales: loud, bubbly noise, heard during inspiration<br>Found in clients with pneumonia (not cleared by coughing)<br>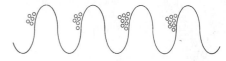 |
| | | Rhonchus: small airway noise<br>Sibilant rhonchus (wheeze): musical noise like squeak<br>May occur during inspiration or expiration, but usually louder during expiration<br>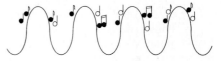 |
| | | Sonorous rhonchus (wheeze): low, loud, coarse sound like snore; may occur at any point of inspiration or expiration; usually means obstruction of trachea or large bronchi (coughing may clear sound)<br>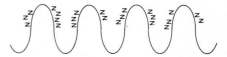 |
| | | Pleural friction rub: dry, rubbing or grating sound usually caused by inflammation of pleural surfaces; heard throughout inspiration and expiration; loudest over lower anterior lateral surface<br>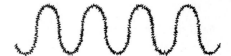 |
| **4.** Evaluate vocal resonance of spoken voice if any abnormalities in tactile fremitus; use one of following techniques:<br>  **a.** Bronchophony: use stethoscope (diaphragm) to listen throughout posterior chest as client says "ninety-nine" | Muffled response: "nin-nin" | Sound increased in loudness and clarity: "ninety-nine"<br>Found in consolidation or compression of lung |

## Clinical guidelines—cont'd

| THE STUDENT WILL: | TO IDENTIFY: | |
| --- | --- | --- |
| | NORMAL | DEVIATIONS FROM NORMAL |
| **b.** Whispered pectoriloquy: client instructed to whisper "one, two, three"; use stethoscope to listen throughout posterior chest | Muffled sounds: "one, two, three" | Clarity and loudness of sounds: "one, two, three"<br>Found in consolidation or compression of lung |
| **c.** Egophony: use stethoscope to listen to posterior chest; ask client to say "e-e-e" | Muffled sound: "e-e-e" | Change in intensity and pitch of sound: "a-a-a"<br>Caused by consolidation |
| **Palpation of anterior chest** | | |
| **1.** Move anterior to client to evaluate anterior thorax and lungs | | |
| **2.** Use one or two hands to palpate skin and thorax of anterior chest | | |
| **3.** Evaluate: | | |
| **a.** Skin texture and temperature, manubrium, suprasternal notch, sternal angle, second rib, body of sternum, costochondral junctions, costal angle, ribs, and chest wall stability | Smooth, warm skin<br><br>Stable, nontender chest wall and landmarks<br>Well-developed musculature | Dry or moist skin<br>Poor skin turgor<br>Crepitation<br>Thorax deformities<br>Pectus excavatum (funnel chest), characterized by depression deformity of lower sternum<br>May impair breathing or cause compression of heart<br>Pectus carinatum (pigeon chest), characterized by outward deformity of sternum<br>Increase in AP diameter<br>Unequal muscle development, unstable chest wall, masses, tenderness |
| **b.** Tracheal position | Midline | Lateral tracheal deviation |
| **4.** Use palmar surface of one hand to assess vocal fremitus; examiner should place hand over equal positions of both lung fields of superior anterior chest and the anterolateral chest wall (Avoid areas with heavy breast tissue.) | Varies from person to person because of intensity and pitch of voice<br>Bilaterally equal<br>Mild vibratory sensation<br>Most intense area of vibratory sensation should be upper medial chest area, lateral to sternum | Increased fremitus<br>Decreased fremitus<br>Unequal fremitus |
| **5.** Instruct client to repeat "one, two, three" or "how now brown cow" | | |
| **Percussion of anterior chest** | | |
| **1.** Instruct client to pull shoulders backward and to sit straight while anterior chest is percussed | | |
| **2.** Percuss downward, comparing one side to other; avoid percussion over breast tissue or bony surface (Fig. 8-14)<br>(If the examiner has difficulty percussing anterior chest while client is sitting, defer this part of examination until client is lying down.) | Resonance throughout lung fields<br>Flat sounds over sternum or heavy breast tissue<br>Dull sounds over heart or liver<br>Tympany over stomach (Fig. 8-15) | Hyperresonance<br>Dullness over lung field |

|  | TO IDENTIFY: |  |
|---|---|---|
| **THE STUDENT WILL:** | **NORMAL** | **DEVIATIONS FROM NORMAL** |

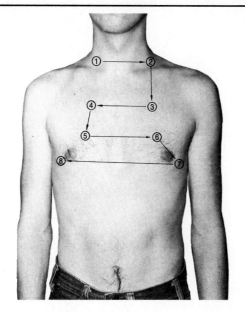

**FIG. 8-14.** Sequence for systematic percussion of the thorax.

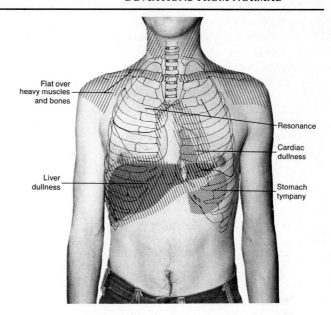

**FIG. 8-15.** Percussion tones of the anterior chest.

### Auscultation of anterior chest

1. Ausculate anterior chest from apex to base; client may be sitting or lying; use same techniques as for posterior thorax auscultation

Vesicular breath sounds over anterior peripheral lung fields
Bronchial breath sounds over trachea
Bronchovesicular breath sounds over large bronchioles (Fig. 8-16)

Bronchial breath sounds over peripheral lung fields
Bronchovesicular breath sounds over peripheral lung fields
Adventitious sounds, including rales (fine, medium, coarse), rhonchi (sonorous, sibilant), and pleural friction rub

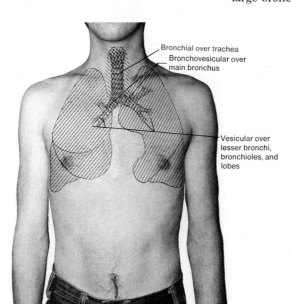

**FIG. 8-16.** Auscultatory sounds of the anterior chest.

## Clinical guidelines—cont'd

| THE STUDENT WILL: | TO IDENTIFY: | |
| --- | --- | --- |
| | NORMAL | DEVIATIONS FROM NORMAL |
| **2.** Evaluate anterior chest resonance of spoken voice if any abnormalities in tactile fremitus; use same techniques as for posterior chest | | |
| **a.** Bronchophony: instruct client to say "ninety-nine"; evaluate with stethoscope | Muffled response: "nin-nin" | Sound increased in loudness and clarity: "ninety-nine" |
| **b.** Whispered pectoriloquy: instruct client to whisper "one, two, three"; evaluate with stethoscope | Muffled response: "one, two, three" | Clarity and loudness of sounds: "one, two, three" |
| **c.** Egophony: instruct client to say "e-e-e" | Muffled response: "e-e-e" | Change in intensity and pitch of sounds: "a-a-a" |

### Evaluation of lateral thorax and lungs

**1.** Instruct client to abduct arm overhead so that lateral chest may be percussed and auscultated (Fig. 8-17)

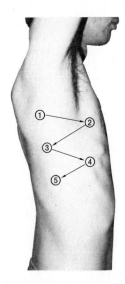

**FIG. 8-17.** Lateral percussion and auscultation position.

| | | |
| --- | --- | --- |
| **2.** Percuss down each lateral thorax | Resonance over lung area<br>Dull sound as percussion reaches liver (on right) and spleen (on left) | Hyperresonance or dullness over lung fields |
| **3.** Auscultate down each lateral thorax | Vesicular breath sounds | Bronchovesicular or bronchial breath sounds<br>No breath sounds |

## Clinical strategies

1. For evaluation of the thorax and lungs, the client must be undressed. This means bra or undershirt off. During inspection of overall respiratory response, the client should be sitting with the gown dropped to the waist.

2. During inspection, first stand back and observe the client. It has been stated that once the examiner touches the client, the client's observable details are no longer seen. This is an essential concept and deserves foremost consideration. During observation, carefully analyze the client's posture, breathing difficulties, breathing style, audible sounds, and any other factors that reflect the client's breathing attempts. For example, a client with breathing difficulties may lean forward to breathe (Fig. 8-18).

3. Although inspection of the front and back is done together, the other assessment techniques—palpation, percussion, and auscultation—are first done in the back and then in the front (or reverse, if you prefer).

4. When palpating, use both hands simultaneously: one hand on the right chest wall and the other on the left chest wall. The purpose is to check symmetry, comparing the findings on one side with those on the other.

5. Any abnormalities identified must be described and defined by intercostal space and distance from sternum, spine, axillary lines, etc.

6. The techniques of percussion are the same whether one is percussing the thorax, heart, liver, or abdomen. However, the tones elicited in those areas are different. Percussion tones represent vibrations from 4 to 5 cm deep. As the beginning examiner learns the technique of percussion, considerable practice will be required until the five tones (resonance, hyperresonance, dullness, flatness, and tympany) are easily recognized. Only after the examiner has memorized the tones and their normal location is there hope of identifying abnormal findings. Following is a description of current percussion techniques:

   a. Place the left hand flat on the posterior chest wall and slightly spread fingers. The distal phalanx of the middle (pleximeter) finger should be firmly pressed on the chest wall. The other fingers should very gently rest on the thorax.

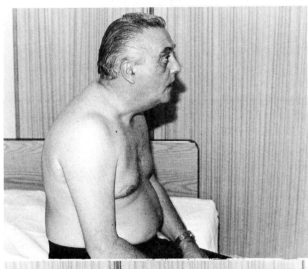

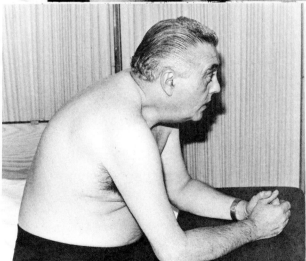

**FIG. 8-18.** Client with breathing difficulty may lean forward to breathe easier.

---

**SAMPLE RECORDING**

Respiration rate 14; regular rhythm without noted difficulty.
Diaphragmatic breathing.
Bilaterally equal excursion.
Client sitting erect, slight kyphosis noted.
Skin intact and warm; no bulging, retractions, tenderness, or asymmetry of chest wall noted.
Thorax oval; AP diameter < lateral diameter.
Tactile fremitus bilaterally equal.
Diaphragmatic excursion 4 cm (1½ inches) bilaterally.
Resonant percussion tone throughout.
Vesicular breath sounds bilaterally throughout.
Few fine basilar rates heard on right, which did not clear with cough.

b. The middle finger of the right hand becomes the hammer (plexor), which taps the interphalangeal joint of the pleximeter.
c. The success of the technique of percussion depends on several elements, including the following (Fig. 8-19):
  (1) The downward snap of the plexor *must* be sharp and rapid.
  (2) The downward snap of the plexor *must* be a wrist action and *not* a forearm or shoulder motion.
  (3) The *tip* of the plexor finger *must* be used, not the finger pad.
  (4) Once the plexor has struck the pleximeter, quickly remove the plexor (this ensures pure quality of tone).
  (5) One location should be tapped several times to ensure clear interpretation of the tone elicited.
  (6) *Short* fingernails are essential. Otherwise the examiner is more likely to use the finger pad of the plexor and not the fingertip.

  (7) Loudness of the tone does not ensure good quality. The examiner should practice the percussion techniques until a light percussion tapping elicits an appropriate tone.
7. When percussing the back, it is helpful to have the client sit with the shoulder drooping slightly forward. This pulls the scapulae laterally and allows increased access to the lung field.
8. When percussing the anterior chest wall, have the client sit with shoulders pulled back. For women with large breasts, percuss the anterosuperior lung fields with the client sitting, then have her recline to a 45-degree angle with hands up and behind the head. This positioning allows percussion access to the inferoanterior lung fields (Fig. 8-20).
9. When percussing for excursion on the posterior chest wall, it is helpful for the examiner as well as the client to hold their breath.
10. Auscultation requires the use of a stethoscope. Because there are many different types of stethoscopes, the ability to accurately assess auscultatory sounds depends partially on the quality of the instrument. Following are characteristics of good stethoscopes and auscultatory techniques:
  a. Characteristics of high-quality stethoscopes:

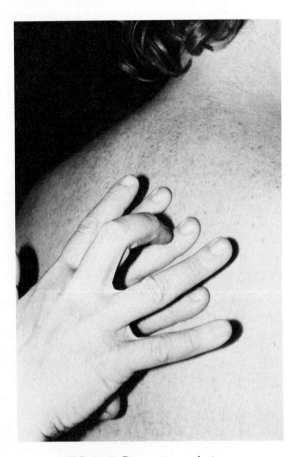

**FIG. 8-19.** Percussion technique.

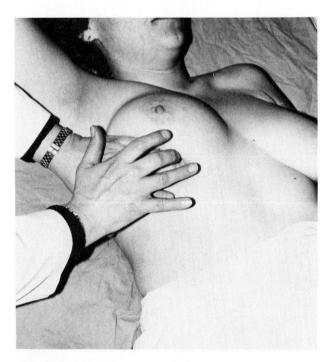

**FIG. 8-20.** Anterior thorax percussion technique for a large-breasted woman.

(1) Use a diaphragm that will pick up high-pitched (breath) sounds and a bell that will pick up low-pitched sounds (heart murmurs).

(2) The diaphragm and bell sound have enough weight to lay firmly on the chest wall when placed there.

(3) The diaphragm should be covered with a factory manufactured diaphragm cover, not a piece of x-ray film.

(4) The bell should have a small rubber or plastic ring around its tip to ensure a secure fit against the chest wall.

(5) The tubing may be in one or two pieces. The human ear is unable to detect sound differences between one-tubing and two-tubing stethoscopes. Thick, stiff, and heavy tubing conducts sound better than thin, elastic, or very flexible tubing. Do not use hospital tubing.

(6) The length of the stethoscope tubing should be between 30.5 and 46 cm (12 and 18 inches).

(7) Earpieces can make the difference between hearing or not hearing a sound. The examiner should choose the largest earpieces that will snugly fit into the ears. The ability of the earpieces to occlude outside noise is the important consideration.

b. Auscultory techniques:

(1) The earpieces should point toward the examiner's nose to snugly fit in the auditory canal.

(2) The examiner should try not to touch or allow the tubing to touch rubbing surfaces during auscultation. This will cause extra noise.

(3) The examiner should hold the head of the stethoscope between the index and middle fingers to stabilize it during auscultation (Fig. 8-21).

(4) When using the diaphragm, exert firm pressure to ensure solid contact with the chest wall.

(5) In using the bell, care must be taken not to flatten the underlying skin by pressing the bell too firmly. The bell must be lightly and evenly placed on the skin. There must be total skin contact around the bell edge. The bell functions by picking up vibratory sensations of the surface tissue in response to the visceral vibrations. If the tissue is stretched too much by firm pressure, vibrations are inhibited and the bell actually converts to a diaphragm.

11. Before auscultating the breath sounds, it is appropriate to give instruction on how to breathe. The client should breathe deeply and slowly through the mouth. Stand in front and demonstrate. Nasal breathing is not encouraged because nasal turbulence interferes with clear auscultation of the thorax.

12. When auscultating the posterior chest, again have the client sit with shoulders drooping slightly forward. When listening for breath sounds, move from apices to bases. Compare one side with the other as you move down the posterior wall. Avoid auscultation over bone. Be sure to listen to each spot for at least two inspirations and expirations. This will ensure a clearer interpretation of the sound heard.

13. During auscultation of the anterior chest, the client should be sitting straight. Auscultation is begun above the clavicle and should again move

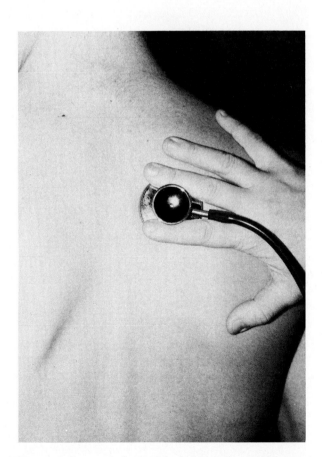

**FIG. 8-21.** Proper technique for holding the stethoscope.

down the chest wall while one side is compared with the other. For large-breasted women the breasts can be displaced upward and laterally for access to the lower anterior lung fields.

14. When auscultating the chest, evaluate the quality of breath sound, compare inspiration length with expiration length, and listen for any abnormalities. Describe what you hear.

15. If you hear adventitious sounds on auscultation, instruct the client to cough. See if the sounds are cleared by a cough.

16. Do not forget to palpate, percuss, and auscultate the lateral chest walls. Compare one side with the other.

### History and clinical strategies: the pediatric client

1. Because many childhood illnesses frequently involve the respiratory system, the thorax and respiratory function of children deserve thorough evaluation.

2. The techniques of pediatric evaluation are the same as for the adult. The results of assessment will depend on cooperation from the child and the examiner's ability to gently assess the child.

3. Coughs and colds seem to accompany the growing child. History data should be gathered about the same elements as discussed for the adult client. An allergic history should also be gathered. If the child is less than 2 years of age and is beginning to eat new foods, the examiner should gather a thorough nutritional history as well.

4. Children with asthma or bronchitis histories should be questioned with regard to the overall progression of that condition. Data should be gathered regarding:
   a. Frequency and duration of the problem
   b. Current care techniques
   c. Precipitating factors
   d. Current medications
   e. Relationship of problem to activities and playing
   f. How does child view the problem?
   g. What does child think is possible in terms of self-help?

5. Any child with a sudden onset of coughing or choking should be expected to have aspirated a foreign object until proved otherwise. The examiner should inquire about the child's playing activities before the current problem (e.g., was he playing with *toys* such as beads, a car with removable wheels, or pieces of a game that could have been put into his mouth). *Great* skill must be employed to gather the information needed without the child becoming frightened and answering "no" to every question asked.

*Food aspiration* is another cause for sudden coughing or breathing problems. Common aspirated objects are peanuts, popcorn, carrot pieces, hot dogs, or peas. All these tend to block and not dissolve if accidentally aspirated. Although it is difficult to determine, some parents may admit that they were force feeding a child before the coughing episode or that the child had food and was playing or running around the house before the coughing period.

6. The respiratory rate of children is obviously faster than that of the adult. Sometimes the parent may bring the child for evaluation because "he is breathing funny." If this occurs, the examiner must collect a detailed history, including a thorough evaluation of the possibility of poisoning or ingestion of a toxic substance. Many times the presenting complaint of salicylate poisoning is a child with rapid, panting respirations.

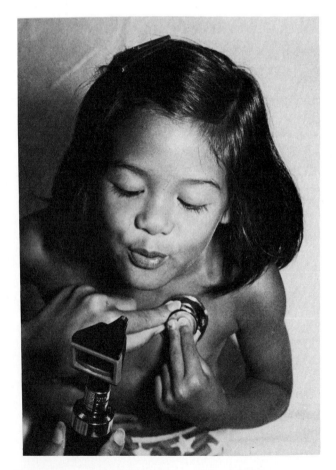

FIG. 8-22. Auscultating the lungs while child blows out otoscope light. (From Whaley, L.F., and Wong, D.L.: Nursing care of infants and children, ed. 2, St. Louis, 1983, The C.V. Mosby Co.)

7. For examination the child should be naked to the waist and sitting on the parent's lap or the examining table. Infants are laid on the examination table.
8. The child must be breathing quietly for breath sounds to be evaluated. As soon as the child is old enough to cooperate, he should be instructed to breathe deeply through his mouth. One technique to facilitate this is to instruct the child to take a deep breath and "blow" out the examiner's penlight

or otoscope (Fig. 8-22) while the examiner listens to the child's chest with the stethoscope in the other hand.
9. There has been much written about stridor and retraction evaluation in children. We want to stress that the emphasis of this text is the clinical assessment of "normal" for both children and adults. If the examiner identifies retractions, wheezing, stridor, or persistent coughing, the child should be referred to a physician for further evaluation.

## Clinical variations: the pediatric client

| CHARACTERISTIC OR AREA EXAMINED | NORMAL | DEVIATIONS FROM NORMAL |
|---|---|---|
| **1.** Anterior and posterior chest | | |
| **a.** Skin color, thorax, and lips | Pink, well oxygenated<br>Babies' skin may become mottled if they are chilled | Cyanosis, pallor<br>Spider nevi<br>Dilated veins over lower thorax |
| **b.** Nail beds, nail configuration | Smooth<br>Flat surface | Clubbing of nail and distal finger |
| **c.** General appearance | Relaxed posture | Apprehensive<br>Tense forward posture<br>Restless<br>Nostrils flaring<br>Supraclavicular retractions<br>Intercostal retractions<br>Use of accessory muscles during breathing |
| **d.** Chest wall configuration | Symmetrical<br>Equal muscular development | |
| **e.** AP diameter of chest | Newborns have rounded chest wall configuration where AP diameter equals transverse diameter<br>By age 6 years AP and lateral diameter ratio should reach toward adult normal of 1:2 or 5:7 | Children with rounded rib cage after age 6 years (may be found in children with cystic fibrosis or asthma) |
| **f.** Chest wall configuration | | |
| 1. Anterior | Symmetrical<br>Flat sternum<br>45° costal angle<br>Harrison groove may be normally found in some children: horizontal groove at level of diaphragm; with breathing there may be slight flaring below groove<br>Bilaterally equal musculature<br>Shoulders equal<br>Clavicles equal | Pectus carinatum (pigeon chest)<br>Pectus excavatum (funnel chest)<br>Costal angle larger than 45° or 50°<br>Harrison groove, with marked flaring below groove, should be considered abnormal<br>Asymmetry<br>Asymmetry<br>Asymmetry |
| 2. Posterior | Straight spinal processes (C7, T1 through T12)<br><br>Symmetrical scapulae<br>Downward and equal slope of ribs | Spinal curvature<br>Scoliosis<br>Kyphosis (humpback)<br>Asymmetry |

## Clinical variations: the pediatric client—cont'd

| CHARACTERISTIC OR AREA EXAMINED | NORMAL | DEVIATIONS FROM NORMAL |
|---|---|---|
| 2. Breathing pattern | Abdominal and nasal breathing during infancy<br>Gradual change until age 6 or 7 years; then girls become mostly thoracic breathers and boys become abdominal breathers<br>Newborn may demonstrate Cheyne-Stokes breathing; this should normally disappear by age 4 weeks | Seesaw breathing where thorax and abdomen alternate during breathing<br>Respiratory grunting<br><br>Abnormal, irregular breathing pattern Cheyne-Stokes |
| 3. Rate of respiration | Ratio of respirations to pulse 1:4<br>Newborn: 30 to 50 resp/min<br>6 months: 20 to 40 resp/min<br>1 year: 20 to 40 resp/min<br>3 years: 20 to 30 resp/min<br>6 years: 16 to 22 resp/min<br>10 years: 16 to 20 resp/min<br>17 years: 14 to 20 resp/min | Any respiration rates that fall short of or exceed stated normal rates |
| 4. Depth of respirations (This is an important quality to evaluate in children.) | Respiratory depth guide to be used when child is lying supine: examiner takes hand and holds it in front of child's nose; breathing normally felt at following distances*: | Breathing may become deeper and labored in cases of metabolic acidosis such as Kussmaul respirations |
| | *Child's age*    *Depth of respiration*<br>1 month    2 inches<br>3 months    3 inches<br>6 to 12 months    4 inches<br>2 years    6 inches<br>3 to 4 years    8 inches<br>5 to 6 years    9 inches<br>8 to 10 years    10 inches | Breathing becomes evident during metabolic alkalosis as body conserves carbon dioxide<br>Decreased depth could also be evidence of airway obstruction |
| 5. Posterior chest palpation (May need to use one or two fingers instead of all fingers.) | | |
|   **a.** Skin | Smooth, warm | Dry or moist skin<br>Poor skin turgor |
|   **b.** Bone, muscle structure | Symmetrical, straight spine, nontender | |
|   **c.** Chest wall stability | Stable ribs, nontender | |
| 6. Vocal fremitus: instruct child to speak as adult was instructed or evaluate when child is crying | Varies from person to person because of intensity and pitch of voice<br>Bilaterally equal mild vibratory sensation<br>Most intense area to feel vibration is upper posterior chest wall medial to scapulae | *Increased fremitus* or increased vibratory sensation as seen in pneumonia or consolidation of lung<br>*Decreased fremitus* or decreased vibratory sensation when there is decreased production of sound (air blockage) or increase in space vibration must pass before it reaches skin surface |
| 7. Lateral chest wall excursion | Bilaterally equal expansion of ribs during deep inspiration; thumbs move equally away from spine<br>Nonpainful breathing<br>No coughing | Unequal excursion or pain with deep inspiration |

*From Barness, L.A.: Manual of pediatric physical diagnosis, ed. 5. Copyright © 1980 by Year Book Medical Publishers, Inc., Chicago. Used by permission.

| CHARACTERISTIC OR AREA EXAMINED | NORMAL | DEVIATIONS FROM NORMAL |
|---|---|---|
| 8. Posterior chest wall percussion: requires lighter pressure than adult technique | More resonant than adult | Hyperresonance in older child |
| | Some children may display hyperresonant tone | Dullness over lung field |
|    a. "Direct" single finger tapping percussion may elicit clearer tone in very small child | Older children: *resonance* | |
| | Flat sound over bone or heavy muscle | |
| | Dull sound over viscera or liver | |
| 9. Diaphragmatic excursion percussion: not routinely done in small child; when done in older child, use same technique as for adult | Resonance should be heard first; changes to a *dull* tone at bottom of lungs | Unusually high diaphragmatic excursion level may be present in children with pleural effusion or atelectasis |
| | Indicates level of diaphragm | |
| | Should occur around tenth rib | |
| | Amount of downward excursion will depend on size of child | |
| 10. Posterior chest auscultation: use either *small* diaphragm or *small* rubber-edged bell stethoscope; all edges of either must have "good" contact with child's chest wall; use same technique as for adult | Louder than adult | Bronchial breath sounds |
| | Bronchovesicular breath sounds normally heard in infant and small child because of thin chest wall with poorly developed musculature | Bronchovesicular breath sounds in older child (over age 6 or 7 years) |
| | Vesicular breath sounds like adult's as child grows older | Adventitious sounds such as fine rales, medium rales, coarse rales, sibilant rhonchi, sonorous rhonchi, and pleural friction rub |
| 11. Vocal resonance: not routinely evaluated in children; when evaluation is desired, use same technique as for adult | | |
| 12. Anterior chest palpation | | |
|    a. Skin | Smooth warm skin | Dry or moist skin |
| | | Poor skin turgor |
| | | Cold or hot skin |
|    b. Bone, muscle structure | | Crepitation |
|    c. Chest wall stability | Stable, nontender chest wall and landmarks | Thorax deformities: pectus excavatum (funnel chest) characterized by depression deformity of lower sternum; may impair breathing or cause compression of heart |
| | Well-developed musculature | Pectus carinatum (pigeon chest) characterized by outward deformity of sternum |
|    d. Tracheal position | Midline | Lateral tracheal deviation |
| 13. Vocal fremitus palpation | Varies from person to person because of intensity and pitch of voice | Increased fremitus |
| | Bilaterally equal | Decreased fremitus |
| | Mild vibratory sensation | |
| | Most intense area of vibratory sensation should be upper medial chest area, lateral to sternum | Unequal fremitus |
| 14. Anterior chest percussion: may use direct or indirect palpation technique | More resonant than in adult; some small children may demonstrate hyperresonant tone | Hyperresonance in older children or dullness over lung fields |
| | Dull sound over heart and liver; liver starts at approximately fifth interspace on right at midclavicular line | |
| | Tympany over stomach | |

## Clinical variations: the pediatric client—cont'd

| CHARACTERISTIC OR AREA EXAMINED | NORMAL | DEVIATIONS FROM NORMAL |
|---|---|---|
| 15. Anterior chest auscultation | Bronchovesicular breath sounds normally heard throughout peripheral lungs of smaller child | Bronchial breath sounds over peripheral lung |
| | Vesicular breath sounds throughout peripheral lungs of older child | Bronchovesicular over peripheral lung fields in older child |
| | Bronchial breath sounds heard over trachea | |
| | Bronchovesicular breath sounds heard over large bronchioles | Adventitious sounds such as fine, medium, and coarse rales, sibilant and sonorous rhonchi, and pleural friction rub |
| 16. Vocal resonance of anterior chest (not normally evaluated in children); when evaluation is desired, use same techniques as for adult | | |
| 17. Lateral thorax and lungs | Resonance over lung area | Hyperresonance or dullness over lung fields |
| | Dull sound as percussion reaches liver (on right) and spleen (on left) | |
| | Vesicular breath sounds | Bronchovesicular breath sounds |
| | | No breath sounds |

## History and clinical strategies: the geriatric client

1. The examiner should not assume that aging is automatically accompanied by respiratory disease. The literature reports that physical changes occur with aging; however, the "normal," healthy elderly individual is usually free of chronic respiratory symptoms. Many of the changes that occur may not be clinically remarkable or may not alter or interfere with the client's life-style. Following are some major changes that occur:
   a. Decrease in muscular strength of the chest wall muscles
   b. Possible stiffening and decreased expansion of chest wall (calcification at the rib articulation points may be involved)
   c. Decrease in vital capacity and increase in residual volume
   d. Decrease in elastic lung recoil and increased lung distensibility; alveoli and bronchioles stretched (enlarged)
   e. Loss of some of the interalveolar septa (folds), resulting in a decrease in alveolar surface available for gas exchange
   f. Underventilation of the alveoli in the lower lung fields
   g. Increase in the mucous production cells in the bronchioles

As with all other changes, these alterations take place at different rates with different individuals. Physical conditioning and general physical health are two very important variables that affect the efficiency of respiratory function. Obese, sedentary, or immobilized individuals have less opportunity to maintain physical fitness and are more vulnerable to respiratory disability.

In summary, it often takes more energy for the older individual to expand the chest wall to carry through the function of respiration. Many elderly clients do not experience dyspnea unless they exceed the ordinary mild to moderate exertion demands that they are accustomed to. Sudden intense activity can result in shortness of breath. Heavy or unusually demanding exercise can create problems. With aging changes a diminished functional reserve occurs, creating a higher vulnerability to respiratory distress or infection. Elderly people should be cautious about exposure to colds, flu, or other infections.

2. The symptoms of cough, dyspnea on exertion, and breathlessness have been covered in the adult section (pp. 203 to 204).
3. Chest pain may be diminished in an older client. Pleuritic pain may not be reported or sensed as

intensely as it would be in a younger person. If chest pain does exist, be certain to examine the client for fractured ribs (sustained from a fall or coughing) as well as arthritic changes in the rib cage.

4. It is a good idea to inquire about the effects of weather on the client. Some people have an increase in respiratory infections in cold, damp weather.
5. Ask about the incidence of colds, flu, and whether the number and/or severity of the episodes has been increasing.
6. The incidence of chronic respiratory disease is higher among the elderly population. Chronic bronchitis, emphysema, lung cancer, and tuberculosis are four of the major health problems. (Pulmonary edema associated with heart disease is covered in Chapter 9.) In addition to cough, dyspnea on exertion, chest pain, and breathlessness, chronic health problems can include:
   a. History of smoking (see adult *Health history* section for specific questions)
   b. Periodic bouts of low-grade fever
   c. Night sweats

d. Remarkable weight change in last 6 months or year
e. New problems with fatigue
f. Any sensations in the chest other than pain (e.g., feeling of heaviness)
g. Family history of any respiratory problems
h. Daily activities altered or decreased because of problems with fatigue, shortness of breath, or discomfort

7. Risk factors for respiratory disability with elderly individuals include:
   a. History of smoking
   b. History of frequent respiratory infections
   c. Immobilization or marked sedentary habits
   d. History of chronic exposure to environmental pollutants
   e. Difficulty swallowing
   f. Indication of weakened chest muscles (e.g., general physical disability, inability to cough or breathe deeply)
   g. Family history of respiratory disability
8. *Note:* It may be difficult for some clients to breathe deeply or to hold breath on command during the physical assessment.

## Clinical variations: the geriatric client

| CHARACTERISTIC OR AREA EXAMINED | NORMAL | DEVIATIONS FROM NORMAL |
|---|---|---|
| **1.** Anterior and posterior chest | | |
| **a.** Skin color and lips and nail beds | Pink, well oxygenated | Cyanosis, pallor |
| | Dark-skinned clients' mucous membranes and nail beds appear pink and well oxygenated | Spider nevi |
| **b.** Nail configuration | 160° angle at nail bed | Clubbing (angle disappears) |
| **c.** General appearance | Relaxed posture | Apprehensive |
| | (Note elderly client's general condition of physical fitness: muscle weakness associated with general physical disability or sedentary life-style may affect client's ability to use respiratory muscles and to expand the chest.) | Tense, forward posture |
| | | Restless |
| | | Nostrils flaring |
| | | Supraclavicular retractions |
| | | Intercostal retractions |
| | | Use of accessory muscles during breathing (*Note:* Pursed-lip breathing—chiefly expiration—is compensatory pattern associated with chronic obstructive pulmonary disease.) |
| **d.** Chest wall configuration | Symmetrical landmarks | Asymmetry of landmarks |
| | Downward and equal slope of ribs | Horizontal ribs |
| | Bilaterally equal muscular development (may be slightly more muscle development on client's dominant side) | |

## Clinical variations: the geriatric client—cont'd

| CHARACTERISTIC OR AREA EXAMINED | NORMAL | DEVIATIONS FROM NORMAL |
|---|---|---|
| | Subcutaneous fat is often decreased, and bony prominences are more marked | |
| | Costal angle less than 90° | Costal angle greater than 90° |
| | (*Note:* Kyphosis [Fig. 8-23] is a fairly common problem with elderly clients. Dorsal scoliosis may exist, accompanied by tracheal deviation. Loss of normal spinal curvature in the dorsal and lumbar regions may occur with arthritis.) | (*Note:* Chronic marked stooping or bending forward may affect lung expansion in localized areas.) |

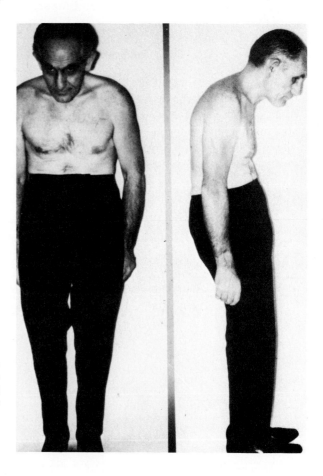

FIG. 8-23. Kyphosis. (*Note:* Increased thoracic curvature is accompanied by loss of normal lumbar curvature.) (From Prior, J.A., Silberstein, J.S., and Stang, J.M.: Physical diagnosis: the history and examination of the patient, ed. 6, St. Louis, 1981, The C.V. Mosby Co.)

| CHARACTERISTIC OR AREA EXAMINED | NORMAL | DEVIATIONS FROM NORMAL |
|---|---|---|
| **e.** Anteroposterior diameter of chest in relation to lateral diameter | 1:2 to 5:7 ratio | Barrel chest (Fig. 8-4) |
| | Kyphosis is often accompanied by increased anteroposterior diameter | |
| **2.** Breathing pattern | Client is able to close mouth and breathe through nose | Mouth breathing |
| | Diaphragmatic (male) | |
| | Thoracic (female) | |
| | Quiet, smooth, even breathing, relatively passive in nature | Noisy breathing |
| | | Breathing appears labored or painful; accompanied by grunting noises; inspiration interrupted by pain |
| | During inspiration chest expands, costal angle increases, and diaphragm descends and flattens | Irregular breathing patterns such as |

| CHARACTERISTIC OR AREA EXAMINED | NORMAL | DEVIATIONS FROM NORMAL |
|---|---|---|
| | (*Note:* With elderly clients the vital capacity is reduced, and general chest expansion may be somewhat reduced. Calcification at rib articulation points may contribute to decreased chest expansion. These alterations may not be clinically evident.) | Cheyne-Stokes: periods of deep, rapid breaths alternating with periods of apnea<br>Obstructive breathing pattern: expiration period prolonged and labored; may alternate with periods of shallow breathing |
| 3. Rate of respiration | 12 to 20 respirations per minute<br>(*Note:* Anxiety or exertion will increase rate.) | Hyperpnea: increase in rate and depth<br>Tachypnea: increased and relatively shallow respirations<br>Bradypnea: decrease in rate<br>Many heavy sighing respirations may exist in depressed or disturbed emotional states<br>(*Note:* Some elderly clients with a chronic respiratory disturbance may present a general uncoordinated breathing pattern: varying in rate, depth, and chest expansion. The exertion of moving from chair to examining table, of undressing, or sitting up from a lying position may disrupt a breathing pattern. Monitor the client's response to mild exertion.) |
| 4. Posterior chest palpation<br>  **a.** General surface characteristics | Skin feels warm, smooth<br>(*Note:* Elderly clients chill easily in a cool environment.) | Excessively dry or moist skin<br>Poor skin turgor<br>Cold or hot skin<br>Crepitation |
|   **b.** C 7 and T 1 spinal processes | May be quite prominent<br>Kyphosis may be present<br>Spine straight, nontender | Curved spine, tender on palpation |
|   **c.** Scapulae and surrounding musculature | Symmetrical location | Asymmetry<br>Asymmetrical muscle atrophy |
|   **d.** General chest wall | Stable ribs, nontender | Tenderness<br>Masses<br>Crepitation |
| 5. Respiratory excursion | Bilaterally equal expansion of ribs during inspiration (thumbs move equally away from the spine)<br>(*Note:* Elderly client may have some difficulty breathing as deeply as a younger individual.) | Unequal excursion |
| 6. Vocal fremitus response | Response varies among individuals because of intensity and pitch of voice<br>Bilaterally equal mild vibratory sensation<br>Most intense vibrations at upper posterior chest wall medial to scapulae | Increased fremitus: increased vibratory sense accompanies consolidation of lung or portion of lung<br>Decreased fremitus: occurs with decreased production of sound (air blockage) or increase in air space or muscle/tissue space between client's lung and examiner's hands (e.g., emphysema) |
| 7. Entire posterior chest percussion | Resonance throughout lung fields | Hyperresonance found over emphysematous lung |

## Clinical variations: the geriatric client—cont'd

| CHARACTERISTIC OR AREA EXAMINED | NORMAL | DEVIATIONS FROM NORMAL |
|---|---|---|
| **a.** Intensity | Moderately loud | Very loud |
| **b.** Pitch | Low | Very low pitch |
| **c.** Duration | Long | Longer |
| **d.** Quality | Hollow | Booming |
| | (*Note:* Some elderly clients manifest an increased distensibility of lungs and may respond with normal hyperresonance on percussion. However, all beginning examiners should refer hyperresonant responses to a physician.) | Dullness over lung: occurs when fluid or solid tissue replaces normal lung tissue; or fluid in the pleural space |
| | | To identify consolidation, consolidated area must be at least 2 to 3 cm in diameter |
| 8. Diaphragmatic excursion percussion | Diaphragmatic dullness to percussion usually occurs at about tenth rib; level may be slightly higher on right | Asymmetrical response |
| | | Diaphragm lower than usual in severe emphysema |
| | Downward excursion (bilateral) should measure approximately 3 to 5 cm (1 to 2 inches), depending on size, age, and general physical condition of client | Diaphragm higher than usual if there is increase (of any form) of intraabdominal pressure |
| | | Severe limited excursion of diaphragm |
| 9. Posterior chest auscultation (*Note:* Elderly client may have difficulty breathing deeply and holding breath on command.) | Vesicular breath sounds heard over almost all of posterior lung fields | Bronchial breath sounds over peripheral lung |
| | Bronchovesicular breath sounds over right upper posterior lung field | Bronchovesicular breath sounds over peripheral lung |
| | | Adventitious sounds, including: |
| | | Rales: discrete noncontinuous sounds produced by secretions in tracheobronchial tree, usually heard in inspiration |
| | | Fine rales: high-pitched crackling noise heard toward end of inspiration; sound originates in alveoli |
| | | Medium: lower, more moist sound, occurring earlier in inspiration and originating in bronchioles and small bronchi |
| | | Coarse: loud, bubbling sound occurring in larger air passages, can sometimes be cleared with cough |
| | | Rhonchi (wheezes): continuous sounds produced in narrowed air passages may be more prominent on expiration |
| | | Sibilant: high-pitched musical sound occurring on inspiration or expiration, originating in smaller air passages |
| | | Sonorous: low, loud, coarse sound originating in trachea or large bronchi; coughing may alter sound |
| | | Pleural friction rub: dry, rubbing or grating sound usually caused by inflammation of pleural surfaces |

| CHARACTERISTIC OR AREA EXAMINED | NORMAL | DEVIATIONS FROM NORMAL |
|---|---|---|
| 10. Vocal resonance bronchophony: client instructed to say "ninety-nine" | Auscultation sounds muffled: "nin-nin" | Sound increased in loudness and clarity: "ninety-nine" |
| 11. Anterior chest palpation:<br>a. Skin texture and temperature, manubrium, suprasternal notch, sternal angle, second rib, body of sternum, costochondral junctions, costal angle, ribs, and chest wall stability | Smooth, warm skin<br>Stable, nontender chest wall and landmarks<br>Symmetrical musculature<br>Decreased subcutaneous fat | Dry or moist skin<br>Poor skin turgor<br>Cold or hot skin<br>Crepitation<br>Thorax deformities:<br>Pectus excavatum (funnel chest): characterized by depression deformity of lower sternum; may impair breathing or cause compression of heart<br>Pectus carinatum (pigeon chest): characterized by outward deformity of sternum; increase in AP diameter<br>Unequal muscle development, unstable chest wall, masses<br>Tenderness on palpation (fairly common with arthritic clients at rib articulation points) |
| b. Tracheal position | Midline (position may be altered in scoliosis) | Lateral tracheal deviation |
| 12. Vocal fremitus response | Varies from person to person because of intensity and pitch of voice<br>Bilaterally equal mild vibratory sensation<br>Most intense area of vibratory sensation is upper medial chest area, lateral to sternum | Increased fremitus<br>Decreased fremitus<br>Unequal fremitus |
| 13. Anterior chest percussion | Resonance throughout lung fields<br>Flat sounds over sternum or heavy breast tissue<br>Dull sounds over heart or liver<br>Tympany over stomach | Hyperresonance<br>Dullness over lung field |
| 14. Anterior chest auscultation | Vesicular breath sounds over anterior peripheral lung fields<br>Bronchial breath sounds over trachea<br>Bronchovesicular breath sounds over large bronchioles | Bronchial breath sounds over peripheral lung fields<br>Bronchovesicular breath sounds over peripheral lung fields<br>Adventitious sounds such as rales (fine, medium, coarse), rhonchi (sonorous, sibilant), and pleural friction rub |
| 15. Anterior chest vocal resonance<br>a. Bronchophony | Muffled response: "nin-nin" | Sound increased in loudness and clarity: "ninety-nine" |
| 16. Lateral thorax percussion | Resonance over lung area<br>Dull sound as percussion reaches liver (on right) and spleen (on left) | Hyperresonance or dullness over lung fields |
| 17. Lateral thorax auscultation | Vesicular breath sounds | Bronchovesicular breath sounds<br>No breath sounds |

**Cognitive
self-assessment**

Mark each statement "T" or "F."

1. _____ The right lung comprises two lobes, and the left lung comprises three lobes.
2. _____ During inspiration the diaphragm descends and flattens.
3. _____ Biot breathing may be seen in healthy persons.
4. _____ The ratio of respiratory rate to pulse rate normally is 1:6.
5. _____ The nipple line is the common landmark for identifying the midclavicular line for all patients, with the exception of large-breasted women.
6. _____ In palpating for rib identification, the initial rib felt below the clavicle is the first rib.

7. Complete the following table.

| Breath sounds | Comparison of duration: inspiration vs. expiration (use < and >) | Sample location |
|---|---|---|
| Vesicular | Inspiration _____ expiration | _____ |
| Bronchovesicular | Inspiration _____ expiration | _____ |
| Bronchial | Inspiration _____ expiration | _____ |

8. The trachea bifurcates at about the level of the:
   ☐ a. cricoid cartilage
   ☐ b. manubrium
   ☐ c. costal angle
   ☐ d. sternal angle
   ☐ e. sternum
9. Tactile fremitus will be *decreased* with:
   ☐ a. pneumonia (consolidation of lung)
   ☐ b. chronic obstructive diseases
   ☐ c. area of atelectasis
   ☐ d. pneumothorax
   ☐ e. large airway obstruction
   ☐ f. all the above
   ☐ g. all except e
   ☐ h. a, c, and d
   ☐ i. all except b
   ☐ j. all except a
10. The best place to feel for tactile fremitus is:
    ☐ a. the lower lateral chest wall
    ☐ b. high in the axillary lateral chest wall
    ☐ c. the posterior lower chest wall
    ☐ d. over the scapulae—posterior chest wall
    ☐ e. over the anterior chest, second or third ribs near the sternum
11. When percussing the posterior chest for inspiratory-expiratory excursion, one would expect to *normally* measure which of the following excursion distances?
    ☐ a. Over 6 cm ($2\frac{1}{2}$ inches)
    ☐ b. 4 to 6 cm ($1\frac{1}{2}$ to $2\frac{1}{2}$ inches)
    ☐ c. 3 to 5 cm (1 to 2 inches)
    ☐ d. 2 to 4 cm ($\frac{3}{4}$ inch to $1\frac{1}{2}$ inches)
    ☐ e. Below 3 cm (1 inch)

12. A client with increased density of the lung caused by pneumonia would be expected to have which of the following lung percussion tones?
    - ☐ a. Resonance
    - ☐ b. Hyperresonance
    - ☐ c. Tympany
    - ☐ d. Dullness
    - ☐ e. Flatness

13. Bronchial breath sounds are normal when heard:
    - ☐ a. over the posterior lateral chest at the level of the scapulae
    - ☐ b. between the scapulae
    - ☐ c. over the trachea
    - ☐ d. in the anterior chest upper lateral areas
    - ☐ e. nowhere throughout the chest

14. A wheeze during expiration is most likely:
    - ☐ a. sibilant rhonchi
    - ☐ b. sonorous rhonchi
    - ☐ c. pleural friction rub
    - ☐ d. fine rales
    - ☐ e. medium rales

15. A high-pitched crackling noise heard toward the end of inspiration is most likely:
    - ☐ a. sibilant rhonchi
    - ☐ b. sonorous rhonchi
    - ☐ c. pleural friction rub
    - ☐ d fine rales
    - ☐ e. medium rales

**PEDIATRIC QUESTIONS**

16. The *normal* newborn may demonstrate which of the following breathing patterns?
    - ☐ a. Cheyne-Stokes
    - ☐ b. Biot
    - ☐ c. Kussmaul respirations
    - ☐ d. Stertorous respirations
    - ☐ e. Tachypnea
    - ☐ f. b and d
    - ☐ g. a and b
    - ☐ h. a, c, and d
    - ☐ i. all except e
    - ☐ j. all the above

17. When examining a 6-month-old child, the nurse must evaluate respiratory rate and depth as well as breath sound and percussion quality. Which of the following would indicate a *normal* response?

|  | Respiration rate | Expiratory distance | Breath sound | Percussion tone |
|---|---|---|---|---|
| ☐ a. | 52 | 3 inches | Vesicular | Hyperresonant |
| ☐ b. | 18 | 2 inches | Bronchovesicular | Resonant |
| ☐ c. | 22 | 5 inches | Vesicular | Hyperresonant |
| ☐ d. | 32 | 4 inches | Bronchovesicular | Hyperresonant |
| ☐ e. | 36 | 6 inches | Bronchovesicular | Resonant |

18. When evaluating the vocal fremitus in a small child, which of the following client participation sounds would be most helpful?
    - ☐ a. Crying
    - ☐ b. No noise
    - ☐ c. Babbling
    - ☐ d. Whispering

19. *One* of the following examples demonstrates an abnormal finding requiring physician referral. Identify the child needing referral.
    - ☐ a. Twelve-year-old boy, respiration rate 18/min, vesicular breath sounds over periphery of lungs, resonant percussion tones over lung fields
    - ☐ b. Nine-year-old girl, thoracic breathing, respiration rate 18/min, vesicular breath sounds over periphery of lungs, resonant percussion tones over lung fields
    - ☐ c. Six-month-old girl, abdominal breathing, respiration rate 37/min, bronchovesicular breath sounds, hyperresonant percussion tone
    - ☐ d. One-year-old boy, abdominal breathing, respiration rate 20/min, bronchovesicular breath sounds throughout lung fields, resonant percussion tones
    - ☐ e. Two-year-old girl, abdominal breathing, respiration rate 44/min, bronchovesicular breath sounds through lung fields, hyperresonant percussion tones

**GERIATRIC QUESTIONS**

20. The aging process of the lungs usually involves:
    - ☐ a. decreased residual volume
    - ☐ b. decreased vital capacity
    - ☐ c. decreased chest wall compliance
    - ☐ d. decreased force of elastic recoil of the lungs
    - ☐ e. decreased anteroposterior chest diameter
    - ☐ f. all the above
    - ☐ g. a, c, and e
    - ☐ h. a and d
    - ☐ i. b, c, and d
    - ☐ j. none of the above

21. Some of the risk factors for respiratory disability in elderly people include:
    - ☐ a. smoking
    - ☐ b. difficulty swallowing
    - ☐ c. history of frequent respiratory infections
    - ☐ d. immobility
    - ☐ e. decreased physical fitness
    - ☐ f. all the above
    - ☐ g. all except b
    - ☐ h. a, c, and e
    - ☐ i. a and d

22. In the older adult total lung capacity:
    - ☐ a. is markedly diminished by 80 years of age
    - ☐ b. increases significantly
    - ☐ c. does not change significantly

## SUGGESTED READINGS
### General

Barber, J.M., Stokes, L.G., and Billings, D.M.: Adult and child care: a client approach to nursing, ed. 2, St. Louis, 1977, The C.V. Mosby Co., pp. 765-774.

Bates, B.: A guide to physical examination, ed. 3, Philadelphia, 1983, J.B. Lippincott Co., pp. 125-165.

DeGowin, E., and DeGowin, R.: Bedside diagnostic examination, ed. 3, New York, 1976, Macmillan Publishing Co., Inc., pp. 259-322.

Judge, R.D., and Zuidema, G., editors: Methods of clinical examination: a physiologic approach, Boston, 1974, Little, Brown & Co., pp. 105-140.

Littman, D.: Stethoscopes and auscultation, Am. J. Nurs. **72**(7):1238-1241, 1972.

Malasanos, L., and others: Health assessment, ed. 2, St. Louis, 1981, The C.V. Mosby Co., pp. 298-320.

Nordmark, M.T., and Rohweder, A.W.: Scientific foundations of nursing, ed. 3, Philadelphia, 1975, J.B. Lippincott Co., pp. 53-77.

Patient assessment: examination of the chest and lungs, Am. J. Nurs. **76**(9):1-23, 1976.

Traver, G.: Assessment of thorax and lungs, Am. J. Nurs. **73**(3):466-471, 1973.

### Pediatric

Alexander, M., and Brown, M.S.: Physical examination. XII. Chest and lungs, Nursing '75 **5**(1):44-48, 1975.

Barness, L.: Manual of pediatric physical diagnosis, ed. 5, Chicago, 1981, Year Book Medical Publishers, Inc, pp.110-144.

Johnson, T., Moore, W., and Jeffries, J., editors: Children are different: developmental physiology, ed. 2, Montreal, 1978, Ross Laboratories, pp. 127-133.

Lowery, G.H.: Growth and development of children, ed. 6, Chicago, 1973, Year Book Medical Publishers, Inc., p. 186.

Prior, J.A., Silberstein, J.S., and Stang, J.M.: Physical diagnosis: the history and examination of the patient, ed. 6, St. Louis, 1981, The C.V. Mosby Co., pp. 481-483.

### Geriatric

Burnside, I.M., editor: Nursing and the aged, New York, 1981, McGraw-Hill Book Co., pp. 234-236, 242-244.

Caird, F.I., and Judge, T.G.: Assessment of the elderly patient, London, 1977, Pitman Medical Publishing Co. Ltd., pp. 26-30.

Campbell, E.J., and LeFrak, S.: How aging affects the structure and function of the respiratory system, Geriatrics **33**(6):68-74, 1978.

Carotenuto, R., and Bullock, J.: Physical assessment of the gerontologic client, Philadelphia, 1980, F.A. Davis Co., pp. 69-79.

Steinberg, F.U., editor: Care of the geriatric patient, ed. 6, St. Louis, 1983, The C.V. Mosby Co., pp. 9-11, 105-117.

ASSESSMENT OF THE

# Cardiovascular system

## VOCABULARY

**angina pectoris** Paroxysmal pain in chest, often associated with myocardial ischemia; pain patterns and severity vary among individuals; pain sometimes radiates to neck, jaw, or left arm; may be accompanied by choking or smothering sensations.

**arteriosclerosis** General term denoting hardening and thickening of the arterial walls. Atherosclerosis is one type of arteriosclerosis.

**atherosclerosis** The formation of plaques within arterial walls resulting in thickening of the walls and narrowing of the lumen; end organs supplied by these vessels receive diminished circulation.

**atrial fibrillation** Rapid, involuntary, random atrial contractions that cause rapid, irregular ventricular contractions and diminished cardiac output; this arrhythmia results from chaotic electrical impulses within the atrial myocardium.

**atrial flutter** Rapid atrial rhythm (approximately 300 per minute) that may or may not cause ventricular tachycardia, depending on the degree of A-V (atrioventricular) blocking.

**auscultatory gap** A phenomenon sometimes experienced by an examiner listening for blood pressure sounds; temporary silent interval between systolic and diastolic sounds that may cover a range of 40 mm Hg; commonly occurs with hypertensive clients with a wide pulse pressure.

**bigeminal pulse** Abnormal pulse characterized by a strong beat and a weaker one in close succession, followed by a pause when no beat is felt; pulse is irregular in rhythm; associated with premature contractions, digitalis toxicity, or a partial heart block.

**bisferiens pulse** Abnormal pulse characterized by two main peaks; occurs with aortic stenosis and/or regurgitation.

**bradycardia** An abnormally slowed heart rate, usually under 50 beats per minute. *Note:* Conditioned athletes often manifest a normally slowed rate of 50 beats, or slightly less, per minute.

**bruit** Audible murmur (a blowing sound) heard in auscultating over a peripheral vessel or an organ.

**coarctation** Stricture or narrowing of the wall of a vessel.

**diastole** Period of time within the cardiac cycle in which ventricles are relaxed and filling with blood.

**ectopic** Describes an event that occurs in an unusual manner or form; in reference to the heart, it could pertain to an extra beat or contraction.

**embolus** A foreign object (composed of air, fat, or clustered cellular elements) that circulates through the blood and usually lodges in a vessel, causing some degree of occlusion.

**gallop rhythm** Audible extra heart sound in the diastolic interval. A *protodiastolic* sound, or *ventricular* gallop, is heard shortly after $S_2$. A late diastolic sound is called a *presystolic,* or *atrial,* gallop. A *summation* gallop is a combination of four sounds within a cycle and includes both protodiastolic and presystolic sounds.

**heave** Palpable diffuse, sustained lift of the chest wall or a portion of the wall.

**hepatojugular reflux** A phenomenon, indicating right heart failure, in which venous pressure rises when the upper abdomen is compressed for 30 to 45 seconds; upon upper right quadrant compression, increased prominence of the jugular vein is noted.

**holosystolic (pansystolic)** Pertaining to the entire systolic interval; usually refers to an audible murmur.

**Homans sign** Calf pain associated with rapid dorsiflexion of the foot, often indicative of thrombophlebitis.

**hyperkinetic** Hyperactive.

**hypovolemic** Pertaining to decreased blood volume; usually refers to a state of shock resulting from massive blood loss and inadequate tissue perfusion.

**"inching"** Recommended method for moving the stethoscope over the precordium while listening for heart sounds; small, sliding movements (vs. lifting and lowering stethoscope from side to side) may enable the listener to hear more sounds.

**infarct** Localized area of tissue necrosis caused by prolonged anoxia.

**intermittent claudication** Condition characterized by symptoms of pain, aching, cramping, and localized fatigue of the legs that occur while walking but can be quickly relieved by rest (2 to 5 minutes); discomfort occurs most often in the calf but may arise in the foot, thigh, hip, or buttock; caused by prolonged ischemia.

**ischemia** Diminished blood supply to an organ or body part.

**Korotkoff sounds** Sounds heard during the taking of blood pressure; an inflated cuff encircles a limb and obstructs normal blood flow through the arteries; as the cuff is released, turbulent blood flow creates a series of sounds that enable the listener to determine systolic and diastolic pressures.

**NSR (normal sinus rhythm)** The heart rate that originates within sinoatrial (S-A) node in right atrium; average adult heart beats 72 to 78 times per minute while at rest.

**palpitation** Sensation of pounding, fluttering, or racing of the heart; can be a normal phenomenon or caused by a disorder of the heart.

**paradoxical pulse** Diminished pulse amplitude on inspiration and increased amplitude on expiration; an exaggeration of a normal response to respiration; often associated with obstructive lung disease.

**PMI (point of maximum impulse)** Specific area of the chest where the heart beat is palpated most clearly; usually the apical impulse, a brief systolic beat in the fourth-fifth intercostal space, 7 to 9 cm left of the midsternal line.

**precordium** Area of the chest that overlies the heart and adjacent great vessels.

**pulse deficit** A discrepancy between the ventricular rate auscultated over the heart and the arterial rate palpated over the radial artery; caused by a ventricle that contracts with a partially filled chamber and is unable to produce a palpable pulse with each beat.

**pulse pressure** The difference between systolic and diastolic pressures, usually within the range of 30 to 40 mm Hg; tends to increase as systolic pressure rises with arteriosclerosis of the large vessels (specifically the aorta); can be altered with vigorous exercise, fever, or other disease states.

**pulsus alternans** Alternating pulse; abnormal pulse characterized by a regular rhythm in which a strong beat alternates

with a weaker one; sometimes differences in amplitude are subtle and more easily distinguished during taking of blood pressure; associated with severe hypertension, coronary artery disease, and left ventricular failure.

**sinus arrhythmia** Normal pulse pattern commonly occurring in some children and young adults; characterized by speeding up of the pulse rate on inspiration and slowing down on expiration.

**systole** Period of time within the cardiac cycle in which the ventricles are contracted and ejecting blood into the aorta and pulmonary artery.

**tachycardia** Rapid heart rate (usually over 100 beats per minute); normally occurs with exercise, excitement, anxiety, or fever, but can also indicate abnormal states such as anemia, heart failure, or shock.

**thrill** Palpable murmur described as feeling like the throat of a purring cat.

**thrombophlebitis** An inflammation of a vein often associated with clot formation; can be induced by trauma, prolonged immobility, postoperative venous stasis, infection, or blood hypercoagulation disorder.

**thrombus** Blood clot attached to the inner wall of a vessel; usually causes some degree of occlusion.

## Cognitive objectives

At the end of this chapter the learner will demonstrate knowledge of assessment of the cardiovascular system by the ability to do the following:

1. Identify the characteristics and phases of Korotkoff sounds.
2. Record a blood pressure, identifying the variables of auscultatory gap, first and second diastolic pressures, and pulse pressure.
3. Point out the common variables that alter blood pressure in healthy individuals.
4. Identify the characteristics of arterial pulse that an examiner notes with inspection and palpation.
5. Name the causes attributed to selected variations of arterial pulse characteristics.
6. State the major differences between observable signs of chronic venous insufficiency and chronic arterial insufficiency.
7. Identify the major differences between carotid and jugular pulsation.
8. Point out some major characteristics of the normal jugular veins and jugular venous pressure.
9. Describe the major characteristics and causes of leg varicosities.
10. Identify and locate the anatomical positions of the heart, the major components of the heart, and adjacent great vessels.
11. Identify some major characteristics of normal signs elicited during inspection and palpation of the precordium.
12. Explain the appropriate purpose and use of the bell and diaphragm of the stethoscope.
13. Identify the origin of the first and second heart sounds.
14. Describe the major auscultatory characteristics of the first and second heart sounds in terms of:
    a. Location
    b. Intensity
    c. Frequency
    d. Timing
    e. Splitting
15. Identify the origin and major characteristics of the third and fourth heart sounds.
16. Recognize the following precordial auscultatory areas and identify selected auscultatory events in each area:
    a. Aortic area
    b. Pulmonary area
    c. Third left interspace
    d. Tricuspid area
    e. Apical area
17. Point out the following six characteristics of cardiac murmurs that must be described during their assessment:
    a. Timing: systole, diastole, continuous
    b. Location: using precordial landmarks and/or distance in centimeters from a landmark
    c. Radiation: described in centimeters, landmarks
    d. Intensity: grades 1 through 6, or loud, medium, soft
    e. Pitch: high, medium, low
    f. Quality: blowing, harsh, rumbling, crescendo, decrescendo
18. Identify the origin and selected major characteristics of systolic and diastolic murmurs.
19. Recognize selected major characteristics of "innocent" murmurs.
20. Identify selected common cardiovascular variations in pediatric and geriatric clients.
21. Use the terms in the vocabulary section.

## Clinical objectives

At the end of this chapter the learner will perform a systematic assessment of the cardiovascular system, demonstrating the ability to do the following:

1. Obtain a pertinent health history from a client.
2. Palpate and auscultate arterial blood pressure.
3. Assess carotid, radial, femoral, popliteal, dorsalis pedis, and posterior tibial pulses through inspection and palpation for:
   a. Rate
   b. Rhythm
   c. Amplitude
   d. Variations in amplitude
   e. Contour
   f. Symmetry
4. Conduct a predesignated maneuver to test for arterial sufficiency in extremities.
5. Evaluate and describe jugular venous pressure.
6. Inspect and describe jugular pulsation quality.
7. Inspect, palpate, and describe the appearance of superficial veins and surface characteristics of the legs.
8. Maneuver the foot and describe the results of an assessment for calf pains.
9. Inspect and palpate the extremities for arterial and venous sufficiency.
10. Observe and describe the client's general condition (at rest) in terms of:
    a. Positioning and comfort
    b. Ease of respirations (in supine or 30- to 45-degree position)
    c. General skin color
11. Inspect and palpate the anterior chest precordium, sternoclavicular, aortic, pulmonary, right ventricular, apical, epigastric, and ectopic areas for:
    a. Contour
    b. General movement

c. Pulsations

d. Heaves or lifts

12. Palpate and describe the results of assessment of the apical impulse for:

a. Amplitude

b. Duration

c. Location

d. Diameter

13. Locate and auscultate the following sites with a stethoscope bell and diaphragm:

a. Aortic area

b. Pulmonary area

c. Third left interspace

d. Tricuspid area

e. Apical area

14. Describe the results of cardiac auscultation in terms of:

a. Rate

b. Rhythm

c. $S_1$: location, intensity, frequency, timing, and splitting

d. $S_2$: location, intensity, frequency, timing, and splitting

e. Systole: relative duration

f. Diastole: relative duration

15. Identify additional systolic or diastolic sounds in terms of:

a. Timing

b. Location

c. Radiation

d. Intensity

e. Pitch

f. Quality

16. Auscultate and describe cardiac sounds while the client is supine, turned to left decubitus position, and sitting up.

17. Summarize the results with a written description of findings.

## Health history additional to screening history

1. If the client complains of leg pains (cramps), inquire about specific situations or activities that worsen or relieve the problem.

a. *Arterial insufficiency* results in pain that worsens with activity, particularly prolonged exercise (e.g., walking). The pain is usually quickly (within 2 minutes) relieved with cessation of movement (standing). Pain may occasionally occur when limbs are elevated and be relieved with dangling of feet. Claudication distance should be specified. Determine how many average city blocks (or yards, numbers of stairs, etc.) a client walks before pain occurs. Remember that variables such as a hilly terrain, walking in start-stop heavy traffic areas, environmental temperature, and pace of walking affect exertion intensity. Signs and symptoms indicating a severe problem are:

(1) Sudden decrease in claudication distance

(2) Diminished or absent pulses or cold, mottled, or bluish extremities

(3) Cutaneous changes, such as reddened pressure areas, ulcers, taut shiny skin

(4) Pain not relieved by rest

Pain is most commonly located in the calf but may be in the lower leg or dorsum of the foot. Hip, buttock, or thigh pain may be present. The client should provide a clear description of the pain (e.g., numbness, feeling of cold, burning, tingling, sharp cramp, aching). Risk factors include family history of diabetes, vascular disease, or heart disease, hyperlipidemia, hypertension, and smoking.

b. *Venous insufficiency* pain intensifies with prolonged standing or sitting in one position. Relief often occurs by elevating the leg, lying down, or exercise (walking). Edema often accompanies the problem. Varicosities may be present. Discomfort may be increased at the end of the day. Pain is commonly located in the calf and lower leg. It may be described as an aching, tiredness, or feeling of fullness. Risk factors include occupation involving prolonged sitting or standing, family or client history of varicosities, overweight, constrictive clothing (e.g., garters, girdles), pregnancy, history of thrombophlebitis, chronic systemic disease (e.g., heart disease, cirrhosis, hypertension).

c. Neurologically caused pain exhibits fewer predictable patterns. The pain often occurs at night and awakens the client. The pain may be associated with exercise or movement, but nothing in particular relieves it. There is usually no edema, cyanosis, cold extremities, or marked cutaneous changes associated with it. The pain may locate in the calf. A family or client history of diabetes mellitus should always be inquired about.

d. There may be other causes for leg pain, such as the following:

(1) New type of shoe (e.g., very high heels, "negative heel" shoes)

(2) Foot problems (with inadequate shoe support)

(3) Participation in new type of exercise or increased exercise

(4) Problems with back and pain radiating to legs (more information in Chapter 14)

(5) Recent injury

e. Clients who complain of leg pain at night should clarify what specifically relieves it (e.g., rubbing leg, walking, dangling) and the duration of pain.

f. All leg pain complaints should be treated with a full symptom analysis. The preceding descriptions may help the examiner to categorize a profile.

2. The following questions concern heart disease and hypertension:

a. Have you experienced any visual changes? Loss of consciousness? Headaches? Marked weakness or fatigue?

b. Are there any new or marked stress factors in your life (home, work, family, friends)?

c. Have you noticed a weight change in the last 6 months?

d. Do you feel dizzy? Does your body position affect the dizziness? (Postural hypotension might affect the client's safety in the home.) Have you ever fallen down?

e. If orthopnea and paroxysmal nocturnal dyspnea are present, inquire about sleep habits.

f. If edema is present, inquire about the times of day when it is most apparent (e.g., first thing in the morning vs. late afternoon or evening).

g. Inquire closely about medications being consumed. (If nitroglycerin or other "prn" preparations are being taken, determine how often per day.) Review over-the-counter medications carefully. Some antacid medications contain large amounts of sodium. Many cold preparations (antitussives, decongestants), nose drops, nasal sprays, and weight control preparations contain sympathomimetic amines.

## EXERTION/EXERCISE PROFILE (SAMPLE FORM)

| | Sleeping | Lying down | Sitting | Light exercise* | Moderate exercise† | Moderately heavy exercise‡ | Other§ |
|---|---|---|---|---|---|---|---|
| Hr/day | 8 | 3 to 4 | 4 | 3 | 2 to 3 | | Twenty-eight stairs (climbs b.i.d.) |
| Hr/wk | | | | | 5 to 6 (short walks to shopping center) | 5 to 6 (heavy housework; occasional long walks) | |
| Hr/mo | | | | | | | |
| Symptoms and problems | None | Feels tired if unable to take AM and PM naps | None | None | None (but carries out daily routines at slow pace) | Occasional SOB; must rest after heavy housework | Feels "winded" midway at landing; rests 2 min |

*Walking from one room to another, fixing small meals, etc.

†Light housework, making bed, sweeping floor, dusting, office work, short walks (flat surface), etc.

‡Scrubbing floors, sexual intercourse, long walks (specify amount), stair climbing (specify flights), lifting, construction work, etc.

§Long periods of standing, exercise programs, jogging, stair climbing (may be recorded as unusual activity if many flights are climbed frequently).

h. Inquire closely about dietary habits. Consider calorie, cholesterol, and salt intakes.

i. For clients with a history of heart disease, severe hypertension, or vascular disease, it may be helpful to establish an exertion/exercise profile. Definitions of light, moderate, or heavy exercise can be established in advance by the examiner or agency or can be defined for individual clients. The profile can be renewed periodically to follow the client's progress. (See sample form on p. 238.)

j. Chronic pain, shortness of breath, fatigue, or other symptoms must be related to reduction or change in functions of daily living. For example, dyspnea increases with stair climbing, and a client might live four flights up in an apartment building. Many people have to walk to the gro-

cery store every day. Interference with sleep, work environment, physical demands, and family relationships should be explored.

3. Chest pain profile. Table 9-1 is not intended to be a complete guide to differential diagnosis. Gastrointestinal and musculoskeletal problems can mimic angina. It will, however, provide some ideas about specific questions to pose.

4. Risk factors for cardiovascular disease:
   a. Family history of diabetes mellitus, heart disease (especially under age 60), hypertension, or vascular disease.
   b. Client history of hyperlipoproteinemia, diabetes, hypertension, obesity, heavy cigarette smoking, lack of physical exercise, stressful life-style ("stressful" must be carefully defined by client)
   c. Age (increasing incidence over 30 years)

**TABLE 9-1.** Chest pain profile*

|  | ANGINA PECTORIS | ESOPHAGITIS | MUSCULOSKELETAL PROBLEMS |
|---|---|---|---|
| Precipitated by | Effort (usually emotion, exercise, eating) | Eating<br>Nervousness | Motion, especially neck movement<br>Hyperventilation<br>Coughing |
| Duration | 10 to 15 min | Variable (up to several hours) | Variable |
| Alleviated by | Stopping activity or rest (often in 2 to 3 min)<br>Nitroglycerin | Eructation<br>Sitting upright<br>Eating<br>Antacids | Heat<br>Analgesic<br>Change of position |
| Worsening of pain | Soon after rising (AM)<br>After heavy meal | Any time (especially at night) | Bedtime or after day of exertion |
| Onset | Often remembers date (pain seldom continues over 5 years without developing abnormal exercise ECG) | Uncertain | Uncertain |
| Disease | Myocardial infarction, diabetes, hypertension, rheumatic heart disease, obesity, indigestion | Indigestion | Trauma |

*Data from Warner-Chilcott Laboratory, AEGIS Production: Differential diagnosis of chest pain, New York, 1967, American Heart Association. Wasson, J., Walsh, B.T., Tompkins, R., and Sox, H.: The common symptom guide, New York, 1975, McGraw-Hill Book Co.

## Clinical guidelines

| THE STUDENT WILL: | TO IDENTIFY: | |
| --- | --- | --- |
| | NORMAL | DEVIATIONS FROM NORMAL |
| **1.** Assemble equipment:<br>  **a.** Stethoscope<br>  **b.** Sphygmomanometer | | |
| **2.** Palpate, then auscultate brachial artery to determine arterial blood pressure in both arms (See *Clinical strategies* for description of procedure for measuring blood pressure.) | Varies with sex, body weight, time of day<br>Other variables that can be somewhat controlled by examiner are listed in *Clinical strategies* | |
| | Upper limits (adult):<br>  140 mm Hg systolic<br>  90 mm Hg diastolic<br>  30 to 40 mm Hg pulse pressure | Elevated systolic ( ↑ 140)*<br>Elevated diastolic ( ↑ 90)*<br>Widened pulse pressure<br>Narrow pulse pressure<br>Low systolic ( ↓ 90)<br>Low diastolic ( ↓ 60) |
| | Pressure in both arms is same or does not vary more than 5 to 10 mm Hg systolic | Significant ( ↑ 5 to 10 mm Hg) discrepancy in pressure readings between upper extremities |
| **3.** Measure blood pressure while client is standing (as well as lying) if client offers history or complaint of syncope or dizziness or is taking antihypertensive medications | On standing, client may manifest drop of maximum of 10 to 15 mm Hg (systolic) and 5 mm Hg (diastolic) | Significant decrease of systolic (more than 15 mm Hg) or diastolic (more than 5 mm Hg) and/or symptoms of dizziness |
| **4.** Measure blood pressure in both legs if pedal, popliteal, and femoral pulses are weak or absent (See *Clinical strategies* for technique.) | Popliteal artery auscultation reveals systolic pressure 5 to 15 mm Hg higher than brachial artery measurement; diastolic reading is same or slightly lower | Systolic pressure is lower in leg(s) than in arms |
| **5.** Palpate both carotid arteries<br>  **a.** Use flat surface of first three finger pads<br>  **b.** Place fingers between trachea and sternocleidomastoid muscle under mandible<br>  **c.** Client should flex neck and rotate head slightly toward side being examined (Fig. 9-1) | | |

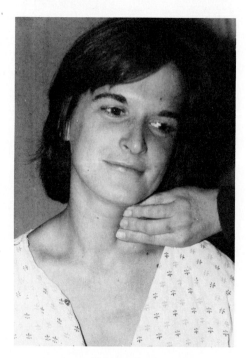

**FIG. 9-1.** Palpating for carotid pulse.

*If pressure is elevated, especially if accompanied by rapid pulse, repeat in 30 minutes.

| THE STUDENT WILL: | TO IDENTIFY: | |
| --- | --- | --- |
| | NORMAL | DEVIATIONS FROM NORMAL |
| **d.** Palpate one artery at a time for: | | |
| 1. Rate | 60 to 90 beats/min (conditioned athletes may be as low as 50/min) | ↑ 90/min (tachycardia) (*Note:* Recent exertion, smoking, or anxiety will elevate pulse.) ↓ 60/min (bradycardia) |
| 2. Rhythm | Regular (*Note:* Slight transient increase in rate during inspiration, especially in clients under 40 years.) | Irregular, without any pattern (e.g., atrial fibrillation) Regularity with occasional pauses or extra beats (e.g., premature contractions) Coupled beats (e.g., bigeminal pulse)* |
| 3. Pulse amplitude and contour | Upstroke smooth, rounded, prompt | Upstroke exaggerated or bounding Pulse weak, small, or thready; peak prolonged |
| 4. Amplitude pattern† | Series of pulse strokes unvaried in amplitude or contour | Upstrokes vary (e.g., strong and weaker beats alternate [pulsus alternans]) Force of beat reduced during inspiration (paradoxical pulse) |
| 5. Symmetry | Symmetrical response (i.e., both carotid pulses manifest same rate, rhythm, amplitude, and contour) | Asymmetrical response |
| 6. Arterial wall contour and consistency | Soft and pliable | Increased resistance to compression; beaded or tortuous |

**6.** Using finger pads of first three fingers, palpate:
   **a.** Both radial pulses at medial aspect of wrist (Fig. 9-2)
   **b.** Both femoral pulses, immediately inferior to inguinal ligament, midway between anterior superior iliac spine and pubic tubercle (*Note:* Firmer compression may be necessary for accurate palpation of obese clients.) (Fig. 9-3)

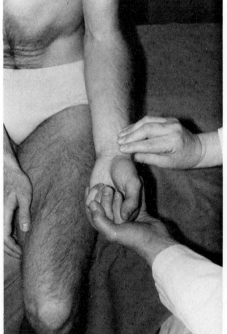

**FIG. 9-2.** Radial artery palpation.

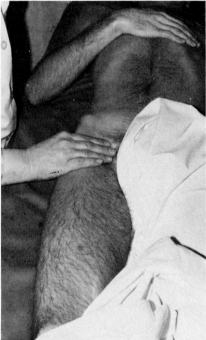

**FIG. 9-3.** Femoral artery palpation.

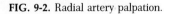

*An irregular, rapid, or slow pulse should be palpated simultaneously with auscultation of the apical pulse. Any difference between apical and peripheral pulse rate should be noted. If pulse irregularity is patterned (occurs in repeated sequences), note whether irregularity occurs during (1) inspiration or expiration and (2) systole or diastole.
†Pulse *amplitude* can be varied or uneven, and pulse *rate* can remain regular or may be irregular.

# Clinical guidelines—cont'd

| THE STUDENT WILL: | TO IDENTIFY: | |
| --- | --- | --- |
| | NORMAL | DEVIATIONS FROM NORMAL |

c. Both popliteal pulses: press fingers firmly into popliteal fossae (Fig. 9-4)

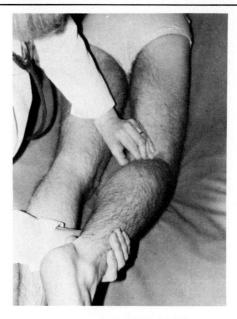

**FIG. 9-4.** Popliteal artery palpation.

d. Both dorsalis pedis pulses: press lightly over dorsum of foot; foot should be moderately dorsiflexed (Fig. 9-5)

e. Both posterior tibial pulses: curve fingers behind and slightly inferior to medial malleolus of ankle (Fig. 9-6)

(*Note:* Dorsalis pedis pulses may be difficult to find or absent in some normal individuals.)

(*Note:* Posterior tibial pulses may also be absent in some normal individuals.)

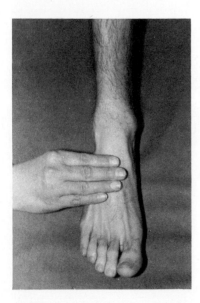

**FIG. 9-5.** Dorsalis pedis artery palpation.

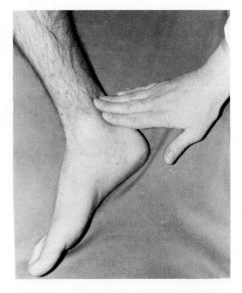

**FIG. 9-6.** Posterior tibial artery palpation.

| THE STUDENT WILL: | TO IDENTIFY: | |
| --- | --- | --- |
| | NORMAL | DEVIATIONS FROM NORMAL |
| 7. Palpate all pulses for: | | |
| a. Symmetrical response | All pulses should be full, strong, and symmetrical | Any asymmetry in force or pulse contour |
| b. Arterial wall contour and consistency | Soft and pliable | Increased resistance to compression; beaded or tortuous |
| 8. Conduct the following maneuver if arterial insufficiency is suspected: | | |
| a. With client lying down, elevate client's legs 30 cm (12 inches) above heart level | | |
| b. Ask client to move feet up and down at ankles for 60 seconds | Extremities (feet) exhibit mild pallor | Marked pallor of one or both feet |
| c. Have client sit up and dangle legs | Original color returns in about 10 seconds | Delayed color return or mottled appearance (Fig. 9-7) |
| (This maneuver can also be conducted with arms and hands.) | Veins in feet fill in about 15 seconds | Delayed venous filling |
| | | Marked redness of dependent feet |
| 9. Evaluate venous pressure by inspecting both sides of client's neck as he lies at 30° to 45° angle; elevate chin slightly and tilt away from side being examined | | |

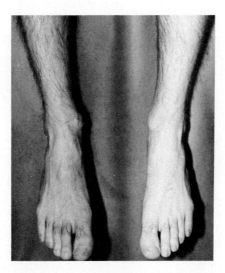

**FIG. 9-7.** Arterial insufficiency with contrasting pallor of foot in dependent position. Note increased venous filling on normal foot.

# Clinical guidelines—cont'd

| | TO IDENTIFY: | |
|---|---|---|
| **THE STUDENT WILL:** | **NORMAL** | **DEVIATIONS FROM NORMAL** |
| **10.** Identify highest point at which jugular vein blood level or pulsations can be seen, using sternal angle as reference point for "zero" level; estimate jugular venous pressure (JVP) in centimeters | JVP should not rise more than 3 cm (1 inch) above level of sternal angle* (Fig. 9-8) | JVP exceeds 3 cm above level of manubrium† (Fig. 9-9)<br>Note if other veins in neck, shoulder, and upper chest are distended |

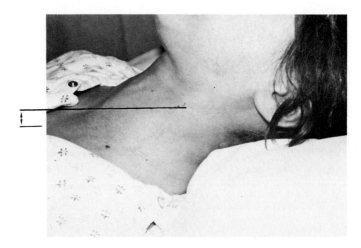

FIG. 9-8. Normal jugular venous pressure in external jugular vein. Blood level is less than 3 cm above the sternal angle.

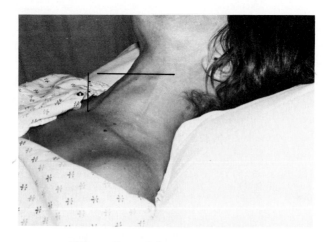

FIG. 9-9. Distended external jugular vein.

| | | |
|---|---|---|
| **11.** Inspect jugular pulsations for quality | Regular<br>Soft and undulating<br>Level of pulsation decreases with inspiration<br>Pulsation increases in recumbent position | Fluttering or oscillating<br>Irregular rhythm<br>Unusually prominent waves |

*If jugular vein is difficult to locate, ask client to lie flat for a few minutes. Neck vein (particularly external jugular) should distend with client in this position.

†If venous pressure is elevated (vein is distended up to neck), raise client's head until highest jugular pulsation can be detected. Record distance in centimeters above sternal angle *and* angle at which client is reclining.

| THE STUDENT WILL: | TO IDENTIFY: NORMAL | DEVIATIONS FROM NORMAL |
|---|---|---|
| 12. Inspect and palpate legs for presence and/or appearance of superficial veins | Distention in dependent position<br>Venous valves may appear as nodular bulges<br>Veins collapse with elevation of limbs | Distended veins in anteromedial aspect of thigh and lower leg or on posterolateral aspect of calf from knee to ankle (Fig. 9-10) |

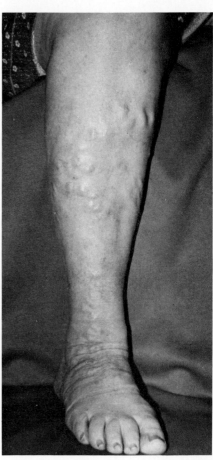

**FIG. 9-10.** Distended veins on lower leg with nodular bulges.

| | | |
|---|---|---|
| 13. Inspect and palpate thigh and calf for surface characteristics | Legs symmetrical<br>Nontender<br>No excess warmth | Swelling (or one leg, especially calf, appears larger than other)*<br>Tenderness on palpation<br>Warmth<br>Redness |
| 14. Sharply dorsiflex client's foot (with knee slightly flexed) to assess calf pain response | No pain | Pain (Homans sign) |
| 15. Inspect and palpate extremities for evidence of adequate arterial supply | Absence of hair over digits or dorsum of hands and feet may be normal<br><br>Skin pink and warm, nonedematous | Reduced or absent peripheral hair (over digits and dorsum of hands and feet)<br><br>Thin, shiny, taut skin<br>Cold extremities (in warm environment)<br>Mild edema |

*If swelling is suspected, both thighs and calves should be measured with a tape to ensure accuracy.

## Clinical guidelines—cont'd

| THE STUDENT WILL: | TO IDENTIFY: | |
| --- | --- | --- |
| | NORMAL | DEVIATIONS FROM NORMAL |
| **16.** Inspect and palpate extremities for evidence of venous sufficiency | | Marked pallor or mottling when extremity is elevated |
| | | Digit tips ulcerated |
| | | Stocking anesthesia |
| | | Tenderness on palpation |
| | | Peripheral cyanosis |
| | | Edema (pits on pressure), bilateral or unilateral* |
| | | Pigmentation around ankles (See Fig. 3-2.) |
| | | Thickening skin |
| | | Ulceration (especially around ankles) |
| **17.** Observe client's general condition while lying supine or at elevation of 30° to 45° | | |
| **a.** Positioning, comfort | Relaxed posture, without discomfort | Pain, coughing, or choking; "smothering" feeling; inability to lie flat for extended period |
| **b.** Respirations | Even and deep | Respirations uneven, shallow, gasping; inadequate exchange |
| **c.** Skin color | Pink/brown | Cyanosis, grayish pallor |
| | | Mottling |

*Edema should be measured against a bony prominence (over ankle or tibia). Record the following:
  1. Type
     a. Pitting (Fig. 9-11)
     b. Nonpitting
  2. Extent and location
     a. Ankle and foot
     b. Ankle only
     c. Foot to knee, etc.
     d. Hands and fingers
  3. Degree of pitting
     a. 0 to 0.6 cm (0 to ¼ inch)—mild
     b. 0.6 to 1.3 cm (¼ to ½ inch)—moderate
     c. 1.3 to 2.5 cm (½ to 1 inch)—severe
  4. Symmetrical or unilateral response

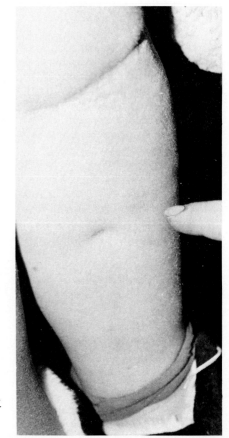

**FIG. 9-11.** Moderate pitting edema at midcalf.

| THE STUDENT WILL: | TO IDENTIFY: | |
|---|---|---|
| | NORMAL | DEVIATIONS FROM NORMAL |
| | | Note color around lips, neck, upper chest |
| **d.** Nail color and configuration | Pink | Cyanotic |
| | 160° angle at nail bed | Clubbing (angle disappears) |
| **18.** Inspect and palpate anterior chest | | |
| **a.** Precordium | | |
| 1. Contour | Rounded, symmetrical | Kyphosis |
| | | Sternal depression |
| | | Any asymmetry |
| 2. General movement: use palmar surface of hand and finger pads (Fig. 9-12) | Even respiratory movements (precordium may lift slightly in thin people) | Entire chest heaving or lifting with heartbeat |
| **19.** Inspect and palpate the following specific areas (Fig. 9-13): | | |
| **a.** Sternoclavicular area for pulsations | Slight or absent | Bounding |
| **b.** Aortic area (right second intercostal space adjacent to sternum) for pulsations | None | Pulsation, thrill (*Note:* Low-frequency vibrations can often be more easily felt than heard.) |
| **c.** Pulmonary area (left second intercostal space adjacent to sternum) for pulsations | None | Pulsation, thrill |
| **d.** Right ventricular area (left and right fifth intercostal space close to sternum) for heave or lift | May be present in hyperkinetic, thin, or pregnant adults | Diffuse lift or heave, pulsations |

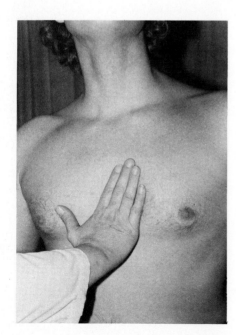

**FIG. 9-12.** Palpation over precordium. Note use of palmar surface of hand and finger pads.

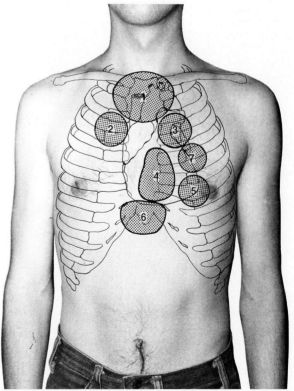

**FIG. 9-13.** Palpation areas for cardiac examination: *1*, sternoclavicular; *2*, aortic; *3*, pulmonary; *4*, anterior pericardium (right ventricular); *5*, apical; *6*, epigastric; *7*, ectopic.

## Clinical guidelines—cont'd

| THE STUDENT WILL: | TO IDENTIFY: | |
| --- | --- | --- |
| | NORMAL | DEVIATIONS FROM NORMAL |
| **e.** Apical area (fifth intercostal space, 5 to 7 cm [2 to 3 inches] from midsternal line) (Fig. 9-14) for: | | |
| 1. Pulsation | May be present | |
| 2. Amplitude | Tapping | Thrusting |
| 3. Duration | First third to half systole | Sustained throughout systole |
| 4. Location | Fourth or fifth intercostal space, 5 to 7 cm from midsternal line* | Displaced left lateral or down |
| 5. Diameter | 1 to 2 cm (⅓ to ½ inch) | Over 2 cm (½ inch) |

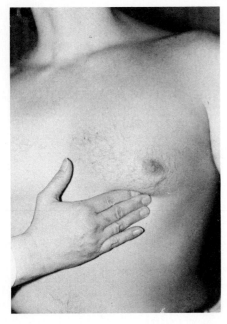

**FIG. 9-14.** Palpation for pulse at apical area. Finger pads are more sensitive to light pulsations.

| | | |
| --- | --- | --- |
| **f.** Epigastric area for pulsations: slide fingers up under rib cage | Aortic pulsation with forward thrust<br>Right ventricular pulsation with downward thrust | Bounding pulsation |
| **g.** Ectopic area (midway between pulmonary and apical areas) for pulsations | None | Outward pulsation |
| **20.** Auscultate the following specific areas (Fig. 9-15) (*Note:* Even though auscultation areas are pictured as separate locations, examiner should "inch" from one area to next.); use both diaphragm and bell to listen to all areas | | |
| **a.** Aortic area (second right interspace) | | |
| **b.** Pulmonary area (second left interspace) | | |
| **c.** Third left interspace | | |

*Note: Apical pulse location may displace slightly laterally if client turns to the left side.

| THE STUDENT WILL: | NORMAL | DEVIATIONS FROM NORMAL |
|---|---|---|

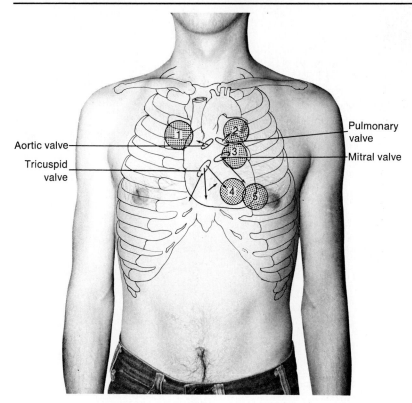

Aortic valve
Tricuspid valve
Pulmonary valve
Mitral valve

**FIG. 9-15.** Anatomical and auscultatory valve areas: *1,* aortic area; *2,* pulmonary area; *3,* third left interspace; *4,* tricuspid area; *5,* mitral area.

| | | |
|---|---|---|
| **d.** Tricuspid area (fifth left interspace near sternum) | | |
| **e.** Apical area (fifth left interspace medial to midclavicular line) | | |
| 1. Rate | 60 to 90 beats/min (conditioned athletes or "seasoned" joggers may have normally slower rate) | Over 90<br>Under 60 |
| 2. Rhythm | Regular | Irregular (without any pattern)<br>Sporadic extra beats or pauses |
| 3. $S_1$ sound | | |
| a. Location | Usually heard at all sites | |
| b. Intensity | Often louder at apex (muscle, fat tissue, and air will diminish sound; rapid rate will accentuate sound) | Accented<br>Diminished (muffled)<br>Varying intensity with different beats (e.g., complete heart block) |
| c. Frequency | Usually lower in pitch than $S_2$ | Frequency (pitch) becomes higher with accented intensity |
| d. Timing | Almost synchronous with carotid impulse<br>Slightly longer in duration than $S_2$ | |
| e. Splitting | May be heard occasionally in tricuspid area<br>Normal $S_1$ splitting sound usually varies from beat to beat: occasionally single sound, occasionally narrow split | $S_4$ sound sometimes mistaken for $S_1$ splitting |

## Clinical guidelines—cont'd

| THE STUDENT WILL: | TO IDENTIFY: NORMAL | DEVIATIONS FROM NORMAL |
|---|---|---|
| 4. S₂ sound | | |
| a. Location | Usually heard at all sites | |
| b. Intensity | Often louder at base (intensity diminished with fat, muscle, or air) | Increased intensity, usually in aortic (e.g., arterial hypertension) or pulmonary area (e.g., pulmonary hypertension) |
| c. Frequency | Usually higher in pitch than S₁ | Decreased intensity |
| d. Timing | Sound shorter in duration than S₁ | |
| e. Splitting | Commonly heard in pulmonary area (on inspiration) in young adults | Wide splitting (e.g., right bundle branch block) <br> Fixed splitting <br> Paradoxical splitting (e.g., left bundle branch block) |
| 5. Systole | | |
| a. Duration | Shorter than diastole at normal heart rate (60 to 90 beats/min) | |
| b. Sounds | S₁ sound duration brief; silent interval | Early systolic ejection click: <br> Aortic—heard at base and apex <br> Pulmonary—heard in pulmonary area <br> Middle and late systolic clicks (e.g., mitral valve deformity) heard at left sternal border <br> Clicks high pitched and sharp in sound |
| 6. Diastole | | |
| a. Duration | Longer than systole at normal rate (60 to 100 beats/min) <br> Shortens in duration as rate increases | |
| b. Sounds | S₂ duration brief <br> Silent interval | |
| (1) S₃ | *Young adults* | *Older adults* |
| (a) Location | Apex | Apex (may signify heart failure) |
| (b) Intensity | Dull, low pitched | Dull, low pitched |
| (c) Timing | Early in diastole (normal S₃ sounds often disappear when client sits up) | Early in diastole |
| (2) S₄ | | |
| (a) Location | | Medial to apex |
| (b) Intensity | Rarely heard in normal client | Higher pitch |
| (c) Timing | | Late diastole (may be confused with split S₁) |
| (3) Other sounds | | *Opening snap* <br> At apex <br> Higher pitch <br> Very early in diastole |
| 7. Murmurs | ("Innocent" murmurs in children and young adults) | |
| a. Timing | Usually early systolic, but characteristics are hard to differentiate from pathological sounds | Systolic: early, middle, late; continuous <br> Diastolic: early, middle, late; continuous |
| b. Location | Usually at pulmonary area, apex, or medial to apex | Area where sound is heard may be small and confined or may cover most of precordium <br> Describe in terms of precordial landmarks and centimeters distance from landmarks |

| THE STUDENT WILL: | TO IDENTIFY: | |
| --- | --- | --- |
| | NORMAL | DEVIATIONS FROM NORMAL |
| c. Radiation | | Describe in relation to landmarks and centimeters distance |
| d. Intensity | Soft, usually below grade 3<br>Varies with position and respiration | Grades 1 to 6, or loud, medium, soft<br>Stable, or varies with respiration and position |
| e. Pitch | | High, medium, low |
| f. Quality | | Blowing, harsh, rumbling<br>Crescendo<br>Decrescendo |
| 8. Other sounds | | Pericardial friction rub (to-and-fro rubbing sound, usually heard during systole and diastole; sound usually is increased when client sits up and leans forward) |
| **21.** Auscultate over each carotid artery with bell of stethoscope (Fig. 9-16) to listen for possible bruits | Faint heart sounds are heard | Unilateral blowing or swishing sound (localized obstruction of carotid artery)<br>Bilateral blowing or swishing sound (referred murmur sound from heart, or hyperkinetic state) |

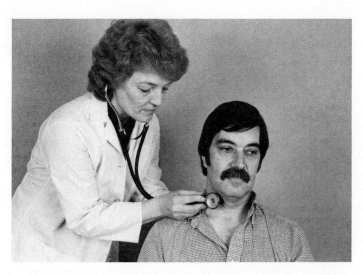

**FIG. 9-16.** Auscultation over the carotid arteries. Examiner lightly places stethoscope bell over area.

| | | |
| --- | --- | --- |
| **22.** Repeat palpation and auscultation maneuvers with client | | |
| **a.** Lying in left decubitus position | | Left decubitus position may enable examiner to pick up $S_3$ and $S_4$ sounds not heard in prone position |
| **b.** Sitting | | Sitting and leaning forward may highlight aortic murmurs not heard in prone position |

## Clinical strategies

1. Procedure for measuring arterial blood pressure (arm):
   a. Client should be comfortably seated, in a partially raised position or lying down.
   b. Arm should be stabilized at heart level with the elbow slightly flexed.
   c. Arm should be uncovered; shirt sleeves should be removed, not rolled up, if they are at all constrictive.
   d. Cuff:
      (1) Contains an inflatable bladder; width of this bladder should be 40% of circumference of arm (measure at midpoint between elbow and shoulder).
      (2) Bladder should be centered over the artery.
      (3) Lower edge should be placed 2 to 5 cm (1 to 2 inches) above the antecubital space.
      (4) Should be completely deflated when applied.
      (5) Should be snugly and smoothly wrapped around the arm.
      (6) Tubing will rest at the medial aspect of the arm (Fig. 9-17).
   e. Examiner should be positioned comfortably so that:
      (1) Aneroid or mercury gauge can be viewed at close range (closer than 90 cm [3 feet]).
      (2) Aneroid gauge can be viewed straight on (avoiding an oblique view) (Fig. 9-18).
      (3) Mercury column top is viewed at eye level.
   f. If a mercury manometer is used, it should be placed on a flat surface.

   g. Examiner should palpate the brachial or radial artery and inflate the cuff 30 mm Hg above the point where the pulse is no longer palpated (Fig. 9-18).
   h. Deflate the cuff slowly (2 to 3 mm Hg per heartbeat) and note onset of pulse.
   i. Apply the stethoscope bell to the previously palpated brachial artery. The bell should be applied as lightly as possible but with no space between the skin and stethoscope. The stethoscope should not be in contact with the cuff or clothing.
   j. Inflate the cuff 30 mm Hg above the point where the previously palpated pulse was obliterated. Deflate slowly (2 to 3 mm Hg per heartbeat).
   k. Note (1) onset of first sound, (2) muffling (or change in character) of sound, and (3) disappearance of sound. (*Note:* In 1980 the Postgraduate Education Committee for the American Heart Association recommended that the diastolic reading be interpreted and recorded at the disappearance of sound for adults.)
   l. If the blood pressure procedure must be repeated to clarify results, wait a minimum of 60 seconds to repeat. (Deflate cuff completely.)
   m. Note variables that can alter client's blood pressure: eating, drinking, or smoking within 30 minutes before measurement is taken, exercise, anxiety, cold environment, pain or discomfort, exertion, bladder distention.

2. Procedure for measuring arterial blood pressure (thigh):
   a. Client should be lying prone.
   b. Leg should be stabilized and uncovered (no restrictive clothing bunched or rolled at upper thigh).
   c. Cuff:
      (1) Should be wider and longer than that used for client's arm (e.g., an 18 to 20 cm bag).
      (2) Should be applied over midthigh so that the bladder is centered over the posterior aspect.
   d. Examiner must be positioned so that the aneroid or mercury gauge can be viewed at close distance. The mercury column should be at eye level.
   e. Examiner should palpate the popliteal fossa and locate the pulsation.
   f. Place the stethoscope over the artery and proceed as with brachial pressure maneuvers.

---

### SAMPLE RECORDING

*Pulses, pressures:* Carotid, radial, femoral, dorsalis pedis, and posterior tibial pulses symmetrical, strong, and regular. No bruits. Jugular venous pressure at the level of the sternal angle while client elevated at 30°.

*Extremities:* Warm, without pallor, cyanosis, edema. No varicosities or calf tenderness. Homans sign negative.

*Precordium/heart:* No thrills, heaves, or pulsations other than PMI barely palpable at fifth left ICS, 8 cm from midsternal line. AP = RP. $S_1$ and $S_2$ are brief and clear. No extra sounds or murmurs.

---

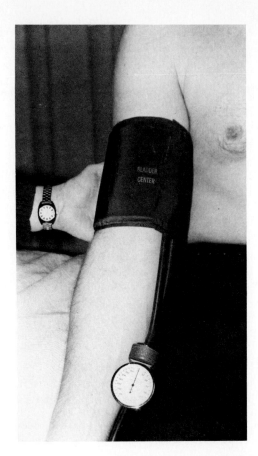

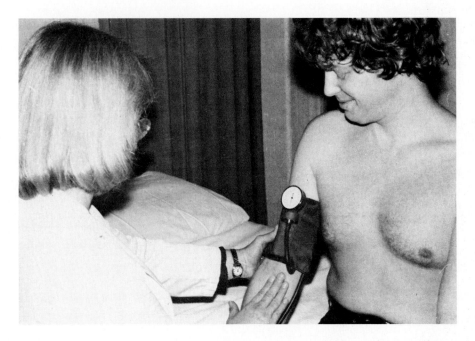

**FIG. 9-17.** Arterial blood pressure measurement. Note the following: (1) bladder is centered over artery; (2) lower edge of cuff is 3 cm above antecubital space; (3) deflated cuff is wrapped snugly and smoothly around arm; (4) tubing rests at medial aspect of arm.

**FIG. 9-18.** Blood pressure measurement. Examiner views gauge "straight on" within a 90 cm range. Examiner palpates brachial artery before auscultation maneuver.

g. *Note:* Examiner can anticipate that popliteal systolic arterial pressure will register higher (5 to 15 mm Hg) than brachial systolic pressure.

h. Diastolic pressure is usually the same or slightly lower.

3. If jugular pulsations are difficult to find, have the client lie flat for maximum venous distention. It is recommended that the internal jugular vein be viewed for registering venous pressure. However, it is often difficult to locate because of its anatomical placement (Fig. 9-19). Note the location of the carotid artery in relation to the jugular veins. Be certain not to confuse the arterial with the venous pulsations. Venous pulsations (a) are less vigorous (of an undulating quality), (b) can be eliminated by pressing over the clavicle, (c) increase in intensity when the client is recumbent, and (d) are rarely palpable.

4. Inspect and palpate the extremities carefully. Foot pulses (dorsalis pedis) are sometimes difficult or impossible to find. *Note:* A cold environment may alter the appearance and temperature of extremities.

5. It is important to inspect the client carefully before proceeding with palpation and auscultation. Stand back and view the entire person. Establish a general picture of posture, comfort, character of respiration, tension, and general skin color.

6. Inspect the precordium *carefully*. Beginners sometimes tend to miss the obvious because they are anxious to auscultate. View the entire anterior chest. It is possible that the whole chest could be heaving. Then let your eyes focus on each inspection site described in the guidelines.

7. Good lighting is necessary for good inspection.

8. It is vital that the examiner develop a system for cardiac palpation and auscultation. There are a number of choices: moving from base to apex, apex to base, alternating diaphragm and bell, having the client sit first or lie down first, etc. Establish the mechanics, then develop a listening and concentration system. The characteristics of rate, rhythm, $S_1$, $S_2$, systole, diastole, and extra sounds are described in the guidelines. Each entity must be evaluated separately. It is impossible to hear everything at once.

9. When auscultating, avoid "jumping" from one site to another. "Inch" the endpiece along the route. This maneuver helps avoid missing important sounds.

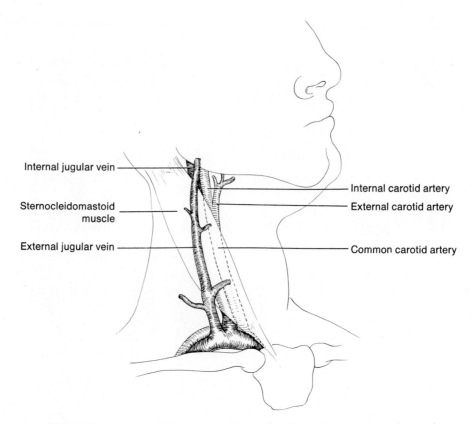

**FIG. 9-19.** Anatomical placement of carotid and jugular vessels in the neck.

10. Stabilize the endpiece on the chest by letting your fourth and fifth fingers, or your wrist, rest on the adjacent chest wall. This will prevent sliding and extraneous noise. Use light pressure with the bell and a firmer pressure with the diaphragm.
11. Often heart sounds are better heard if the client breathes out and holds the expiration. Asking the client to breathe out and to lean forward while in a sitting position is helpful.
12. For women with large breasts, displace the breast upward with one hand and palpate or auscultate with the other. Some clients can assist in displacement.
13. It is sometimes helpful to place a hand on the client's shoulder to steady him while he is sitting.

## History and clinical strategies: the pediatric client

1. There are basically two types of cardiovascular disease in children. The first is a *congenital* problem with the heart itself or its pumping mechanisms. The second type, called *acquired,* occurs as the result of a systemic disease, such as rheumatic fever.
2. The examiner must use every sense available to evaluate the child's cardiovascular system. The obvious decompensating characteristics such as cyanosis, peripheral edema, and dyspnea will be recognized early and easily. But it is the subtle, early signs and symptoms that the examiner must be continuously watchful for. Early warning symptoms of a *potential* cardiovascular problem *may be:*
   a. Infant who becomes tired of sucking and must rest periodically before able to finish
   b. Infant who has tachycardia and tachypnea while eating
   c. Child who is reported to tire frequently during playing (In this case it is important to clarify how much and what kinds of activities cause fatigue: an hour of playing tag vs. a short walk.)
   d. Child who is reported to "turn blue" with prolonged crying episodes
   e. Child who requires several rest/sleep periods during the day beyond what is normal for the age
   f. Child who repeatedly complains that he does not want to go out and play because he cannot keep up with the others or because he becomes short of breath or tired when he plays
   g. Child who assumes a knee-chest position during sleeping; or squats instead of sits when playing or watching television
   h. Child who complains of leg pains with running (inquire as to how much running causes pains and what pains actually feel like)
   i. Excessively labored breathing in an infant during defecation
   j. Child who is falling behind the normal growth and development schedule
   k. Child with a history of frequent headaches or nosebleeds accompanying a rise in blood pressure and/or leg cramping
   Although any single symptom listed above may not be caused by a cardiovascular dysfunction, it warrants full investigation of additional subjective and objective data.
3. Cardiovascular evaluation of the child extends far beyond examination of the heart. The evaluation should begin as the examiner first sees the child. The overall health, nutritional state, color, ease of respirations, and general overt qualities of the child should communicate information about the child's cardiovascular function.
4. The blood pressure of children under the age of 1 year may be difficult to obtain because of improper cuff size or excessive baby fat or simply because the child is extremely wiggly. The examiner can be assured that if the infant is screaming and pink, the blood pressure is substantial. It is the lethargic or ill-appearing infant who demands a blood pressure recording. If the examiner has difficulty obtaining an audible blood pressure, the "flush technique" may be used. Following are the steps:
   a. Elevate the child's arm to drain its blood.
   b. Wrap a 2-inch elastic bandage from the fingertips to the elbow.
   c. Apply a blood pressure cuff (no more than two thirds or less than half the length of the upper arm).
   d. Pump the cuffing to about 120 mm Hg.
   e. Lower the infant's arm and remove the bandage.
   f. Slowly deflate the cuff.
   g. The point where there is a "flush" of the arm from white to pink is taken as the reading. This is generally considered to be the median reading between systolic and diastolic.
5. Following are general guidelines for obtaining blood pressure readings in children:
   a. Every child 18 months and older should be screened for hypertension. This means that the child's blood pressure should be evaluated during every well-child examination.
   b. Equipment for obtaining pediatric blood pressures is the same as for the adult. The cuff should not be larger than two thirds or smaller

than half the length of the child's arm between the elbow and shoulder. Proper size cuffs are mandatory for adequate evaluation of children. Pediatric cuffs are available in $2\frac{1}{2}$ and 5 inch sizes. (See Table 9-2.)

   c. The American Heart Association states that the muffling of the blood pressure tone in children should actually be considered the diastolic reading.

   d. Crying or sudden jerking may alter the child's blood pressure between 5 and 10 mm Hg. The child should be evaluated during a quiet period.

   e. Every child should have at least one or two thigh screening blood pressure measurements during early childhood to rule out a vast difference between upper and lower extremity pressure (a sign of coarctation of the aorta).

6. Fever in a child will normally increase the child's pulse. For every degree of fever, the pulse may increase 8 to 10 beats/min.

7. In physically examining the child's cardiovascular system, the techniques of inspection, palpation, and auscultation are normally used. Percussion may be used by the experienced examiner with the older child, but, generally, small patients poorly tolerate the procedure.

8. All techniques require that the child be undressed to the underwear and sitting on the table (infants may be held). It is helpful for cooperative children to recline to a 45-degree angle during examination. If that is impossible, a supine position is preferable to an upright position because more cardiovascular "sounds" are generally heard with the child lying down.

9. Auscultating the hearts of infants and toddlers is a true feat. The child must be quiet during the examination. Crying, talking, or pulling at the stethoscope tubing will defeat the process. The examiner is encouraged to examine the cardiovascular system early during the examination before the child becomes frightened, bored, or cold.

10. As will be discussed in subsequent clinical guidelines, a child's chest should be auscultated in the same spots as an adult's heart. Because of the rapidity of a child's heart rate, the examiner may need to listen to each selected area for a fairly long time to feel comfortable in describing the findings. Some parents may become concerned because of the long listening time, therefore it is suggested that the examiner explain to the parent that a long listening time is not a cause for concern.

11. If the examiner identifies any unusual findings, suggestive history, extra noises, or murmurs, it is recommended that the child be referred to a physician for further verification. The beginning examiner should *not* attempt to define a murmur as "functional" or an extra odd heart sound as insignificant. It is the examiner's duty at this time to identify normal findings and to recognize and refer abnormal or suggestive findings. The cardiovascular health of a young child is too valuable to provide an experimental opportunity for the examiner.

**TABLE 9-2.** Guidelines for choosing correct width of blood pressure cuff for children

| AGE (yr) | CUFF WIDTH (cm) |
|---|---|
| Less than $1\frac{1}{2}$ | 4.5 |
| $1\frac{1}{2}$ to 2 | 8 |
| 2 to 10 | 9.5 |
| Older than 10 | 12 |

Data from Waring, W.W., and Jeansonne, L.O.: Practical manual of pediatrics: a pocket reference for those who treat children, ed. 2, St. Louis, 1982, The C.V. Mosby Co.

# Clinical variations: the pediatric client
## ASSESSMENT OF PRESSURES, PULSES, AND THE PERIPHERAL VASCULAR SYSTEM

| CHARACTERISTIC OR AREA EXAMINED | NORMAL | | | DEVIATIONS FROM NORMAL | |
|---|---|---|---|---|---|
| **1.** Blood pressure: technique described under *Clinical strategies* <br> **a.** Sitting or lying, depending on age | | *Mean systolic\** *(±2 S.D.)* | *Mean diastolic\** *(±2 S.D.)* | Elevated blood pressures are those that exceed the following readings† | |
| | Newborn | 80 ± 16 | 46 ± 16 | 3 to 6 yr‡ | >110/70 |
| | 2 mo to 1 yr | 89 ± 29 | 60 ± 10 | 6 to 9 yr‡ | >120/75 |
| | 1 yr | 96 ± 30 | 66 ± 25 | 10 to 13 yr‡ | >130/80 |
| | 2 yr | 99 ± 25 | 64 ± 25 | 14 yr‡ | |
| | 3 yr | 100 ± 25 | 67 ± 23 | M | >133/82 |
| | 4 yr | 99 ± 20 | 65 ± 20 | F | >128/84 |
| | 5 to 6 yr | 94 ± 14 | 55 ± 9 | 15 yr§ | |
| | 6 to 7 yr | 100 ± 15 | 56 ± 8 | M | >137/85 |
| | 7 to 8 yr | 102 ± 15 | 56 ± 8 | F | >128/84 |
| | 8 to 9 yr | 105 ± 16 | 57 ± 9 | 16 to 19 yr§ | |
| | 9 to 10 yr | 107 ± 17 | 57 ± 9 | M | >140/85 |
| | 10 to 11 yr | 111 ± 17 | 58 ± 10 | F | >128/84 |
| | 11 to 12 yr | 113 ± 18 | 59 ± 10 | | |
| | 12 to 13 yr | 115 ± 19 | 59 ± 10 | | |
| | 13 to 14 yr | 118 ± 19 | 60 ± 10 | | |
| | (Fig. 9-20 shows normal blood pressure percentiles for boys and girls.) | | | | |

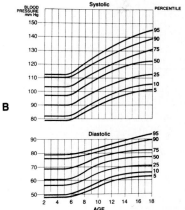

**FIG. 9-20.** Blood pressure percentiles. **A,** Boys (right arm, seated). **B,** Girls (right arm, seated). (From the National Heart, Lung, and Blood Institute's Task Force on Blood Pressure Control in Children: Pediatrics **59**(suppl. 5, part 2):797-820, 1977.)

*Data from Haggerty, R.J., Maroney, M.W., and Nadas, A.S.: Am. J. Dis. Child. **92**:536, 1956, Copyright 1973, American Medical Association.
†Data from Londe, S., and Goldring, D.: Am. J. Cardiol. **37**:650, 1976.
‡Supine reading.
§Seated reading.

# Clinical variations: the pediatric client—cont'd

**ASSESSMENT OF PRESSURES, PULSES, AND THE PERIPHERAL VASCULAR SYSTEM—cont'd**

| CHARACTERISTIC OR AREA EXAMINED | NORMAL | DEVIATIONS FROM NORMAL |
|---|---|---|
| | Pressure in both arms is same or does not vary more than 5 to 10 mm Hg | Significant (>5 to 10 mm Hg) discrepancy in pressure readings between upper extremities |
| **b.** Standing | (Not routinely done with children. If problem is suspected, have child stand up. Follow adult guidelines.) | |
| | Pulse pressure between 20 and 50 mm Hg throughout childhood | Narrowing of pulse pressure seen with aortic stenosis |
| | | Widening of pulse pressure may be seen in children with patent ductus arteriosus or aortic regurgitation |
| **c.** Thigh measurement: technique same as adult | In child less than 1 year systolic pressure in thigh should equal that of arm | Systolic pressure in thigh measurement is *lower* than systolic arm measurement (sign of coarctation of aorta) |
| | In child over 1 year systolic pressure in thigh greater than that in arm by 10 to 40 mm Hg; diastolic pressure in thigh equals that in arm | |
| **2.** Carotid artery palpation | | |
| **a.** Rate | *Age\**        *Rate/min\** <br> Newborn    120 to 170 <br> 12 mo      80 to 160 <br> 2 yr        80 to 130 <br> 3 yr        80 to 120 <br> 4 yr        80 to 120 <br> 6 yr        75 to 115 <br> Beyond 6 yr   70 to 110 | Any findings beyond limits stated <br> Increases may be caused by factors such as toxicity, fever, excitement, and respiratory distress <br> Decreases may be caused by heart block, digitalis poisoning, sepsis, *Salmonella* infection |
| **b.** Rhythm | Regular <br> Sinus arrhythmia: pulse rate will speed up with inspiration and slow down with expiration; makes pulse seem irregular in rhythm; to further evaluate, instruct child to hold breath while you continue to feel pulse; rate should become regular | Irregular pulse unrelated to breathing† |

*Data from Barness, L.: Manual of pediatric physical diagnosis, ed. 5. Copyright © 1980 by Year Book Medical Publishers, Inc., Chicago. Used by permission; Haggerty, R.J., Maroney, M.W., and Nadas, A.S.: Am. J. Dis. Child. **92**:536, 1956.

†An irregular (rapid or slow) pulse should be palpated simultaneously with auscultation of the apical pulse. Any difference between apical and peripheral pulse rate should be noted. If pulse irregularity is patterned (occurs in repeated sequences), note whether irregularity occurs during (1) inspiration or expiration and (2) systole or diastole.

| CHARACTERISTIC OR AREA EXAMINED | NORMAL | DEVIATIONS FROM NORMAL |
|---|---|---|
| | Carefully watch respirations in infant to evaluate if pulse rhythm fluctuates with breathing | |
| | Common in children over age 3 years | |
| | Especially prominent at puberty | Extrasystoles or PVCs heard for first |
| | Extrasystoles or premature ventricular contractions (PVC) *may* be normal in healthy child; will feel like skipped beat; emotional factors may trigger; exercise will usually cause disappearance | time in ill child; child with known cardiac disease; or child with suggestive or questionable history |
| c. Pulse amplitude | Pulse upstroke smooth, rounded, and prompt | Upstroke exaggerated, bounding, weak, thready |
| d. Amplitude pattern | Series of pulse strokes unvaried in amplitude or contour | Upstrokes vary, for example, strong and weaker beats alternate (pulsus alternans) |
| e. Symmetry | Symmetrical response (i.e., both carotid pulses manifest same rate, rhythm, amplitude, and contour) | Asymmetrical response |
| f. Arterial wall contour | Soft and pliable | Increased resistance to compression, beaded or tortuous |
| 3. Radial artery palpation | (Pulses in nos. 4 to 6 may or may not be evaluated, depending on the age and overall health of the child. Any child with known cardiovascular disease or suggestive symptomatology should receive a thorough evaluation. Other children are normally screened by evaluating carotid, femoral, radial, and apical pulses. Criteria for evaluation have been listed previously.) | Significant difference between radial and femoral pulses |
| 4. Popliteal pulse palpation | | Weak or absent femoral pulses may indicate coarctation of aorta |
| 5. Dorsalis pedis pulse palpation | | |
| 6. Posterior tibial pulse palpation | | |
| 7. Femoral pulse palpation | | |
| 8. Evaluation of venous pressures (Not routinely done in well children.) | Jugular veins may be visible but should not pulsate or appear engorged | Noted pulsations of neck or engorgement |
| 9. Evidence of adequate arterial supply | Warm, pink, nonedematous extremities | Thin, shiny, taut skin |
| | Mottling (if infant is in cool environment and has been uncovered for some time) | Cold or mottled extremities in warm environment |
| | | Edema* |
| | | Marked pallor |
| | | Tenderness of skin |
| 10. Evidence of adequate venous sufficiency | | Peripheral cyanosis |
| | | Edema* |
| | | Thickening of skin |

*Often one associates heart failure with peripheral edema. In children, however, the signs of heart failure are quite different. Signs may include a rapid respiratory rate in the supine position followed by slight dyspnea, liver enlargement, venous engorgement, orthopnea, pulsus alternans, and a gallop rhythm. Only very late in its course are signs of pulmonary or peripheral edema noticeable (Barness, 1980).

## Clinical variations: the pediatric client—cont'd
**ASSESSMENT OF THE HEART AND PRECORDIUM**

| CHARACTERISTIC OR AREA EXAMINED | NORMAL | DEVIATIONS FROM NORMAL |
|---|---|---|
| **1.** General appearance | | |
| **a.** Positioning, comfort | Playing Relaxed posture, without discomfort | Client experiencing pain, coughing or choking, "smothering" feeling (unable to lie flat for extended period) |
| **b.** Respirations | Even and deep | Respirations uneven, shallow, gasping Inadequate exchange |
| **c.** Skin color | Pink/brown | Cyanosis, grayish pallor Mottling Note color around lips, neck, upper chest |
| **d.** Nail color and configuration | Pink 160° angle at nail bed | Cyanotic Clubbing (angle disappears) |
| **2.** Anterior chest precordium | | |
| **a.** Contour | Rounded, symmetrical | Kyphosis Sternal depression Any asymmetry |
| **b.** General movement | Even respiratory movements (precordium may lift slightly in thin people) | Areas of bulging, or entire chest heaving or lifting with heartbeat Appearance of thrill across chest wall |
| **3.** Inspection and palpation (Child should be sitting and leaning forward.) | | |
| **a.** Sternoclavicular area pulsations | Slight or absent | Bounding |
| **b.** Aortic area (second right intercostal space beside sternum) pulsations | None | Pulsation, thrill (*Note:* Low-frequency vibrations can often be more easily felt than heard.) |
| **c.** Pulmonary area (second and third left intercostal spaces near sternum) pulsations | May feel some slight pulsations following physical activity | Thrill or strong pulsations that continue even when patient is at rest |
| **d.** Right ventricular area (third, fourth, and fifth intercostal spaces to right and left over sternum); note difference from adult | Very thin children may feel slight palpations | Systolic thrill, strong pulsations Heaves |
| **e.** Apical area (PMI) (infants and small children: fourth intercostal space to left of midclavicular line; after age 7 years, fifth intercostal space to right of the midclavicular line) | | |
|    1. Pulsation | May be present May be difficult to palpate in children under 2 years | |
|    2. Amplitude | Tapping | Thrusting |
|    3. Duration | First third to half systole | Sustained throughout systole |
|    4. Location | As described | Displaced lateral left or down |
|    5. Diameter | 1 to 1.5 cm ($\frac{1}{3}$ inch) | Over 2 cm ($\frac{3}{4}$ inch) |
| **f.** Epigastric area (at sternal angle) pulsations | Aortic pulsation with forward thrust Right ventricular pulsation with downward thrust | Bounding pulsation |

| CHARACTERISTIC OR AREA EXAMINED | NORMAL | DEVIATIONS FROM NORMAL |
|---|---|---|
| **g.** Ectopic area (space between pulmonary and aortic area) pulsations | None | Outward pulsations |
| **4.** Auscultation (child sitting) | | |
| **a.** Aortic area (location as discussed) | | |
| **b.** Pulmonary area (location as discussed) | | |
| **c.** Third left intercostal space | | |
| **d.** Tricuspid area (fifth interspace near sternum to right in young children; to left in older children) | | |
| **e.** Apical area (location as discussed) | | |
|   1. Rate | As previously discussed | As previously discussed |
|   2. Rhythm | Described under pulses | Described under pulses |
|   3. Pitch | Higher pitch/shorter duration than in adult | |
|   4. $S_1$ sound | | |
|     a. Location | Usually heard at all sites | |
|     b. Intensity | Often louder at apex (Muscle, fat tissue, and air will diminish sound; rapid rate will accentuate sound.) | Accented<br>Diminished (muffled)<br>Varying intensity with different beats (e.g., complete heart block) |
|     c. Frequency | Usually lower in pitch than $S_2$ | Frequency (pitch) becomes higher with accented intensity |
|     d. Timing | Almost synchronous with carotid impulse<br>Slightly longer in duration than $S_2$ | |
|     e. Splitting | May be heard occasionally in tricuspid area<br>Normal $S_1$ splitting sound usually varies from beat to beat, occasionally a single sound, occasionally a narrow split | $S_4$ sometimes mistaken for $S_1$ splitting |
|   5. $S_2$ sound | | |
|     a. Location | Usually heard at all sites<br>May be loudest in pulmonary area | |
|     b. Intensity | Often louder at base<br>Intensity diminished with fat, muscle, or air | Increased intensity, usually in aortic area (e.g., arterial hypertension) or pulmonary area (e.g., pulmonary hypertension)<br>Decreased intensity |
|     c. Frequency | Usually higher in pitch than $S_1$ | |
|     d. Timing | Sound shorter in duration than $S_1$ | |
|     e. Splitting | Commonly heard in pulmonary area (on inspiration) in child<br>Equal quality and intensity of sound | Wide splitting (e.g., right bundle branch block)<br>Fixed splitting<br>Paradoxical splitting (e.g., left bundle branch block)<br>Area of apex |

# Clinical variations: the pediatric client—cont'd
ASSESSMENT OF THE HEART AND PRECORDIUM—cont'd

| CHARACTERISTIC OR AREA EXAMINED | NORMAL | DEVIATIONS FROM NORMAL |
|---|---|---|
| 6. Systole | | |
|    a. Duration | Shorter than diastole at normal heart rate | |
|    b. Sounds | $S_1$ sound duration brief; silent interval | Early systolic ejection click: aortic—heard at base and apex pulmonary—heard in pulmonary area |
| | | Middle and late systolic clicks (e.g., mitral valve deformity) heard at left sternal border |
| | | Clicks high pitched and sharp in sound |
| 7. Diastole | | |
|    a. Duration | Longer than systole at normal rate | |
| | Shortens in duration as rate increases | |
|    b. Sounds | $S_2$ duration brief | |
| | Silent interval | |
| 8. $S_3$ sound | May be normal in children (may occur in as many as 30% of all children) | |
|    a. Location | Apex | |
|    b. Intensity | Different intensity from second sound, dull, low in pitch | |
|    c. Timing | Early in diastole | |
| 9. $S_4$ sound | Never normal | |
|    a. Location | | Medial to apex |
|    b. Intensity | | Higher pitch |
|    c. Timing | | Late diastole (may be confused with split $S_1$) |
| | | Opening snap: at apex; higher pitch; very early in diastole |
| 10. Other sounds | | Pericardial friction rub: scratchy, high pitched, grating sound, unaffected by change in respirations |
| **f.** Murmurs | "Innocent" murmurs | "Organic" murmurs |
|    1. Timing | Usually early systolic | Systolic or diastolic at any point during or continuous |
|    2. Location | Second or third intercostal space along left sternal border | |
|    3. Position in which heard | Usually supine | Heard in all positions |
|    4. Duration | Short | Longer |
|    5. Quality | Soft and musical | Louder, blowing, harsh, rumbling |
|    6. Intensity | Soft (grades 1, 2) | Loud (grades 3, 4, 5) |
|    7. Affected by exercise | Yes | Constant |
| **5.** Repeat palpation and auscultation with child lying and in left decubitus position | | |

## History and clinical strategies: the geriatric client

The incidence of cardiovascular disease is higher in elderly individuals than in younger adults. However, the examiner should not assume that all elderly people are suffering from hypertension, cardiac or coronary artery disease, or vascular impairment.

The heart size of an older client who is not hypertensive or manifesting a heart disease often becomes smaller. Cardiac enlargement is usually associated with hypertension or other disease within the heart or vessels.

At rest, cardiac output decreases by 30% to 40% by 65 to 70 years of age. However, general organ atrophy and reduced exertion decrease the need for blood flow. Several authors have stated that the aging heart functions well under *normal* conditions but may not be able to respond efficiently to increased circulatory needs associated with extreme stress, blood loss, tachycardia, unusual exertion, or fever.

Although the process of arteriosclerosis advances with age, the amount of circulatory inadequacy at any given age is not predictable. This process may not cause symptoms or signs in many individuals.

Signs or symptoms associated with cardiovascular disease in the elderly are often the same as those manifested in younger adults. (Refer to the history portion of the adult cardiovascular section for related questions.)

Following are special needs, concerns, and responses of older adults in relation to cardiovascular problems.

1. Angina pectoris. In some instances the elderly individual may not experience chest pain to the extent that a younger person does. Dyspnea or palpitation on exertion may be reported as an initial symptom. Chest pain radiation may be reported as a "tightness" in the chest, neck, or shoulder. The pain radiation pattern is usually the same as with younger adults.
2. Confusion or slowed mental function may be an early sign of low cardiac output. Note that confusion (even in mild form) alters the client's ability to provide an accurate account of symptoms.
3. Other early symptoms of cardiac distress are fatigue, light-headedness, or weakness.
4. Explore complaints such as "fatigue," "out of breath," and "tired" carefully. They are sometimes used interchangeably to indicate dyspnea. The precise amount of exertion that precedes the symptom should be described. Note that shortness of breath may indicate many problems other than heart disease. Sedentary elderly people with limited cardiac reserve may complain of breathless-

ness. Clarify whether shortness of breath interferes with sleep. If insomnia or wakefulness coexists with the dyspnea, clarify the number of times the client awakens each night and exactly what is done to deal with the symptom.
5. Coughing and wheezing may be indicative of heart disease, particularly if the onset is sudden or recent.
6. Dizziness, syncope, palpitations, or transient ischemia attacks may be associated with arrhythmias. Chest pain may accompany these symptoms.
7. Transient ischemial attacks are usually of limited duration (15 to 20 minutes) and are indicated by a variety of symptoms or signs. Dizziness, confusion, unilateral weakness or numbness, and aphasia are some of the complaints. These episodes often leave little or no aftereffects and frequently precede a stroke. Carotid arterial atherosclerosis can contribute to these "attacks." A history of "spells" or "attacks" should be a signal for immediate referral to a physician.
8. A complaint of hemoptysis may be associated with congestive heart failure or a pulmonary embolism.
9. Edema of both legs is often associated with heart disease. Clarify the pattern of swelling with the client in terms of frequency and time of day when it is most pronounced.
10. Weakness, bradycardia, hypotension, and confusion may indicate an excess of potassium, which sometimes occurs in conjunction with therapeutic measures for heart disease.
11. Weakness, fatigue, muscle cramps, and a variety of arrhythmias may be indicative of a low potassium level.
12. Digitalis toxicity may be indicated by anorexia, nausea, vomiting, diarrhea, headache, yellow vision, arrhythmias, or mental confusion.
13. Hypertension. Some authors state that the systolic pressure may normally rise gradually as an individual ages. Other authorities feel that the average systolic pressure is not altered by age. Most authors agree that the diastolic pressure does not change markedly with aging. The Joint National Committee on Detection, Evaluation, and Treatment of High Blood Pressure recommended in 1976 that blood pressures of individuals over 50 years of age in the range of 140/90 to 160/95 be rechecked in 6 to 9 months. The final diagnosis of hypertension is usually based on a number of blood pressure readings taken over a period of weeks or months. An elderly individual's blood pressure may fluctuate widely from one assessment to another (particularly the systolic pressure).

Most of the time, hypertension is asymptomatic. Severe hypertension may produce symptoms of headache (dull, in the morning), memory impairment, visual changes, epistaxis, angina pectoris, and dyspnea on exertion.

One of the major problems associated with hypertension is maintaining client compliancy with prescribed therapy. The following questions might be helpful in assessing the hypertensive client:

a. How much of a problem is hypertension for you in terms of:
   (1) Symptoms
   (2) Interference with activities of daily living
   (3) Taking medications
b. Do you feel the prescribed therapy is effective?
c. Do you have any difficulty with the therapy (e.g., fear of addiction to drugs, side effects of drugs, false hope that drugs will "cure" the problem, only wishing to take medication when hypertensive symptoms occur)?
d. Have you had any experience with other family members (or close friends) who had hypertension?

14. If the examiner is assessing a client who offers a history of chronic heart or vascular disease, the effects of disability or symptoms, the client's coping skills and state of "chronicity" should be explored. (Review questions in Chapter 1 under *Activities of daily living assessment* and *Psychosocial history*.) The overall concerns to be covered are:
   a. The client's understanding of his health state
   b. The client's comprehension of his therapy
   c. The client's overall *feelings* about his state of health and the success of the therapy
   d. Interference with activities of daily living

e. The client's self-assessment of his and his family's coping ability

15. Risk factors (indicating more rigorous monitoring or treatment) for borderline hypertensive clients include:
   a. Left ventricular hypertrophy
   b. Other target organ damage (e.g., kidney, eyes, brain)
   c. High serum cholesterol
   d. Diabetes mellitus
   e. Smoking
   f. Family history of hypertension with complications
   g. Being a male

16. Risk factors for diagnosed coronary atherosclerosis clients include:
   a. Hypertension
   b. Obesity (an excess of 30% over ideal weight)
   c. Smoking
   d. Diabetes mellitus
   e. Marked stress factors in life-style
   f. Cardiotoxic drugs (e.g., antidepressants, phenothiazines)
   g. Inactivity
   h. Erratic strenuous exercise

17. *Note:* Some elderly clients have difficulty complying with examiner requests for body positioning or breathing patterns during the physical assessment. It may be impossible for an individual to lie flat for any extended period. It may be difficult to fully exhale and to hold the exhalation for the required period of examiner listening time. The examination may have to proceed more slowly, and the practitioner should be aware of variables contributing to and indicators of client discomfort (e.g., arthritis, emphysema, pulmonary congestion, kyphosis).

# Clinical variations: the geriatric client
ASSESSMENT OF PRESSURES, PULSES, AND THE PERIPHERAL VASCULAR SYSTEM

| CHARACTERISTIC OR AREA EXAMINED | NORMAL | DEVIATIONS FROM NORMAL |
|---|---|---|
| 1. Blood pressure (*Note:* For an initial examination the examiner should record blood pressure.)<br><br>  **a.** In both arms while client is lying down<br>  **b.** Client standing up during measurement | Normal (adult) upper limits:<br>  Systolic—140 mm Hg<br>  Diastolic—90 mm Hg<br>  Pulse pressure—30 to 40 mm Hg<br>Some authorities state that maximum systolic pressure of 160 mm Hg may be within normal limits if:<br>  1. It remains stable over period of time<br>  2. Client has no symptoms or evidence of end organ damage<br>  3. Client is checked regularly (every 6 to 9 months)* | Low systolic (↓ 90)<br>Systolic pressure over 160 mm Hg<br><br>Systolic pressure between 140 and 160 mm Hg with accompanying risk factors:<br>  1. Left ventricular hypertrophy<br>  2. Evidence of other end organ damage (e.g., kidneys, eyes, brain)<br>  3. High serum cholesterol<br>  4. Diabetes mellitus<br>  5. Smoking<br>  6. Family history of hypertension with complications<br>  7. Male sex |
| | Most authorities agree that maximum diastolic pressure level is 90 to 95 mm Hg† | Diastolic pressure exceeding 90 mm Hg<br>Low diastolic pressure (↓ 60)<br>Widened pulse pressure<br>(*Note:* Widened pulse pressure is fairly common because of decreased elasticity of aorta.)<br>Narrow pulse pressure |
| | Pressures in both arms same or do not vary more than 5 to 10 mm Hg systolic<br>On standing, client may manifest drop of maximum of 10 to 15 mm Hg systolic and 5 mm Hg diastolic | Significant (↑ 5 to 10 mm Hg) discrepancy in pressure readings between upper extremities<br>Significant decrease of systolic (more than 15 mm Hg) or diastolic (more than 5 mm Hg) pressure and/or symptoms of dizziness |
|   **c.** Measurement of blood pressure in both legs if pedal, popliteal, and femoral pulses are weak or absent | Popliteal artery auscultation reveals systolic pressure 5 to 15 mm Hg higher than brachial artery measurement<br>Diastolic reading same or slightly lower | Systolic pressure lower in leg(s) than in arms |
| 2. Palpation of carotid, radial, femoral, popliteal, dorsalis pedis, and posterior tibial pulses for:<br>  **a.** Rate | 60 to 90 beats/min (*Note:* The heart normally slows in rate with aging because of increase in vagal tone. Some individuals may normally manifest a rate of 50 beats/min; however, patients with slow heart rates should be referred for further evaluation.) | ↑ 90 minute (tachycardia)<br>(*Note:* Recent exertion, smoking, anxiety will elevate pulse.)<br>  ↓ 60 minute (bradycardia)<br>(*Note:* Bradycardia and atrial fibrillation are two of most common irregularities encountered; associated with "sick sinus syndrome." Often dizziness, syncope, or transient ischemia attacks accompany above signs.) |

*If pressure is elevated (especially if accompanied by rapid pulse), repeat in 30 minutes.
†A nurse, physician, or agency protocol should be established to determine systolic and diastolic pressures warranting referral. *Note:* Systolic pressure may show a wide variation at different times. Several measurements should be taken (over a period of weeks) to determine accuracy.

## Clinical variations: the geriatric client—cont'd

**ASSESSMENT OF PRESSURES, PULSES, AND THE PERIPHERAL VASCULAR SYSTEM—cont'd**

| CHARACTERISTIC OR AREA EXAMINED | NORMAL | DEVIATIONS FROM NORMAL |
|---|---|---|
| **b.** Rhythm | Regular<br>(*Note:* Infrequent ectopic beats are fairly common. However, all patients with irregularities should be referred for further evaluation.) | Irregular (without any pattern, e.g., atrial fibrillation)<br>Regularity with occasional pauses or extra beats (e.g., premature contractions)<br>Coupled beats (e.g., bigeminal pulse)* |
| **c.** Amplitude and contour | Pulse upstroke is often more rapid in older adults<br>Should be smooth and rounded | Upstroke exaggerated or bounding<br><br>Pulse weak, small, or thready; peak prolonged |
| **d.** Amplitude pattern | Series of pulse strokes is unvaried in amplitude or contour | |
| **e.** Symmetry | All pulses are symmetrical (i.e., manifest same rate, rhythm, amplitude, and contour) | Asymmetrical response |
| (*Note:* If client has a history of hypertension, palpate femoral and brachial arteries at the same time.) | Femoral and brachial pulses occur at approximately same time with equal amplitude | Delayed, diminished femoral pulse (in comparison with brachial pulse) |
| **3.** Arterial wall contour and consistency | Arterial wall thickens; loses elasticity with aging, resulting in some increased resistance to compression<br>(*Note:* Dorsalis pedis pulses may be difficult to find or absent in some normal individuals.)<br>(*Note:* Posterior tibial pulses may also be absent or decreased in some normal individuals.) | |
| **a.** Conduct following maneuver if arterial insufficiency is suspected:<br>1. With client lying down, elevate legs 30 cm (12 inches) above his heart level | | |
| 2. Ask client to move feet up and down at ankles for 60 seconds | Extremities (feet) exhibit mild pallor | Marked pallor of (one or both) feet |
| 3. Have client sit up and dangle legs (This maneuver can also be conducted with arms and hands.) | Original color returns in about 10 seconds<br>Veins in feet fill in about 15 seconds | Delayed color return or mottled appearance<br>Delayed venous filling<br>Marked redness of dependent feet |

*An irregular (rapid or slow) pulse should be palpated simultaneously with auscultation of the apical pulse. Any difference between apical and peripheral pulse rate should be noted. If pulse irregularity is patterned (occurs in repeated sequences), note whether irregularity occurs during (1) inspiration or expiration or (2) systole or diastole.

| CHARACTERISTIC OR AREA EXAMINED | NORMAL | DEVIATIONS FROM NORMAL |
|---|---|---|
| **4.** Jugular venous pressure (JVP) (client sitting at 30° to 45° angle) | JVP should not rise more than 3 cm above level of sternal angle | JVP exceeds 3 cm above level of manubrium* <br><br> Note whether other veins in neck, shoulder, and upper chest are distended |
| **a.** Inspection of jugular pulsations for quality | Regular <br> Soft and undulating <br> Level of pulsation decreases with inspiration <br> Pulsation increases in recumbent position | Fluttering or oscillating <br> Irregular rhythm <br> Unusually prominent waves |
| **5.** Inspection and palpation of arms and legs for presence and/or appearance of superficial veins | Distention in dependent position <br> Venous valves may appear as nodular bulges <br> Veins collapse with elevation of limbs <br> (*Note:* Vessels may appear tortuous or distended in elderly clients.) | Distended veins in anteromedial aspect of thigh and lower leg or on posterolateral aspect of calf from knee to ankle |
| **6.** Inspection and palpation of thigh and calf for surface characteristics | Legs symmetrical <br> Nontender <br> No excess warmth | Swelling (or one leg, especially calf, appears larger than other) <br> Tenderness on palpation <br> Warmth <br> Redness <br> (*Note:* If swelling is suspected, both thighs and calves should be measured with tape for accuracy.) |
| **a.** Sharp dorsiflexion of client's foot (with client's knee slightly flexed) to assess calf pain response | No pain | Pain elicited (Homans sign) |
| **7.** Inspection and palpation of extremities for evidence of adequate arterial supply | Absence of hair over digits or dorsum of hands and feet may be normal <br> Skin pink and warm, nonedematous <br> (*Note:* Extremities may feel cool to touch in a cool environment. Loss of subcutaneous fat contributes to increased response to cool environment.) | Reduced or absent peripheral hair (over digits and dorsum of hands and feet) <br> Thin, shiny, taut skin <br> Cold extremities (in warm environment) <br> Mild edema <br> Marked pallor or mottling on elevating extremity <br> Digit tips ulcerated <br> Stocking anesthesia <br> Tenderness on palpation <br> Peripheral cyanosis |
| **8.** Inspection and palpation of extremities for evidence of venous sufficiency | | Edema (pits on pressure), bilateral or unilateral† <br> Pigmentation around ankles (see Fig. 3-2) <br> Thickening skin <br> Ulceration (especially around ankles) |

*If venous pressure is elevated (vein is distended up to neck), raise client's head until highest jugular pulsation can be detected. Record distance in centimeters above sternal angle and angle at which client is reclining.

†Edema should be measured against a bony prominence (over ankle or tibia). Record the following:

1. Type
   a. Pitting
   b. Nonpitting
2. Extent and location
   a. Ankle and foot
   b. Ankle only
   c. Foot to knee, etc.
   d. Hands, fingers
3. Degree of pitting
   a. 0 to 0.6 cm (0 to ¼ inch)—mild
   b. 0.6 to 1.3 cm (¼ to ½ inch)—moderate
   c. 1.3 to 2.5 cm (½ to 1 inch)—severe

# Clinical variations: the geriatric client—cont'd
## ASSESSMENT OF THE HEART AND PRECORDIUM

| CHARACTERISTIC OR AREA EXAMINED | NORMAL | DEVIATIONS FROM NORMAL |
|---|---|---|
| 1. Observation of general condition while client is lying supine or at elevation of 30° to 45° | | |
|   **a.** Positioning, comfort | Relaxed posture, without discomfort | Client experiencing pain, coughing or choking, "smothering" feeling (unable to lie flat for extended period) |
|   **b.** Respirations | Even and deep | Respirations uneven, shallow, gasping Inadequate exchange |
|   **c.** Skin color | Pink/brown | Cyanosis, grayish pallor Mottling Note color around lips, neck, upper chest |
|   **d.** Nail color and configuration | Pink 160° angle at nail bed | Cyanotic Clubbing (angle disappears) |
| 2. Inspection and palpation of anterior chest | | |
|   **a.** Precordium | | |
|     1. Contour | Kyphosis and scoliosis are fairly common in elderly people; may distort normal rounded symmetrical contour and contribute to heart displacement | All asymmetry should be noted in summary |
|     2. General movement | Even respiratory movements (precordium may lift slightly in thin people) | Entire chest heaving or lifting with heartbeat |
| 3. Inspection and palpation of following areas: | | |
|   **a.** Sternoclavicular area pulsations | Slight or absent | Bounding |
|   **b.** Aortic area (right second intercostal space adjacent to sternum) pulsations | None | Pulsation, thrill (*Note:* Low-frequency vibrations can often be more easily felt than heard.) |
|   **c.** Pulmonary area (left second intercostal space adjacent to sternum) pulsations | None | Pulsation, thrill |
|   **d.** Right ventricular area (left and right fifth intercostal space close to sternum) heave or lift | May be present in hyperkinetic, thin adults | Diffuse lift or heave, pulsations |
|   **e.** Apical area (left fifth intercostal space 5 to 7 cm [2 to 2¾ inches] from midsternal line) for: | | |
|     1. Pulsation | May be present | |
|     2. Amplitude | Tapping | Thrusting |
|     3. Duration | First third to half systole | Sustained throughout systole |
|     4. Location | Fourth or fifth intercostal space, 5 to 7 cm from midclavicular line* | Displaced left lateral or down |
|     5. Diameter | 1 to 2 cm | Over 2 cm |
|   **f.** Epigastric area (slide fingers up under rib cage) pulsations | Aortic pulsation with forward thrust Right ventricular pulsation with downward thrust | Bounding pulsation |

*Note: Apical pulse location may displace slightly laterally if client turns to left side.

| CHARACTERISTIC OR AREA EXAMINED | NORMAL | DEVIATIONS FROM NORMAL |
|---|---|---|
| **g.** Ectopic area (midway between pulmonary and apical areas) pulsations | None | Outward pulsation |
| **4.** Auscultation of following specific areas: | | |
| **a.** Aortic area (second right interspace) | | |
| **b.** Pulmonary area (second left interspace) | | |
| **c.** Third left interspace | | |
| **d.** Tricuspid area (fifth left interspace near sternum) | | |
| **e.** Apical area (fifth left interspace medial to midclavicular line) for: | | |
| 1. Rate | 60 to 90 beats/min (*Note:* The heart normally slows in rate with aging because of increase in vagal tone.) Some individuals may normally manifest rate of 50 beats/min; however, patients with slow heart rates should be referred for further evaluation | Over 90 beats/min Under 60 beats/min |
| 2. Rhythm | Regular (*Note:* Infrequent ectopic beats are fairly common with aging. However, all patients with irregularities should be referred.) | Irregular (without any pattern) Sporadic extra beats or pauses |
| 3. S₁ sound<br>  a. Location | Usually heard at all sites | |
|   b. Intensity | Often louder at apex (muscle, fat tissue, and air will diminish sound; rapid rate will accentuate sound) | Accented Diminished (muffled) Varying intensity with different beats (e.g., complete heart block) |
|   c. Frequency | Usually lower in pitch than $S_2$ | Frequency (pitch) becomes higher with accented intensity |
|   d. Timing | Almost synchronous with carotid impulse Slightly longer in duration than $S_2$ | |
|   e. Splitting | May be heard in tricuspid area (normal S, splitting sound usually varies from beat to beat: occasionally single sound, occasionally narrow split) | $S_4$ sometimes mistaken for $S_1$ splitting |
| 4. S₂ sound<br>  a. Location | Usually heard at all sites | |
|   b. Intensity | Often louder at base (intensity diminished with fat, muscle, or air) | Increased intensity, usually in aortic area (e.g., arterial hypertension) or pulmonary area (e.g., pulmonary hypertension) Decreased intensity |

# Clinical variations: the geriatric client—cont'd

**ASSESSMENT OF THE HEART AND PRECORDIUM—cont'd**

| CHARACTERISTIC OR AREA EXAMINED | NORMAL | DEVIATIONS FROM NORMAL |
|---|---|---|
| c. Frequency | Usually higher in pitch than $S_1$ | |
| d. Timing | Sound shorter in duration than $S_1$ | |
| e. Splitting | Occasionally heard in pulmonary area (on inspiration) | Wide splitting (e.g., right bundle branch block)<br>Fixed splitting<br>Paradoxical splitting (e.g., left bundle branch block) |
| 5. Systole | | |
| a. Duration | Shorter than diastole at normal heart rate (60 to 90 beats/min) | |
| b. Sounds | $S_1$ sound duration brief, silent interval | Early systolic ejection click:<br>aortic—heard at base and apex<br>pulmonary—heard in pulmonary area<br>Middle and late systolic clicks (e.g., mitral valve deformity) heard at left sternal border<br>Clicks high pitched and sharp in sound |
| 6. Diastole | | |
| a. Duration | Longer than systole at normal rate (60 to 90 beats/min)<br>Shortens in duration as rate increases | |
| b. Sounds | $S_2$ duration brief<br>Silent interval | |
| (1) $S_3$ | Absent | May signify heart failure |
| (a) Location | | At apex |
| (b) Intensity | | Dull, low pitched |
| (c) Timing | | Early in diastole (best heard when client is in left lateral decubitus position, with bell of stethoscope) |
| (2) $S_4$ | Absent<br>(*Note:* Some authorities state that $S_4$ sounds are fairly common in the elderly and may just indicate decreased left ventricular compliance. However, all patients with extra sounds should be referred for evaluation.) | May indicate left ventricular hypertrophy or myocardial ischemia |
| (a) Location | | Usually at apex or medial to apex |
| (b) Intensity | | Slightly higher in pitch than $S_3$ |
| (c) Timing | | Late diastole (may be confused with split $S_1$)<br>Best heard when client is in left lateral decubitus position, with bell |
| c. Other sounds | None | Opening snap: at apex or left sternal border; higher pitch; very early in diastole |

| CHARACTERISTIC OR AREA EXAMINED | NORMAL | DEVIATIONS FROM NORMAL |
|---|---|---|
| 7. Murmurs | | |
|   a. Systolic | Most authorities agree that soft, early systolic murmurs may be "functional" in elderly clients; commonly found, and caused by aortic lengthening, tortuosity, and sclerotic changes<br>Best heard in aortic area or at base of heart; however, all clients with murmurs should be referred for further evaluation | Loud aortic (ejection) murmurs that radiate into the neck may indicate obstructive aortic disease<br>Systolic murmurs heard at apex may indicate mitral calcification |
|   b. Diastolic | Diastolic murmurs are always abnormal | |
|   c. Timing | | Systolic—early, middle, late, continuous<br>Diastolic—early, middle, late, continuous |
|   d. Location | | Area where sound is heard may be small and confined or may cover most of precordium (Describe in terms of precordial landmarks and distance in centimeters from landmarks.) |
|   e. Radiation of sound | | (Describe in terms of landmarks and distance in centimeters.) |
|   f. Intensity | | Loud, medium, soft or grades 1 through 6<br>Stable, or varies with respiration or position |
|   g. Pitch | | High, medium, low |
|   h. Quality | | Blowing, harsh, rumbling<br>Crescendo<br>Decrescendo |
| 8. Other sounds | | Pericardial friction rub: to-and-fro rubbing sound, usually heard during systole and diastole; sound usually increased when client sits up and leans forward |
| **5.** Auscultation over carotid arteries | Faint heart sounds | Unilateral bruit (swishing sound) caused by obstruction or partial obstruction of carotid artery<br>Bilateral bruit resulting from referred heart murmur sound (particularly aortic systolic) or hyperkinesis |
| **6.** Repeat palpation and auscultation maneuvers with client (a) lying in left decubitus position and (b) sitting | | |

**Cognitive
self-assessment**

1. Which of the following statements are true about Korotkoff sounds?
   - ☐ a. At phase one the arterial intraluminal pressure is the same as the cuff pressure.
   - ☐ b. At phase two the sounds are replaced by a bruit.
   - ☐ c. Systolic pressure is recorded at the beginning of phase two.
   - ☐ d. Muffling of the sounds (phase four) is thought by many authorities to be the most accurate indicator of diastolic pressure for children.
   - ☐ e. The adult diastolic pressure is recorded when Korotkoff sounds are no longer heard.
   - ☐ f. c, d, and e
   - ☐ g. all the above
   - ☐ h. all except c
   - ☐ i. all except b
   - ☐ j. b and d

2. Which of the following statements are true about arterial blood pressure?
   - ☐ a. A difference of 5 to 10 mm Hg systolic pressure between arms is within normal limits.
   - ☐ b. The systolic pressure in the upper extremities is usually about 10 mm Hg higher than in the lower extremities.
   - ☐ c. A narrow cuff on an obese arm will yield a false low value.
   - ☐ d. Standing might lower the systolic pressure by 10 to 15 mm Hg in a healthy individual.
   - ☐ e. A wide cuff on a very small arm will yield a false low value.
   - ☐ f. a, b, and e
   - ☐ g. a, c, and d
   - ☐ h. all except c
   - ☐ i. a, d, and e
   - ☐ j. a, b, and c

3. Identify the variables that might alter a healthy client's blood pressure.
   - ☐ a. Age, sex, and weight
   - ☐ b. Circadian rhythm
   - ☐ c. Stress or anxiety
   - ☐ d. Food intake
   - ☐ e. Cuff/arm ratio
   - ☐ f. a, c, and e
   - ☐ g. all the above
   - ☐ h. all except b
   - ☐ i. all except d

4. You are auscultating Mrs. Jones's arterial blood pressure and hear a tapping sound at 210 mm Hg that continues until the mercury reaches 195. Then there is silence until the mercury reaches 185, at which time the tapping resumes and gradually intensifies. At 140, the loud, sharp sounds become muffled. At 110, the sounds disappear. How would you record this pressure?
   - ☐ a. 210/140
   - ☐ b. 210/110
   - ☐ c. 210/185/140
   - ☐ d. 195/185/110
   - ☐ e. 210/140/110

5. Which statement(s) is/are true about Mrs. Jones's blood pressure?
   - ☐ a. She has a wide pulse pressure.
   - ☐ b. She has a narrow pulse pressure.
   - ☐ c. She manifests an auscultatory gap.
   - ☐ d. At 140 mm Hg the cuff pressure first fell below the arterial intraluminal pressure.
   - ☐ e. At 110 mm Hg the cuff pressure first fell below the arterial intraluminal pressure.
   - ☐ f. a, c, and d
   - ☐ g. b, c, and d
   - ☐ h. a, c, and e
   - ☐ i. b and e
6. Identify the *true* statements about the following types of arterial pulses.
   - ☐ a. Anxiety can create a bounding pulse.
   - ☐ b. Aortic rigidity and atherosclerosis can create a bounding pulse.
   - ☐ c. Obstructive lung disease can cause a paradoxical pulse.
   - ☐ d. Pulsus alternans is evidence of left-sided heart failure.
   - ☐ e. The normal pulse contour is smooth and rounded.
   - ☐ f. a and d
   - ☐ g. a, c, and e
   - ☐ h. b and c
   - ☐ i. all the above
   - ☐ j. a, b, and e
7. Bates describes the differences between carotid and jugular pulsations. Which of the following statements are true about carotid pulsations?
   - ☐ a. They are rarely palpable.
   - ☐ b. Pulsation is not affected by inspiration.
   - ☐ c. Pulsation is not affected by position.
   - ☐ d. Pulsation usually increases in a recumbent position.
   - ☐ e. Soft, undulating quality with two or three outward thrust components.
   - ☐ f. b, d, and e
   - ☐ g. b and c
   - ☐ h. b and d
   - ☐ i. a and d
   - ☐ j. all except d
8. Which statement(s) is/are true about the jugular veins and jugular venous pressure?
   - ☐ a. The internal jugular vein connects, without valves, to the right atrium.
   - ☐ b. Jugular pulsation can usually be obliterated by moderate pressure at the scapular base of the neck.
   - ☐ c. Neck veins frequently distend when a healthy client is in a supine position.
   - ☐ d. The sternal angle is the common reference point for measuring jugular venous pressure.
   - ☐ e. Pregnancy usually increases jugular venous pressure.
   - ☐ f. all the above
   - ☐ g. all except e
   - ☐ h. b and d
   - ☐ i. a, b, and c

9. Mr. Jones's feet are cool to touch. You have asked him to elevate both legs about 30 cm (12 inches) above his body for approximately 60 seconds. Both feet manifest a mild pallor. Then you ask him to sit up and dangle his legs. His normal (pink) skin color returns to his toes in about 15 seconds. Which statement(s) is/are true about what you have observed?
   - ☐ a.  Venous insufficiency should be suspected.
   - ☐ b.  Arterial insufficiency should be suspected.
   - ☐ c.  The results are within normal limits.
   - ☐ d.  The leg-raising drained the feet of most of the venous blood.
   - ☐ e.  The leg-raising drained the feet of most of the arterial blood.
   - ☐ f.  c and d
   - ☐ g.  a and d
   - ☐ h.  b and d
   - ☐ i.  c and e
   - ☐ j.  none of the above

10. Which statement(s) is/are true about varicosities in the legs?
    - ☐ a.  Varicose means "dilated, swollen."
    - ☐ b.  Varicosities can result from proximal obstruction in the pelvic vein.
    - ☐ c.  Varicosities can result from inherent weakness in the saphenous vessel wall.
    - ☐ d.  The great and small saphenous veins may both be involved.
    - ☐ e.  The valves in the communicating veins between superficial and deep veins may be incompetent.
    - ☐ f.  a, b, and d
    - ☐ g.  c and e
    - ☐ h.  a and c
    - ☐ i.  all the above
    - ☐ j.  all except d

11. Which of the following statements is/are true about the heart?
    - ☐ a.  The heart lies within the mediastinum.
    - ☐ b.  The base of the heart is normally found in the fifth intercostal space.
    - ☐ c.  Most of the anterior cardiac surface consists of the right ventricle.
    - ☐ d.  The left ventricle makes up a small portion of the anterior cardiac surface.
    - ☐ e.  In a normal, average individual two thirds of the heart lies to the left of the midsternal line.
    - ☐ f.  all the above
    - ☐ g.  all except b
    - ☐ h.  all except c
    - ☐ i.  a, c, and d

12. Which of the following statement(s) is/are true?
    - ☐ a.  Low-frequency vibration sounds might be palpated more easily than they can be auscultated.
    - ☐ b.  A fever could create a palpable right ventricular impulse.
    - ☐ c.  When the client rolls to the left side, the apical impulse is laterally displaced.
    - ☐ d.  The normal apical impulse is palpated in an area 3 to 4 cm in diameter.
    - ☐ e.  The normal apical impulse is sustained during the first third to half of systole.
    - ☐ f.  a, c, and e

    ☐ g. c, d, and e
    ☐ h. all except e
    ☐ i. b and c
    ☐ j. all except d

13. Which of the following conditions would *not* produce right ventricular heave?
    ☐ a. Anxiety
    ☐ b. Pulmonary stenosis
    ☐ c. Pregnancy
    ☐ d. Aortic stenosis
    ☐ e. Anemia

14. Which of the following statement(s) is/are true?
    ☐ a. In auscultation of the heart, most low-pitched sounds are diastolic filling sounds or murmurs.
    ☐ b. Low-pitched sounds are often best heard when the client is supine.
    ☐ c. Auscultation should be performed with both the bell and the diaphragm.
    ☐ d. Loudness, quality, and pitch of a sound may vary with the age and build of a client.
    ☐ e. Auscultation is performed only when the client is lying down.
    ☐ f. all except e
    ☐ g. all the above
    ☐ h. all except b
    ☐ i. all except a
    ☐ j. c and d

15. Which of the following statement(s) is/are true?
    ☐ a. Heart murmurs are of longer duration than heart sounds.
    ☐ b. Heart murmurs originate within the heart itself.
    ☐ c. Heart murmurs originate within the great vessels.
    ☐ d. Most "innocent" murmurs are faint or under grade 3 intensity.
    ☐ e. "Innocent" murmurs are usually soft ejection murmurs.
    ☐ f. a, b, and d
    ☐ g. all except e
    ☐ h. all the above
    ☐ i. a, c, and d

16. Which of the following statement(s) is/are true?
    ☐ a. Aortic regurgitation causes a diastolic murmur.
    ☐ b. Pulmonic regurgitation causes a diastolic murmur.
    ☐ c. Mitral stenosis causes a diastolic murmur.
    ☐ d. Tricuspid stenosis causes a diastolic murmur.
    ☐ e. a and b
    ☐ f. none of the above
    ☐ g. all the above
    ☐ h. c and d

17. A systolic ejection murmur occurs:
    ☐ a. at the mitral or tricuspid valves
    ☐ b. at the pulmonary or aortic valves

18. A systolic regurgitant murmur occurs:
    ☐ a. at the mitral or tricuspid valves
    ☐ b. at the pulmonary or aortic valves

Identify the characteristics of an arterial pulse that an examiner notes when palpating (as identified in the *Clinical guidelines*), beginning with:
Rate
Rhythm

19. _____

20. _____

21. _____

22. _____

23. Label the cardiac chambers, valves, and vessels as shown in the accompanying illustration.

   a. _____      h. _____

   b. _____      i. _____

   c. _____      j. _____

   d. _____      k. _____

   e. _____      l. _____

   f. _____      m. _____

   g. _____

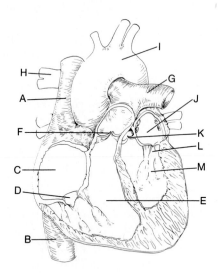

24. The first heart sound is caused by closure of _____and _____valves. It occurs at the beginning of: Systole? Diastole?

25. The second sound results from _____and _____valve closure. It occurs at the beginning of: Systole? Diastole?

Each statement describes a sign related to chronic venous insufficiency (CVI) or chronic arterial insufficiency (CAI). Fill in the blanks with either CVI or CAI.

26. _____ Extremity pulse diminished or absent

27. _____ Extremity cool

28. _____ Pigmentation and/or ulceration around ankles

29. _____ Loss of hair over foot and toes

30. _____ Marked pedal edema (with pitting)

31. _____ Extremity turns "dusky red" in dangling (dependent) position

32. _____ Thin, shiny, taut skin (over extremity)

The following statements describe characteristics of the first heart sound (S₁) or the second heart sound (S₂). Assign "a" (S₁) or "b" (S₂) to each statement.

33. _____ Usually sounds louder at the apex of the heart.
34. _____ Splitting heard near the pulmonary area.
35. _____ Slightly higher frequency than the other sound.
36. _____ Almost synchronous with carotid impulse.
37. _____ Splitting heard in the tricuspid area.
38. _____ Exercise shortens the P-R interval and results in a louder sound.
39. _____ A right bundle branch block causes delay of pulmonary valve closure and results in splitting.

The following statements describe characteristics of the third heart sound (S₃) or the fourth heart sound (S₄). Assign "a" (S₃) or "b" (S₄) to each statement.

40. _____ The sound originates in early diastolic rapid ventricular filling and wall vibration.
41. _____ The sound originates in late diastole rapid ventricular filling.
42. _____ Known as a presystolic gallop.
43. _____ Known as a protodiastolic gallop.
44. _____ Very commonly heard in normal children and young adults.
45. _____ Often signifies myocardial failure in older adults.

Match the sounds in column B with the locations in column A (as shown on the accompanying illustration) where they can best be heard.

**Column A**

46. _____ Aortic area
47. _____ Pulmonary area
48. _____ Third left intercostal space
49. _____ Tricuspid area
50. _____ Apical area

**Column B**

a. S₁—mitral valve closure
b. Aortic and pulmonary murmurs
c. S₂ splitting
d. Aortic stenosis—sound of hypertension
e. Split S₁, ventricular septal defect

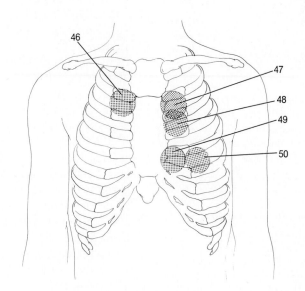

51. When examining 5-year-old John M., the examiner identifies the following findings:

    History: healthy child
    Pulse: 88 regular
    BP: 102/52
    Peripheral circulation good
    Heart sounds $S_1$, $S_2$ regular
    Extra sound consistently heard just following $S_2$ sound (split? $S_3$?)
    Murmur identified in systole: child was sitting; had soft short sound; remained audible following 30-second jumping exercise

    The examiner should:
    ☐ a. record the finding as a probable functional murmur and recheck the child in 8 weeks
    ☐ b. consider the cardiovascular examination normal; reevaluate child at next regularly scheduled well-child visit
    ☐ c. send the child *immediately* to the physician for further evaluation
    ☐ d. schedule the child for an ECG and stress test
    ☐ e. send the child for physician evaluation fairly soon, at a time convenient for both parties

52. Steven is a 7-year-old black boy. During his examination the nurse evaluated his pulse and blood pressure, which were normal. Which of the following readings would it have been?
    ☐ a. BP 94/40; pulse 88
    ☐ b. BP 128/72; pulse 84
    ☐ c. BP 112/78; pulse 74
    ☐ d. BP 102/48; pulse 102
    ☐ e. BP 120/62; pulse 94

53. At which of the following ages should routine blood pressure screening be initiated?
    ☐ a. 18 months
    ☐ b. 3 years
    ☐ c. 5 years
    ☐ d. 6 years
    ☐ e. 10 years

54. In auscultating the chest of a 4-year-old healthy child, all the following signs may be considered *normal* except one. Identify the abnormal finding.
    ☐ a. Sinus arrhythmia
    ☐ b. Single PVC
    ☐ c. $S_1$ split
    ☐ d. $S_3$ sound
    ☐ e. $S_4$ sound

55. In elderly people, cardiac output:
    ☐ a. decreases by 30% to 40% over a 40- to 50-year span
    ☐ b. is the same as in younger adults unless there is disease present
    ☐ c. may not respond adequately during severe stress
    ☐ d. may not respond adequately to tachycardia
    ☐ e. increases because of normal left ventricular enlargement and increasing peripheral resistance
    ☐ f. none of the above
    ☐ g. d and e
    ☐ h. a, c, and d

56. Pulses in geriatric clients:
    - ☐ a. may normally be slower than the average pulse of adults
    - ☐ b. are normally irregular and rapid
    - ☐ c. are normally irregular and slow
    - ☐ d. are less symmetrical in timing and amplitude than younger adult pulses
57. The systolic pressure in an older individual:
    - ☐ a. may be slightly higher because elderly people are often more excitable
    - ☐ b. may be slightly higher than the young adult because of elasticity changes in the large arteries
    - ☐ c. may be slightly lower than in the young adult because of loss of subcutaneous fat
    - ☐ d. is within 5 to 10 mm Hg of 120 range unless the client is hypertensive

---

## SUGGESTED READINGS

### General

Bates, B.: A guide to physical examination, ed. 3, Philadelphia, 1983, J.B. Lippincott Co., pp. 157-209, 304-306, 309-323.

Judge, R.D., and Zuidema, G., editors: Methods of clinical examination: a physiologic approach, ed. 3, Boston, 1974, Little, Brown & Co., pp. 141-199.

Kirkendall, W.M., and others: Recommendations for human blood pressure determination by sphygmomanometers, Dallas, 1980, Communication Division, American Heart Association.

Malasanos, L., and others: Health assessment, ed. 2., St. Louis, 1981, The C.V. Mosby Co., pp. 142-159, 321-347.

Nordmark, M.T., and Rohweder, A.W.: Scientific foundations of nursing, ed. 3, Philadelphia, 1975, J.B. Lippincott Co., pp. 15-52.

Patient assessment: abnormalities of the heartbeat, Programmed instruction, Am. J. Nurs. **77:**4, 1977.

Patient assessment: auscultation of the heart, Part II, Programmed instruction, Am. J. Nurs. **77:**2, 1977.

Patient assessment: examination of the heart and great vessels, Part I, Programmed instruction, Am. J. Nurs. **76:**11, 1976.

Patient assessment: pulses, Programmed instruction, Am. J. Nurs. **79:**1, 1979.

Prior, J.A., Silberstein, J.S., and Stang, J.M.: Physical diagnosis; the history and examination of the patient, ed. 6, St. Louis, 1981, The C.V. Mosby Co., pp. 242-303.

Walker, H.K., and others: Clinical methods: the history, physical and laboratory examinations, Boston, 1976, Butterworth, Inc., pp. 154-196.

### Audiovisual materials

Blue Hill Educational Systems, Inc. (videotape cassettes), New York, 1976.
  Tape 12A. Cardiovascular system: peripheral circulation (1 hr)
  Tape 12B. Cardiovascular system: the heart (1 hr)
  Tape 12C. Cardiovascular system: the heart (1 hr)
  Tape 12D. Cardiovascular system: the heart (½ hr)
Concept Media Filmstrips: Physical assessment: heart and lungs, Costa Mesa, Calif., 1976.
  Tape 5: Initial assessment of the heart
  Tape 6: Auscultation of heart sounds
Warner-Chilcott Laboratory, AEGIS Production: Differential diagnosis of chest pain, New York, 1967, American Heart Association.

### Pediatric

Alexander, M., and Brown, M.S.: Pediatric history taking and physical diagnosis for nurses, ed. 2, New York, 1979, McGraw-Hill Book Co., pp. 186-213.

Barness, L.: Manual of pediatric physical diagnosis, ed. 5, Chicago, 1981, Year Book Medical Publishers, Inc., pp. 110-144.

Brown, M.S., and Alexander, M.: Physical examination. II. Examining the heart, Nursing '74 **4**(12):41-47, 1974.

Haggerty, R.J., Maroney, M.W., and Nadas, A.S.: Essential hypertension in infancy and childhood, Am. J. Dis. Child. **92:**536, 1956.

Johnson, T.R., Moore, W.M., and Jeffries, J.E., editors: Children are different: developmental physiology, ed. 2, Columbus, Ohio, 1978, Ross Laboratories, pp. 136-141.

Pillitteri, A.: Nursing care of the growing family: a child health text, Boston, 1977, Little, Brown & Co., pp. 551-556.

Waring, W.W., and Jeansonne, L.O.: Practical manual of pediatrics: a pocket reference for those who treat children, ed. 2, St. Louis, 1982, The C.V. Mosby Co.

### Geriatric

Babu, T.N., and others: What is "normal" blood pressure in the aged? Geriatrics **32**(1):73-76, 1977.

Caird, F.I., and Judge, T.G.: Assessment of the elderly patient, London, 1977, Pitman Medical Publishing Co., Ltd., pp. 31-39.

Carotenuto, R., and Bullock, J.: Physical assessment of the gerontologic client, Philadelphia, 1980, F.A. Davis Co., pp. 83-100.

Foster, S., and Kousch, D.C.: Controlling high blood pressure: promoting patient adherence, Am. J. Nurs. **78**(5):829-832, 1978.

Harris, R.: Cardiopathy of aging: are the changes related to congestive heart failure? Geriatrics **32**(2):42-46, 1977.

Luisada, A.A.: Using noninvasive methods to study the aging heart, Geriatrics **32**(2):58-61, 1977.

Mead, W.F.: The aging heart, Am. Fam. Phys. **18**(2):73-80, 1978.

Steinberg, F.U., editor: Care of the geriatric patient, ed. 6, St. Louis, 1983, The C.V. Mosby Co., pp. 92-104.

Ward, G.W., Bandy, P., and Fink, J.W.: Controlling high blood pressure: treating and counseling the hypertensive patient, Am. J. Nurs. **78**(5):824-828, 1978.

# 10

## ASSESSMENT OF THE

# Breasts

### VOCABULARY

**areola**  A circular, dark pigmented area around the nipple of the breast.

**Cooper ligaments**  Suspensory ligaments of the breast.

**gynecomastia**  Condition characterized by abnormally large mammary glands in the male.

**inverted nipple**  Nipple that is turned inward.

**mastitis**  An inflammation of the breast.

**Paget disease**  Condition characterized by an excoriating or scaling lesion of the nipple, extending from an intraductal carcinoma of the breast.

**peau d'orange**  Dimpling of the skin that resembles the skin of an orange.

**pectoralis major muscle**  One of the four muscles of the anterior upper portion of the chest.

**retraction**  Shortening or drawing backward of the skin.

**sebaceous gland**  An oil-secreting gland of the skin.

**striae**  Colorless lines caused by mechanical stretching of the skin.

**supernumerary nipple**  Extra nipple.

**tail of Spence**  Upper outer tail of the breast that extends into the axillary region.

**Montgomery tubercles**  Small sebaceous glands located on the areola of the breast.

## Cognitive objectives

At the end of this chapter the learner will demonstrate knowledge of assessment of the breasts by the ability to do the following:

1. Identify the lymphatic system associated with the breasts and discuss lymphatic drainage patterns.
2. List inspection criteria associated with examination of the breasts.
3. List palpation criteria associated with examination of the breasts.
4. Identify client positions for examination of the breasts.
5. Describe selected signs and/or symptoms that would warrant physician referral or further investigation.
6. List instruction techniques associated with breast self-examination.
7. Identify the appropriate times of the month for women to perform breast self-examination.
8. Point out maturational variations associated with the breasts and their assessment.
9. Identify selected variations for pediatric and geriatric clients.
10. Use the terms in the vocabulary section.

## Clinical objectives

At the end of this chapter the learner will perform a systematic assessment of the breasts, demonstrating the ability to do the following:

1. Obtain a pertinent health history from the client.
2. Demonstrate and record results of inspection of the breasts while the client is seated and lying down. This assessment should include:
   a. General breast assessment
      (1) Size
      (2) Symmetry
      (3) Contour
      (4) Appearance of skin (color, texture, venous patterns)
      (5) Moles or nevi
   b. Areolar area
      (1) Size
      (2) Shape
      (3) Surface characteristics
   c. Nipples
      (1) Direction
      (2) Size and shape
      (3) Color
      (4) Surface characteristics
      (5) Discharge
3. Demonstrate and record results of palpation of the breasts while the client is seated and lying down, including:
   a. General breast assessment
      (1) Firmness
      (2) Tissue qualities
   b. Nipples
      (1) Elasticity
      (2) Tissue qualities
      (3) Discharge
   c. Lymphatic assessment
      (1) Supraclavicular and infraclavicular nodes
      (2) Central and lateral axillary nodes
      (3) Pectoral, scapular, and subscapular nodes
      (4) Brachial, intermediate, and internal mammary nodal chains
4. Demonstrate and record appropriate inspection and palpation of the male breasts.
5. Demonstrate instructional techniques and rationale in teaching self-examination of the breasts.

## Health history additional to screening history

1. By synthesizing historical data, genetic factors, and information about exposure to carcinogenic agents, compile a risk profile for the client. Table 10-1 shows the assessment criteria that will help to develop a breast cancer risk profile for women living in the United States. Use these data to develop a profile for *every* female client assessed. If the examiner determines that the client has a basically high-risk profile, then thorough examination, breast self-examination instruction techniques, and regular reevaluation periods become vitally important.
2. If the client has a symptomatic complaint of the breasts (e.g., pain, tenderness, lump, nipple discharge, skin rashes, or changes in size or shape of the breasts, a thorough investigation must be made. In addition to the steps stated in the symptom analysis section (Chapter 1), the following questions should be asked:
   a. How long has the lump or thickening been present?
   b. Have there been recent changes in breast characteristics, such as pain, tenderness, size, shape, overlying skin characteristics? Describe.
   c. If there is pain, is it described as stinging, pulling, burning, or drawing?
   d. Is the pain unilateral or bilateral?
   e. Is the pain or discomfort localized, or does it spread?
   f. Does the lump or discomfort change in size or character with menses?
   g. Has the client been involved in any strenuous activity that could contribute to the breast discomfort?

h. Does the client complain of nipple discharge? If so, inquire about:
  (1) Duration of problem
  (2) Drainage characteristics, including color, consistency, odor, amount
  (3) Times present (always, before menses, other)
  (4) Drug therapy such as oral contraceptives, phenothiazines, digitalis, diuretics, or steroids

i. Continued questioning should include items from the risk profile assessment criteria in Table 10-1.

3. Does the client examine her own breasts regularly? Has she been taught the breast self-examination? At what part of the month does she examine her breasts? Have client explain the technique she uses. The box on p. 283 contains the American Cancer Society evaluation guidelines for detection of breast cancer in asymptomatic women.

**TABLE 10-1.** Assessment criteria for development of a breast cancer risk profile

| QUESTIONS FOR CLIENT | HIGH-RISK CRITERIA | LOW-RISK CRITERIA |
|---|---|---|
| Age | Women over 40 years of age | Women under 25 years of age |
| Race | Whites; affluent blacks | Low-income whites; low-income blacks |
| Ethnic ancestry | Northern European, Jewish ancestry | Latin or Mediterranean ancestry; American Indians, Orientals |
| Hemisphere | Western | Eastern |
| Climate | Cold | Warm |
| Income (high, medium, low) | High and middle income | Lower incomes |
| Home location past 10 years (city, town, rural community) | Large cities, industrial cities, especially in Northeast | Medium cities, small towns, rural areas |
| Breast cancer in family that occurred before menopause (inquire about mother, sisters, maternal grandmother, maternal aunts, maternal first cousins) | Positive response to any of these if they occurred before menopause | Negative response to any of these; positive response if it occurred after menopause |
| Menarche and menopause history: early, late | Early menstruation, late menopause | Late menstruation, early menopause |
| Chronic psychological stress | Yes | No |
| Obesity | Yes | No |
| Obesity-diabetes-hypertension triad | Yes | No |
| Low-dietary-fat intake | No | Yes |
| History of breast abnormalities (may include fibrocystic disease, adenomas, mastitis, breast abscesses, or breast injury) | Positive response to any items listed; other abnormalities | Negative response to any items listed |
| Diet history: whether it is high in animal proteins and fats or high in vegetable consumption and low in animal proteins and fats; caffeine | Diet high in animal proteins and/or animal fats  High consumption of caffeine | Diet mostly vegetarian or low in animal proteins and/or animal fats (e.g., Seventh Day Adventists)  Low consumption of caffeine |
| Reproductive and sexual histories | Late beginning of sexual activity  No history of sexual activity | Early beginning of sexual activity |
| Children | No children | Has had children |
| Breast-fed children | No breast-feeding | Has breast-fed children |
| Age when children were born | Delivered first child after age 35 years | Delivered first child before age 20 years |

Data from Leis, H.P., Jr.: Epidemiology of breast cancer: identification of the high-risk woman. In Gallager, H.S., and others, editors: The breast, St. Louis, 1978, The C.V. Mosby Co.; Kushner, R.: Breast cancer risks for U.S. women. In Martin, L.L.: Health care of women, Philadelphia, 1978, J.B. Lippincott Co.

## EVALUATION GUIDELINES FOR DETECTION OF BREAST CANCER IN ASYMPTOMATIC WOMEN

- Women 20 years of age and older should perform breast self-examination every month.
- Women 20 to 40 should have a physical examination of the breast every three years, and women over 40 should have a physical examination of the breast every year.
- Women between the ages of 35 and 40 should have a baseline mammogram.
- Women under 40 should consult their personal health care provider about the need for mammography.

- Women over 40 should have a mammogram every one to two years when feasible.
- Women over 50 should have a mammogram every year when feasible.
- Women with personal or family histories of breast cancer should consult their health care provider about the need for more frequent examinations, or about beginning periodic mammography before the age of 40.

From American Cancer Society: CA **32**(4):226-230, 1982.

# Clinical guidelines
## ASSESSMENT OF THE FEMALE BREASTS

| THE STUDENT WILL: | TO IDENTIFY: | |
| | NORMAL | DEVIATIONS FROM NORMAL |
| --- | --- | --- |
| 1. Instruct client to *sit* comfortably and erect on side of cart; *arms should be at side;* gown should be around waist so that breasts may be fully evaluated (Fig. 10-1) | | |

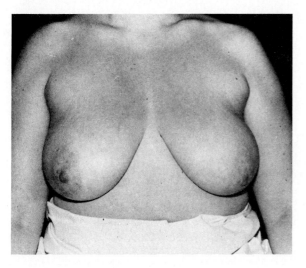

**FIG. 10-1.** Breasts ready for inspection.

## Clinical guidelines—cont'd
ASSESSMENT OF THE FEMALE BREASTS—cont'd

| | TO IDENTIFY: | |
|---|---|---|
| THE STUDENT WILL: | NORMAL | DEVIATIONS FROM NORMAL |

**2.** Inspect and bilaterally compare:

   **a.** Breasts

| | | |
|---|---|---|
| 1. Size | Varies | |
| 2. Symmetry | Bilaterally equal | Recent unilateral increase in size, marked asymmetry |
| | Slight asymmetry (Fig. 10-2) | |
| 3. Contour | Smooth, convex, even pattern | Dimpling, retraction |
| | | Interruption of convex pattern |
| | | Fixation |

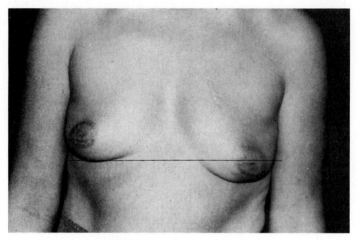

**FIG. 10-2.** Breast asymmetry.

| | | |
|---|---|---|
| 4. Skin color | Even throughout | Hyperpigmentation |
| | | Erythema |
| 5. Skin texture | Smooth, elastic, movable, striae | Thickened, rough |
| | | Lesions or thickening |
| | | Edema (peau d'orange) (Fig. 10-3) |

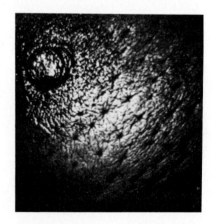

**FIG. 10-3.** Peau d'orange. (From Gallagher, H.S.: Leis, H.P., Jr., Snyderman, R.K., and Urban, J.A., editors: The breast, St. Louis, 1978, The C.V. Mosby Co.)

| THE STUDENT WILL: | TO IDENTIFY: | |
| --- | --- | --- |
| | NORMAL | DEVIATIONS FROM NORMAL |
| 6. Venous patterns | Bilaterally similar | Localized, unilateral increase in vascular pattern |
| 7. Moles, nevi | Long history of presence<br>Nonchanging<br>Nontender | Newly developed or changed<br>Tender |
| **b.** Areolar area | | |
| 1. Size | Bilaterally equal | Unequal |
| 2. Shape | Round or oval | Other than round or oval |
| 3. Surface characteristics | Smooth, bilaterally similar, Montgomery tubercles (Fig. 10-4) | Masses, lesions<br>Color pigment changes<br>Unilateral pigment change |

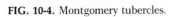

**FIG. 10-4.** Montgomery tubercles.

| | | |
| --- | --- | --- |
| **c.** Nipples | | |
| 1. Direction | Bilaterally equal in pointing direction (Fig. 10-5, *A*)<br>Supernumerary nipples | Asymmetrical deviations (Fig. 10-5, *B*) |

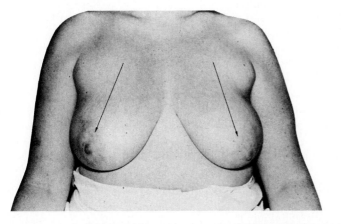
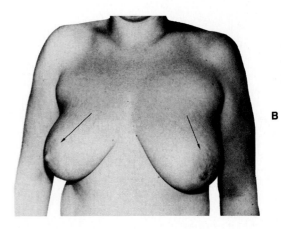

A        B

**FIG. 10-5. A,** Symmetrical breasts (note nipple position). **B,** Lateral deviation of right breast (note nipple position).

# Clinical guidelines—cont'd
**ASSESSMENT OF THE FEMALE BREASTS—cont'd**

| THE STUDENT WILL: | TO IDENTIFY: | |
| --- | --- | --- |
| | NORMAL | DEVIATIONS FROM NORMAL |
| 2. Size, shape | Bilaterally equal<br>Long-standing inversion (unilateral or bilateral) (Fig. 10-6, *A*) | Asymmetrical<br>Recent inversion or retraction (unilateral or bilateral) (Fig. 10-6, *B*) |

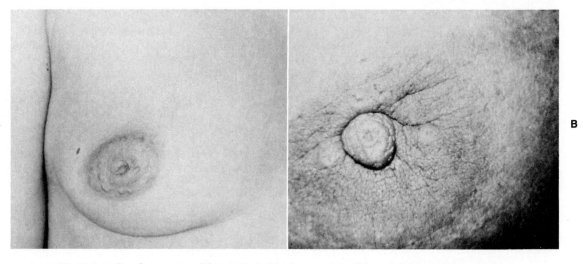

FIG. 10-6. **A,** Simple inversion of the nipple. **B,** Nipple retraction. (**B** from Gallagher, H.S., and others, editors: The breast, St. Louis, 1978, The C.V. Mosby Co.)

| | | |
| --- | --- | --- |
| 3. Color | Homogeneous | Edema, redness<br>Bilaterally unequal<br>Pigment changes |
| 4. Surface characteristics | Smooth, may be slightly wrinkled<br>Skin intact | Ulceration, crusting<br>Erosion, scaling<br>Wrinkled, dry, cracking, with lesions |
| 5. Discharge (if present, describe odor, color, amount, consistency) | Absent | Serous, bloody, odorous, purulent discharges (Fig. 10-7) |

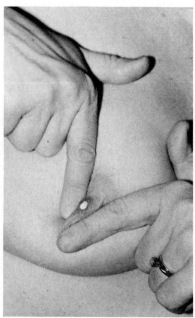

FIG. 10-7. Nipple discharge.

| THE STUDENT WILL: | TO IDENTIFY: | |
| --- | --- | --- |
| | NORMAL | DEVIATIONS FROM NORMAL |

**3.** Inspect breasts while client is *seated with arms abducted overhead* (Fig. 10-8), to observe and bilaterally compare all items previously listed, as well as:

   **a.** Bilateral pull on suspensory ligaments — Equal; breasts bilaterally symmetrical — Asymmetry / Shortening or appearance of attachment of either breast (fixation)

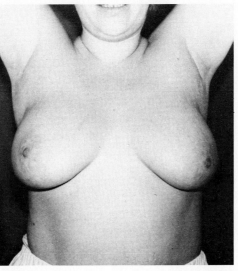

FIG. 10-8. Inspect breasts with client's arms extended overhead.

**4.** Inspect breasts while client is *seated and leaning over,* to observe (Fig. 10-9) and bilaterally compare:

   **a.** Symmetry — Breasts hang equally / Smooth skin contour — Asymmetry / Bulging retraction

   **b.** Bilateral pull on suspensory ligaments — Equal; breasts bilaterally symmetrical — Shortening or appearance of attachment of either breast (fixation)

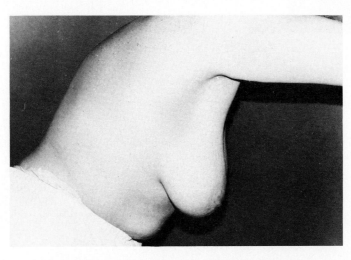

FIG. 10-9. Inspect breasts with client leaning forward.

## Clinical guidelines—cont'd
### ASSESSMENT OF THE FEMALE BREASTS—cont'd

| | TO IDENTIFY: | |
| --- | --- | --- |
| THE STUDENT WILL: | NORMAL | DEVIATIONS FROM NORMAL |

5. Inspect breasts while client is *seated and pushing hands onto hips or pushing palms together* (Fig. 10-10) and contracting pectoral muscles, to observe and bilaterally compare all items as previously listed

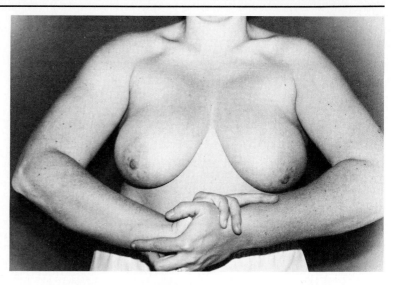

FIG. 10-10. Inspect breasts while client flexes pectoral muscles.

6. Palpate each breast in a systematic clockwise direction; client is seated with arms at sides (Fig. 10-11)

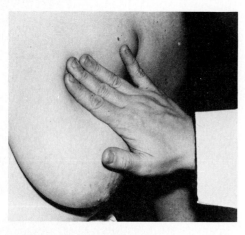

FIG. 10-11. Examiner using finger pads to examine breasts.

7. Palpate and bilaterally compare:
   **a.** Four quadrants, tail of breast, and areolar area for:

| | | |
| --- | --- | --- |
| 1. Firmness | Bilaterally equal<br>With aging or poor bra support, sagging of breast tissue may occur | Asymmetry |
| 2. Tissue qualities (see *Clinical strategies* for further description) | Smooth, diffuse tissue bilaterally<br>Nodular, bilateral granular consistency<br>Premenstrual engorgement<br>Elastic, nontender<br>Firm mammary ridge found along each breast at approximately 4 to 8 o'clock position | Tenderness unrelated to menstrual cycle<br>Unilateral pain or tenderness, unilateral mass<br>Heat of tissue |

| THE STUDENT WILL: | TO IDENTIFY: | |
| --- | --- | --- |
| | **NORMAL** | **DEVIATIONS FROM NORMAL** |

**b.** Nipple
    1. Elasticity and tissue characteristics
    2. Discharge (note color, odor, consistency, amount)
**c.** Lymph nodes associated with lymphatic drainage system (Fig. 10-12); location and characteristics of lymph nodes, including supraclavicular and infraclavicular, central and lateral axillary, pectoral, subscapular, scapular, brachial, intermediate, and internal mammary chains (Fig. 10-13)

Bilaterally equal, nontender
Smooth, skin intact
Absent

Nonpalpable

Tender, friable tissue, cracks, bleeding
Lesions, dryness, crusting, erosion
Present; serous, bloody, purulent, odorous
Palpable
Note:
1. Location
2. Size
3. Contour
4. Consistency
5. Discreteness
6. Mobility
7. Tenderness

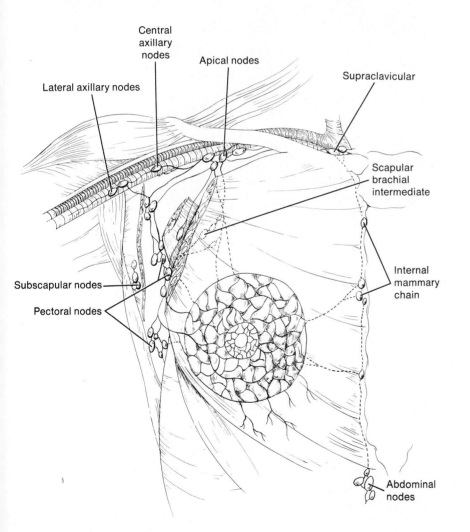

FIG. 10-12. Lymphatic drainage of the breast.

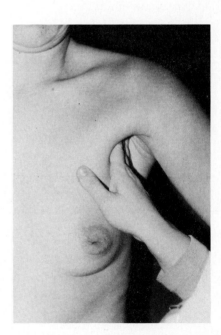

**FIG. 10-13.** Palpating axillary lymph nodes.

## Clinical guidelines—cont'd
### ASSESSMENT OF THE FEMALE BREASTS—cont'd

| THE STUDENT WILL: | TO IDENTIFY: NORMAL | DEVIATIONS FROM NORMAL |
|---|---|---|
| 8. Instruct client to remain *sitting* and *raise both arms over head;* may be most comfortable for client to grasp hands and rest them on top of head; repeat and compare bilaterally the palpation of: | | |
|   **a.** Four quadrants of each breast | Criteria as previously described | Criteria as previously described |
|   **b.** Tail of each breast | | |
|   **c.** Areolar area | | |
|   **d.** Nipple | | |
|   **e.** Lymph nodes | | |
| 9. Instruct client to lie supine with arm of breast to be examined resting over head (Fig. 10-14); place small towel under shoulder and back of breast to be examined (this displaces breast tissue more diffusely over chest wall) | | |

**FIG. 10-14.** Positioning for breast examination. Note placement of towel.

| | | |
|---|---|---|
| 10. Inspect: | | |
|   **a.** Breasts, noting: | Criteria as previously described | Criteria as previously described |
|     1. Symmetry | | |
|     2. Contour | | |
|     3. Skin color | | |
|     4. Skin texture | | |
|     5. Venous patterns | | |
|     6. Moles, nevi | | |
|   **b.** Areolar area surface characteristics | | |
|   **c.** Nipple characteristics | | |
| 11. Palpate each breast in systematic clockwise direction; carefully evaluate: | | |
|   **a.** Four quadrants of each breast | Criteria as previously described | Criteria as previously described |
|   **b.** Tail of each breast | | |
|   **c.** Areolar area | | |
|   **d.** Nipple | | |
|   **e.** Lymph nodes | | |

# Clinical guidelines—cont'd

## ASSESSMENT OF THE MALE BREASTS

| THE STUDENT WILL: | TO IDENTIFY: | |
| --- | --- | --- |
| | NORMAL | DEVIATIONS FROM NORMAL |
| 1. Inspect male client's breasts while he is seated, arms resting at sides | | |
| 2. Inspect nipple and areolar area; compare bilaterally | Intact, smooth<br>Bilaterally equal color<br>Flat tissue<br>Smooth, nontender<br>Skin intact, nontender | Ulcerated<br>Masses, swelling<br>Discolorations<br>Tenderness<br>Unilateral or unequal swelling or masses (Fig. 10-15) |
| 3. Palpate client's breast and areolar area while he is seated, arms resting at sides; note skin texture, tissue consistency; compare bilaterally | | |

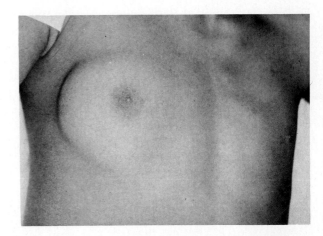

**FIG. 10-15.** Adult gynecomastia (diffuse type). (From Gallagher, H.S., Leis, H.P., Jr., Snyderman, R.K., and Urban, J.A., editors: The breast, St. Louis, 1978, The C.V. Mosby Co.)

4. Palpate lymphatic system associated with the breast (similar to female breast assessment)

## Clinical strategies

1. Complete breast examination requires that the breast be evaluated in numerous positions. This facilitates pull on the suspensory ligaments that will most likely demonstrate retraction or dimpling of an affected breast. To summarize the previous clinical guidelines, the evaluation positions include:
   a. Inspection: client sitting, arms at side; sitting, arms above head; sitting or standing, leaning over; sitting, hands pressed onto hips
   b. Palpation: client sitting, arms at side; sitting, arms above head
   c. Palpation: client lying, arm above head
   The total time required to completely evaluate the breasts should be between 5 and 10 minutes.
2. Symmetry is a key consideration in the assessment of the breasts. There should be a comparison of one side with the other throughout the assessment process.
3. For proper breast assessment, the client must be undressed to the waist. She must be encouraged to uncover both breasts at once so that they may be viewed together and compared. The examiner is not doing the client a favor by allowing her to uncover only one breast at a time.
4. Room lighting, for examination of the breast, is very important. The illumination should be overhead and adequate to shed an even light over all breast surfaces. Recognizing subtle coloring or surface characteristic changes of the breasts may depend on the lighting of the examination room.
5. The male client must be evaluated with the same sensitivity as the female client. Male breast cancer accounts for about 1% of all cancer of the breast. Beyond that, there are numerous other disease or inflammatory processes that can cause gynecomastia or areolar inflammation (Fig. 10-15).
6. When palpating the breast, the examiner must learn to use the sensitive finger pads of the palmar surface of the hand (Fig. 10-11). The examiner must inch along the breast surface, using a rotating exploratory manner. Try *not to lift* the fingers off the breast when moving from one point to the next. The examination technique should smoothly and continually move forward.
7. It is most beneficial to first do a complete light palpation and then repeat the procedure, changing to a deeper, heavier palpation. Most authorities state that the light exploratory palpation will yield more information than the deeper palpation.
8. For women with very large breasts, the palpation component of the seated examination is best performed when the examiner immobilizes the breast underneath with one hand while examining the above surface with the other hand. This bimanual palpation technique must assist in the detection of small mobile masses not picked up by other techniques.
9. If the examination takes place right before the client's menstrual period and her breasts are tender and engorged, make arrangements for the client to return after the end of her period for a thorough breast assessment.

**TABLE 10-2.** Physical findings helpful in the differential diagnosis of a breast lump

| PHYSICAL FINDINGS | FAVORS MALIGNANCY | FAVORS BENIGNANCY |
| --- | --- | --- |
| Hard, dominant lump | Single, definite | Multiple, indistinct |
| Firm, palpable, radiating ducts | No help | Indicates cystic disease |
| Venous engorgement | Unilateral | Bilateral |
| Nipple deviation | Unilateral | Bilateral, symmetrical |
| Nipple excoriation | Unilateral | Bilateral |
| Skin dimpling | Present | Absent |
| Chest wall fixation | Present | Absent |
| Peau d'orange | Present | Absent |
| Bloody discharge | Present | Absent |
| Axillary or supraclavicular nodes | Present | Absent |
| Freely movable mass | No help | Typical of fibroadenoma |
| Tenderness | No help | May indicate cystic mass |
| Inflammation, heat | Ominous in nonlactating or nonpostpartum breast | Abscess in lactating or postpartum breast |

From Nance, F.: Clin. Obstet. Gynecol. **18**(2):188, 1975.

10. During the examination of the nipples, the examiner should gently express the nipple with the index fingers of both hands and slowly strip the nipple between the fingers as they slide from the areola to the tip of the nipple. Palpation of the nipple should also include an exploration for small masses or duct thickening. If nipple discharge is present, note if it is coming from a single duct opening or multiple ones.

11. Although it is relatively simple to palpate the areas where the lymph nodes are located, it is another issue to relate the lymph nodes with their drainage significance. Following is an outline of the patterns for breast lymphatic drainage. (See Fig. 10-12.)
    a. Lymphatic drainage of superficial breast tissue
       1. Mammary chain (located along medial and superior borders of breast tissue; drainage occurs toward opposite breast)
       2. Scapular
       3. Brachial    }   All located in upper outer quadrant of breast; drainage occurs toward axillary nodes
       4. Intermediate
    b. Lymphatic drainage of deep breast tissue
       1. Supraclavicular
       2. Apical nodes or subclavicular or infraclavicular
       3. Central axillary
       4. Lateral axillary
       5. Pectoral (anterior)
       6. Subscapular (posterior)

       All these lymph nodes drain the breast. The most common drainage patterns are toward the *lateral axillary* (drains arm), *subscapular,* and *supraclavicular chains.* The medial and inferior deep breast tissue may also drain into the abdominal region.
    c. Areolar lymphatic drainage (areolar and nipple areas)
       1. Central axillary
       2. Apical nodes or subclavicular or infraclavicular
       3. Superior mammary chain

       Drainage of the areolar area involves an upward movement, toward the subclavicular and supraclavicular regions.

12. When dealing with a symptomatic breast problem, the examiner should start the evaluation procedure with the unaffected breast.

13. If the examiner identifies a lump or mass in the breast, it should be evaluated according to the following criteria:
    a. Location according to clock orientation and distance from the nipple
    b. Size
    c. Contour and shape—margin regularity versus irregularity
    d. Consistency (soft, firm, rough)
    e. Discreteness (difficulty determining borders)
    f. Mobility
    g. Tenderness (marked or absent)
    h. Erythema of overlying skin
    i. Tissue characteristics over mass (bulging, dimpling)

14. In compiling the data associated with a breast mass or breast problem, the examiner must determine the urgency of the client's problem. Table 10-2 presents the physical findings related to benign and malignant breast masses and thus will help the examiner evaluate the data collected during physical assessment.

15. Work hard to develop a systematic assessment method. As with all of the body systems, a patterned assessment process reduces the likelihood of missing a significant finding.

## Techniques and strategies for teaching breast self-examination

One in every thirteen women in the United States will develop breast cancer. In 1983 alone, over 114,000 new cases were discovered. Although it is impossible to prevent cancer of the breast, every health care provider must assume the position that it is possible to detect a breast mass early and to initiate prompt treatment. Each examiner must incorporate teaching breast self-examination techniques into the examination procedures because most breast masses will be detected by the women themselves. The American Cancer Society states that 85% of all women who are treated promptly for early breast cancer do recover.

The examiner can facilitate client education and health maintenance by (1) developing a risk profile for the client and sharing the data collected and by (2) teaching breast self-examination techniques.

The teaching program should include both an informal and a structured presentation. The informal component will take place as the examiner is actually checking the client's breasts. Each step should be explained as it is being done. Involve the client in the process. If the client understands what is being done and why, compliance is likely to increase.

The formal component involves scheduling 10 to 15 minutes with the client to systematically discuss the anatomy of the breast, the sequence of the examination techniques, the anticipated findings, the appropriate times of the month to examine the breasts, and what the client should do about abnormal or questionable findings.

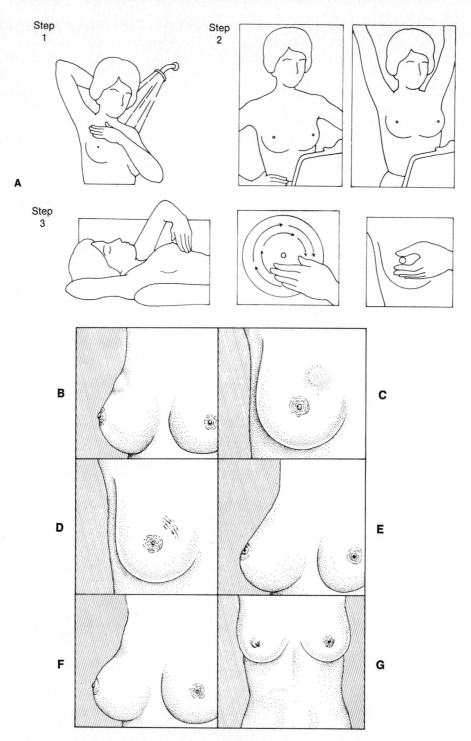

**FIG. 10-16. A,** Steps in breast self-examination. Inspect and palpate breasts *(1)* in the shower, *(2)* before a mirror, and *(3)* lying down. In all positions use the palmar surface of the examining fingers to inch along the breast tissue. Examine each breast using a circular movement until you are confident that the tail of the breast and all four quadrants have been evaluated. Gently express each nipple. Observe for discharge and bleeding. During inspection and palpation look for the following: swelling or elevated area **(B),** redness or inflammation **(C),** puckering or dimpling **(D),** nipple pulled inward **(E),** depression or sunken area **(F),** and nipple pulled askew compared with the other nipple **(G).** (Courtesy American Cancer Society: Teaching breast self-examination, Instructional material no. 77-1R-50M, no. 2015-LE, June 1977.)

The following sequence of information provides the examiner with an instructional overview of breast self-examination*:

1. Breast cancer facts
   a. Over 114,000 new cases of breast cancer were discovered in the United States in 1983.
   b. Over 37,000 women die from breast cancer each year.
   c. Up to 85% of women who receive prompt treatment for early breast cancer recover.
   d. Breast cancer is the leading cause of death from cancer in women, accounting for 26% of all female cancer deaths.
   e. Breast cancer is the leading cause of death from all causes among women from 40 to 44 years of age.
   f. Breast cancer usually begins as a lump or thickening in the breast.
   g. About 90% of all breast lumps are found by the women themselves.
   h. About 80% of all breast lumps are benign.
2. Age of women who should examine breasts: *all* women from menarche through old age.
3. Best time of month to examine breasts
   a. Menstruating women: sixth to seventh day of menstrual period; at this time the breasts are least engorged or tender.
   b. Pregnant women: pick single day of each month; the birthdate is generally used.
   c. Postmenopausal women: pick a single day of each month; again, the birthdate is usually a convenient number to remember.

*Data from American Cancer Society: Teaching breast self-exami-
nation, Instructional material no. 77-1R-50M-6/77, no. 2015-LE;
Silverberg, E., and Lubera, J.A.: CA **33**(1):2-25, 1983.

4. Breast anatomy the client must know
   a. Lymph nodes and locations associated with breast self-examination
   b. The four quadrants, the tail, the mammary ridge
   c. Areolar area
   d. Nipple
   e. Tissue characteristics: tenderness, nodular
5. Steps in teaching breast self-examination (Fig. 10-16); instructions for client
6. What to do if lump or abnormality is identified
   a. Note time of month in relation to menses.
   b. Assist client to make appointment with physician for further evaluation.

## History and clinical strategies: the pediatric client

Although the breasts should be inspected during each well-child visit as part of the chest examination, there are basically two time periods when the examiner systematically evaluates the breasts: (1) following the birth of the child and during the newborn period; and (2) as a girl reaches puberty and her breasts begin to develop. Because the clinical guidelines for inspection and palpation remain the same for both the child and the adult, this section of the chapter has been developed to provide information about breast development and clinical strategies when approaching the pediatric client.

Often the neonate's breasts may be enlarged for 1 to 2 months. This is a simple hypertrophic breast, which is normal. Characteristics include flat nipple, small areola, and a small amount of milky discharge. Deviations requiring referral include hypertrophy extending beyond 3 months, redness, heat, or firmness around the nipple, and increased pigmentation around the areola.

Boys who are stocky or heavy may experience some hypertrophy of breast tissue. This may be a normal finding but many times is of great concern to the boy. He should be assured that, as he grows and thins, the hypertrophy will disappear. The examiner should assess the breasts to rule out actual breast development, tenderness, masses, redness, or inflammation. At puberty, true gynecomastia is normal for some boys, but for others it may be a symptom of a systemic disease process. Refer these boys for further evaluation.

As breast tissue in girls begins to develop, there will usually be protrusion of the nipple first. Breasts in girls normally develop between the ages 10 years 8 months and 13 years 6 months. Menarche occurs in most girls at about 12 years 3 months (Fig. 10-17). Table 10-3 summarizes the physical development of girls. If there is no evidence of breast or other puberty development by age 13 years, the girl should be re-

**TABLE 10-3.** Maturational sequence in girls

| STAGE | BREAST DEVELOPMENT | DEVELOPMENT DESCRIPTION |
|---|---|---|
| 1 | | Preadolescent |
| 2 | | Breast and papilla elevated as small mound; areolar diameter increased |
| 3 | | Breast and aerola enlarged; no contour separation |
| 4 | | Areola and papilla form secondary mound |
| 5 | | Mature; nipple projects areolar part of general breast contour |

From Tanner, J.M.: Growth at adolescence, ed. 2, Oxford, England, 1962, Blackwell Scientific Publications, Ltd.

ferred to a physician. Once menarche has begun, the examiner should employ the same breast examination techniques as for the adult client. The young client will need much reassurance and assistance to feel comfortable during the breast examination.

Following are educational factors that may help the client feel more comfortable during examination of the breasts:

1. Breasts may develop at different ages; this is based on hereditary and hormonal characteristics and has nothing to do with the client's femininity.

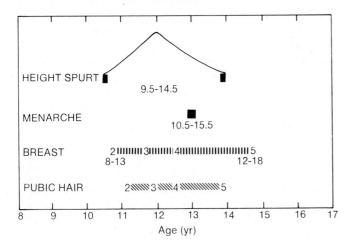

**FIG. 10-17.** Summary of maturational development of girls. For explanation of numbers 2 through 5, see Table 10-3; summary numbers on table (e.g., 9.5-14.5) indicate average or common range for development characteristic. (From Marshall, W.A., and Tanner, J.M.: Arch. Dis. Child. **44:**291, 1969.)

2. The right and left breasts may not develop at the same rate.
3. Assess the client's understanding of breast development and menarche.
4. Begin educational instruction regarding care of the breasts, qualities of a supportive bra, and breast self-examination techniques.

### History and clinical strategies: the geriatric client

The elderly client is subject to the same risk factors and physical change parameters as the younger client. The incidence of breast cancer (among women) rises steadily after the age of 40 and continues throughout the aging process. Breast self-examination remains an important consideration for older women.

The physical changes in the breasts that accompany aging follow:

1. Adipose tissue often increases (even if subcutaneous fat decreases over extremities).
2. In some women subcutaneous fat may decrease in the breasts.
3. Breast glandular tissue atrophies.
4. Suspensory ligaments relax and the breasts appear elongated or pendulous.
5. Chronic cystic disease diminishes after menopause.

In summary, breast palpation is often easier to accomplish because the nodular, glandular palpatory sensation associated with the breast glandular tissue in younger women is diminished. Breast lumps become even more significant in older clients. Refer to the adult section in this chapter for assessment guidelines.

---

## Cognitive self-assessment

1. The lymphatic system of the breasts drains to *two* major sites. These are:
   - ☐ a. axillary
   - ☐ b. internal mammary
   - ☐ c. supraclavicular
   - ☐ d. abdominal
   - ☐ e. pectoral
   - ☐ f. a and c
   - ☐ g. c and e
   - ☐ h. b and e
   - ☐ i. a and b
   - ☐ j. b and d

2. All the following inspection findings are *normal except one*. Identify the *abnormal* findings.
   - ☐ a. Slight breast asymmetry
   - ☐ b. Deviated nipple
   - ☐ c. Venous pattern seen on both breasts

☐ d. Inverted nipples (bilateral)

☐ e. Montgomery tubercles

3. All the following palpation criteria are *normal except one*. Identify the *abnormal* finding:

☐ a. Diffuse nodularity

☐ b. Mammary ridge

☐ c. Palpable supraclavicular lymph node

☐ d. Bilateral tenderness

☐ e. Soft tissue bilaterally

4. Which of the following women should be referred to a physician for further evaluation?

☐ a. A 26-year-old with multiple nodules palpated in each breast.

☐ b. A 48-year-old who has a 6-month history of reddened and sore left nipple and areolar area.

☐ c. A 35-year-old with asymmetrical breasts and inversion of nipples since birth of second child 8 years ago.

☐ d. A 15-year-old with minimal breast development.

☐ e. A 64-year-old with very slight ulcerated area at tip of right nipple; no masses, tenderness, or lymph nodes palpated.

☐ f. all except c

☐ g. a, c, and d

☐ h. b, d, and e

☐ i. a and c

☐ j. b and e

5. When palpating lymph nodes associated with drainage of the breasts, the examiner must palpate:

☐ a. along the sternum

☐ b. supraclavicular and subclavicular area

☐ c. pectoral area

☐ d. axillary area

☐ e. lower thoracic area under breast

☐ f. all the above

☐ g. all except a

☐ h. all except c and e

☐ i. all except c

☐ j. all except a and e

Mark each statement "T" or "F."

6. _____ It is not necessary to examine an asymptomatic 20-year-old woman in both sitting and lying positions.

7. _____ Nipples normally point slightly down and laterally.

8. _____ Engorgement and an orange peel appearance of the breast tissue is a normal premenstrual finding.

9. _____ A supernumerary nipple is considered a precancerous state, and the client should be referred to a physician.

10. _____ Because of the vastness of breast tissue, large-breasted women should only receive breast palpation in a supine position.

11. _____ Nipple inversion is always considered a cancerous sign.

12. _____ As the breasts become engorged premenstrually, dimpling of breast tissue may normally occur.

13. _____ It is just as important for a 25-year-old woman to perform breast self-examination as it is for a 75-year-old woman.

14. _____ In an older woman breast tissue that is found to be nodular is considered normal.

15. _____ About 90% of all breast lumps were first detected by women themselves.

16. _____ The presence of nipple discharge is usually indicative of an underlying malignancy.

**PEDIATRIC QUESTIONS**

17. Of the following children, *one* has an abnormal finding during the breast examination and should be referred. Identify the child with the abnormal finding.
    - ☐ a. John is a 9-day-old boy who has bilateral hypertrophy of the breast. A slight amount of milky-colored nipple discharge is observed.
    - ☐ b. Bonnie is a 1-month-old girl who has bilateral hypertrophy of the breast. There is no nipple discharge.
    - ☐ c. Amy is a 3-month-old female who has bilateral hypertrophy of the breast. There is no nipple discharge.
    - ☐ d. Michael is a 12-year-old husky boy who has recently developed bilateral hypertrophy of the breast. There is no nipple discharge.
    - ☐ e. Marilyn is a 13-year-old girl who is concerned because, unlike all of her friends, she has had no breast development.

18. Which of the following 15-year-old girls should receive breast self-examination instructions?
    - ☐ a. Nancy: well developed; negative family history for breast cancer
    - ☐ b. Cindy: just beginning breast development; negative family history for breast cancer
    - ☐ c. Judy: has small breasts; both her aunt and grandmother have had breast cancer
    - ☐ d. Lynn: average breast development appropriate for age; has just started menstruating; mother has fibrocystic disease
    - ☐ e. Karen: very large breasted; started menstruating at age 12 years; negative family history for breast cancer
    - ☐ f. a, b, and e
    - ☐ g. all except d
    - ☐ h. b, c, and e
    - ☐ i. all the above
    - ☐ j. none of the above

**SUGGESTED READINGS**
**General**

American Cancer Society: Mammography 1982: a statement of the American Cancer Society, CA **32**(4):226-230, 1982.

American Cancer Society: Teaching breast self-examination, Instructional material no. 77-1R-50M-6/77, no. 2015-LE.

Bates, B.: A guide to physical examination, ed. 3, Philadelphia, 1983, J.B. Lippincott Co., pp. 210-227.

DeGowin, E., and DeGowin, R.: Bedside diagnostic examination, ed. 3, New York, 1976, Macmillan Publishing Co., Inc., pp. 248-259.

Gallager, H.S., and others, editors: The breast, St. Louis, 1978, The C.V. Mosby Co.

Judge, R.D., and Zuidema, G., editors: Methods of clinical examination: a physiologic approach, Boston, 1974, Little, Brown & Co., pp. 261-269.

Malasanos, L., and others: Health assessment, ed. 2, St. Louis, 1981, The C.V. Mosby Co., pp. 275-288.

Martin, L.L.: Health care of women, Philadelphia, 1978, J.B. Lippincott Co., pp. 302-333.

Prior, J.A., Silberstein, J.S., and Stang, J.M.: Physical diagnosis: the history and examination of the patient, ed. 6, St. Louis, 1981, The C.V. Mosby Co., pp. 228-241.

Silverberg, E., and Lubera, J.A.: A review of American Cancer Society estimates of cancer cases and deaths, CA **33**(1):2-25, 1983.

**Pediatric**

Barness, L.: Manual of pediatric physical diagnosis, ed. 5, Chicago, 1981, Year Book Medical Publishers, Inc., p. 100.

Daniel, W.A., Jr.: Adolescents in health and disease, St. Louis, 1977, The C.V. Mosby Co., pp. 29-38.

Marshall, W.A., and Tanner, J.M.: Variations in the pattern of pubertal changes in boys, Arch. Dis. Child. **45**:22, 1970.

Pillitteri, A.: Nursing care of the growing family: a child health text, Boston, 1977, Little, Brown & Co., pp. 218, 310.

Tanner, J.M.: Growth at adolescence, ed. 2, Oxford, England, 1962, Blackwell Scientific Publications, Ltd.

**Geriatric**

Carotenuto, R., and Bullock, J.: Physical assessment of the gerontologic client, Philadelphia, 1980, F.A. Davis Co., pp. 81-82.

Malasanos, L., and others: Health assessment, ed. 2, St. Louis, 1981, The C.V. Mosby Co., p. 627.

Martin, L.L.: Health care of women, Philadelphia, 1978, J.B. Lippincott Co., pp. 209, 331.

ASSESSMENT OF THE

# Gastrointestinal system, abdomen, and rectal/ anal region

## VOCABULARY

**ascites** The accumulation of serous fluid in the peritoneal cavity.

**ballottement** Technique of palpating a floating structure by bouncing it gently and feeling it rebound.

**borborygmi** The audible abdominal sounds produced by hyperactive intestinal peristalsis.

**diastasis recti** Lateral separation of the two halves of the rectus abdominis muscle.

**flank** Part of the body between the bottom of the ribs and the upper border of the ilium.

**flatulence** Presence of excessive amounts of gases in the stomach or intestine.

**guarding** Protective withdrawal or positioning of a body part.

**linea alba** White line of connective tissue in the abdomen extending from sternum to pubis.

**McBurney point** Point of specialized tenderness in acute appendicitis, situated on a line between the umbilicus and the right anterosuperior iliac spine, about 1 or 2 inches above the latter.

**Murphy sign** Sign of gallbladder disease consisting of pain on taking a deep breath when the examiner's fingers are pressing on the approximate location of the gallbladder.

**pilonidal fistula (or sinus)** An abnormal channel containing a tuft of hair, situated most frequently over or close to the tip of the coccyx but also occurring in other regions of the body.

**Poupart ligament** Inguinal ligament.

**pyrosis** Burning sensation in the epigastric and sternal region with the raising of acid liquid from the stomach; also called heartburn.

**rebound tenderness** Sign of inflammation in the peritoneum in which pain is elicited by sudden withdrawal of a hand pressing on the abdomen.

**Riedel lobe** Tongue-shaped mass of tissue projecting from the right lobe of the liver.

**shifting dullness** Change in the dull sounds heard with palpation; at first the dull sound is heard in one location, then in a different location.

**striae** Streaks of linear scars that often result from rapidly developing tension in the skin; also called stretch marks.

**tenesmus** Spasmodic contraction of the anal or vesical sphincter with pain and a persistent desire to empty the bowel or bladder; involves involuntary, ineffective straining efforts.

**tympanites** Distention of the abdomen caused by pressure of gas in the intestine or the abdominal cavity.

**verge (anal)** The external ring opening of the anus.

## Cognitive objectives

At the end of this chapter the learner will demonstrate knowledge of assessment of the gastrointestinal system and the abdomen by the ability to do the following:

1. Describe five activities or conditions that contribute to client comfort and relaxation in preparation for an abdominal examination.
2. Describe the location of the major abdominal organs in terms of abdominal quadrants.
3. Identify the major abdominal organs in terms of location, relative size, and relationship to adjacent structures by completing an illustration.
4. Recognize normal findings associated with inspection of the abdominal surface, configuration, and pulsations.
5. Identify the rationale for performing auscultation of the abdomen before performing percussion and palpation.
6. Recognize normal findings associated with auscultation of the abdomen.
7. Identify normal findings associated with percussion of the abdomen.
8. Recognize the major characteristics of a normal liver span and location.
9. Identify the major characteristics of a normal spleen location and accessibility through percussion and palpation.
10. Describe the method for effective percussion and palpation of liver and spleen borders.
11. Give three reasons for performing light palpation of the abdomen.
12. Describe three reasons for performing deep palpation of the abdomen.
13. Recognize the major palpable characteristics of liver, kidney, small bowel, and pancreatic masses.
14. Identify abdominal areas that might be normally tender on deep palpation.
15. Recognize normal drainage patterns of the superficial inguinal nodes.
16. Identify specific examiner behaviors that will minimize client discomfort and enhance efficiency of the rectal examination.
17. Point out major characteristics of structures within the anal and rectal canals.
18. Identify selected common variations for pediatric and geriatric clients.
19. Apply the terms in the vocabulary section.

## Clinical objectives

At the end of this chapter the learner will perform a systematic assessment of the abdomen and the inguinal area, demonstrating the ability to do the following:

1. Obtain a pertinent health history from a client.
2. Inspect the abdominal surface for:
   a. Skin color
   b. Surface characteristics
   c. Presence of scars
   d. Venous network pattern
   e. Umbilicus contour, placement, and surface characteristics
   f. Abdominal contour and symmetry
   g. Surface motion: peristalsis and pulsations
   h. General movement with respirations
3. Auscultate all four quadrants and the epigastrium for:
   a. Presence and timing of bowel sounds
   b. Presence and creation of vascular sounds
4. Percuss all four quadrants of the abdomen and describe the tone(s) elicited in specific areas.
5. Percuss the upper and lower liver borders and estimate the midclavicular liver span and descent on inspiration.
6. Percuss in the left midaxillary line for splenic dullness or absence of dullness.
7. Percuss the gastric bubble and estimate its size.
8. Lightly palpate all four quadrants for:
   a. Tenderness
   b. Guarding
   c. Surface characteristics
   d. Masses
9. Deeply palpate all four quadrants for normal and abnormal tenderness and masses.
10. Deeply palpate at the right costal margin for:
    a. Liver border
    b. Contour
    c. Tenderness
11. Deeply palpate at the left costal margin for the splenic border.
12. Deeply palpate the abdomen for the right and left kidneys.
13. Deeply palpate the midline epigastric area for aortic pulsation.
14. Lightly palpate the inguinal regions for:
    a. Horizontal and vertical lymph nodes
    b. Contour
    c. Consistency
    d. Delimitation
    e. Tenderness
    f. Redness
    g. Size
15. Inspect and palpate the sacrococcygeal and perianal areas for surface characteristics and tenderness.
16. Inspect and palpate the anus for:
    a. Sphincter tone
    b. Tenderness
    c. Surface characteristics

17. Palpate the distal rectal walls for surface characteristics.
18. Summarize results with a written description of findings.

## Health history additional to screening history

1. Nutritional assessment. The screening questions, outlined in the original data base (Chapter 1), provide the examiner with basic information about the client's food intake (through the use of a 24-hour recall chart), the client's weight measurement and stability, and major variables that might alter intake pattern. These data can be analyzed to assure the client and examiner that daily nutritional needs are being met in terms of the basic four food groups.

    If food consumption or weight problems exist, further assessment is warranted.
    a. The 24-hour recall intake record can be extended to cover a week's intake (to give an overview of day-to-day variations).
    b. The final data can be analyzed in terms of recommended daily dietary allowances for calories, proteins, fats, carbohydrates, vitamins, and minerals.
    c. Further variables that might affect food intake should be explored:
       (1) A survey of food preferences and dislikes
       (2) Family routines and values (e.g., food portions, eating times, control of food purchase and service, insistence on having a "clean plate," family values regarding ideal weight or appearance)
       (3) Cultural and religious values (e.g., forbidden foods, foods that are served frequently)
       (4) Psychological variables (e.g., depression, anxiety, compulsive eating habits)
       (5) Physical status (e.g., ill health, allergies or food idiosyncracies, mouth or dental problems, alterations in physical activity)
       (6) Access to food (e.g., transportation, type and availability of grocery store)
       (7) Personal habits or life-style (e.g., use of convenience foods because of limited time or interest in cooking, frequent dining out, night occupation and unusual eating schedule, dormitory or rooming house controls, disorganized life-style with no regular eating or shopping patterns, constant use of "fast food" restaurants for lunch or dinner, frequent entertaining or feasting on weekends and holidays, sedentary life-style with frequent snacks)
       (8) Eating behaviors (e.g., rapid eating, nibbling food all day, skipping meals, late-night snacks)
       (9) Self-imposed dietary additions or restrictions (e.g., vitamin/mineral supplements, food supplements, vegetarian diet, low-calorie diet, low-carbohydrate diet, other diet forms)
       (10) Body image profile (self-assessment of satisfaction with present weight, weight distribution, recall of peer reaction to client's appearance)
       (11) General knowledge of basic four food requirements, shopping within a budget, and content of fat, sugar, and proteins in basic foods
2. Abdominal pain may be reported as "indigestion," "heartburn," "stomachache," or other vague descriptions that need clarification and a full symptom analysis by the examiner. The client may experience pain that is diffuse and may be unable to specifically locate the discomfort. The pain may be precisely located and/or it may radiate to adjacent or remote areas. The discomfort may feel superficial or very deep. Referred pain often occurs as the pain intensifies. The following referral patterns may be helpful in eliciting information from the client (Fig. 11-1).
3. Indigestion. Various interpretations might include a feeling of fullness, heartburn, mild diffuse discomfort, excessive belching, flatulence, nausea, a bad taste, loss of appetite, or severe pain. The client must clarify the following:
    a. Location of feeling or pain (if possible); radiation of pain (to arms, shoulders)
    b. Symptoms associated with food intake (e.g., immediately before? immediately after? delayed response?)
    c. Amount and type of food associated with discomfort
    d. Associated symptoms (e.g., vomiting, headache, diarrhea)
    e. Associated problems (e.g., anxiety, sleeplessness)
    f. Time of day or night that symptom most often occurs
    g. Does body position or activity cause or relieve pain?
4. Nausea. Might be described as an upset stomach, queasy stomach, a need to vomit, a fullness or tightness in the throat. Associated symptoms such as dizziness, increased salivation, headache, and weakness need to be explored. Again, onset, duration, and patterns should be clarified. Are there any notable stimuli (e.g., particular foods, odors,

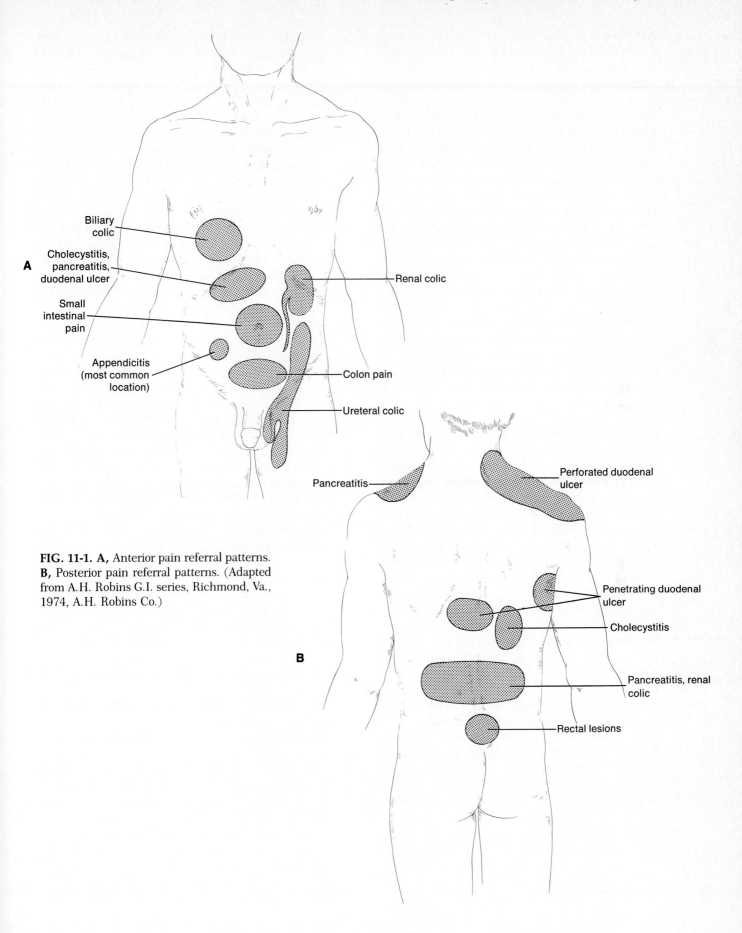

**FIG. 11-1. A,** Anterior pain referral patterns. **B,** Posterior pain referral patterns. (Adapted from A.H. Robins G.I. series, Richmond, Va., 1974, A.H. Robins Co.)

times of day, activity)? Does it occur with a certain meal? Before or after food intake? Is it associated with vomiting? If so, how?

5. Vomiting. To what extent is it associated with abdominal pain, nausea, retching? Are there other associated symptoms (e.g., fever, headache, diarrhea)? Clarify the timing between food intake and a vomiting episode. Once the symptom has been fully analyzed, the estimated quantity, color, consistency, odor, and taste should be established. If vomiting has occurred repeatedly, find out if the appearance of the vomitus has changed. Ask if there has been a weight loss. Determine whether fluid intake has been maintained, increased, or decreased. Specify which solids or liquids can be retained.

6. Heartburn. The location is usually substernal. Ask if pain radiates to other areas (e.g., chest, neck, shoulders, back, or arms). Ask if body movement or position change alters the pain (e.g., bending over, sitting up, or lying down). Ask about specific food irritants (e.g., spices, coffee, alcohol). Establish the time of day or night when discomfort is most noticeable.

7. Appetite changes. A loss or gain of appetite should be explored in terms of particular foods that have been eliminated or added as well as an estimate of the quantity of food that has been changed. Careful inquiry about average weight and recent (last 3 to 9 months) loss or gain is important. Inquire about associated symptoms or situations that might interfere with appetite (e.g., increased stress, abdominal pain, bowel habit changes, other illnesses, or deliberate attempts to reduce caloric intake). Comparing a sample of a previous "normal" 24-hour intake with a present 24-hour intake might be helpful. (*Note:* Recent oral or dental problems can affect appetite.)

8. Diarrhea. The number of stools per day (24-hour period) or week should be established. Clarify whether this present pattern represents a change in bowel habits. If so, note the onset. Associated symptoms such as fever, nausea, vomiting, abdominal pain, abdominal distention, flatus, intermittent cramping, marked peristalsis, explosive diarrhea, or urgency to evacuate should be explored. The consistency, color, quantity, and odor of each stool should be noted. Does the client notice accompanying mucus, blood, or food particles with the stool? Is there nocturnal diarrhea? Has the client been taking antibiotics? Has there been a weight loss? Has the diarrhea interfered with activities of daily living?

9. Constipation. Usually defined as decreased number of stools, marked difficulty or pain with passage of stools, and/or excessive dryness or hardness of stools. Again the number of stools per day or week must be established. The date and time of the most recent stool should be noted. Establish whether this is a *change* of bowel habit. If so, was the onset sudden or gradual? Have the stools changed in size (smaller, thinner, larger)? Does the client feel that there is stool remaining in the rectum? Have there been any food intake changes recently (quantity or type of foods)? Has fluid intake been altered? Other associated abdominal or general symptoms should be inquired about. For example, has the client been depressed?

10. Anal discomfort. May be described in terms of itching, pain on defecation, a painful lump, or a stinging or burning sensation. Clarify whether body position (e.g., lying down or standing erect) alters the pain. Ask about the color, form, size, and consistency of stools. Ask if the client has noticed mucus or blood (streaks over stool, droplets on toilet paper, discoloration of water in the toilet bowl) at the time of bowel movement. Itching often interferes with sleep. Clarification of duration and daily patterns of itching is important.

11. General considerations for gastrointestinal symptom analysis:
    a. It is very important to list all medications that the client is taking in addition to careful exploration of medicines, enemas, or any self-help treatments that the client has been using.
    b. Severity of the symptom is often best determined by the client's account of symptom interference with activities of daily living (e.g., loss of sleep, marked eating habit change, loss of time at work, or alteration of daily tasks).
    c. The final accuracy of the description of the severity, duration, rhythmicity, and patterns of the pain depend greatly on the client's ability to articulate subjective sensations and a personal pain threshold and the examiner's ability to maintain a balance between nondirective and selective probing approaches.

# Clinical guidelines

| THE STUDENT WILL: | TO IDENTIFY: | |
|---|---|---|
| | NORMAL | DEVIATIONS FROM NORMAL |

**Abdomen**

1. Assemble necessary equipment:
   a. Stethoscope
   b. Small ruler
   c. Marking pencil
2. Position client comfortably in a supine position, making sure:
   a. Client's bladder recently emptied
   b. Arms on chest or at sides
   c. Small pillow under head
   d. Client's knees slightly flexed, supported by small pillow
   e. Client draped over breasts and at pubis
3. Take additional measures to ensure client comfort:
   a. Make sure room is warm
   b. Have warm hands, short fingernails, warm stethoscope
   c. Instruct client to breathe slowly through mouth if he appears anxious
   d. Offer explanations of examiner activity as assessment progresses

| THE STUDENT WILL: | NORMAL | DEVIATIONS FROM NORMAL |
|---|---|---|
| 4. Observe general behavior of client | Appears relaxed<br>Facial muscles relaxed<br>Lying quietly<br>Respirations even and slow | Marked restlessness<br>Marked immobility or rigid posture<br>Knees drawn up<br>Facial grimacing<br>Respirations rapid, uneven, or grunting |
| 5. Inspect the abdominal surface for: | | |
|   a. Skin color | May be paler than other parts because of lack of exposure | Jaundice<br>Redness (inflammation)<br>Lesions, bruises, discoloration, cyanosis (localized at umbilicus or generalized) |
|   b. Surface characteristics | Smooth, soft<br>Silver-white striae (usually lower abdomen) (See Fig. 3-5.) | Rashes, lesions<br>Glistening, taut appearance<br>Pink, red striae<br>Purplish striae |
|   c. Scars (configuration, location, length) | | |
|   d. Venous network | Very faint fine network may be visible | Prominent venous pattern<br>Engorgement of veins around umbilicus |
|   e. Umbilicus | | |
|     1. Placement | Centrally located | Displaced upward, downward, or laterally |
|     2. Contour | Usually sunken, may protrude slightly | Visible hernia around or slightly above umbilicus |
|     3. Surface characteristics | Smooth, noninflamed | Inflamed |

## Clinical guidelines—cont'd

| THE STUDENT WILL: | TO IDENTIFY: | |
| --- | --- | --- |
| | NORMAL | DEVIATIONS FROM NORMAL |
| **f.** Contour | Flat<br>Rounded (Fig. 11-2)<br>Scaphoid (concave profile) (Fig. 11-3) | Distended<br>Marked concavity associated with general wasting signs or anteroposterior rib expansion (Fig. 11-4) |

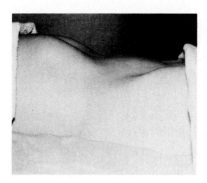

**FIG. 11-2.** Rounded abdominal contour.

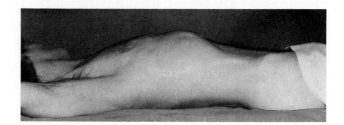

**FIG. 11-3.** Scaphoid abdominal contour.

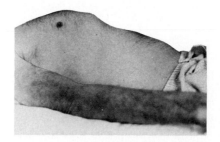

**FIG. 11-4.** Marked concavity below costal margin associated with increased anteroposterior chest diameter.

| | | |
| --- | --- | --- |
| **g.** Symmetry (*Note:* Examiner must view abdomen at eye level from the side, as well as from behind client's head.) | Evenly rounded with maximum height of convexity at umbilicus | Distention of upper or lower half<br>Visible masses or bulges in any area of abdominal surface |
| **h.** Surface motion | | |
| 1. Peristalsis | Usually not visible | Visible |
| 2. Pulsation | Upper midline pulsation may be visible in thin people | Marked pulsation |
| **i.** General movement with respirations | Smooth, even movements<br>Female exhibits chiefly costal movement<br>Male exhibits chiefly abdominal movement | Grunting, labored<br>Respirations accompanied by restricted abdominal movement |

| THE STUDENT WILL: | TO IDENTIFY: | |
| --- | --- | --- |
| | NORMAL | DEVIATIONS FROM NORMAL |
| **6.** Instruct client to take a deep breath and hold it | Contour remains smooth and symmetrical | Bulges or masses appear |
| **7.** Instruct client to raise head without using arms for support | Rectus abdominis muscles prominent<br>Midline bulge may appear ( Fig. 11-5) | Appearance of bulges through muscle layer |

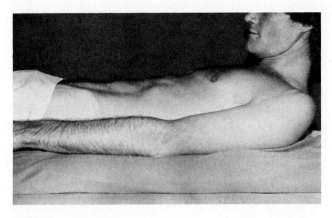

**FIG. 11-5.** Rectus abdominis muscles become prominent when head and neck are raised. Note that superficial masses will rise with muscles.

| | | |
| --- | --- | --- |
| **8.** Auscultate all four abdominal quadrants and the epigastrium, using diaphragm of stethoscope and pressing lightly | | |
|    **a.** Presence and timing of bowel sounds | Usually 5 to 34/min<br>Irregular in timing | Absence of sound established after 5 minutes of listening<br>Note sounds that are infrequent |
|    **b.** Quality of sounds | Gurgles, clicks<br>Quality of sound varies greatly | High-pitched, tinkling noises |
|    **c.** Arterial vascular sounds concentrated in epigastric area, in area surrounding umbilicus, over liver, and at posterior flank | | Bruits (usually high-pitched, soft "swishing" sound, and systolic in timing)<br>(*Note:* Bruit will continue as client is moved into various positions.) |
|    **d.** Bell of stethoscope will pick up lower (venous) sounds | | Venous hum (lower in pitch, softer, and continuous sound) |
|    **e.** Friction rub | | Infrequently heard sound, associated with respirations (soft, and may be confused with normal breath sounds)<br>Rubs most often heard over spleen or liver |

## Clinical guidelines—cont'd

| THE STUDENT WILL: | TO IDENTIFY: | |
| --- | --- | --- |
| | NORMAL | DEVIATIONS FROM NORMAL |
| **9.** Percuss lightly in all four quadrants (*Note:* Develop a system or route for percussion process, as shown in Fig. 11-6); note tone | General distribution of tympany (depending on amount of air and solid material in bowel)<br>Suprapubic dullness heard over distended bladder | Marked dullness in local area |

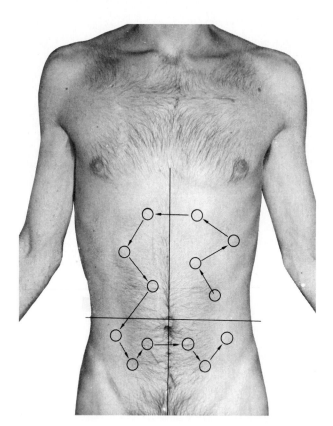

**FIG. 11-6.** Suggested percussion route for the abdomen.

| | | |
| --- | --- | --- |
| **a.** Liver percussion<br>　1. Percuss upward at right midclavicular line, beginning below level of umbilicus; continue percussing over tympanic area until dull percussion rate indicates liver border; note location of lower liver border with marker | Lower border of liver usually at costal margin or slightly below | Lower border of liver exceeds 2 to 3 cm ($^{3}/_{4}$ to 1 inch) below costal margin |
| 　2. Percuss downward at right midclavicular line, beginning from area of lung resonance, and continue until dull percussion rate indicates upper liver border; note location of upper liver border with marker (Fig. 11-7) | Upper border of liver usually begins in fifth to seventh intercostal space | Upper border lowered<br>Dullness extending above fifth intercostal space |

| THE STUDENT WILL: | TO IDENTIFY: | |
|---|---|---|
| | **NORMAL** | **DEVIATIONS FROM NORMAL** |

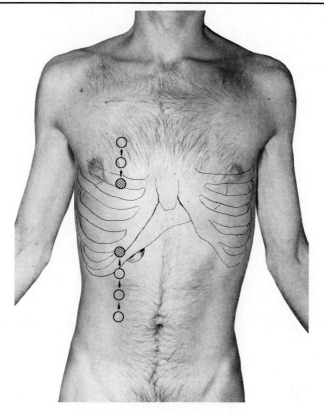

**FIG. 11-7.** Liver percussion route.

| THE STUDENT WILL: | NORMAL | DEVIATIONS FROM NORMAL |
|---|---|---|
| 3. Estimate midclavicular liver span | 6 to 12 cm (2½ to 4½ inches)<br>Normal liver span usually greater in men than women and in taller individuals | Span exceeds 12 cm (4½ inches) |
| 4. Additional liver percussion maneuvers | | |
| a. Percuss upward then in downward direction over right midaxillary line | Liver dullness may be felt in fifth to seventh intercostal space | Dull percussion exceeds limits of fifth to seventh intercostal space |
| b. Percuss upward then in downward direction over midsternal line and estimate midsternal liver span | Normal midsternal liver span ranges from 4 to 8 cm (1½ to 3 inches) | Span exceeds 8 cm (3 inches) |
| c. Instruct client to take a deep breath and hold it; then percuss upward in right midclavicular line again; estimate liver descent | Lower border of liver should move inferiorly by 2 to 3 cm | Liver does not move with inspiration, or movement less than 2 cm |

## Clinical guidelines—cont'd

| THE STUDENT WILL: | TO IDENTIFY: | |
| --- | --- | --- |
| | NORMAL | DEVIATIONS FROM NORMAL |
| **b.** Spleen percussion<br> 1. Percuss down lower left thoracic wall in posterior midaxillary region beginning from an area of lung resonance to costal margin (Fig. 11-8) | Small area of splenic dullness may be heard at sixth to tenth rib, or tone may be tympanic (colonic) | Dullness extends above sixth rib or covers large area between sixth rib and costal margin |

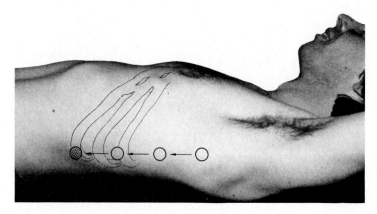

**FIG. 11-8.** Spleen percussion route.

| | | |
| --- | --- | --- |
| 2. Percuss lowest intercostal space in left anterior axillary line before and after client takes a deep breath (Fig. 11-9) | Area usually tympanic | Tympany changes to dullness on inspiration<br>Enlarged spleen is brought forward on inspiration to produce dull percussion note |

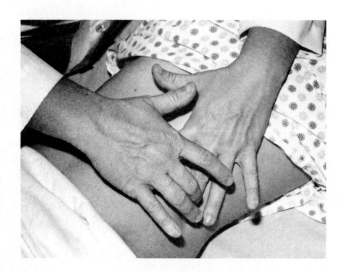

**FIG. 11-9.** Percussion at lowest intercostal space in left anterior axillary line before and after client takes a deep breath.

| | | |
| --- | --- | --- |
| 3. Percuss over left lower rib cage | Gastric "bubble" tympanic and varies in size | |

| THE STUDENT WILL: | TO IDENTIFY: | |
| --- | --- | --- |
| | NORMAL | DEVIATIONS FROM NORMAL |

**10.** Abdominal palpation
   **a.** Lightly palpate all four quadrants with pads of fingertips (Fig. 11-10, *A*)

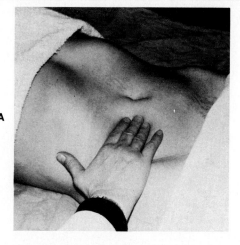

FIG. 11-10. **A,** Light abdominal palpation with distal pads of fingers.

| THE STUDENT WILL: | NORMAL | DEVIATIONS FROM NORMAL |
| --- | --- | --- |
| 1. Tenderness | Not present | Cutaneous (superficial areas of hypersensitivity) |
| 2. Muscle tone | Abdomen relaxed<br>Muscular resistance may be seen in anxious client | Involuntary resistance (muscles cannot be relaxed by voluntary effort) |
| 3. Surface characteristics | Smooth; consistent tension felt by examiner | Masses (superficial)<br>Localized areas of rigidity or increased tension |
| **b.** Continue palpation of all four quadrants using moderate pressure with flat and sides of hand (Fig. 11-10, *B*) | (*Note:* This intermediate maneuver is performed as a method of gradually approaching deep palpation without alarming client and stimulating muscular resistance. If onset of resistance is noted, use a lighter touch and proceed again.) | |

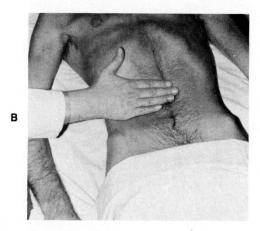

FIG. 11-10, cont'd. **B,** Abdominal palpation with moderate pressure; examiner uses flat and side of hand.

## Clinical guidelines—cont'd

| THE STUDENT WILL: | TO IDENTIFY: | |
| --- | --- | --- |
| | NORMAL | DEVIATIONS FROM NORMAL |
| 1. Tenderness | None | Present |
| 2. Masses | None | Present |
| 3. General tone and location of major structures | Abdominal surface feels smooth, and tension under palpating hand feels consistent throughout | Localized areas of rigidity or increased tension |

c. Deeply palpate all four quadrants; one of two methods may be used
  1. Distal flat portions of fingers (finger pads) are pressed gradually and deeply into palpation areas (Fig. 11-10, *C*)

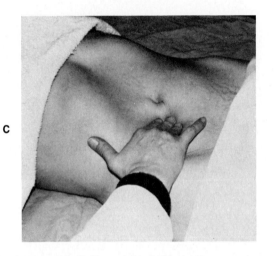

**FIG. 11-10, cont'd. C,** Deep abdominal palpation; examiner uses flat surface of distal pads of fingers.

  2. Bimanual: lower hand rests lightly on surface and upper hand exerts pressure for deep palpation (Fig. 11-10, *D*)

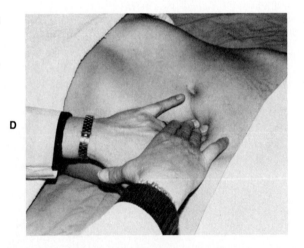

**FIG. 11-10, cont'd. D,** Deep abdominal palpation using bimanual technique.

| | | |
| --- | --- | --- |
| a. Tenderness | Often present in midline near xiphoid process | Present in local or generalized areas |
| | Often present over cecum | Client response to pain may be muscle guarding and/or facial grimace, pulling away from examiner |
| | May be present over sigmoid colon | |

| THE STUDENT WILL: | TO IDENTIFY: | |
| --- | --- | --- |
| | NORMAL | DEVIATIONS FROM NORMAL |
| b. Masses | Aorta often palpable at epigastrium and pulsates in forward direction<br>Borders of rectus abdominis muscles<br>Feces in ascending or descending colon<br>Sacral promontory | Masses that descend on inspiration<br>Pulsatile masses<br>Laterally mobile masses<br>Fixed masses |
| 3. Palpate with fingertips around umbilicus for:<br>a. Bulges<br>b. Nodules<br>c. Umbilical ring | Umbilical ring round with no irregularities or bulges<br>Umbilicus may be inverted or slightly everted | Masses, bulges<br><br>Umbilical ring may be incomplete or may feel soft in center |

**11.** Specific organ identification
  **a.** Liver palpation
    1. Deeply palpate at right costal margin before and during deep inspiration and after complete expiration; left hand is placed under eleventh and twelfth ribs; right hand is parallel to right costal margin (Fig. 11-11)

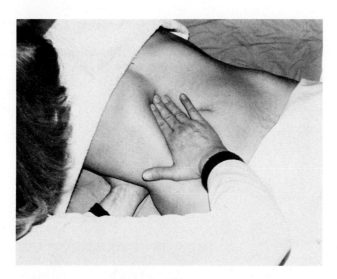

**FIG. 11-11.** Liver palpation with left hand under eleventh and twelfth ribs and right hand parallel to right costal margin.

| THE STUDENT WILL: | NORMAL | DEVIATIONS FROM NORMAL |
| --- | --- | --- |
| a. Liver border and contour<br>(*Note:* If border is felt, repeat palpation/inspiration maneuver at medial and lateral sites of costal border for better estimate of contour.) | Liver often not palpable<br>Liver often "bumps" against fingers on inspiration (especially in thin clients) | (*Note:* Very enlarged liver may lie under examiner's hand as it extends downward into abdominal cavity.) |
| b. Liver border surface<br>c. Liver tenderness<br>(*Note:* Both hands can be "hooked" over right costal margin as examiner faces client's feet to palpate liver border on deep inspiration.) | Border feels smooth<br>None | Irregular surface or edge<br>Tenderness elicited<br>(*Note:* Client's inspiration may be abruptly halted if pain exists.) |

## Clinical guidelines—cont'd

| | TO IDENTIFY: | |
|---|---|---|
| **THE STUDENT WILL:** | **NORMAL** | **DEVIATIONS FROM NORMAL** |

**b.** Spleen palpation
  1. While standing at client's right side, palpate the spleen by placing left hand over client's left costovertebral angle and exerting pressure to move the spleen anteriorly; right hand is pressed gently under left anterior costal margin (Fig. 11-12)

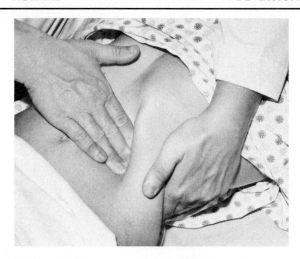

FIG. 11-12. Palpation of the spleen. Note that examiner's left hand is pressing spleen anteriorly.

  2. Instruct client to take a deep breath and then to exhale. As client exhales, examiner's hand should follow tissue contour under border of ribs in an attempt to palpate the spleen edge.
  3. Repeat procedure with client lying on right side with legs and knees somewhat flexed; stand to client's right and place left hand over client's left costovertebral angle; right hand is pressed under left anterior costal margin (Fig. 11-13)

Spleen not normally palpable

Spleen palpated (as firm mass that bumps against examiner's fingers)

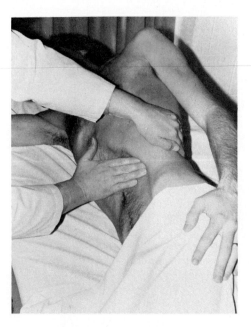

FIG. 11-13. Spleen palpation.

| THE STUDENT WILL: | TO IDENTIFY: | |
| --- | --- | --- |
| | NORMAL | DEVIATIONS FROM NORMAL |

**c.** Kidney palpation
  1. Left kidney
     a. Examiner stands to client's right; client returns to supine position
     b. Examiner's left hand is placed at left posterior costal angle; right hand is placed at client's left anterior costal margin
     c. Client is instructed to take a deep breath and to exhale completely. As the client exhales, the examiner elevates client's left flank with left hand and palpates deeply with right hand (Fig. 11-14)

Occasionally lower pole of the kidney can be felt in thin clients
Contour smooth, and no tenderness on palpation

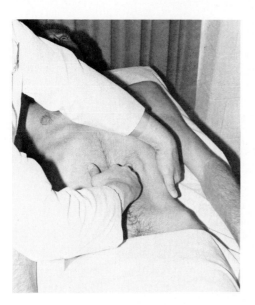

**FIG. 11-14.** Left kidney palpation.

  2. Right kidney
     a. Same maneuver is repeated on client's right side; examiner remains at client's right, elevates posterior costal margin with left hand, and palpates deeply at anterior margin with right hand

Lower pole of right kidney may be palpated (on inspiration) as smooth, firm, and nontender

## Clinical guidelines—cont'd

| | TO IDENTIFY: | |
| THE STUDENT WILL: | NORMAL | DEVIATIONS FROM NORMAL |
| --- | --- | --- |
| **d.** Inguinal nodes | | |
|    1. Lightly palpate (with finger pads) inguinal areas just below inguinal ligament and inner aspect of upper thigh at the groin (Fig. 11-15) for horizontal and vertical inguinal nodes | | |
|      a. Presence | Small, mobile<br>Nontender nodes often present | Enlarged, tender |
|      b. Contour | Smooth or nonpalpable | |
|      c. Consistency | Soft or nonpalpable | Hard |
|      (*Note:* Femoral pulses can also be palpated at this time. Techniques and palpable qualities are covered in Chapter 9.) | | |

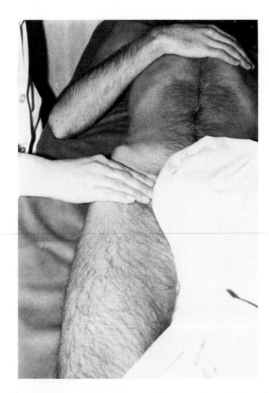

**FIG. 11-15.** Palpation of inguinal area; finger pads applied just below inguinal ligament.

| THE STUDENT WILL: | TO IDENTIFY: | |
| --- | --- | --- |
| | NORMAL | DEVIATIONS FROM NORMAL |
| **12.** Jar kidneys to evaluate tenderness | | |
|    **a.** Approach from behind as client is seated; identify right and left costovertebral angles | | |
|    **b.** Strike each angle with ulnar surface of right fist (Fig. 11-16) | Client perceives jar or thud | Tenderness elicited |

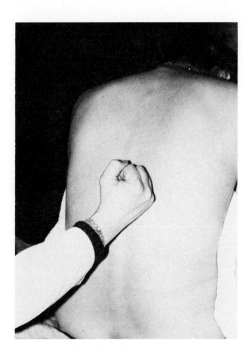

**FIG. 11-16.** Fist percussion over costovertebral angle.

*Special maneuvers*
1. If fluid within the abdomen is suspected:
    a. As the client remains in a supine position, fluid associated with ascites will pool in the lateral (flank) areas. Lines can be drawn on the abdomen to indicate the midline tympany percussion area in contrast to lateral dullness.
    b. If the client turns to the right side, the tympanic sound will shift toward the upper (left) side. As the fluid pools in the right side, the area of dullness will rise toward the midline.
    c. As the client turns to the left lateral position, the fluid will migrate to the left side and the left dullness will rise toward the midline.
2. Small amounts of free fluids can be identified if the client assumes an elbow-knee position. The fluid will pool in the periumbilical region, and the area of dullness can be identified through percussion.
3. If the client is experiencing pain, the examiner should test for rebound tenderness: Press firmly over an area of the abdomen that is remote from the area of discomfort. Release the hand suddenly. If the client experiences a sharp stabbing pain at the site of original discomfort, this can be interpreted as rebound tenderness.

## Clinical guidelines—cont'd

| THE STUDENT WILL: | TO IDENTIFY: | |
|---|---|---|
| | NORMAL | DEVIATIONS FROM NORMAL |

**Rectal/anal region**

1. Evaluate anal and rectal region

| THE STUDENT WILL: | NORMAL | DEVIATIONS FROM NORMAL |
|---|---|---|
| **a.** Inspect sacrococcygeal and perianal areas while client is lying on left side with right hip and knee flexed<br>1. Skin and surface characteristics | Surface smooth and clear | Lumps, rash, inflammation, scars, pilonidal dimpling, tuft of hair at pilonidal area |
| **b.** Palpate coccygeal area for tenderness | No tenderness | Tender |
| **c.** Spread buttocks with both hands; inspect anus for:<br>1. Surface characteristics (penlight can be used) | Increased pigmentation<br>Coarse skin | Inflammation<br>Lesions<br>Scars<br>Skin tags<br>Fissures<br>Lumps<br>Swelling<br>Excoriation<br>Hemorrhoids<br>Mucosal bulging |
| **d.** Ask client to strain down; place gloved and lubricated finger at anal opening; as sphincter relaxes, slowly insert finger pointing toward client's umbilicus | | |
| **e.** Ask client to tighten sphincter around finger to assess sphincter tone | Sphincter tightens evenly around finger with minimal discomfort to client | Hypotonic sphincter<br>Hypertonic sphincter, with marked tenderness |
| **f.** Rotate finger to examine anal muscular ring for surface characteristics | Smooth, even pressure on finger | Nodules<br>Irregularities |
| **g.** Insert finger farther to palpate all four rectal walls<br>(*Note:* Prostate examination is covered in Chapter 12.) | Continuous, smooth surface with minimal discomfort to client | Nodules<br>Masses<br>(*Note:* The cervix is sometimes palpable on the anterior wall; do not mistake for a mass.)<br>Tenderness |
| **h.** As finger is extracted, note characteristics of any stool<br>1. Color | Brown | Presence of blood, pus<br>Black, tarry stool<br>Pale or yellow |
| 2. Consistency | Soft | Light tan or gray |

## Clinical strategies

1. Much has been said in textbooks about helping the client to feel comfortable before an abdominal examination. It is extremely difficult to complete an assessment if the abdominal muscles are not relaxed. The basic comfort measures described in the guidelines are essential; however, the examiner must be sensitive to the client's state of anxiety and should be prepared to be flexible with examination procedures if the client remains tense.

   a. If palpation stimulates muscle tension, it might be helpful to lighten the touch and to proceed more slowly.

   b. The abdominal examination can be delayed until later in the assessment when the client might feel more comfortable.

   c. Be certain that the client is draped as fully as possible.

   d. It is sometimes difficult to examine the abdomen while the client is talking; clients tend to lift and bob their heads as they converse. However, it is often soothing to have the examiner talking quietly, describing the procedures, perhaps reviewing the client's history.

2. This statement has appeared in other chapters, but it is worth repeating: *Look before you touch.* Once an individual begins using other senses, the impact of the visual sense diminishes. It is helpful to circle around the examining table and to view the abdomen carefully from all angles for surface and contour characteristics.

3. It is helpful for the examiner to *visualize* organs or major structures within the abdominal cavity during inspection, auscultation, percussion, and palpation of the abdomen (Fig. 11-17 and Table 11-1). This mental picture heightens the tactile sense.

**TABLE 11-1.** Structures of the abdominal cavity

| Right upper quadrant | Left upper quadrant |
|---|---|
| Liver | Stomach |
| Gallbladder | Spleen |
| Duodenum | Left kidney |
| Pancreas | Pancreas |
| Right kidney | Splenic flexure of colon |
| Hepatic flexure of colon | |
| **Right lower quadrant** | **Left lower quadrant** |
| Cecum | Sigmoid colon |
| Appendix | Left ovary and tube |
| Right ovary and tube | |

**Superpubic midline**
Bladder
Uterus

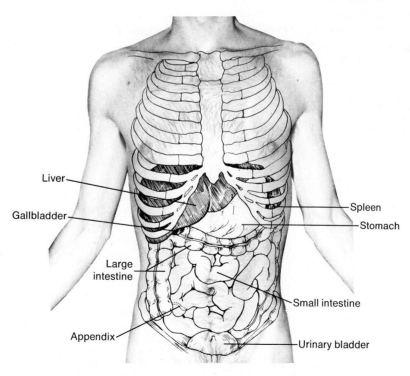

**FIG. 11-17.** Major structures of abdominal cavity.

---

**SAMPLE RECORDING**

*Abdomen:* Rounded and symmetrical with centrally placed umbilicus. No lesions, rashes, discolorations, scars, inflammation, or visible peristalsis. Normal bowel sounds; no bruits or venous hums. Tympanic percussion tones throughout. Abdomen relaxed and without tenderness or masses. Liver 10 cm in right midclavicular line. Spleen and kidneys not palpated. No CVA tenderness.

*Rectal and anal region:* Sacrococcygeal, perianal, and anal surfaces present no lesions, rash, inflammation, masses, or hemorrhoids. Good sphincter tone. Anal and distal rectal mucosa smooth and without masses.

---

4. The examiner should inquire about a history of pain or discomfort *before* beginning palpation. If discomfort is described and located, begin the palpation in another region of the abdomen.
5. The beginning examiner must establish early and consistent routines for carrying out the mechanics of the assessment. Most individuals examine the abdomen from the client's right side. Making this decision early in the learning period is extremely helpful in expediting assessment skills.
6. If lesions, scars, masses, or fluid levels (lines) are identified, it is often easier and clearer to draw a picture of the finding and indicate dimensions and location rather than to attempt a description of it.

## History and clinical strategies: the pediatric client

1. Nutritional assessment. Entire textbooks have been written about the nutritional assessment of children. A basic list of nutritional questions has already been presented in Chapter 1. In addition to this, the examiner must be alert to common nutritional concerns associated with the child.
   a. Obesity is a common problem for children. Questions about a child's overweight situation should include those presented in the adult nutritional assessment section as well as those that follow:
      (1) Family history regarding obesity problems
      (2) Age of the child when overweight problems began
      (3) Whether the child is concerned about his overweight state
      (4) Whether the child understands the relationship between foods consumed and weight gained (For example, a story is told about one teenage girl who consumed three cases of liquid diet supplement every day to cancel the 1000 calories she consumed by eating three meals.)
   b. Toddler nutrition. Many parents of toddlers will express concern that their child's eating patterns have changed. The examiner must gather a food consumption profile from the past week as well as assess the child physically. If the child shows normal progression of height, weight, and maturational development, the examiner should try to decrease parental anxiety by sharing growth and development progression facts as well as normal development eating changes of the toddler.
   c. Adolescent nutrition. Studies have shown that less than 50% of all teenagers in the United States eat breakfast every day. This usually arouses concern among parents who state that their teenager is not eating correctly.

      Although the examiner should develop a profile of the adolescent's nutritional style and food consumption, unless a problem arises such as overweight, underweight, anemia, fatigue, or systemic disease, there may be little the examiner can do to change the adolescent's style of food consumption.

      It is important to assess the adolescent's knowledge of good nutrition and to supply educational facts where necessary.
   d. Anorexia nervosa. This disease, referred to as a "socially acceptable" form of suicide, is becoming more common in the United States. Its assessment is included at this point because of the close correlation with adolescent nutrition. A hypothetical profile of a child affected by anorexia nervosa follows:

      The individual is usually a female teenager from an upper middle class family. Her parents, who may be perfectionists, are successful and view themselves as being well adjusted and supportive. Both her mother and father have made many personal sacrifices for the child. The girl is popular and successful. Throughout her life she has conformed to the wishes of her parents. Hardly ever has she expressed her own wishes or translated her own desires into actions.

      Anorexia nervosa is such a serious situation that the examiner must explore its potential with all very thin teenagers, especially those whose parents express a concern that the teenager has lost too much weight or will not eat. Although there is usually some significant event that triggers the situation, usually the first symptom to appear will be weight loss. As the anorexia nervosa cycle continues, the examiner will find the parent and the teenager in battle about eating, food, and weight loss. The more the parent harps, the more serious the situation becomes.

The examiner should use the following questions to gather data. Any teenager who appears at risk should be referred immediately.
(1) Is the client less than 25 years of age?
(2) Has there been a weight loss of more than 25% of the client's original weight?
(3) Does the client express an intractable or negative attitude about gaining weight or eating?
(4) Are there any other physical problems present?
(5) Are any of the following factors pertinent (a cluster of at least four is considered high risk)?
　(a) Distorted body image
　(b) Periods of amenorrhea
　(c) Periods of hyperactivity
　(d) History of being overweight
　(e) Denial of hunger
　(f) Denial of fatigue
　(g) History of self-induced vomiting to stay thin
　(h) Morbid fear of obesity
　(i) Preoccupation with food

2. Abdominal pain in the child is extremely difficult to assess. If the examiner asks the child if the palpation hurts or to point to the spot where it hurts, the child will usually comply and provide a response indicating discomfort or pain. More important, the examiner should rely on objective findings to assist in assessing the pain. Factors such as different pitch in a cry, a grimace or change in facial expression, or sudden protective movement by arms and legs are helpful indications.

3. A history of abdominal pain in the older child may have many causes. Some of the most common are anxiety, constipation, urinary tract infections, parasite invasion, or irritated bowel. The examiner should carefully question the child or parent about each of these.

4. Pinworms may be common in children, especially those who frequently have dirty hands and have their hands in their mouths. The child may complain of abdominal pain or nighttime rectal itching. The parent should be encouraged to observe the child's rectal area with a flashlight at night as the child sleeps. The worms are most likely to be seen at that time. If the parents suspect pinworms, a specimen should be obtained for analysis. The best technique for this is to put cellophane tape, sticky side up, on the end of a tongue blade and gather the specimen as close to the anal opening as possible.

5. For crawling infants and toddlers the examiner should inquire about pica. Common items eaten are plaster, dirt, paint chips, grass, and blanket fuzz. Although it is normal for children to put nonfood items into their mouths, most learn by age 2 years what is and is not edible.

6. Constipation is a common problem during childhood, especially during the toilet training period. If this is a problem, the examiner should inquire about the following:
　a. How long the problem has existed
　b. Family history of similar problems or diseases affecting bowels
　c. Whether toilet training has been associated with the problem
　d. How many stools per day and week the child usually has (and within the past week)
　e. Current family or home stresses (describe)
　f. Food, juice, and water consumption during the last 48 hours
　g. What parent has done about problem
　h. How parent feels about problem

7. Symptoms such as indigestion, nausea, vomiting, and diarrhea should be explored as detailed in the adult history section.

8. The approach to the pediatric client is extremely important in attempting to assess the abdomen. The abdomen may be the place to start the entire physical examination of the child, but if the examiner moves in with both hands to palpate the abdomen of an 18-month-old, this is bound to fail. The following approach may be helpful for assessing the young infant and child. By age 5 years the child should be ready to cooperate more fully.
　a. Undress the infant or child to diaper and have him on the parent's lap. Do not attempt to examine the small child's abdomen by placing him on the examination table. The child may tense, fight, or cry.
　b. Observe the child's abdomen as he sits or lies on the parent's lap.
　c. Instruct the parent to stand the child up for observation of the abdominal contour and "pot belly" appearance. This is also a time to observe for umbilical bulging or hernia.
　d. For auscultation, percussion, and palpation, the child may be laid in the parent's lap with the

child's legs extending onto the examiner's lap.

e. There is some disagreement as to the sequence of pediatric abdominal assessment elements. Should it be: (1) inspection, (2) auscultation, (3) percussion, and (4) palpation; or (1) inspection, (2) auscultation, (3) palpation, and (4) percussion? Some authorities suggest that percussion is a frightening procedure and should be done last. Try it both ways and then decide for yourself.

f. Even for a small infant the position that facilitates a soft abdomen is one in which both the knees and the neck are flexed. This is easy to achieve as the parent holds the child.

g. Because of the soft examination surface during palpation, it is helpful in both young and older children for the examiner to place the left hand under the child's back and palpate downward with the right hand directly over the same surface. This facilitates a ballottement approach to assessing the abdominal contents. Be gentle but firm during palpation.

h. An internal rectal examination is not routinely performed for the well child because of the invasiveness of the technique. If there is an obvious problem, such as constipation, that requires an internal rectal examination, the examiner should proceed with the same guidelines as for the adult. An ill child with an abdominal complaint should be referred for further evaluation.

i. It will be most helpful to undress the child and make some introductory attempts to touch the child during the history session. Another technique involves letting the child play with the examiner's stethoscope while the initial history and physical assessment is occurring.

j. If the examiner has a question about a finding but because of the parent's soft lap is unable to adequately assess, a last choice is to move both the parent and the child to the examination table. The child should be placed on the examination table, and the parent should assist in holding the child.

k. For the most part the abdomen is easy to assess early during the examination process, before the child becomes upset. If, however, the child is crying during the initial part of the examination, delay the assessment.

l. Crying tenses the abdominal muscles and interferes with accurate assessment.

m. Giving the infant a bottle during the abdominal examination is fine and will, in fact, assist in quieting the child and relaxing the abdominal muscle wall. Caution should be taken to avoid vigorous deep palpation in a child who has just consumed a large bottle of milk, juice, or formula.

n. Older children are generally eager to cooperate but may pose two new problems: ticklishness and firm abdominal muscles.

   (1) Ticklishness may be overcome by gentle continued contact with the child's skin. The sensation should decrease. If not, the examiner may place the child's hand under the examiner's hand.

   (2) A firm abdomen will be a problem in older children and especially in teenage boys. A pillow under the head and flexion of the knees may help to relax the abdominal muscles.

o. Tenseness of the abdominal wall in all children may be a problem, especially if the child is afraid. The examiner should attempt to engage the child in small talk to take the child's mind off the examination. Although it is important for the examiner to observe the child's facial response during palpation of the abdomen, the examiner should try to avoid direct eye contact with the child continuously. This alone may increase tenseness of the child as well as the abdomen.

## Clinical variations: the pediatric client

| CHARACTERISTIC OR AREA EXAMINED | NORMAL | DEVIATIONS FROM NORMAL |
|---|---|---|
| **Abdomen** | | |
| **1.** Inspection | | |
|    **a.** Skin color | May be paler than other parts because of lack of exposure | Jaundice<br>Redness (inflammation)<br>Lesions, bruises, discoloration, cyanosis (localized at umbilicus or generalized) |
|    **b.** Surface characteristics | Smooth, soft<br>Note scars, striae | Rashes, lesions<br>Glistening, taut appearance<br>Pink or red striae<br>Purplish striae |
|    **c.** Venous network | Very faint fine network may be visible, mostly during infancy | Prominent venous pattern<br>Engorgement of veins around umbilicus |
|    **d.** Umbilicus | Centrally located<br>Newborn: should dry within 5 days; should drop off within 2 weeks with dry base remaining; cord should contain two arteries and one vein | Drainage from navel after cord falls off<br>Babies with cords containing one artery have high incidence of congenital anomalies<br>Inflamed, bluish, or nodular appearance |
|    *Note:* Is hernia present during crying only or also at quiet times? Note how size changes. | Surface smooth, noninflamed<br>Umbilical hernia common, especially in blacks<br>Considered normal in white children until 2 years of age, black children until 7 years of age (by 1 month of age hernia should attain its maximum size)<br>Hernia may vary from few millimeters to 3 cm (1 inch) | Umbilical hernia extending beyond 2 years of age in white children, beyond 7 years of age in black children<br><br><br>Child with hernia over 2 cm (¾ inch) should be referred for further assessment<br>Hernia that continues to grow after 1 month of age requires referral |
|    **e.** Contour | Infant, toddler: rounded "pot belly" both standing and lying (Fig. 11-18) | Scaphoid abdomen in infant or toddler<br>Generalized distention |

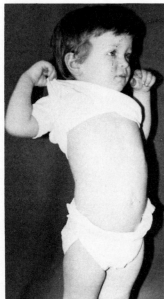

**FIG. 11-18.** Toddler displaying "pot belly" profile.

## Clinical variations: the pediatric client—cont'd

| CHARACTERISTIC OR AREA EXAMINED | NORMAL | DEVIATIONS FROM NORMAL |
|---|---|---|
| | School age: may show some pot belly (lordotic stance) until age 13 years when standing; when child is lying, abdomen should appear scaphoid (Fig. 11-19) | |

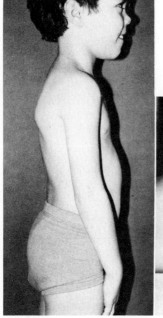
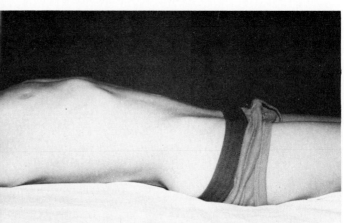

FIG. 11-19. **A,** "Pot belly" stance of preschool-age child. **B,** Scaphoid contour of school-age child.

| CHARACTERISTIC OR AREA EXAMINED | NORMAL | DEVIATIONS FROM NORMAL |
|---|---|---|
| **f.** Symmetry | Evenly rounded with maximum height of convexity at umbilicus | Distention of upper or lower half<br>Visible masses or bulges in any area of abdominal surface |
| **g.** Surface motion<br> 1. Peristalsis<br> 2. Pulsations | Usually not visible<br>Upper midline pulsation may be visible in thin children | Marked peristalsis<br>Marked pulsation |
| **h.** Movement with respirations | Until approximate age 7 years, children are abdominal breathers; after age 7 years boys exhibit chiefly abdominal movement, girls exhibit chiefly costal movement | Grunting, labored respirations accompanied by restricted abdominal movement |
| **i.** Tenseness of abdominal muscles | Diastasis recti abdominis condition in which two recti muscles do not approximate each other; common in black children; should disappear during preschool years<br>May be 1 to 5 cm (½ to 2 inches) wide | Same condition with evidence of accompanying hernia<br>Problem continues in school-age child |

| CHARACTERISTIC OR AREA EXAMINED | NORMAL | DEVIATIONS FROM NORMAL |
|---|---|---|
| **2.** Auscultation | | |
|   **a.** Bowel sounds | Usually 5 to 34/min<br>Irregular in timing | Absence of sound established after 5 minutes of listening; note sounds that are infrequent |
|     1. Quality | Gurgles, clicks (quality of sound varies greatly) | High-pitched, tinkling noises<br>May sound like metallic tinkling |
|   **b.** Vascular sounds | | Bruits (usually high-pitched, soft "swishing" sound, and systolic in timing)<br>(*Note:* Bruit will continue as client is moved into various positions.)<br>Murmur near umbilical area<br>Venous hum (lower in pitch, softer, and a continuous sound) |
|   **c.** Friction rub | | Infrequently heard sound, associated with respirations (soft and may be confused with normal breath sounds)<br>Rubs most often heard over spleen or liver |
| **3.** Percussion | | |
|   **a.** General tone | General distribution of tympany (depending on amount of air and solid material in bowel)<br>Suprapubic dullness heard over distended bladder<br>Children's abdomens frequently sound louder in tympany tones than those of adults primarily because children often swallow more air during swallowing and eating | Marked dullness in local area |
|   **b.** Liver tone and span | Upper liver border usually percussed at approximately sixth rib or interspace anteriorly and at ninth rib posteriorly<br>Lower liver border usually percussed at approximately costal margin or 2 to 3 cm (¾ to 1 inch) lower<br>Average: 5 years of age—7 cm (2¾ inches); 12 years of age—9 cm (3½ inches) | Upper border lower<br>Dullness extending above fifth intercostal space<br>Lower border of liver exceeds 2 to 3 cm below costal margin<br><br>Span that exceeds these limits |
|   **c.** Spleen tone and span | May hear small area of dullness above ninth interspace along left midaxillary line<br>In young infants and children: may extend to 1 to 2 cm below costal margin | Dullness extends above sixth rib or covers large area between sixth rib and costal margin<br>Spleen in any ill-appearing child that extends below costal margin<br>Spleen in children over 1 year of age that extends below costal margin |
| **4.** Palpation | | |
|   **a.** Light and moderate palpation | | |
|     1. Tenderness | Not present | Cutaneous (superficial areas of hypersensitivity) |
|     2. Muscle tone | Abdomen relaxed<br>Muscular resistance may accompany anxious child | Involuntary resistance (muscles cannot be relaxed by voluntary effort) |

## Clinical variations: the pediatric client—cont'd

| CHARACTERISTIC OR AREA EXAMINED | NORMAL | DEVIATIONS FROM NORMAL |
|---|---|---|
| 3. Surface characteristics | Smooth; consistent tension felt by examiner | Masses (superficial)<br>Localized areas of rigidity or increased tension |
| 4. Umbilical area | Note size of umbilical hernia if present | Tenderness |
| **b.** Deep palpation: (be gentle; use one hand) | | |
| 1. Tenderness | Often present in midline near xiphoid process<br>Often present over cecum<br>May be present over sigmoid colon | Present in local or generalized areas<br>Client response to pain may be with muscle guarding and/or facial grimace, pulling away from examiner |
| 2. Masses | Aorta often palpable at epigastrium and pulsates in forward direction<br>Borders of rectus abdominis muscles<br>Feces in ascending or descending colon | Masses that descend on inspiration<br>Pulsatile masses<br>Laterally mobile masses<br>Fixed masses<br>Wilms tumor located adjacent to vertebral column; does not extend across midline |
| 3. Umbilical ring | Umbilicus may be inverted or slightly everted<br>Umbilical ring round, with no irregularities or bulges | Umbilical ring may be incomplete or may feel soft in center<br>Masses, bulges |
| **c.** Organ identification | | |
| 1. Liver palpation | | |
| a. Border location | 0 to 6 months: palpable 0 to 3 cm below costal margin<br>6 months to 4 years: palpable 1 to 2 cm below costal margin<br>Over 6 years: palpable 1 to 2 cm or not palpable below right costal margin | Greater than 2 cm below right costal margin |
| b. Tenderness | None | Tenderness elicited<br>(*Note:* Client's inspiration may be abruptly halted if pain exists.) |
| 2. Spleen palpation | May feel at costal margin or slightly under ribs in small children<br>Only tip (feeling like tongue) should be palpable | Able to palpate more than tip<br>Palpable spleen in older child who also appears ill or has multiple other symptoms |
| 3. Kidney palpation | Palpated periodically, not always<br>Lies adjacent to vertebral column<br>Descends slightly with inspiration<br>Most likely able to palpate lower pole of right kidney; smooth contour | |
| 4. Bladder palpation | Frequently palpated as smooth mass extending midline, somewhere between pubis and umbilical area<br>Ability to palpate should disappear after urination | Bladder distention after voiding |
| 5. Inguinal nodes | | |
| a. Presence | Small, mobile<br>Nontender nodes often present | Enlarged, tender |
| b. Contour | Smooth or nonpalpable | |
| c. Consistency | Soft or nonpalpable | Hard |
| **d.** Kidney jarring to evaluate costovertebral angle tenderness | Client perceives jar or thud<br>No tenderness elicited | Tenderness elicited |

| CHARACTERISTIC OR AREA EXAMINED | NORMAL | DEVIATIONS FROM NORMAL |
|---|---|---|
| **Anal/rectal region** | | |
| **1.** Evaluation of anal and rectal region | | |
|   **a.** Inspection | | |
|     1. Skin surface characteristics | Surface smooth and clear | Lumps, rash, inflammation, scars, pilonidal dimpling, tuft of hair at pilonidal area |
|   **b.** Palpation of coccygeal area for tenderness | No tenderness | Tender |
|   **c.** Inspection of anus | | |
|     1. Surface characteristics | Increased pigmentation<br>Coarse skin | Inflammation<br>Lesions<br>Scars<br>Skin tags<br>Fissures<br>Lumps<br>Swelling<br>Excoriation |
|   **d.** Internal rectal examination not routinely done in children unless ill or specific problem exists; when performed, follow same guidelines as for adult client | | |

## History and clinical strategies: the geriatric client

1. Nutritional assessment. Many authorities state that maintaining adequate nutritional intake is a major problem for the older adult. This problem is not confined to chronically ill individuals or to low-income persons. Following are risk factors for poor nutritional intake patterns:
   a. Living alone
   b. Physical disability (e.g., diminished vision, neurological deficits, decreased mobility, arthritic changes, diminished strength, general symptoms of fatigue, dyspnea, or pain)
   c. Depression; anxiety
   d. Mouth or dental problems
   e. Swallowing or choking problems
   f. Sedentary life-style (particularly if associated with boredom, depression, or obesity)
   g. Obesity (usually accompanied by long-standing overeating habits)
   h. Limited access to markets (especially if client is unable to drive, if stores are within walking distance and require daily trips, or if client must rely on driving services of others)
   i. Limited cooking facilities or capability (often results in increased use of convenience foods or "empty" calories)
   j. Limited income (this problem exists in all income ranges; fixed incomes do not reflect inflation trends)
   k. Numerous food idiosyncracies or general loss of senses of taste and smell
   l. Confusion (even mild, transient states of confusion will interrupt eating patterns)
   m. Misconceptions about nutritional requirements (e.g., belief that fewer nutrients are required for the elderly)

n. Special diets prescribed (especially if difficult to purchase or to prepare or if taste is less desirable)

o. Medications (prescribed or over-the-counter drugs may cause gastrointestinal side effects such as dry mouth, anorexia, nausea, sedation, "heartburn") (*Note:* Aspirin is frequently the source of gastrointestinal symptoms.)

p. Alcohol or drug abuse

The questions described in the original data base will help the examiner to elicit information related to the variables that alter food and fluid intake.

The actual *amounts* or *types* of food that are routinely consumed are sometimes difficult to assess because many older adults eat erratically (numerous meals are taken in small amounts scattered over a 24-hour period, or eating habits vary widely from day to day). A 24-hour recall may not reflect true eating patterns. A diary, covering a week or a month of food consumption, may be helpful if the client is sufficiently motivated to follow through with recording. Several appointments devoted to nutritional assessment may be necessary if the examiner suspects intake is inadequate.

2. Elimination assessment. Authorities state that elderly clients frequently express numerous problems associated with elimination and that individuals may be preoccupied with bowel movement regularity to the extent that it can alter daily living functions. Problems may be described as a "spastic" or "irritable" colon, colitis, "gas on the stomach," constipation, or diarrhea. Clarification of symptoms is necessary. Constipation and diarrhea are discussed in the adult history section of this chapter. If long-standing problems exist, inquire carefully about the client's effort to treat himself. Risk factors associated with bowel elimination problems follow:

a. Hemorrhoids

b. Taking of laxatives (clarify whether this is a long-standing or recent habit)

c. Recent dietary changes: reduced intake; elimination of certain foods

d. Dietary intake with insufficient bulk

e. Limited fluid intake

f. Depression (often associated with constipation)

g. Anxiety

h. Physical immobility

i. Weakened abdominal muscles

j. Medication side effects or abuse (prescribed or over the counter, e.g., iron, antibiotics, tranquilizers, antacids)

3. Hiatus hernia is a common problem with adults over age 70. The diaphragmatic muscle weakens, and the lower portion of the esophagus slides from the abdominal cavity into the thoracic cavity. The gastroesophageal sphincter does not constrict efficiently, and gastric contents regurgitate into the lower esophagus. Epigastric pain and burning are common complaints, especially at night or during prolonged periods in a supine position.

4. Major aging changes associated with the gastrointestinal system include:

a. Decrease in total volume of acid secretion

b. Decreased hunger contractions

c. Delayed gastric emptying

d. Diminished tone of bowel wall

e. Decreased peristalsis

f. Decreased abdominal muscle strength

g. Decreased anal sphincter tone

5. Other special problems related to aging are the following:

a. Diminished esophageal swallow reflex, especially in the lower third of the esophagus; may result in difficulty swallowing (choking) or dilation of the lower esophagus with retention of food in this area.

b. Increased swallowing of air, often associated with anxiety; may result in frequent eructation, abdominal distention, or flatus.

c. Atrophic gastritis and diminished gastric acid content may be associated with diminished absorption of vitamin $B_{12}$ (pernicious anemia). Malabsorption of iron can also occur in an alkaline gastric medium.

d. Medications may decrease gastric secretions or gastrointestinal motility.

e. Diverticulosis, an outpouching of a weakened area of the bowel wall, is a common condition with the elderly. It is frequently asymptomatic but may be associated with decreased intestinal contractions and resulting flatulence and heartburn.

In many instances the changes just listed do not produce any signs or symptoms that are significant to the client or the examiner. These changes take place at different rates with different individuals and are not predictable on a chronological basis. However, all symptoms should be explored carefully and not assumed to be a "functional" disorder by the examiner. Elderly clients may manifest less pain and less abdominal rigidity in acute or chronic conditions. Details related to the major symptoms are covered in the adult section of this chapter.

# Clinical variations: the geriatric client

| CHARACTERISTIC OR AREA EXAMINED | NORMAL | DEVIATIONS FROM NORMAL |
|---|---|---|
| **1.** General behaviors of client | Appears relaxed<br>Facial muscles relaxed<br>Lying quietly<br>Respirations even and slow | Marked restlessness<br>Marked immobility or rigid posture<br>Knees drawn up<br>Facial grimacing<br>Respirations rapid, uneven, or "grunting" |

**Abdomen**

| CHARACTERISTIC OR AREA EXAMINED | NORMAL | DEVIATIONS FROM NORMAL |
|---|---|---|
| **1.** Inspection of abdominal surface | | |
|   **a.** Skin color | May be paler than other parts because of lack of exposure | Jaundice<br>Redness (inflammation)<br>Lesions, bruises, discoloration, cyanosis (localized at umbilicus or generalized) |
|   **b.** Surface characteristics | Smooth, soft<br>Silver-white striae (usually lower abdomen) | Rashes, lesions<br>Glistening, taut appearance |
|   **c.** Scars (configuration, location, length) | | |
|   **d.** Venous network | Faint fine network may be visible | Prominent venous pattern<br>Engorgement of veins around umbilicus |
|   **e.** Umbilicus | | |
|     1. Placement | Centrally located | Displaced upward or downward |
|     2. Contour | Usually sunken, may protrude slightly | Visible hernia around or slightly above umbilicus |
|     3. Surface | Smooth, noninflamed | Inflamed |
|   **f.** Contour | Flat<br>Rounded<br>Scaphoid (concave profile)<br>(*Note:* elderly individuals may have increased fat deposits over abdominal area even though subcutaneous fat is decreased over extremites.) | Distention (common distress signal in elderly clients)<br>Marked concavity associated with general wasting signs or associated with anteroposterior rib expansion |
|   **g.** Symmetry | Evenly rounded with maximum height of convexity at umbilicus | Distention of upper or lower half<br>Visible masses or bulges in any area of abdominal surface |
|   **h.** Surface motion | | |
|     1. Peristalsis | Usually not visible | Visible |
|     2. Pulsation | Upper midline pulsation may be visible in thin people | Marked pulsation |
|   **i.** General movement with respirations | Smooth, even movements<br>Women exhibit chiefly costal movement<br>Men exhibit chiefly abdominal movement | Grunting, labored<br>Respirations accompanied by restricted abdominal movement |
| **2.** Instruct client to take a deep breath and hold it | Contour remains smooth and symmetrical | Bulges or masses appear |
| **3.** Instruct client to raise head without using arms for support | Rectus abdominis muscles prominent<br>Midline bulge may appear | Appearance of bulges through muscle layer |
| **4.** Auscultatory bowel sounds | Usually 5 to 34/min<br>Irregular in timing | Absence of sound established after 5 minutes of listening<br>Note sounds that are infrequent |
|   **a.** Quality | Gurgles, clicks<br>Quality of sound varies greatly | High-pitched, tinkling noises |

## Clinical variations: the geriatric client—cont'd

| CHARACTERISTIC OR AREA EXAMINED | NORMAL | DEVIATIONS FROM NORMAL |
|---|---|---|
| **5.** Vascular sounds | | |
| **a.** Arterial: concentrate in epigastric area, in area surrounding umbilicus, over liver, and at posterior flank | | Bruits (usually high-pitched, soft, swishing sound, and systolic in timing) (*Note:* Bruit will continue as client is moved into various positions.) |
| **b.** Venous | | Venous hum (lower in pitch, softer, and continuous sound) |
| **6.** Friction rubs | | Infrequently heard sound associated with respirations (soft, and may be confused with normal breath sounds) |
| **7.** Percussion tones over entire abdomen | General distribution of tympany (depending on amount of air and solid material in bowel) Suprapubic dullness heard over distended bladder | Marked dullness in local area |
| **8.** Liver | | |
| **a.** Lower border percussion | Lower border of liver usually at costal margin or slightly below; however, if elderly client has distended lungs, liver border will descend 1 to 2 cm into abdominal cavity | Lower border of liver exceeds 2 to 3 cm below costal margin |
| **b.** Upper border percussion | Upper border of liver usually begins in fifth to seventh intercostal space Upper border may descend 1 to 2 cm if liver has lowered with diaphragm, associated with distended lungs | Upper border lowered Dullness extending above fifth intercostal space |
| **c.** Midclavicular liver span | 6 to 12 cm (2½ to 4½ inches) Normal liver span usually greater in men than women, and greater in taller individuals | Span exceeds 12 cm |
| **d.** Right midaxillary liver percussion | Liver dullness may be felt in fifth to seventh intercostal space | Dull percussion note exceeds limits of fifth to seventh intercostal space |
| **e.** Midsternal liver span | Ranges from 4 to 8 cm (1½ to 3 inches) | Span exceeds 8 cm |
| **f.** Liver descent with deep inspiration (*Note:* Deep inspiration may be difficult for elderly client.) | Lower border of liver should move inferiorly by 2 to 3 cm | Liver does not move with inspiration, or movement less than 2 cm |
| **9.** Spleen percussion | | |
| **a.** At left posterior midaxillary line | Small area of splenic dullness may be heard at sixth to tenth rib, or tone may be tympanic (colonic) | Dullness extends above sixth rib, or dullness covers large area between sixth rib and costal margin |
| **b.** At lowest left intercostal space in anterior axillary line (performed after client takes deep breath) | Area usually tympanic | Tympany changes to dullness on inspiration (An enlarged spleen is brought forward on inspiration to produce a dull percussion note.) |
| **10.** Percussion of gastric "bubble" in left lower rib cage | Tympanic and varies in size | |

| CHARACTERISTIC OR AREA EXAMINED | NORMAL | DEVIATIONS FROM NORMAL |
|---|---|---|
| 11. Palpation | | |
|    **a.** Muscle tone | (*Note:* Elderly clients often manifest a more lax abdominal tone.) | Involuntary resistance<br>Elderly clients may not manifest rigidity response to extent that younger client does; rigidity may be replaced by distention |
|    **b.** Tenderness | Not present on light or moderate palpation<br>Deep palpation may cause discomfort in midline near xiphoid process<br>Over cecum<br>Over sigmoid colon | Cutaneous (superficial areas of hypersensitivity) or deep pain response in local or generalized area |
|    **c.** Surface characteristics | Smooth | Induration<br>Nodules<br>Rough texture |
|    **d.** General tone and location of major structures | Abdomen surface feels smooth, and tension under palpating hand feels consistent throughout | Localized areas of rigidity, distention, or increased tension |
|    **e.** Masses | Aorta often palpable at epigastrium and pulsates in forward direction<br>Borders of rectus abdominis muscles<br>Feces in ascending or descending colon<br>Sacral promontory | Masses that descend on inspiration<br>Pulsatile masses<br>Laterally mobile masses<br>Fixed masses<br>Aortic pulsations directed laterally |
|    **f.** Umbilicus | Umbilical ring round, with no irregularities or bulges<br>Umbilicus may be inverted or slightly everted | Masses, bulges<br>Umbilical ring may be incomplete or may feel soft in center |
| 12. Specific organ identification | | |
|    **a.** Liver palpation | | |
|       1. Border and contour | Liver often not palpable<br>Liver often "bumps" against fingers on inspiration (especially with thin clients)<br>Liver commonly palpated 1 to 2 cm below costal margin in clients with distended lungs and lowered diaphragm | (*Note:* Greatly enlarged liver may lie under examiner's hand as it extends downward into abdominal cavity.) |
|       2. Border surface | Smooth | Irregular, nodular surface or edge |
|       3. Tenderness | None | Tenderness elicited<br>(*Note:* Client's inspiration may be abruptly halted if pain exists.) |
|    **b.** Spleen palpation | Spleen not normally palpable | |
|    **c.** Kidney palpation | Kidneys rarely palpated in elderly clients<br>Lower pole of right kidney may be felt in very thin clients; if palpated, contour smooth and no associated tenderness | |
|    **d.** Inguinal nodes (horizontal and vertical) | | |
|       1. Presence | Small, mobile<br>Nontender nodes often present | Tender, enlarged |
|       2. Contour | Smooth or nonpalpable | |
|       3. Consistency | Soft or nonpalpable | |

## Clinical variations: the geriatric client—cont'd

| CHARACTERISTIC OR AREA EXAMINED | NORMAL | DEVIATIONS FROM NORMAL |
| --- | --- | --- |
| (*Note:* Femoral pulses can also be palpated at this time. Techniques and palpable qualities are covered in Chapter 9.) *Note:* Special maneuvers for assessing fluid in abdominal cavity and abdominal pain are conducted in same manner as described in adult section of this chapter (p. 317). | | |

**Anal/rectal region**

| CHARACTERISTIC OR AREA EXAMINED | NORMAL | DEVIATIONS FROM NORMAL |
| --- | --- | --- |
| 1. Inspection of sacrococcygeal and perianal areas for: | | |
|   **a.** Skin and surface characteristics | Surface smooth and clear | Lumps<br>Rash<br>Inflammation<br>Scars<br>Pilonidal dimpling<br>Tuft of hair at pilonidal area |
| 2. Palpation of coccygeal area for tenderness | No tenderness | Tender |
| 3. Inspection of anus for:<br>  **a.** Surface characteristics | Increased pigmentation<br>Coarse skin | Inflammation<br>Lesions<br>Scars<br>Skin tags<br>Fissures<br>Lumps<br>Swelling<br>Excoriation<br>Hemorrhoids<br>Mucosa (pinkish red in color) bulges through anal ring |
| 4. Ask client to strain down to assess sphincter tone | Sphincter tightens evenly around examiner's finger with minimal discomfort to client | Client unable to tighten sphincter around finger or experiences discomfort with tightening |
| 5. Palpation of anal muscular ring for:<br>  **a.** Surface characteristics | Smooth, even pressure on finger | Nodules<br>Irregularities |
| 6. Palpation of all four rectal walls | Continuous smooth surface with minimal discomfort to client | Nodules<br>Masses<br>(*Note:* Cervix is sometimes palpable on anterior wall. Do not mistake for a mass.) |
| (*Note:* Prostate examination is covered in Chapter 12.) | | (*Note:* Elderly clients often have rectal polyps; however, they are soft and sometimes difficult to palpate.) |
| 7. As finger is extracted, note characteristics of any stool<br>  **a.** Color | Brown | Presence of blood, pus<br>Black, tarry stool<br>Pale or yellow stool<br>Mucus on stool surface |
|   **b.** Consistency | Soft | |

# Male genitourinary system

## VOCABULARY

**anuria** Absence of urine production or the inability to produce more than 250 ml of urine per day

**balano-** Combining form denoting the glans penis. EXAMPLE: *Balanitis* means inflammation of the glans penis.

**chordee** Ventral curvature of the penis; congenital anomaly caused by a restrictive band of tissue between the meatus and the glans; usually associated with hypospadias.

**cryptorchism (undescended testis)** Failure of one or both of the testicles to descend into the scrotum.

**dysuria** Difficulty, pain, or burning sensation with urination.

**enuresis** Any involuntary urination, especially during sleep.

**epididymitis** Inflammation of the epididymis (tightly coiled, comma-shaped structure overlying posterolateral surface of testis); infection can be acute or chronic; area is extremely tender, usually involving the scrotal wall and occasionally extending along the spermatic cord.

**epispadias** Congenital defect in which the urinary meatus opens on the dorsum of the penis; opening may be located on the glans, anywhere along the penile shaft, or extend into the pubic symphysis.

**hematuria** The presence of blood in the urine.

**hernia** An abnormal opening in a muscle wall or cavity that permits protrusion of its contents.

*direct inguinal hernia* Protrusion of abdominal contents through external ring of inguinal canal, usually in region superior to the canal.

*indirect inguinal hernia* Protrusion of abdominal contents into internal ring of inguinal canal; contents may remain in the canal, emerge through external ring, or extend downward into scrotal sac; occurs more commonly than direct inguinal herniation.

*femoral hernia* Protrusion of abdominal contents through femoral canal (below inguinal ligament); occurs more often with women than men and is less common than inguinal hernias.

**hydrocele** Nontender, serous fluid mass located within the tunica vaginalis (layered, hollow membrane adjacent to testis); examiner's finger can get above the mass within the scrotum.

**hypospadias** Congenital defect in which the urinary meatus opens on the ventral aspect of the penis; opening may be located in the glans, penile shaft, scrotum, or perineum.

**oliguria** Inadequate production or secretion of urine (usually less than 400 ml in a 24-hour period).

**orchi-** Combining form denoting the testes. EXAMPLE: *Orchitis* means inflammation of one or both of the testes.

**paraphimosis** Condition characterized by the inability to pull the foreskin forward from a retracted position; glans is usually swollen and inflamed.

**phimosis** Tightness of the foreskin that results in an inability to retract it; usually caused by adhesions of the prepuce to the underlying glans.

**pyuria** Presence of white cells (pus) in the urine.

**refractory period** Rest interval following nerve excitation or muscle contraction. EXAMPLE: In sexual intercourse the refractory period is the phase that follows orgasm; it refers to the normal loss of erection after ejaculation and the time required before another ejaculation can occur.

**smegma** Accumulation of bacteria, urine, and cellular debris underneath the foreskin; sometimes associated with phimosis and resulting irritation and inflammation.

**spermatocele (epididymal cyst)** A painless, fluid-filled epididymal mass that contains spermatozoa.

**tenesmus** Rectal or anal spasm characterized by pain and a sensation of urgency; overly vigorous digital examination can cause anal sphincter spasms; rectal tenesmus may be associated with prostatitis and resulting perirectal inflammation.

**torsion (of spermatic cord)** The twisting of the spermatic cord resulting in an infarction of the testis; severe pain, redness, and swelling are present; loss of the testis can be prevented if the condition is diagnosed and treated quickly.

**varicocele** The abnormal tortuosity and dilation of spermatic veins; spermatic cord is described as feeling like a bag of worms; condition is not painful but involves a pulling or dragging sensation.

## Cognitive objectives

At the end of this chapter the learner will demonstrate knowledge of assessment of the male genitourinary system by the ability to do the following:

1. Identify and locate the major internal and external structures of the male genitourinary system.
2. Point out observable and palpable characteristics of normal penis and scrotal contents.
3. Identify major inguinal and lower abdominal structures associated with assessment for hernias.
4. Locate, on a drawing, the three common pelvic area hernia sites.
5. Identify palpable characteristics of the normal prostate gland.
6. Identify common selected variations for pediatric and geriatric clients.
7. Use the terms in the vocabulary section.

## Clinical objectives

At the end of this chapter the learner will perform a systematic assessment of the male genitourinary system, demonstrating the ability to do the following:

1. Obtain a pertinent history from a client.
2. Inspect and palpate the pubic region for:
   a. Hair distribution
   b. Parasites
   c. Surface characteristics
3. Inspect and palpate the penis for:
   a. Surface characteristics
   b. Foreskin
   c. Meatus location
   d. Discharge
   e. Tenderness
4. Inspect and palpate the scrotum and scrotal contents for:
   a. Size and contour
   b. Testes
      (1) Size
      (2) Contour
      (3) Mobility
      (4) Tenderness
   c. Epididymides
   d. Vas deferens
   e. Additional scrotal contents
5. Transilluminate scrotal contents.
6. Evaluate inguinal region for hernias: palpate external inguinal ring and femoral area.
7. Inspect and palpate sacrococcygeal and perianal area for surface characteristics and tenderness.
8. Inspect and palpate the anus for:
   a. Sphincter tone
   b. Tenderness
   c. Surface characteristics
9. Palpate distal rectal walls for surface characteristics.
10. Palpate the prostate gland for:
    a. Size
    b. Contour
    c. Consistency
    d. Tenderness
11. Summarize results with a written description of findings.

## Health history additional to screening history

1. Reproductive functions and sexuality. The examiner should screen all clients for sexual needs or problems by initially posing a broad, nondirective question. The question might be worded in this way: "Do you have any concerns regarding sexual practices or values that you would like to discuss?" This lets the client know that he can share his problems if he wishes to, and it does not direct him toward any specific area of concern. Please note that anyone posing this question should be prepared to follow through with intervention skills in this area.

A more specific detailed assessment will help to clarify general concerns and can supplement the original data base.
   a. Present practices and values
      (1) Are you comfortable with your intimate relationships (with or without sexual activ-

ity)? Do you have difficulty meeting your needs for intimacy (or affection)?

(2) Are you having a sexual relationship with anyone at present?

(3) Do you feel satisfied with this relationship? (For example, do you and your partner share similar feelings about the methods and variety of sexual acts you perform; about the frequency of sex; about the kind and amount of affection displayed; about initiating sex? Do you talk about sexual feelings with your partner? Is there anything you would change about this relationship?

(4) If you do not have a sexual partner, are your sexual needs being met?

(5) Do you have more than one sexual partner? If so, is this a satisfactory arrangement?

(6) How many partners have you had in the past year?

(7) How do you feel about homosexuality (i.e., is it a personal issue with you)?

(8) How do you feel about masturbation?

(9) Have there been any recent changes in your sexual desire (arousal patterns), specific sexual acts or behaviors, frequency of sexual experiences, choice of sexual partners?

(10) Do you and/or your partner(s) use contraception? What method do you use? Do you have questions or difficulty with this?

(11) Do you have any questions about male sexuality, sexual function, female sexuality, sterility, venereal disease, other?

b. Past history

(1) Describe your personal experience with sex education. Was sexuality discussed with family members? Was it discussed openly? Were there others outside the family who informed or influenced you sexually? Explain.

(2) Were your parents affectionate with each other?

(3) What were your early experiences with masturbation; wet dreams; sex play with other children; adolescent relationships; dating (feeling comfortable with girls); petting?

(4) How old were you when you first had sexual intercourse? How did you feel about it?

(5) Have you ever had a homosexual experience? Describe.

(6) How many sexual partners have you had?

c. Genital health

(1) Do you examine your penis and your scrotum (testicles)? How often? (*Note:* It is more helpful to allow the client to demonstrate how he examines himself during the physical assessment rather than to have him describe the procedure.)

(2) Do you have any general concerns about your genitalia (e.g., size, shape, surface characteristics, texture)?

(3) Are you able to pull back (and replace) the foreskin on your penis?

(4) Have you ever noticed any sores, rashes, swelling, lumps, or discharge?

(5) Have you felt any itching, burning, or stinging in your penis?

(6) Are you able to have an erection? Do you have difficulty attaining or maintaining an erection?

(7) Do you experience pain with an erection (either in your penis or scrotum)?

(8) Do you ever have prolonged painful erections? If so, is it associated with sexual arousal?

(9) When you have an erection, does your penis curve downward or to the side?

(10) Do you have any difficulty with ejaculation (e.g., premature, inadequate, painful)?

(11) Describe the fluid that discharges at the time of ejaculation (color, consistency, odor, amount).

(12) Do you ever feel any irregularities, lumps, soreness, or heaviness in your testicles?

(13) Have you ever been treated for (or ever been exposed to) any venereal diseases: gonorrhea, syphilis, herpes simplex, venereal warts? If so, describe symptoms, treatment, follow-up procedures.

(14) Do you take any precautions to prevent exposure to sexually transmitted diseases?

(15) Do you have specific questions or concerns about symptoms or disease transmission?

2. Genitourinary symptoms

a. Urinary frequency. How many times do you void (urinate) in a 24-hour period? Does this frequency involve sleeping hours as well as waking hours? Can you estimate the volume voided each time? Has the volume increased or decreased?

b. Nocturia. How many times do you have to urinate at night? Is this a *change* of habit for you? Has your daytime or nighttime fluid intake changed?

c. Urgency. Does urgency occur with every urination, occasionally, or rarely? Does urgency occur without voiding? Is it associated with other symptoms such as frequency, dysuria, or incontinence?

d. Hesitancy. Do you have to wait a while for your stream to start? Once you have started, can you pass 80% to 90% of your urine in a continuous stream? Do you have to strain to start or to maintain your stream?

e. Flow of urinary stream. Have you had any decrease in the size of your stream? Are you having to stand closer to the toilet to avoid urinating on the floor? (The examiner is concerned with the force as well as caliber of the stream.)

f. Urethral discharge. What color is it? Has the amount of discharge increased or decreased since it started? Is the discharge associated with pain? With urination? Is an unusual odor associated with discharge? Describe.

g. Hernia. If you feel a lump in your scrotum, are you able to push the lump back inside? Does the lump ever change size? How long has it been since you were able to push the lump back inside (a day, a week)? Do you have a heavy feeling or dragging sensation in your scrotum?

## Clinical guidelines

| THE STUDENT WILL: | TO IDENTIFY: | |
| --- | --- | --- |
| | NORMAL | DEVIATIONS FROM NORMAL |
| 1. Assemble equipment | | |
| a. Rectal glove | | |
| b. Lubricant | | |
| c. Penlight | | |
| 2. Inspect and palpate the general pubic region (Palpation of inguinal lymphatics is described in Chapter 11.) | | |
| a. Hair distribution | Variable in adults<br>Diamond-shaped pattern often extending to umbilicus | Patchy growth or loss<br>Absence of hair<br>Female configuration: triangular, with base over pubis |
| b. Parasites | Absent | Nits, pubic lice |
| c. Skin surface characteristics | Smooth, clear | Scars<br>Lower abdominal or inguinal lesions<br>Rash (especially in folds)<br>(*Note:* Tinea cruris ["jock itch"] is a common fungal infection found in the groin. Large, clearly marginated, reddened patches are pruritic and often associated with "athlete's foot." Monilial infections, which are red, eroded patches with scaling and pustules, also are often seen; they are associated with immobility and disability, systemic antibiotics, and immunological deficits.) |
| 3. Inspect the penis | | |
| a. Skin color and surface characteristics | Usually dark<br>Hairless<br>Wrinkled; surface vascularity may be apparent | Reddened<br>Lesions<br>Swelling<br>Nodules |
| b. Foreskin | Uncircumcised: prepuce present and folded over glans (Fig. 12-1)<br>Circumcised: prepuce often absent, or small flaps remains at corona (Fig. 12-2) | |

| THE STUDENT WILL: | TO IDENTIFY: | |
| --- | --- | --- |
| | NORMAL | DEVIATIONS FROM NORMAL |

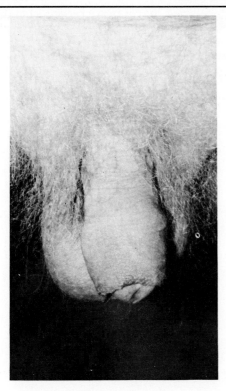

FIG. 12-1. Uncircumcised penis.

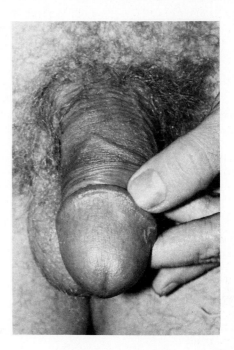

FIG. 12-2. Circumcised penis.

| | | |
| --- | --- | --- |
| **4.** Ask client to retract foreskin if present (Fig. 12-3) | Foreskin retracts easily to expose glans and returns to original position with ease | Failure to retract; discomfort with retraction<br>Difficulty returning prepuce to original position |

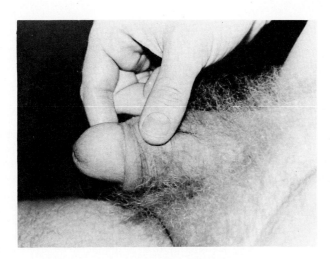

FIG. 12-3. Client retracting foreskin.

## Clinical guidelines—cont'd

| | TO IDENTIFY: | |
| THE STUDENT WILL: | NORMAL | DEVIATIONS FROM NORMAL |
| --- | --- | --- |
| 5. Inspect glans and under prepuce fold | Glans smooth, pink, bulbous<br>Prepuce fold wrinkled, loosely attached to underlying glans, darker in color than glans<br>(*Note:* Circumcised penises have varying lengths of foreskin remaining; some have multiple folds and others have few or none.) | Lesions<br>Crusting under fold or around tip of glans<br>Redness, swelling |
| 6. Inspect urethral meatus for:<br>  **a.** Location<br><br>  **b.** Discharge | <br><br>Central, at distal tip of glans<br><br>Usually not present | <br><br>Dorsal location<br>Ventral location<br>Yellow-green discharge<br>Milky-white discharge<br>Discharge with foul odor |
| 7. Ask client to compress glans anteroposteriorly to open distal end of urethra (Fig. 12-4); inspect for surface characteristics | Pink, smooth<br>No discharge | Reddened, swollen<br>Discharge<br>Crusting |

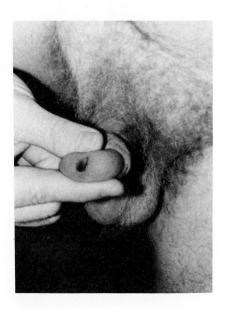

**FIG. 12-4.** Client compressing glans to open urethral meatus.

| | | |
| --- | --- | --- |
| 8. Palpate entire penis between thumb and first two fingers for palpable characteristics; use glove if lesions or discharge is visualized | Nontender<br>Smooth, semifirm consistency | Tenderness<br>Swelling<br>Nodules<br>Induration |
| 9. Ask client to hold penis out of the way; inspect scrotum for size and contour | Sac divided in half by septum<br>Left scrotal sac may be longer than right<br>Size varies: may appear pendulous<br>Scrotal contents contracted when surface temperature cool | |

| THE STUDENT WILL: | TO IDENTIFY: | |
| --- | --- | --- |
| | **NORMAL** | **DEVIATIONS FROM NORMAL** |
| **10.** Lift scrotum to examine underside surface characteristics (spread rugated surface for better view) (*Note:* While viewing surface of scrotum, visualize scrotal contents: placement, proximity, size; tactile maneuvers will be more efficient [Fig. 12-5].) | Deeply pigmented Hairless Rugous surface | Reddened Edematous Rugae not present Rash Lesions |

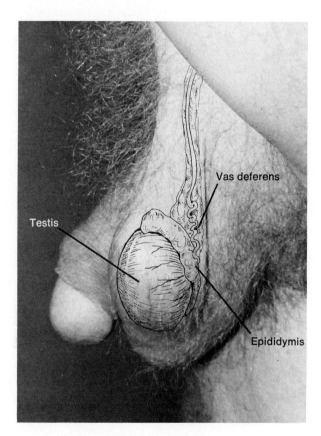

**FIG. 12-5.** Palpable scrotal contents.

| | | |
| --- | --- | --- |
| **11.** Palpate each half of scrotum for surface characteristics | Nontender Thin loose skin over muscular layer | Marked tenderness Swelling, redness (*Note:* Scrotal inflammation can exacerbate quickly into cellulitis and gangrene. If inflammation is present, examine rugated surface carefully for fissures or breaks in the skin. Refer immediately for treatment.) |
| | No pitting | Pitting |

## Clinical guidelines—cont'd

| THE STUDENT WILL: | TO IDENTIFY: | |
| --- | --- | --- |
| | NORMAL | DEVIATIONS FROM NORMAL |

**12.** Palpate testes simultaneous between thumb and first two fingers (Fig. 12-6)

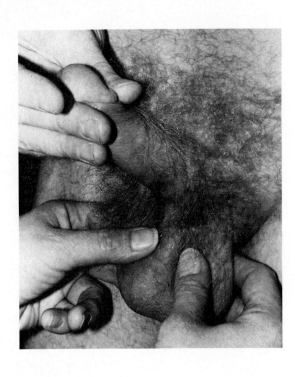

FIG. 12-6. Examiner palpating scrotum.

| THE STUDENT WILL: | NORMAL | DEVIATIONS FROM NORMAL |
| --- | --- | --- |
| **a.** Presence | Present in each sac | Not present |
| **b.** Size | Approximately 4 × 3 × 2 cm (1½ × 1 × ¾ inches) | Enlarged (unilateral/bilateral) Atrophied |
| | Equal in size | |
| **c.** Tenderness | Mildly sensitive to moderate compression | Markedly tender |
| **d.** Contour | Smooth, ovoid | Nodular Irregular |
| **e.** Mobility | Movable | Fixed |
| **13.** Palpate epididymides for palpable characteristics | Nontender | Tender |
| | Usually located on posterolateral surface of each testis | |
| | Discretely palpable | |
| | Comma shaped | Irregular |
| | Smooth | Enlarged Indurated Nodular |
| **14.** Palpate vas deferens for palpable characteristics (use thumb and forefinger) | Nontender | Tender |
| | Discretely palpable from epididymis to external inguinal ring | Tortuous |
| | Smooth and cordlike | Thickened; beaded |
| | Movable | Indurated |

| THE STUDENT WILL: | TO IDENTIFY: | |
| --- | --- | --- |
| | NORMAL | DEVIATIONS FROM NORMAL |
| **15.** Palpate for additional scrotal contents | None | Mass distal or proximal to testis either tender or nontender |
|    **a.** Transilluminate each scrotal sac if mass or irregularity is suspected | Testes and epididymides do not transilluminate | Hydrocele ⎫<br>Spermatocele ⎬ Transilluminate<br>Tumors ⎫<br>Hernias ⎬ Do not transilluminate<br>Epididymitis ⎭ |
| **16.** Evaluate inguinal region for hernia: if possible, client should be standing and examiner sitting | | |
| **17.** Inspect inguinal region for bulges; then ask client to strain, and continue to inspect area | | Bulges at area of external ring, Hesselbach triangle, femoral area |
| **18.** Palpate both right and left inguinal rings: use index finger or little finger of hand on client's corresponding side; client should be standing if possible, and examiner seated (Fig. 12-7); ask client to strain | Finger follows spermatic cord upward to triangular slitlike opening, which may or may not admit finger | Palpable mass touches examiner's fingertip or pushes against side of finger |

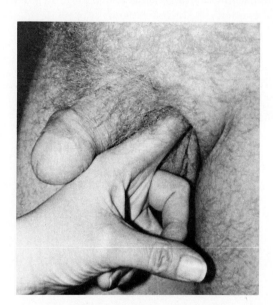

**FIG. 12-7.** Palpation for inguinal hernia.

| | | |
| --- | --- | --- |
| **19.** Palpate each femoral area (fossa ovalis) for bulges; ask client to strain | | Soft bulge emerges at fossa |

## Clinical guidelines—cont'd

| THE STUDENT WILL: | TO IDENTIFY: NORMAL | DEVIATIONS FROM NORMAL |
|---|---|---|
| **20.** Evaluate anal and rectal region (also described in Chapter 11) | | |
| **a.** Inspect sacrococcygeal and perianal areas (client lying on left side with right hip and knee flexed) | | |
| 1. Skin and surface characteristics | Surface smooth and clear | Lumps<br>Rash<br>Inflammation<br>Scars<br>Pilonidal dimpling<br>Tuft of hair at pilonidal area |
| **b.** Palpate coccygeal area for tenderness | No tenderness | Tenderness |
| **c.** Spread buttocks with both hands and inspect anus for: | | Inflammation<br>Lesions<br>Scars |
| 1. Surface characteristics (penlight can be used) | Increased pigmentation<br>Coarse skin | Skin tags<br>Fissures<br>Lumps<br>Swelling<br>Excoriation |
| **d.** Ask client to strain down; place gloved and lubricated finger at anal opening; as sphincter relaxes, slowly insert finger pointing toward client's umbilicus; ask client to tighten sphincter around finger to assess tone | Sphincter tightens evenly around finger with minimal discomfort to client | Hemorrhoids<br>Mucosal bulging<br>Hypotonic sphincter<br>Hypertonic sphincter with marked tenderness |
| **e.** Rotate finger to examiner anal muscular ring for surface characteristics | Smooth, even pressure on finger | Nodules<br>Irregularities |
| **f.** Insert finger further to palpate all four rectal walls | Continuous, smooth surface with minimal discomfort to client | Nodules<br>Masses<br>Tenderness<br>Tenderness |
| **g.** Palpate entire prostate gland (Fig. 12-8) at anterior surface for: | | |
| 1. Size | Approximately 4 cm (1½ inches) in diameter; projecting less than 1 cm into rectum | Enlarged |
| 2. Contour | Symmetrical<br>Bilobed with palpable sulcus | Asymmetrical<br>Median sulcus obliterated |
| 3. Consistency | Firm, smooth | Boggy feeling<br>Irregular<br>Nodules |
| 4. Tenderness | Nontender | Tender |
| **h.** Ask client to strain; palpate area above prostate if possible | | Masses or bulges touch finger |
| **i.** Slowly withdraw finger and examine any fecal material adhering to glove | Stool brown, soft | Presence of blood, pus<br>Black, tarry stool<br>Pale or yellow stool<br>Light tan or gray stool |

| THE STUDENT WILL: | TO IDENTIFY: NORMAL | DEVIATIONS FROM NORMAL |
|---|---|---|

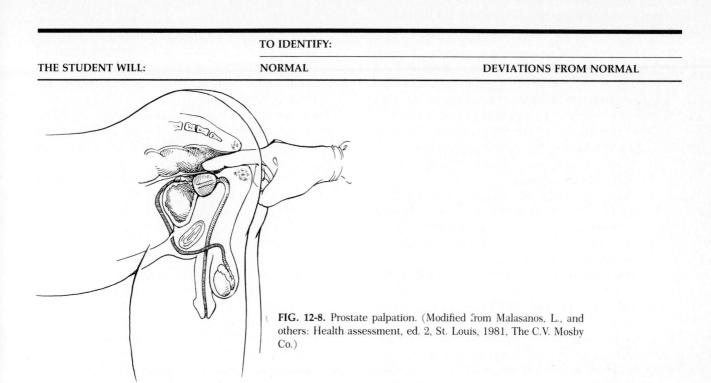

**FIG. 12-8.** Prostate palpation. (Modified from Malasanos, L., and others: Health assessment, ed. 2, St. Louis, 1981, The C.V. Mosby Co.)

## Clinical strategies

1. Several authors discuss the female practitioner's possible emotional discomfort with examination of male genitalia. One way of avoiding discomfort is to be well prepared with the baseline cognitive data. Read carefully about surface, consistency, and contour characteristics of male genitalia. Have a clear mental picture of the size, location, contour, and palpable characteristics of scrotal contents before engaging in physical assessment (Fig. 12-5). It is also helpful to observe an experienced examiner during the process of examination.

2. One author indicates that male genitalia examinations are often deferred for some of the following reasons: "... patient refused.... will do later.... too cold in room.... no time.... patient too nervous.... VIP."* The male genital examination should be considered a routine part of any physical examination.

3. Testicular tumors are often asymptomatic. Educating a client to examine his own genitalia regularly is important. Self-examination on a weekly or a monthly basis is advisable. A regular time and place for self-assessment is helpful. Examination

during the shower or bath might be convenient and simple. Many clients are not familiar with their scrotal contents and do not know what normal structures would feel like. The actual process of the examination is an excellent opportunity to explain the procedure and why it is being done. It is helpful to guide the client through the process of self-examination.

4. The examiner must have short fingernails!

---

### SAMPLE RECORDING

Circumcised penis with no lesions, induration, or discharge. Scrotal contents palpated without tenderness or masses. External inguinal canals palpated without masses, bulges, or tenderness.

Sacrococcygeal, perianal, and anal surfaces present no lesions, rash, inflammation, masses, or hemorrhoids. Good anal sphincter tone. Anal and distal rectal mucosa are smooth with no masses. Bilobed prostate is firm, not enlarged, and nontender to palpation.

---

*Warren, M.M.: Testicular tumors, Continuing Ed., March 1975, p. 31.

## History and clinical strategies: the pediatric client

1. The examiner must assess two types of clients in this area. One will be the infant or little boy and the second the maturing, developing adolescent. Although the techniques of examination are similar, the observations and histories are unique.

2. The examiner must ask the parents of the male infant or little boy the following questions:
   a. Does the child have difficulty voiding?
   b. Is the stream straight?
   c. Does the child's urination stream seem adequate? (That is, is there a very fine high pressure stream or a heavier easy flow?)
   d. Does the child cry and hold his genitalia as if something were hurting?
   e. Has the parent ever noticed any swelling, discoloration, or sores about the penis or scrotum?
   f. Has the child ever had a urinary tract infection?
   g. Does the child have difficulty because of bed-wetting or wetting himself? How much of a problem is this? What has the parent done about it? Any tests for the problem? How does the child feel about the problem? Is there a family history of bed-wetting?
   h. To the parent's knowledge, are the child's testes descended?
   i. Has the child ever been told he has a hydrocele or hernia?
   j. Has the parent ever noticed that the child's scrotum appears to swell or change size with crying or coughing?
   k. Has child ever caused trauma to his genitalia either through injury or during play?

3. For older boys, the examiner will fluctuate between asking significant subjective questions appropriate for the smaller boys and those appropriate for the adult male. Much will depend on the actual maturation, development, and interest of the client. For example, it would be appropriate to ask a mature 16-year-old who is known to be dating, "Do you have any concerns regarding sexual practices or values that you would like to discuss?" Other specific interview questions regarding sexuality are thoroughly discussed in the adult section of this chapter.

4. As boys mature, it should be anticipated that they will have many educational needs regarding what is happening to their own bodies, as well as how to sexually explore with others. The examiner should be alert to these needs and be prepared to develop a beginning profile of the boy's current knowledge and understanding. Not every boy will feel comfortable sharing this information with the examiner, but the examiner should be prepared for and alert to an adolescent asking for clarification and assistance. Profile questions should include items such as:
   a. Has he ever had education classes regarding the changes that boys' bodies go through? If so, is he able to describe the type of material presented?
   b. Were girls involved in the education classes? Did they also study about the changes girls' bodies are undergoing?
   c. How does his family feel about discussing this information at home?
   d. Within his family, who does he talk with about sexual changes and dating?
   e. If he needs information clarified, who does he go to?
   f. Has he ever had any classes or organized discussions about dating, petting, birth control?
   g. What does he know about venereal disease?

5. Most adolescents are not intimidated by direct questioning, as long as it does not appear that someone is pointing a punitive finger toward them. Therefore the level of questoning may relate directly to *normal* activities that the young adolescent may be experiencing, may feel guilty about, or may have incorrect information about, such as homosexual desires, masturbation, sexual fantasies, nocturnal emissions, or erections. The examiner may ask questions such as: "Many fellas your age are experiencing new and normal sensations, such as wanting to touch other boys or having wet dreams at night. Do you have any concerns that I could perhaps provide more information about?"*

6. The examination strategies will vary with age.
   a. Infants through age 2 years should present no problem; the assessment is usually done following the abdominal examination. The examiner simply moves from the abdomen to the genitalia and inguinal area.
   b. Boys 3 to 8 years of age should be examined in their undershorts. After the abdominal examination, matter-of-factly tell the child what is going to happen and then slip down his pants to examine the genitalia and inguinal area. During and following the examination, the ex-

*Daniel (1977) provides an excellent discussion of the normal experimentation of adolescent males.

aminer should reassure the child that everything is perfectly normal and healthy.

  c. For boys over age 8, provide them with a drape, just as you would for an adult. A reassurance of normal findings is also recommended.

7. Evaluation for undescended testes
  a. History. If the parent reports that at one time the testes were found in the scrotum, the testes should not be considered undescended.
  b. Rugae. If the scrotum shows well-formed rugae, it usually means that the testes have descended at some time.
  c. Techniques to force testes into the scrotum (palpation of scrotum should confirm presence)
    (1) Have the child stand; slightly milk the inguinal canal region to pull the testes into the scrotum.
    (2) Have the child sit on a chair or the examination table, feet next to the buttocks, with the knees pulled tight to the chest.
    (3) Have the child sit Indian style (cross-legged); this will relax the cremasteric reflex.
    (4) Child may be placed into very warm water.
  d. Palpate the inguinal canal. If the testis is located in the inguinal canal but cannot be pushed down or if no testis is felt, an undescended testis is very likely.
  e. Boys whose testes have not descended by age 4 years should be referred to a physician.

8. If the testis is palpated momentarily in the scrotum but it quickly slips up into the inguinal canal before adequate assessment, the examiner may block the slippage by gently placing the index finger of the left hand over the inguinal canal and palpating the testis with the right hand.

9. Inguinal hernias are fairly common in children. Generally, the parent will describe a bulge in the child's inguinal region. The inguinal region of a larger boy may be palpated in the same manner as for the adult. For the smaller boy it is better to try to produce the hernia or bulge by external techniques such as the following:
  a. Instruct the child to stand; give him a balloon to blow up.
  b. Have the infant or toddler in a standing position on the examination table. The examiner should place one hand behind the child's back and with the other hand pump in and out on the child's abdomen. The external abdominal pressure may produce the inguinal bulge.
  c. Instruct the child to sit on the examination table and pull his knees to his chest. The examiner then tries to straighten the leg on the questionable side. Again, intraabdominal pressure should fill the hernia sac and produce a bulge.

10. Hydroceles are a common finding in children under 2 years of age. Any child with what appears to be a large scrotum should be evaluated for a hydrocele. To do this, the examiner must darken the examination room and transilluminate the scrotum. A fluid-enlarged scrotum shows a pink, light shadow. With scrotal palpation the examiner is not able to reduce the fluid.

## Clinical variations: the pediatric client

| CHARACTERISTIC OR AREA EXAMINED | NORMAL | DEVIATIONS FROM NORMAL |
|---|---|---|
| **1.** Pubic region | | |
| **a.** Skin surface | Smooth, clear | Scars, rashes, lesions |
| **b.** Hair distribution | Variable as male develops (Table 12-1) | Patchy growth or loss |
| | | Female configuration: triangle with base over pubis |

**TABLE 12-1.** Pubic hair development in males

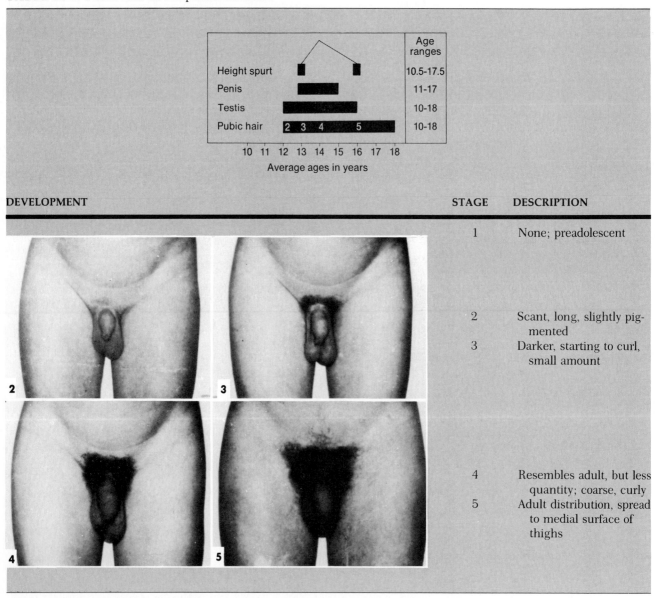

| DEVELOPMENT | STAGE | DESCRIPTION |
|---|---|---|
| | 1 | None; preadolescent |
| | 2 | Scant, long, slightly pigmented |
| | 3 | Darker, starting to curl, small amount |
| | 4 | Resembles adult, but less quantity; coarse, curly |
| | 5 | Adult distribution, spread to medial surface of thighs |

From Tanner, J.M.: Growth at adolescence, ed. 2, Oxford, England, 1962, Blackwell Scientific Publications, Ltd.

| CHARACTERISTIC OR AREA EXAMINED | NORMAL | DEVIATIONS FROM NORMAL |
|---|---|---|
| **2.** Penis | | |
| **a.** Skin color and surface characteristics | Penis size in newborn 2 to 3 cm (¾ to 1¼ inches) long<br>Variable as male develops (Table 12-2) | Reddened<br>Lesions<br>Swelling<br>Nodules |

**TABLE 12-2.** Penis and testes/scrotum development in males

| DEVELOPMENT | STAGE | DESCRIPTION |
|---|---|---|
| | 1 | Penis, testes, and scrotum preadolescent |
| | 2 | Enlargement of scrotum and testes, texture alteration; scrotal sac reddens; penis usually does not enlarge |
| | 3 | Further growth of testes and scrotum; penis enlarges and becomes longer |
| | 4 | Continued growth of testes and scrotum; scrotum becomes darker; penis becomes longer; glans and breadth increase in size |
| | 5 | Adult in size and shape |

From Tanner, J.M.: Growth at adolescence, ed. 2, Oxford, England, 1962, Blackwell Scientific Publications, Ltd.

## Clinical variations: the pediatric client—cont'd

| CHARACTERISTIC OR AREA EXAMINED | NORMAL | DEVIATIONS FROM NORMAL |
|---|---|---|
| **b.** Foreskin | Uncircumcised: prepuce present and folded over glans (Fig. 12-9)<br>Circumcised: prepuce often absent, or small flap remains at corona (Fig. 12-10) | Continually retracted foreskin in uncircumcised male |

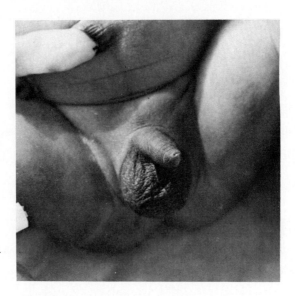

FIG. 12-9. Uncircumcised penis in newborn.

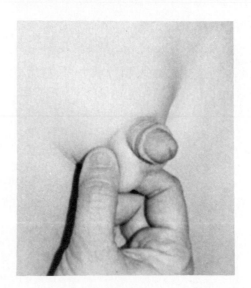

FIG. 12-10. Circumcised penis in small child.

| | | |
|---|---|---|
| 1. Foreskin retraction | For uncircumcised males after age 3 or 4 months (be gentle; if tissue resists, do not force)<br>Foreskin retracts easily to expose glans and returns to original position with ease | Unable to retract, or very tightly attached foreskin of child over 3 months of age<br>Failure to retract; discomfort with retraction<br>Difficulty returning prepuce to original position |

| CHARACTERISTIC OR AREA EXAMINED | NORMAL | DEVIATIONS FROM NORMAL |
|---|---|---|
| **c.** Glans and under prepuce fold | | Lesions<br>Crusting under fold or around tip of glans<br>Redness, swelling<br>Pinpoint opening |
| **d.** Urethral meatus | | |
| 1. Location | Central, at distal tip of glans | Pinpoint opening<br>Dorsal location<br>Ventral location |
| 2. Discharge | Usually not present | Yellow-green discharge<br>Milky white discharge<br>Discharge with foul odor |
| **e.** Penis shaft palpation | Nontender<br>Smooth, semifirm consistency | Tenderness<br>Swelling<br>Nodules<br>Induration |
| **3.** Scrotum | | |
| **a.** Contour | Sac divided in half by septum<br>Left scrotal sac may be longer than right<br>Scrotal contents and scrotum may retract upward with cool temperature | |
| **b.** Size | Size varies; may appear pendulous | Fluctuates in size greatly with crying or coughing<br>Hydrocele common in boys under 2 years of age; nontender mass |
| **4.** Scrotum and testes palpation | Testis present in each sac | Hydrocele, unable to reduce (see *Clinical strategies*)<br>Solid scrotal mass<br>Testes not present in sac (see *Clinical strategies*) |
| **a.** Size | Birth: 1 to 2 cm<br>11 to 18 years: 3.5 to 4.5 cm<br>Equal in size | Unilateral or bilateral testicle size |
| **b.** Tenderness | Mildly sensitive to slight compression | Markedly tender |
| **c.** Contour | Smooth, ovoid | Nodular<br>Irregular |
| **d.** Mobility | Movable | Fixed |
| **5.** Epididymis | Nontender<br>Usually located on posterolateral surface of each testis<br>Discretely palpable<br>Comma shaped<br>Smooth | Tender<br>Irregular shape<br>Enlarged<br>Indurated<br>Nodular |
| **6.** Vas deferens | Nontender<br>Discretely palpable from epididymides to external inguinal ring<br>Smooth and cordlike<br>Movable | Tender<br>Tortuous<br>Thickened; beaded<br>Indurated |
| **7.** Inguinal hernia inspection (see *Clinical strategies*); older boys may palpate right and left inguinal rings *if hernia is suspected;* child should stand and bear down after finger is in place | With little finger, follow spermatic cord upward to triangular slitlike opening; opening may or may not admit finger | Bulges appearing at area of external ring, Hesselbach triangle, femoral area<br>Palpable mass touches examiner's fingertip or pushes against side of finger |

## History and clinical strategies: the geriatric client

1. Sexual functions. Physiological changes occurring in the aging male result in sexual function alterations.
   a. Erections develop more slowly in response to stimulation. Erection time may be longer or may be delayed until shortly before ejaculation.
   b. The erection may feel less full or firm.
   c. Ejaculation is less intense, invoking fewer contractions.
   d. The volume of seminal fluid expelled is lessened. The production of spermatozoa diminishes.
   e. The refractory phase is longer, lasting for about 12 hours to several days.

   Note that the changes described occur gradually and at different rates according to the individual. Despite testosterone level decreases, an elderly man is capable of sexual function indefinitely if he is generally healthy and is within a sexually stimulating environment.

   The questions posed to the adult male regarding his sexual and reproductive functions are generally appropriate for the elderly client (pp. 340-341).

   The questions about early childhood and adolescent experiences may not have as much bearing on present sexual concerns as they would with a younger client. An older man may be preoccupied with his present needs for intimacy and sexual activity. Some of the variables that could alter sexual function follow:
   a. Feelings of being too old or too frail to engage in sexual activity; election to withdraw from all sexual encounters or stimulation
   b. Loss of spouse, isolation, unavailability of a sexual partner, or a sexually restrictive environment
   c. Depression related to sexual or other concerns
   d. Physical illness resulting in fatigue, anxiety about health status, or pain (from arthritis, respiratory or cardiac problems, etc.)
   e. Effects of certain diseases (neurogenic or vascular impairment, diabetes mellitus)
   f. Side effects of medications (e.g., some antihypertensive drugs, sedatives, tranquilizers, alcohol)
   g. Surgery for prostatism (may or may not affect erection status); retrograde ejaculation is a possible concern
   h. Inadequate nutrition
   i. Diminished strength of muscles associated with the act of intercourse
   Several authors have stated that the majority of men requesting help for impotence offer no organic basis for the problem. It is imperative that the examiner be well informed about sexual needs and behaviors of the geriatric client and prepared to follow through with a thorough assessment in this area.

2. Genitourinary symptoms. The symptoms of urinary frequency, nocturia, urgency, hestiancy, abnormal flow of urinary stream, urethral discharge, and scrotal masses are described in the adult section of this chapter. Additional concerns or questions follow:
   a. Nocturnal frequency is a common concern. Ask the client what amount and type of fluids he drinks in the evening. Also, ask if he is taking diuretics.
   b. Incontinence: Was the onset sudden or slow? Does the client feel (or sense) any warning that he has to urinate?

3. Prostatism. Early symptoms include the following:
   a. Hesitancy in initiating stream
   b. Diminished force of stream
   c. Urinary frequency
   d. Nocturia
   These symptoms may be subtle, ignored, or tolerated by the client. The later symptoms of hematuria or urinary tract infection alarm the client. *Note:* The size of the prostate gland (as estimated when palpated) may not be indicative of the degree of obstruction of the urethra. The number and intensity of symptoms offered by the client may not correlate with the estimated palpatory enlargement of the gland.

4. Cancer of the prostate gland is often asymptomatic.

5. Pain associated with genitourinary illness may be ill defined or vague, located in the groin, low back, perineum, abdomen, or flank.

## Clinical variations: the geriatric client

The assessment procedure and physical findings for the geriatric male are the same as for the younger client. The following alterations may be noted:

1. The genital examination should be preceded by an abdominal assessment to palpate and percuss the bladder for fullness (after the client has been asked to urinate), discomfort, or dullness.
2. The scrotal sac may appear elongated or pendulous. Elderly clients sometimes have the problem of sitting on the scrotum, resulting in trauma or excoriation of the surface.
3. The testes may feel slightly softer than in a younger man and may be slightly smaller.
4. The prostate gland may feel larger than in a younger client.

**Cognitive
self-assessment**

Match the lettered structures with the corresponding numbered label.

1. _____ Scrotum          8. _____ Urethral meatus
2. _____ Shaft of penis   9. _____ Prepuce
3. _____ Epididymis      10. _____ Pubis
4. _____ Anus            11. _____ Glans
5. _____ Vas deferens    12. _____ Corona
6. _____ Urethra         13. _____ Testis
7. _____ Bladder         14. _____ Rectum

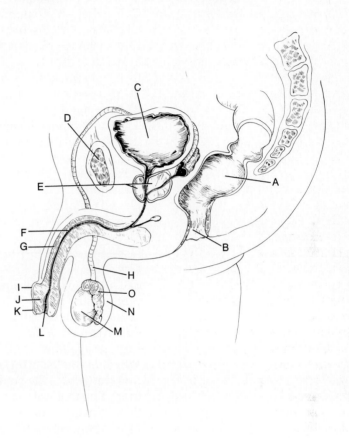

15. The skin of the penis is usually:
    ☐ a. dark red
    ☐ b. moderately deep red
    ☐ c. pale red
16. Scrotal skin is:
    ☐ a. pale
    ☐ b. deeply pigmented
17. Scrotal skin is:
    ☐ a. thick
    ☐ b. thin
18. Testes are usually:
    ☐ a. firm
    ☐ b. soft
19. Testes are approximately _____ in length.
    ☐ a. 4 to 5 cm
    ☐ b. 1 to 2 cm
    ☐ c. 5 to 6 cm

20. Normal testes are _____ sensitive to mild compression.
    - ☐ a. markedly
    - ☐ b. never
    - ☐ c. slightly
21. The epididymides are usually located _____ to the testes.
    - ☐ a. posterolateral
    - ☐ b. anteromedial
22. Which statement(s) is/are true about the normal epididymides?
    - ☐ a. They are slightly tender to palpation.
    - ☐ b. They are nontender to palpation.
    - ☐ c. They are discretely palpable within the scrotum.
    - ☐ d. They may visibly bulge in the posterior portion of the scrotal sac.
    - ☐ e. all except b
    - ☐ f. all except a
    - ☐ g. a and c
    - ☐ h. b and d
23. The vas deferens is usually:
    - ☐ a. taut or fixed to surrounding tissue
    - ☐ b. movable
24. Which of the following structures, if present in the scrotum, would transilluminate?
    - ☐ a. Hydrocele
    - ☐ b. Testis
    - ☐ c. Scrotal hernia
    - ☐ d. Spermatocele
    - ☐ e. Varicocele
    - ☐ f. Epididymal nodule
    - ☐ g. all the above
    - ☐ h. none of the above
    - ☐ i. a and d
    - ☐ j. a, c, and e
25. Which of the following structures or conditions, if present in the scrotum, would usually be described as painful by the client?
    - ☐ a. Spermatocele
    - ☐ b. Epididymitis
    - ☐ c. Hydrocele
    - ☐ d. Testicular tumor
    - ☐ e. Anteverted epididymis
    - ☐ f. all the above
    - ☐ g. none of the above
    - ☐ h. a and d
    - ☐ i. b, c, and e

Match the lettered structures shown at the top of p. 359 with the corresponding numbered label.
26. _____ Spermatic cord
27. _____ Internal inguinal ring
28. _____ External inguinal ring
29. _____ Inguinal canal
30. _____ Anterosuperior iliac spine
31. _____ Fossa ovalis
32. _____ Poupart ligament

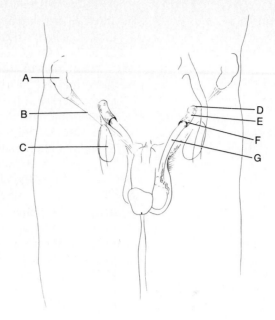

**PEDIATRIC QUESTIONS**

33. The *average* age for the beginning development of pubic hair in males is:
    - ☐ a. 9 years
    - ☐ b. 10 years
    - ☐ c. 11 years
    - ☐ d. 12 years
    - ☐ e. 13 years

34. When examining the uncircumcised male, the examiner should attempt to retract the foreskin after which of the following ages?
    - ☐ a. 6 weeks
    - ☐ b. 2 months
    - ☐ c. 4 months
    - ☐ d. 6 months
    - ☐ e. Never

35. Which of the following techniques should be used to attempt to force the testes back into the scrotum of a boy who is being evaluated for undescended testes?
    - ☐ a. Child should stand; examiner attempts to milk testes into scrotum.
    - ☐ b. Child is sitting on examination table, feet against buttocks, pulling knees tight to chest.
    - ☐ c. Child sits cross-legged (Indian style) to relax cremasteric reflex.
    - ☐ d. Child stands and examiner pushes on child's abdomen.
    - ☐ e. Place child in warm tub of water.
    - ☐ f. all the above
    - ☐ g. a, c, and d
    - ☐ h. all except c
    - ☐ i. all except d
    - ☐ j. b, d, and e

**GERIATRIC QUESTIONS**

36. In older men a palpable scrotal mass:
    - ☐ a. is usually indicative of cancer
    - ☐ b. is common because the testicle hypertrophies and becomes irregular in shape with aging
    - ☐ c. may be a hydrocele
    - ☐ d. none of the above

37. Early symptoms of prostatism:
    - ☐ a. include hesitancy in initiating urine stream
    - ☐ b. include hematuria
    - ☐ c. include inability to maintain an erection
    - ☐ d. none of the above

38. Physiological sexual function changes that normally occur with the aging male include:
    - ☐ a. an extended erection period
    - ☐ b. slow detumescence
    - ☐ c. longer refractory phase
    - ☐ d. decrease in volume of seminal fluid at time of ejaculation
    - ☐ e. loss of ability to maintain erection
    - ☐ f. a and b
    - ☐ g. a and d
    - ☐ h. c and e
    - ☐ i. a, c, and d
    - ☐ j. all except e

---

## SUGGESTED READINGS
### General

Bates, B.: A guide to physical examination, ed. 3, Philadelphia, 1983, J.B. Lippincott Co., pp. 258-272.

Conklin, M., and others: Should health teaching including self-examination of the testes? Am. J. Nurs. **78**(12):2073-2074, 1978.

Diekelmann, N.: Primary health care of the well adult, New York, 1977, McGraw-Hill Book Co., pp. 51-69, 127-137, 139-149, 217-223.

Malasanos, L., and others: Health assessment, ed. 2, St. Louis, 1981, The C.V. Mosby Co., pp. 385-396.

Murray, B.L., and Wilcox, L.J.: Testicular self-examination, Am. J. Nurs. **78**(12):2074-2075, 1978.

Prior, J.A., Silberstein, J.S., and Stang, J.M.: Physical diagnosis: the history and examination of the patient, ed. 6, St. Louis, 1981, The C.V. Mosby Co., pp. 330-345.

Williams, H.A.: Screening for testicular cancer, Pediatric Nursing, pp. 38-40, Sept.-Oct. 1981.

### Pediatric

Alexander, M., and Brown, M.S.: Pediatric history taking and physical diagnosis for nurses, ed. 2, New York, 1979, McGraw-Hill Book Co., pp. 241-253.

Barness, L.: Manual of pediatric physical diagnosis, ed. 5, Chicago, 1981, Year Book Medical Publishers, Inc., pp. 156-162.

Danile, W.A., Jr.: Adolescents in health and disease, St. Louis, 1977, The C.V. Mosby Co., pp. 27-39, 65-71.

Marshall, W.A., and Tanner, J.M.: Variations in the pattern of pubertal changes in boys, Arch. Dis. Child. **45**:13-23, 1970.

Rauh, J., and Brookman, R.: Children are different: developmental physiology. In Johnson, T.R., Moore, W.M., and Jeffries, J.E., editors, Columbus, Ohio, 1978, Ross Laboratories, pp. 26-29.

### Geriatric

Caird, F.I., and Judge, T.G.: Assessment of the elderly patient, London, 1977, Pitman Medical Publishing Co., Ltd., pp. 44-47.

Carotenuto, R., and Bullock, J.: Physical assessment of the gerontologic client, Philadelphia, 1980, F.A. Davis Co., pp. 113-119.

Diekelmann, N.: Primary health care of the well adult, New York, 1977, McGraw-Hill Book Co., pp. 187-199.

Steinberg, F.U., editor: Care of the geriatric patient, ed. 6, St. Louis, 1983, The C.V. Mosby Co., pp. 360-372, 501-509.

ASSESSMENT OF THE

# Female genitourinary system

## VOCABULARY

**adnexa** General term meaning adjacent or related structures. EXAMPLE: The ovaries and fallopian tubes are adnexa of the uterus.

**amenorrhea** The absence of menstruation.

**Bartholin glands** Two mucus-secreting glands located within the posterolateral vaginal vestibule.

**condyloma acuminatum (wart)** A soft, warty, papillomatous projection that appears on the labia and within the vaginal vestibule; viral in origin and sexually transmitted.

**condyloma latum** Slightly raised, moist, flattened papules that appear on the labia or within the vaginal vestibule; a sign of secondary syphilis and sexually transmitted.

**cystocele** Bulging of the anterior vaginal wall caused by protrusion of the urinary bladder through relaxed or weakened musculature.

**dysmenorrhea** Abnormal pain associated with the menstrual cycle. Mild, self-limiting premenstrual pain is considered normal. Pain becomes abnormal when it is severe, disabling, or accompanied by other severe symptoms such as nausea, vomiting, fainting, or intestinal cramping.

**dyspareunia** Pain associated with sexual intercourse. The term is most often applied to female conditions, including vaginal spasms, lack of lubrication, or genital lesions.

**escutcheon** General term meaning a surface that is shield shaped. In female anatomy it denotes the visible surface of the lower abdomen, the mons pubis, and the inverted-triangle–shaped patch of hair covering the area.

**fornix (plural: fornices)** General term designating a fold or an arch-like structure. The vaginal fornix is the ringed recess (pocket) that forms around the cervix as it projects into the vaginal vault; although continuous, this fornix is anatomically divided into the anterior, posterior, and lateral fornices.

**fourchette** A small fold of membrane connecting the labia minora in the posterior part of the vulva.

**-gravida** A combining form that denotes number of pregnancies. EXAMPLE; *Multigravida* designates more than one pregnancy.

**hymenal caruncles** Small, irregular, fleshy projections that are remnants of a ruptured hymen; they are a normal phenomenon and may or may not be present at the vaginal introitus in varied sizes and shapes.

**introitus** General term denoting an opening or the orifice of a cavity or hollow structure. EXAMPLE: vaginal introitus.

**leukorrhea** A white, vaginal discharge; can be a normal phenomenon that occurs (and increases) with pregnancy, birth control medication, or as a postmenstrual phase; can also be an abnormal sign indicating malignancy or infection.

**menarche** Onset of menstruation in adolescence or young adulthood.

**menorrhagia** Abnormally heavy or extended menstrual periods.

**metrorrhagia** Any uterine bleeding that is not related to menstruation. EXAMPLE: A bleeding lesion within the vagina, cervix, or uterus.

**nabothian cyst (retention cyst)** Small white or purplish firm nodule that commonly appears on the cervix; forms within the mucus-secreting nabothian glands, present in large numbers on the uterine cervix.

**oligomenorrhea** Abnormally light or infrequent menstruation.

**-para** Combining form denoting the number of viable births. EXAMPLES: *Nulliparous* means having experienced no viable births (also indicated as *para 0*); *multiparous* designates more than one viable birth.

**pudendum** Collective term denoting the external genitalia; for the female it includes the mons pubis, labia major, labia minora, vaginal vestibule, and vestibular glands.

**rectocele** Bulging of the posterior vaginal wall caused by protrusion of the intestinal contents through relaxed or weakened musculature.

**Skene glands (periurethral)** Mucus-secreting glands that lie just inside the urethral orifice; not visible on examination.

**vaginitis** Inflammation of the vaginal vault; has various causes.

*atrophic* Associated with aging and diminished vaginal lubrication; itching, redness, a thin yellowish discharge, and superficial erosions may be present; leukoplakia or petechiae may appear.

*monilial* Related to a common yeastlike organism (*Candiasis albicans*) normally present in mucous membranes that may cause a superficial infection; presenting symptoms are itching, redness, swelling, a white cheesy discharge, and whitish patches that bleed when scraped off.

*trichomonas* Caused by a protozoan parasite that is sexually transmitted; itching, burning, and a malodorous frothy, yellow-green discharge are commonly seen.

*nonspecific* Presenting symptoms are redness and a thin grayish discharge.

NOTE: Diagnosis of vaginitis is confirmed with smears and cultures of vaginal secretions. Its signs and symptoms may not be as concise or predictable as presented here.

---

## Cognitive objectives

At the end of this chapter the learner will perform a systematic assessment of the female genitourinary system and rectal/anal region, demonstrating the ability to do the following:

1. Identify and locate the major internal and external structures of the female genitourinary system.
2. Point out observable and palpable characteristics of normal external genitalia and perineum.
3. Identify observable and palpable characteristics of normal internal structures:
   a. Vagina
   b. Cervix
   c. Fornices
4. Describe the major characteristics of normal vaginal discharge.
5. Identify the appropriate and effective procedures for using a vaginal speculum.
6. Name specific examiner behaviors that will minimize client discomfort and enhance effectiveness of the pelvic examination.
7. Identify common normal palpable findings elicited during a bimanual examination.
8. Describe common normal deviations of findings related to pelvic examination associated with:
   a. Nulliparous clients
   b. Mulitparous clients
   c. Early pregnant clients
9. Identify major palpable characteristics of the anteverted, retroverted, anteflexed, and retroflexed uterus.
10. Give the reasons for performing a rectovaginal examination.
11. Identify common pediatric and geriatric variations of the female genitourinary system.
12. Use the terms in the vocabulary list.

## Clinical objectives

At the end of this chapter the learner will perform a systematic assessment of the female genitourinary system and rectal/anal region, demonstrating the ability to do the following:

1. Obtain a pertinent history from a client.
2. Inspect the pubic region and external genitalia for:
   a. Hair distribution
   b. Parasites
   c. Inguinal skin surface characteristics
   d. Labia majora surface
   e. Labia minora surface
      (1) Vestibule surface
      (2) Clitoris size and surface
      (3) Urethral meatus contour and surface
   f. Vaginal introitus contour and surface
   g. Perineum surface
   h. Anal surface
3. Palpate external genitalia for:
   a. Labia and vestibule consistency and tenderness
   b. Urethral duct tenderness and discharge
   c. Bartholin gland tenderness, discharge, and swelling
   d. Perineum consistency and tenderness

4. Palpate vaginal introitus and test for bulging (or straining) and urinary incontinence.
5. Perform a vaginal examination and inspect for:
   a. Cervix
      (1) Color
      (2) Position
      (3) Size
      (4) Surface characteristics
      (5) Os configuration
      (6) Discharge color, odor, and texture
   b. Vagina
      (1) Color
      (2) Surface characteristics
      (3) Consistency
      (4) Secretions: color, odor, and texture
6. Obtain specimens for cervical cytological evaluation.
7. Perform a bimanual vaginal examination to identify:
   a. Vaginal wall surface characteristics and tenderness
   b. Cervix
      (1) Size
      (2) Contour
      (3) Consistency
      (4) Surface texture
      (5) Mobility
      (6) Location in vaginal tube
      (7) Os patency
   c. Uterus
      (1) Fundus location, contour, surface consistency, shape, size, mobility, and tenderness
      (2) Isthmus consistency
   d. Adnexa
      (1) Ovary location and surface characteristics
      (2) Masses
      (3) Pulsations
8. Perform a rectovaginal examination to identify:
   a. Rectovaginal septum and pouch characteristics
   b. Tenderness in pouch
   c. Rectal wall surface characteristics
   d. Anal sphincter surface and tone
   e. Tenderness
9. Summarize results with a written description of findings.

## Health history additional to screening history

1. Sexual history. A screening question might be worded in the following manner: "Do you have any sexual difficulties or concerns that you would like to share with me?" or "Are you satisfied with your sexual habits and activities as they occur now?" This gives the client an opportunity to express concerns and does not direct her toward any particular issue. More specific questions might be posed if the client indicates that she wishes to discuss specific sexual matters.
   a. Are your needs for intimacy and affection being met?
   b. Are you sexually active at present?
   c. Are your sexual activities meeting your physical needs?
   d. Do you and your partner talk about sex? Do you generally agree on sexual needs, sexual expression, and modes of behavior?
   e. Do you have any problems with sexual arousal, arousing your partner, or completing a sexual experience satisfactorily?
   f. If particular problems exist, what do you feel is the cause?
   g. Have you attempted to solve the problem? If so, in what way? What was the outcome of these attempts?
   h. Do you have any questions about sexual behavior or sexuality in general that you would like to pose (e.g., concerns about venereal disease, sexual anatomy, orgasm, masturbation, sexual fantasies)?
2. Abnormal bleeding
   a. If associated with menses, it might fall into one of the following categories:
      (1) Too many periods (menstrual interval is less than 19 to 21 days)
      (2) Infrequent menses (menstrual interval is over 37 days)
      (3) Amenorrhea
      (4) Extended menses (duration is over 7 days)
      (5) Intermenstrual bleeding
      (6) Flow pattern increased during menses
   b. Amount of flow (normal or abnormal) is difficult to determine. Inquire about the nature of the *change* in the amount of flow. Ask about the number of pads or tampons used during the heavy flow in a 24-hour period. Find out if the pad or tampon is soaked when it is changed. Do clots accompany the bleeding?
   c. Is there bleeding associated with intercourse? With douching?
3. Premenstrual tension should be defined by the client. Is it associated with headaches? Weight change? Edema? Breast tenderness? Marked (or difficult) mood swings? Does it occur before every period or just occasionally? Are premenstrual problems incapacitating (e.g., do they interfere with activities of daily living)?
4. Vaginal discharge. Discharge is normal with many women and often occurs in cycles with an increase

at midcycle or just before menses. If vaginal discharge is a complaint, establish the *change* that has occurred in terms of estimated amount, color, odor, consistency, and times or intervals of increased discharge.

   a. Are you taking any medications for other problems (especially broad-spectrum antibiotics, metronidazole, or steroids)? Do you take birth control pills?

   b. Do you douche? If so, how often, what solution, and what amount? Were you douching before or after the discharge?

   c. Is the discharge associated with itching? (If itching is present, is there a family or client history of diabetes mellitus?)

   d. Do you wear cotton or ventilated underwear or pantyhose?

   e. Was the onset of the discharge sudden or gradual?

   f. Does your sexual partner have any problem with discharge, itching, rash or lesions, pain?

5. Birth control. If any measure is used, establish the type, the length of time it has been used, and the client's assessment of its effectiveness, convenience, noninterference with sexual activity, and noninterference with the client's general physical and mental health. More specific questions include the following:

   a. Birth control pills. Do you take them regularly? Do you have any symptoms or physical problems associated with taking the pill?

   b. Diaphragm. Are you able to use it each time you have intercourse? Do you use cream (or jelly) every time you use the diaphragm? Do you have any problems inserting, removing, or retaining it? Do you examine your diaphragm periodically for thinning or weak spots, cracks, holes, or tears? How long before intercourse do you insert it? How long do you leave it in place following intercourse? How long ago were you fitted with your diaphragm?

   c. IUD. Do you insert your finger into your vagina to feel for the string periodically? How often? Do you have any problem with bleeding or spotting between periods? Do you have any problem with menstrual cramps?

6. Menopause. If it has been established that the client is approaching, in the midst of, or completing the menopausal phase, a general question about any concerns should be posed. More specific questions include:

   a. Do you recall your mother experiencing menopause? How old was she? Did she describe her experience to you?

   b. Do you have any concerns or problems with menstrual irregularity, mood changes, tension, back pain, hot flashes, painful intercourse, changes in sexual desire or sexual behaviors, other physical changes?

   c. What kind of birth control measures are you using? Describe.

   d. What general feelings do you have about menopause?

7. Pelvic discomfort associated with the menstrual cycle is normal with some women. If the client complains of pain, establish the *change* that has occurred in terms of timing (with menstrual cycle) and location (e.g., vulvar or vaginal, localized in lower abdomen, or general pain). Is the pain associated with intercourse? If so, does it occur at the time of insertion, deep penetration throughout intercourse, and/or is there a residual pain following intercourse?

# Clinical guidelines

| THE STUDENT WILL: | TO IDENTIFY: | |
| --- | --- | --- |
| | NORMAL | DEVIATIONS FROM NORMAL |

1. Assemble equipment:
   a. Gloves
   b. Speculum
   c. Sterile cotton swabs
   d. Glass slides
   e. Wooden spatula
   f. Lubricant
   g. Cytology fixative
   h. Examining lamp
   i. Culture plates for gonorrhea screening
2. Check with client to be certain that bladder has been recently emptied
3. Position draped client in lithotomy position (Fig. 13-1)
   (*Note:* Examiner may assist client in positioning her buttocks at edge of examining table after checking to see that client's feet are secure in stirrups.)

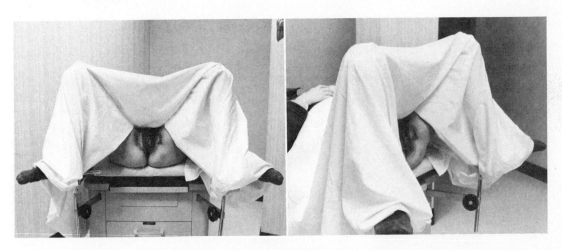

**FIG. 13-1.** Draped client in dorsal lithotomy position.

4. See that equipment is within easy reach and arrange light for good visualization of external genitalia
5. Wear gloves on both hands; warn client that examiner is going to touch her to begin procedure

## Clinical guidelines—cont'd

| | TO IDENTIFY: | |
| --- | --- | --- |
| **THE STUDENT WILL:** | **NORMAL** | **DEVIATIONS FROM NORMAL** |
| **6.** Inspect external genitalia | | |
|    **a.** Hair distribution | Variable in adults<br>Usually inverse triangle with base over pubis; some hair may extend up mid-line toward umbilicus<br>No parasites | Male hair distribution (diamond-shaped pattern)<br>Patchy loss of hair<br>Absence of hair in client over 16 years<br>Nits, pubic lice |
|    **b.** Inguinal and mons pubis skin surface characteristics | Smooth, clear | Scars<br>Inguinal swelling, excoriation, lesions, rash |
|    **c.** Labia majora surface characteristics | Darker pigmentation<br>Shriveled or full<br>Gaping or closed<br>Usually symmetrical<br>Skin surface smooth<br>May appear dry or moist | Inflammation, ulceration<br>Lesions<br>Nodules<br>Marked asymmetry |
| **7.** Spread labia to view: | | |
|    **a.** Inner surface of labia majora; labia minora and surface of vestibule (Fig. 13-2) | Dark pink pigmentation and moist<br>Usually symmetrical | Inflammation<br>Leukoplakia<br>Lesions<br>Nodules<br>Varicosities<br>Marked asymmetry<br>Swelling<br>Excoriation |

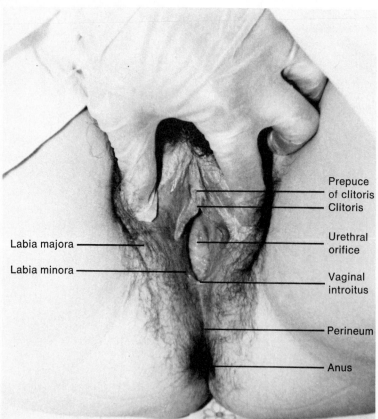

**FIG. 13-2.** Labia spread with thumb and fingers to view external genitalia.

| THE STUDENT WILL: | TO IDENTIFY: | |
| --- | --- | --- |
| | NORMAL | DEVIATIONS FROM NORMAL |

**b.** Clitoris

    1. Size — 2 cm (¾ inch) length visible / 0.5 cm diameter — Enlargement / Atrophy

    2. Surface — Medial aspect covered by prepuce — Inflamed

**c.** Urethral meatus and immediate surrounding tissue surface — Irregular opening or slit / May be close to or slightly within vaginal introitus / Usually located at midline — Discharge from surrounding glands (Skene) or urethral opening / Polyp / Inflammation / Urethral caruncle / Lateral position of meatus

**d.** Vaginal introitus and immediate surrounding tissue surface — Thin vertical slit or large orifice with irregular edges (hymenal caruncles) / Moist tissue — Surrounding inflammation / Profuse vaginal discharge / Swelling / Lesions

**e.** Perineum surface — Smooth or evidence of episiotomy / Scar (midline or mediolateral) may be visible — Inflammation, fistula / Lesions, mass

**f.** Anus surface — Increased pigmentation and coarse skin — Scars, skin tags / Lesions, inflammation / Fissures, lumps / Excoriation

**8.** Palpate external genitalia

    **a.** Labia and vestibule (Fig. 13-3)

        1. Consistency — Soft, homogeneous — Irregular, nodular

        2. Tenderness — Nontender — Tender

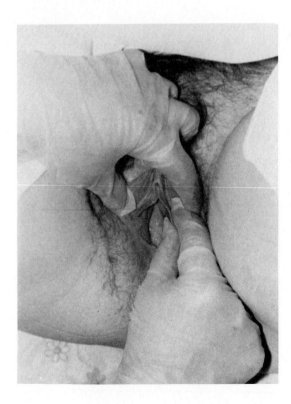

**FIG. 13-3.** Palpation of labia.

## Clinical guidelines—cont'd

|  | TO IDENTIFY: | |
| --- | --- | --- |
| **THE STUDENT WILL:** | **NORMAL** | **DEVIATIONS FROM NORMAL** |
| **b.** Insert index finger in vagina and milk urethral ducts (Fig. 13-4) to test for: | | |
|   1. Tenderness | Nontender | Tenderness |
|   2. Discharge | No discharge | Discharge* |
| **c.** Palpate lateral and posterior areas surrounding introitus (Fig. 13-5) to test for: | | |
|   1. Tenderness | Nontender | Tenderness |
|   2. Discharge | No discharge | Discharge* |
|   3. Surface characteristics | Homogeneous | Swelling |

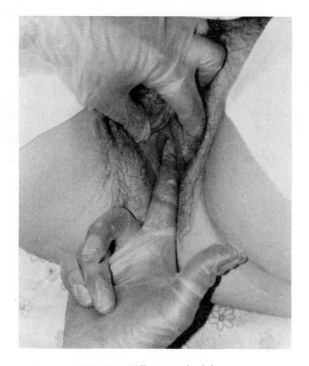

**FIG. 13-4.** Milking urethral duct.

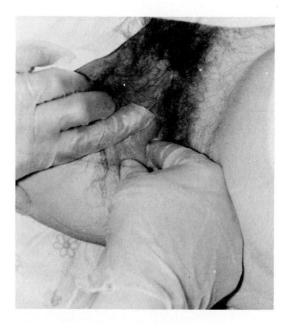

**FIG. 13-5.** Palpation of lateral and posterior areas surrounding vaginal introitus.

| | | |
| --- | --- | --- |
| **d.** Palpate perineum between index finger and thumb (Fig. 13-6) for: | | |
|   1. Consistency | Nulliparous: thick, smooth Multiparous: thin, rigid Scarring | Paper thin |
|   2. Tenderness | Nontender | Tender |

*Prepare a culture of any discharge.

| THE STUDENT WILL: | TO IDENTIFY: | |
| --- | --- | --- |
| | NORMAL | DEVIATIONS FROM NORMAL |

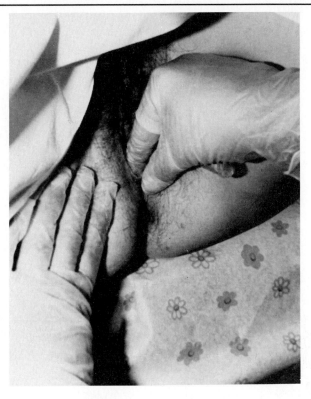

**FIG. 13-6.** Palpating perineum.

| THE STUDENT WILL: | NORMAL | DEVIATIONS FROM NORMAL |
| --- | --- | --- |
| **9.** Ask client to squeeze vaginal orifice around examiner's finger; insert middle and index fingers into vagina; ask client to strain down or bear down to elicit: | Nulliparous client squeezes tightly<br>Multiparous client demonstrates less tone | Client unable to constrict vaginal orifice around examiner's finger |
| **a.** Bulging | No bulging | Cystocele (anterior wall bulging)<br>Enterocele<br>Rectocele (posterior wall bulging)<br>Uterine prolapse (cervix visible on straining, or uterus protrudes on straining) |
| **b.** Incontinence | No urinary incontinence | Urinary incontinence |
| **10.** Select speculum of appropriate size, and warm and lubricate with water (if necessary) | | |

## Clinical guidelines—cont'd

| THE STUDENT WILL: | TO IDENTIFY: | |
| --- | --- | --- |
| | NORMAL | DEVIATIONS FROM NORMAL |

**11.** Place two fingers just inside vaginal introitus and apply pressure over posterior wall (Fig. 13-7); wait for relaxation

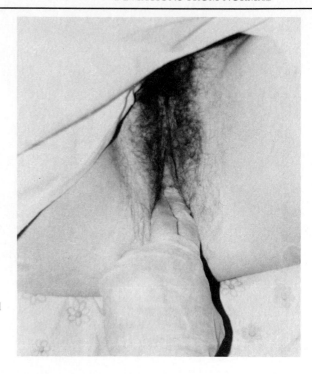

**FIG. 13-7.** Applying pressure in posterior vaginal orifice with two fingers.

| THE STUDENT WILL: | NORMAL | DEVIATIONS FROM NORMAL |
| --- | --- | --- |
| **12.** Insert closed speculum (held at oblique angle) over fingers and direct at 45° angle downward; remove fingers; lock speculum in place (Fig. 13-8) to inspect cervix | | |
| **a.** Color | Pink color evenly distributed | Inflamed |
| | Bluish (in pregnancy) | Pale (associated with anemia) |
| | | Cyanotic (other than pregnancy) |
| | Symmetrical, circumscribed erythema surrounding os may indicate normal condition of exposed columnar epithelium; however, beginning examiners should consider any reddened appearance a problem for consultation | Erythema, especially if patchy or if borders irregular or asymmetrical around os |
| **b.** Position | Midline | Cervix situated laterally |
| | Cervix and os may be pointed in anterior or posterior direction | |
| | May project into vaginal tube 1 to 3 cm (resulting in 1 to 3 cm fornices surrounding cervix) | Projection of over 3 cm (1 inch) into vaginal tube |
| **c.** Size | Usually 2.5 cm (1 inch) diameter | Over 4 cm (1½ inches) diameter |
| **d.** Surface | Smooth | Reddened granular area around os (especially asymmetrical) |
| | Occasional visible squamocolumnar junction (symmetrical reddened circle around os) | Friable tissue |
| | | Red patches, lesions |
| | Nabothian cysts (smooth, round, small, yellowish raised areas) | Strawberry spots |
| | | White patches |

| THE STUDENT WILL: | TO IDENTIFY: | |
| --- | --- | --- |
| | NORMAL | DEVIATIONS FROM NORMAL |

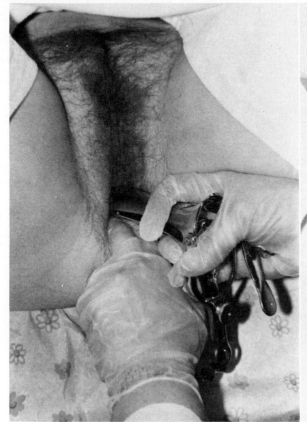

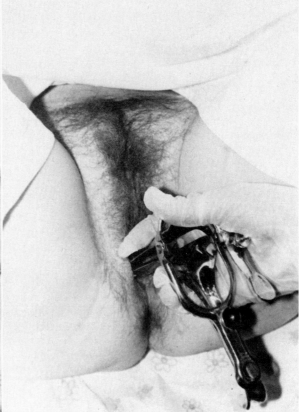

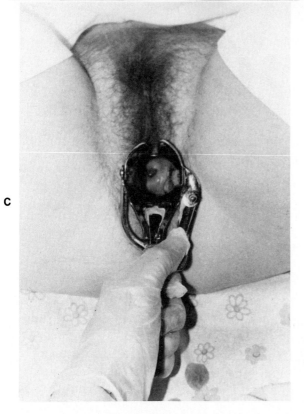

**FIG. 13-8. A,** Closed speculum is inserted over fingers. Insert speculum at an oblique angle if vaginal opening is not relaxed. **B,** Fingers removed; closed speculum is inserted in a downward (45° angle) direction. **C,** Speculum in place, locked, and stabilized. (Note cervix in full view.)

## Clinical guidelines—cont'd

| THE STUDENT WILL: | TO IDENTIFY: | |
| --- | --- | --- |
| | NORMAL | DEVIATIONS FROM NORMAL |
| **e.** Os | Nulliparous: small, evenly round<br>Multiparous: slitlike, may be star shaped or irregular | |
| **f.** Cervical discharge | Mucous plug may be present at os<br>Odorless<br>Creamy or clear<br>Thin, thick, or stringy<br>Discharge often heavier at midcycle or immediately before menstruation | Odor<br>Colored (yellowish, greenish, gray) |
| **13.** Obtain specimens for:<br>　**a.** Papanicolaou smear<br>　**b.** Gonorrheal culture (See *Clinical strategies* if indicated.) | | |
| **14.** Inspect vagina: as unlocked, partially opened speculum is rotated and slowly removed, it tends to close itself | | |
| 　**a.** Color | Pink | Reddened<br>Lesions<br>Pallor (associated with anemia) |
| 　**b.** Surface | Transverse rugae (rugae diminish after vaginal deliveries)<br>Moist, smooth | Leukoplakia<br>Dried<br>Lesions, cracks<br>Bleeding |
| 　**c.** Consistency | Smooth, homogeneous | Nodular<br>Swollen |
| 　**d.** Secretions | Thin<br>Clear or cloudy<br>Odorless | Thick, curdy, frothy<br>Gray, greenish, yellowish<br>Foul odor |
| 　**e.** Amount | Minimal to moderate | Profuse |
| **15.** Perform bimanual vaginal examination | | |
| 　**a.** Rise to standing position; remove glove from one hand, lubricate the other, and insert middle and index fingers into vaginal opening; compress posteriorly; wait for a moment and vaginal opening will relax; insert fingers gradually | | |
| 　**b.** Palpate vaginal wall | | |
| 　　1. Surface | Smooth, homogeneous | Nodules |
| 　　2. Tenderness | Nontender | Tender |
| **16.** Locate cervix with gloved hand; place palmar surface of other hand in abdominal midline, midway between umbilicus and pubis and press lightly toward intravaginal hand | | |

| THE STUDENT WILL: | TO IDENTIFY: | |
|---|---|---|
| | NORMAL | DEVIATIONS FROM NORMAL |

**17.** Palpate cervix and fornices with palmar surface of both fingers (Fig. 13-9)

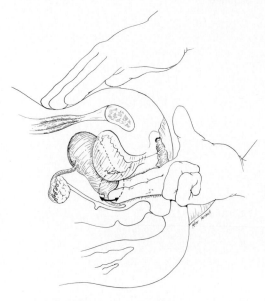

**FIG. 13-9.** Cervical palpation.

| | | NORMAL | DEVIATIONS FROM NORMAL |
|---|---|---|---|
| **a.** | Cervical size | 2.5 to 4 cm | Enlarged |
| **b.** | Contour | Evenly rounded<br>Slightly ovoid | Irregular |
| **c.** | Consistency and surface | Firm (like tip of nose), smooth | Soft, nodular<br>Hard |
| **d.** | Mobility | Cervix moves 1 to 2 cm in each direction without discomfort | Immobile (fixed), or discomfort associated with movement |
| **e.** | Location | Anterior or posterior midline | Laterally displaced |

**18.** Insert one finger gently into cervical os to evaluate:

| | | | |
|---|---|---|---|
| **a.** | Patency | Os admits fingertip 0.5 cm | Os stenosed |
| **b.** | Fornices (pockets surrounding cervical protrusion) | Pliable and smooth<br>Nontender | Hardened, nodular, or irregular surface<br>Tender on palpation |

**19.** Palpate uterus: place intravaginal fingers in anterior fornix; slowly slide abdominal hand toward pubis with flattened fingers pressing downward to evaluate:

## Clinical guidelines—cont'd

| THE STUDENT WILL: | TO IDENTIFY: | |
| --- | --- | --- |
| | NORMAL | DEVIATIONS FROM NORMAL |

**a.** Location of fundus
   1. Anteverted (Fig. 13-10)

Fundus at level of pubis palpated between abdominal and gloved hand; cervix aimed posteriorly
(*Note:* Most women have an anteverted uterus. Fundus should be palpated at level of the pubis.)

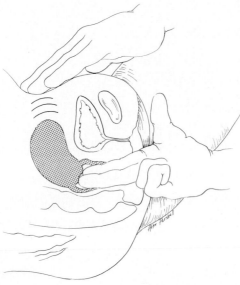

**FIG. 13-10.** Anteverted uterus.

   2. Midposition (Fig. 13-11)

Fundus may not be palpable (depending on amount of abdominal adipose tissue and degree of abdominal muscle relaxation); cervix pointed along axis of vaginal canal

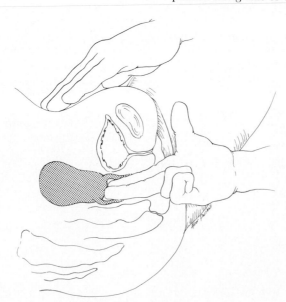

**FIG. 13-11.** Midposition uterus.

| THE STUDENT WILL: | TO IDENTIFY: | |
| --- | --- | --- |
| | **NORMAL** | **DEVIATIONS FROM NORMAL** |
| 3. Anteflexed (Fig. 13-12) | Fundus palpable at pubis between abdominal and gloved hand; cervix pointed along axis of vaginal canal | |

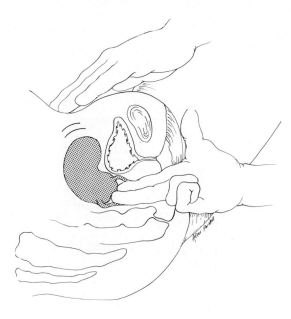

**FIG. 13-12.** Anteflexed uterus.

| 4. Retroflexed (Fig. 13-13) | Fundus not palpable; cervix directed along axis of vaginal canal | |
| --- | --- | --- |

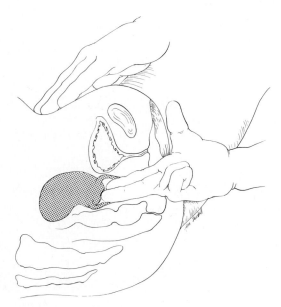

**FIG. 13-13.** Retroflexed uterus.

## Clinical guidelines—cont'd

| THE STUDENT WILL: | TO IDENTIFY: | |
| --- | --- | --- |
| | NORMAL | DEVIATIONS FROM NORMAL |
|     5.  Retroverted (Fig. 13-14) | Fundus not palpable; cervix aimed anteriorly | Enlarged; fundus above level of pubis |
|   **b.**  Contour of fundus | Rounded | Irregular |
|   **c.**  Consistency and surface of uterine wall | Firm, smooth | Soft, nodular<br>Masses |

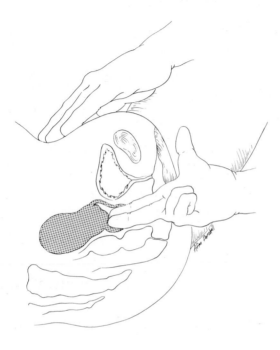

**FIG. 13-14.** Retroverted uterus.

**20.** After fundus is palpated, spread fingers within vagina and press into and upward within posterior, anterior, and lateral fornices to palpate lateral uterine wall

| | | |
| --- | --- | --- |
|   **a.**  Shape and size of uterine wall | Pear shaped, 5.5 to 8 cm long<br>Somewhat enlarged in multiparous client | Nodular<br>Enlarged<br>Tender on palpation |
|   **b.**  Consistency | Smooth | Nodular |

**21.** Gently "bounce" uterus between intravaginal hand and abdominally placed hand for:

| | | |
| --- | --- | --- |
|   **a.**  Mobility | Freely movable | Fixed |
|   **b.**  Tenderness | Nontender | Tender |

**22.** Place outside hand in right lower abdominal quadrant and intravaginal hand in right fornix; slide flat portion of fingers toward intravaginal hand (Fig. 13-15) to evaluate:

| THE STUDENT WILL: | TO IDENTIFY: | |
|---|---|---|
| | NORMAL | DEVIATIONS FROM NORMAL |

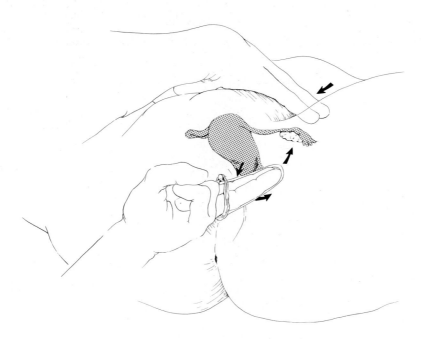

**FIG. 13-15.** Palpation of left adnexal area.

| THE STUDENT WILL: | NORMAL | DEVIATIONS FROM NORMAL |
|---|---|---|
| **a.** Right ovary | Slightly tender on palpation | Markedly tender |
| **b.** Palpable characteristics* | Not always palpable | |
| | Firm, smooth, ovoid | Nodular |
| | Walnut sized | Enlarged |
| | Approximately 4 cm | |
| | Mobile | Immobile mass felt |
| **c.** Other organs, masses, pulsations | Usually no other structures palpable except occasional round ligaments | Masses Nodularity Pulsations Fallopian tubes usually not palpable; if palpated, may indicate problem |
| **23.** Repeat procedure for left side | | |
| **24.** Withdraw fingers from vagina; examine secretions on fingers for: | | |
| **a.** Odor | None | Foul odor |
| **b.** Color | Clear or creamy | Gray, yellow, frothy |
| **c.** Amount | Minimal to moderate | Profuse |
| **25.** Perform a rectovaginal examination: withdraw fingers; change glove; lubricate and reinsert index finger into vagina and middle finger into anus; place other hand on abdomen | | |

*Remember, most palpation is done with the *intravaginal* hand and the palmar surfaces of the fingers.

## Clinical guidelines—cont'd

| THE STUDENT WILL: | TO IDENTIFY: | |
| --- | --- | --- |
| | NORMAL | DEVIATIONS FROM NORMAL |
| **26.** Palpate anterior rectal wall for: | | |
| **a.** Rectovaginal septum characteristics | Thin, smooth, pliable | Thickened, nodular |
| **b.** Rectovaginal pouch characteristics | Smooth | Nodular |
| | Uterine body (occasionally the fundus) may be felt | Tenderness |
| | Nontender | |
| **27.** Rotate finger in rectum to explore rectal wall for surface characteristics | Continuous smooth surface with minimal discomfort | Masses |
| | | Nodules |
| | | Induration |
| | | Tenderness |
| **28.** Withdraw fingers slowly, noting: | Sphincter evenly tight around finger | Sphincter markedly relaxed |
| **a.** Anal sphincter tone | | Nodules, induration, masses |
| **b.** Tenderness | Nontender | Tenderness |
| **29.** Examine gloved finger for stool | If present, brown | Black |
| | | Blood present |

## Clinical strategies

1. Procedure for obtaining Papanicolaou smears
   a. This procedure is performed after the cervix and surrounding tissue have been inspected and while the speculum is still in place in the vagina. The examiner should not apply lubricant to the speculum if the intent is to collect a Pap smear specimen.
   b. The bifid end of the wooden spatula is introduced into the vagina.
   c. The longer projection at the end of the spatula is inserted into the cervical os.
   d. The spatula is then rotated in a full circle, flush against the surrounding cervical tissue (light pressure is sufficient to keep the spatula in contact with the cervix).
   e. The spatula is then withdrawn, and the specimen is spread on a microscopic slide. A single light stroke with each side of the spatula enables the examiner to thin out the specimen over the slide surface. Avoid scraping the slide with back and forth motions.
   f. The slide is labeled and sprayed with a fixative solution or placed in a fixative solution container and labeled.
   g. The rounded end of the spatula is then introduced into the vagina and gently scraped over the posterior fornix area to collect a vaginal pool specimen.
   h. The spatula is withdrawn, and each side is lightly spread over another slide.
   i. This slide is labeled and sprayed or immersed in a fixative solution.
2. Procedure for obtaining a gonorrhea culture specimen
   a. Endocervical culture
      (1) The specimen for this culture can be collected immediately following the Papanicolaou smear procedure.
      (2) A sterile cotton applicator is introduced into the vagina and inserted into the cervical os.
      (3) The examiner holds the applicator in place for 10 to 30 seconds (there is no need to rotate the applicator).
      (4) The applicator is withdrawn and spread (and rotated) in a large **Z** pattern over the medium of a Thayer-Martin plate, or the applicator is placed in a Thayer-Martin culture tube.
      (5) The plate or tube is labeled.
      (6) The examiner must be familiar with agency routines for keeping the specimen warm, cross-streaking, and immediate transport to the laboratory.
   b. Anal culture
      (1) The specimen for this culture is collected after the vaginal speculum has been removed.

(2) The sterile cotton-tipped applicator is inserted about 2.5 cm (1 inch) into the anal canal and rotated in a full circle. The applicator is also moved from side to side while inserted.

(3) The examiner holds the applicator in place for 10 to 30 seconds.

(4) The applicator is withdrawn and spread (and rotated) in a large **Z** pattern over the medium in a Thayer-Martin plate.

(5) The plate is labeled. (*Note:* If the swab contains feces, it must be discarded and another specimen taken.)

(6) The examiner must be familiar with agency routines for keeping the specimen warm, cross-streaking the medium, and transporting the specimen to the laboratory.

3. Mechanics of the pelvic examination

   a. The examiner must make a decision about which hand will insert and hold the speculum; then he or she must decide which will be the intravaginal hand during the bimanual examination. Once the decision is made, the examiner should maintain this routine. Often the dominant hand is more efficient with speculum insertion as well as serving as the internal hand for the bimanual assessment.

   b. The beginning examiner should become familiar with the vaginal speculum before using it in a clinical setting. The metal speculum is very different from the disposable plastic speculum. The plastic speculum base widens as a portion of it moves in an adjacent groove. When the base is stabilized, it goes into place with a resounding snap that often alarms both examiner and client! The metal speculum opens and stabilizes in position with the aid of twisting lever nuts and rods. It is most helpful to "play" with these instruments in advance until the examiner feels comfortable with them (Fig. 13-16).

---

### SAMPLE RECORDING

*External:* Female hair distribution with no masses, lesions, scars, rash, or swelling in inguinal area. Labia, vestibule, urethral meatus are intact without inflammation, swelling, lesions, discharge, or tenderness. No bulging at vaginal orifice. Perineum intact with healed episiotomy scar.

*Internal:* Cervix multiparous, pink, firm, mobile, and midline without lesions.

Vaginal surface rugous and moist without inflammation. No discharge visualized. Nonodorous.

Uterine fundus anterior and firm under symphysis pubis, contour smooth, nontender.

Ovaries and tubes not palpable. No masses or tenderness on palpation.

*Rectovaginal:* Septum smooth and firm. Cul-de-sac and rectum without nodules, tenderness, or masses. Good anal sphincter tone.

---

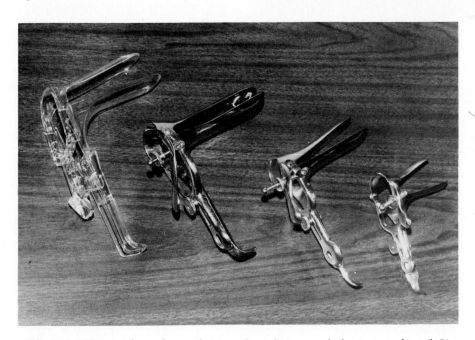

**FIG. 13-16.** Variety of metal specula in graduated sizes, and plastic speculum (left).

4. Promoting client comfort
   a. Inquire about whether the client has had a pelvic examination before and ask if she has any concerns. Showing and explaining instruments, equipment, and the procedure will alleviate some anxiety.
   b. Assist the client in stabilizing her feet in the stirrups (she should wear her shoes). Help her to place her buttocks at the *edge* of the examining table.
   c. A client who is ill or weak may need assistance in maintaining her legs in position (an assistant may be necessary to support the client's legs).
   d. If the client is unable to assume the lithotomy position, an assessment can be accomplished while the client assumes the Sims position.
   e. Be certain that the room is warm and privacy is ensured.
   f. When draping the client, be certain to fully cover her knees with the drape.
   g. Posing questions during the examination is difficult, particularly if you are unable to establish eye contact. However, we have found it helpful to maintain a relaxed dialogue, describing our activities as we do them, so that the client feels included and informed.
   h. Some practitioners carry small hand mirrors and offer the client the opportunity to view her own genitalia with explanations and guidance from the examiner.
   i. If the client becomes tense during the examination, stop the procedure but keep examining hands in place as you urge her to breathe slowly through her mouth and to concentrate on the breathing rhythm.
   j. Be certain all equipment is close at hand before beginning the examination.

## History and clinical strategies: the pediatric client

1. The extent of the gynecological examination of the child will depend on the child's age and presenting complaints. For the well child, during a screening examination, the extent of the examination includes only inspection and palpation of the external genitalia. The vaginoscopy examination is done for a young child only when a problem is anticipated or for a teenager who is sexually active and requests birth control information or who is experiencing abdominal, gynecological, or urinary problems.
2. Because of the complexity of the procedure, the vaginoscopy examination of the young child is beyond the scope of this text. Although it may at times become necessary to perform a speculum examination, it requires special equipment and a well-prepared and knowledgeable practitioner who frequently performs pediatric gynecological examinations.
3. Examining the external genitalia of any child should be anticipated as a stressful event for both the client and her parent, if present. The examiner must explain to the child and the parent exactly what will be done before the examination as well as continue to explain throughout the inspection and palpation of the external genitalia. It may be necessary to explain to the parent that thorough inspection of the child's external genitalia is part of every complete examination.

   The young infant and child will usually participate cooperatively if the examination is completed in a matter-of-fact manner.

   By the time the child reaches 4 to 6 years of age, the examiner will need to spend even more time reassuring the child that the procedure involves only looking at her genitalia and touching her on the outside. If necessary, the examiner should enlist the help of the child by taking the child's hand and having her first touch herself; then the examiner can palpate the genitalia.

   A school-age or young teenage child will not like the examination but will allow it to occur uneventfully. The child's parent may or may not be present during the examination. If the child appears fearful or anxious, the parent may be able to provide comfort. If the child is older, the examiner should be alert to the child's embarrassment because her parent is present. The examiner should confer with the child before the examination and, if appropriate, ask the parent to wait outside.

   As the child begins to mature, she will become very interested in her own body and what she looks like. The examiner may use a mirror to allow the child to look at herself. Education could coincide with the examination.

   Older teenagers deserve to be examined without a parent present if they desire or if the examiner wants to talk with the adolescent alone. As for the younger adolescent, a mirror may be used as an educational tool and to involve the teenager in the actual assessment process.
4. Positioning the child for the examination will depend on the child's age.
   a. Birth to 3 years of age. The child should be on the parent's lap with the child's back reclining at about a 45-degree angle against the parent's chest. The child should feel secure in this position, and the parent can help by holding the child's legs in a frog position up against her

chest. This will allow the examiner full access to the external genitalia. The examiner should be sitting opposite the parent and have an adequate light source.

b. Three to 5 years. Because of the child's size, she will need to be moved to the examination table. If possible, the head of the table should be up about 30 degrees. The child should be resting back on the incline and her legs again held up by her parent in a frog position against her chest. The child does not need to be at the end of the examination table.

c. Six to 15 years. The child should be on the examination table in a modified lithotomy position, lying flat or at an upward slight angle. Her legs must be flexed at the knee, and her heels should be close to her buttocks. The knees are then separated so that the genitalia may be viewed. If the parent is present, he or she should stand near the girl's head and assist in maintaining a spread-knee position. Depending on the child's age and the length of her legs, she may need to be toward the end of the table. If the examiner has difficulty visualizing the genitalia, a small pillow may be placed under the child's hips. Although the conventional gynecological stirrups are extremely convenient for the examiner, they are often frightening to the young adolescent and spaced too widely for comfort.

d. Over age 15 years. The adolescent will require the same lithotomy positioning as the adult. The success and adequacy of this positioning will depend on the examiner's approach to the client.

5. Frequently the examiner performs the first speculum examination for the teenage or young adult client. The first examination is perhaps the client's most important, since during that examination the client is developing perceptions that will remain with her for future examinations. Special preparations the examiner should make follow:

a. Discuss the procedure with the client while she is still dressed.

b. If possible, use illustrations or models to show exactly what will happen and what the examiner will be observing.

c. Prepare all necessary equipment so that once the procedure is started, there will be no interruptions.

d. Use the appropriate size speculum.
(1) There are pediatric and virginal specula that are approximately 1 to 1.5 cm wide. These can be carefully inserted with minimal discomfort.
(2) A small adult speculum may be used if the client is sexually active.

6. The history questioning about the genitourinary system of girls should focus on the following three areas:

a. Urinary functioning. Does the child have any difficulties with voiding, such as urinary incontinence, bed-wetting, inability to maintain a steady stream until the bladder is emptied, burning or urgency with urination? If any of these are present, explore in detail, including family history of similar problems, use of bubble bath, and frequency of urinary tract problems.

b. Vaginal itching or discharge. These are both frequent problems that require in-depth investigation. Common causes of these include inconsistent or inadequate cleansing of the area; foreign bodies such as a toy, toilet tissue, crayons, or coins; sexual abuse or genital fondling. The parent and/or child must be questioned about these possibilities, and the examiner must be careful to consider them during the physical assessment.

c. Maturational changes. Girls over 9 years of age who are also showing breast and pubic hair development should be questioned about whether they have begun menstruation and whether they understand about the developmental changes their bodies are undergoing. Areas of specific investigation include:
(1) The girl's awareness and information about menstruation
(2) The girl's feelings about menstruation
(3) The girl's information regarding sexual activities and techniques to prevent pregnancy

## Clinical variations: the pediatric client

| CHARACTERISTIC OR AREA EXAMINED | NORMAL | DEVIATIONS FROM NORMAL |
|---|---|---|
| 1. Position child as previously discussed | | |
| 2. Careful examination of external genitalia of the infant to make sure it is unambiguous | | Inability to identify labia majora, labia minora, clitoris, urethera, vaginal introitus |
| 3. Inguinal and mons pubis surface characteristics | Smooth, clear surface area<br>Parasites absent | Poor perineal hygiene<br>Scars, swellings, discolorations<br>Excoriated surface<br>Lesions, rash<br>Lice |
| 4. Hair distribution | See Table 13-1 for maturational development | Absence of pubic hair by child's thirteenth birthday |

**TABLE 13-1.** Pubic hair development in females

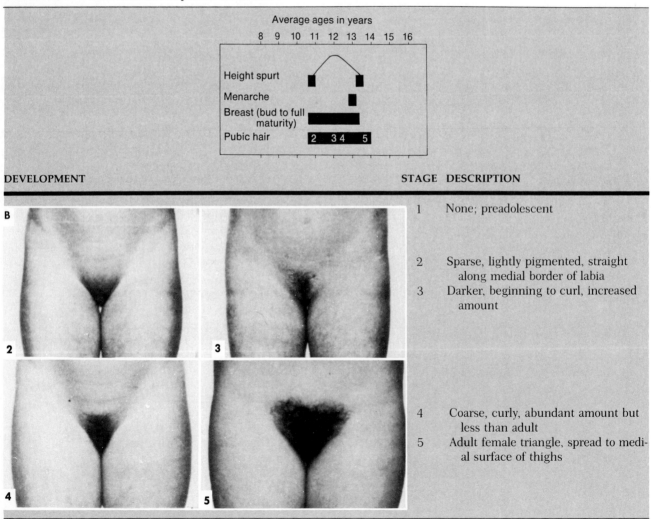

| DEVELOPMENT | STAGE | DESCRIPTION |
|---|---|---|
| | 1 | None; preadolescent |
| | 2 | Sparse, lightly pigmented, straight along medial border of labia |
| | 3 | Darker, beginning to curl, increased amount |
| | 4 | Coarse, curly, abundant amount but less than adult |
| | 5 | Adult female triangle, spread to medial surface of thighs |

From Tanner, J.M.: Growth at adolescence, ed. 2, Oxford, England, 1962, Blackwell Scientific Publications, Ltd.

| CHARACTERISTIC OR AREA EXAMINED | NORMAL | DEVIATIONS FROM NORMAL |
|---|---|---|
| **5.** Labia majora surface characteristics | Pink, smooth surface<br>Symmetrical, dry appearance<br>Becomes prominent and hair covered during puberty | Swelling, redness<br>Discoloration, excoriated or rash surface |
| **6.** Labia minora | Very prominent in infants (may normally protrude from labia majora)<br>By puberty labia minora recede to adult configuration<br>Light pink color in infants and small children, changing to dark pink by puberty<br>Symmetrical | Labia fused by adhesions<br><br>Inflammation, swelling, nodules, varicosities<br>Marked asymmetry<br>Tissue appearing white and thin |
| **7.** Clitoris size | From 3 mm to 1 cm (½ inch) in length, depending on age and maturational development | Enlargement, atrophy<br>Ambiguous appearance |
| **8.** Uretheral meatus and surrounding tissue | Irregular opening or slit<br>Usually located midline; may be close to or slightly within vaginal introitus | Redness, rashes, or lesions<br>Lateral position of meatus<br>Discharge from surrounding Skene glands or urethral opening |
| **9.** Vaginal introitus and immediate surrounding tissue | Moist tissue, even pink color<br>Hymen may or may not be across or partially across vaginal opening; by menarche, opening should be at least 1 cm wide<br>Vaginal opening present | If hymen intact (imperforate hymen), bluish color or bulging behind hymen may mean presence of blood; most commonly found in<br>(1) newborn: will generally reabsorb on own;<br>(2) adolescent: menstrual blood<br>Any time imperforate hymen found, client should be referred<br>Lesions, redness, rashes, swelling |
| **10.** Perineum surface | Smooth, pink | Inflammation, fistula, lesion, mass |
| **11.** Anus | Deeper pigmentation and coarse skin | Lesions, rash, skin tags, inflammation, lumps, excoriation, unclean surface<br>Presence of pinworms |
| **12.** External genitalia palpation<br>  **a.** Labia and vestibule<br>  **b.** Skene glands | <br>Soft, homogeneous, nontender<br>Not visible or palpable | <br>Nodular, tender<br>Tender or swollen glands; presence of discharge |
|   **c.** Bartholin glands | Not visible or palpable | Tender or swollen glands<br>Unilateral swelling<br>Presence of discharge |
|   **d.** Vaginal discharge | Mucoid or sanguineous discharge in newborn<br>Watery discharge present for 2 to 3 years before onset of menstruation<br>Within 1 year following onset of menstruation, discharge as seen in adult | Thick or foul odorous discharge |

*Note:* If speculum examination is required in a small child, she should be referred to a physician. If speculum examination is required in a menstruating adolescent, techniques previously described should be used; findings are similar to those for the adult.

## History and clinical strategies: the geriatric client

1. Sexual history. The elderly woman is capable of sexual functioning during her entire lifetime. Changes associated with aging do occur in the external and internal genitalia, but they happen slowly and at different rates according to the individual. A summary of the aging changes follows:
   a. The vaginal tube becomes shorter and narrower.
   b. Vaginal fluids lessen and may secrete at a slower rate to direct stimulation.
   c. The vaginal walls are thinner and more friable.
   d. Excitement phase: the time and extent of the expansion phase of the vagina is diminished.
   e. Plateau phase: uterine elevation is reduced; vasocongestion of the labia is diminished.
   f. Orgasmic phase: duration of orgasm is lessened, and the number of uterine contractures are fewer. Occasionally the uterine muscles will lapse into spasm, which can be painful.
   g. Resolution phase: this phase is more rapid than in younger women.

   Some of the changes mentioned accelerate if the woman experiences no sexual stimulation for an extended period of time (either with a sexual partner or through masturbation). Lack of a sexual partner can be a problem. Some older women, even though they have sexual needs and a desire for intimacy, are not comfortable with extramarital relationships, masturbation, or other life-style alterations if they have no sexual partner.

   All the intimacy and sex-related questions listed in the adult section of this chapter are appropriate for the elderly woman. Additional questions might be considered if the client indicates that she is interested in pursuing the topic of sexuality.
   a. If you have a male sexual partner, do you feel that he is comfortable with his sexual behaviors, responses, and capabilities?
   b. Do you ever experience pain in response to direct stimulation of the vagina? During orgasm?
   c. Do you have difficulty with urinary frequency or urgency during sexual stimulation?
   d. Do you have other physical problems that interfere with sexual behavior (e.g., painful joints, fatigue, dyspnea, fear of injuring yourself or causing illness)?
   e. Does your partner have any other physical problems that interfere with sexual behaviors?
   f. Are adequate privacy and time available for you to meet your sexual needs?
   g. Do you have any problems with family members objecting to your friendships or sexual habits?

   (*Note:* Some elderly women have consciously made the decision to discontinue sexual activity. An overly enthusiastic practitioner might create conflict and cause embarrassment. Other older females are quite creative and zealous in pursuing needs for sexual fulfillment. Homosexual encounters, masturbation, extramarital experiences, and creative sexual methods with a partner may be part of their life-style. The practitioner should be well informed about elderly individuals' needs and capabilities before pursuing a detailed sexual history.)

2. Symptoms associated with the genitourinary system
   a. Vaginitis and/or vulvitis occur often with immobilization. Poor hygiene practices, urinary incontinence, poor nutrition, and obesity contribute to this problem. Medications (especially antibiotics), systemic diseases (e.g., diabetes or atherosclerosis), and atrophic changes also aggravate a potential inflammation. Any individuals who are immobilized should be examined *regularly* for itching and scratching (with resultant lichenification), redness, yellow or whitish discharge, leukoplakia, petechiae, and vaginal odors.
   b. Vaginitis may occur because of limited vaginal secretions, increased alkaline condition (associated with diminished estrogen output), or pessary irritation. Symptoms are itching, pain during intercourse, general localized soreness, and perhaps a resulting increase in vaginal discharge that may be yellowish or brown and foul in odor.
   c. Uterine cancer is first suspected with postmenopausal bleeding. *Any bleeding episode* is cause for immediate referral to a physician.
   d. Genital prolapse may feel like pressure or heaviness in the genital area. Back pain, attacks of cystitis (urgency, frequency, burning on urination), urinary retention, urinary incontinence, and constipation may accompany this problem. (*Note:* The severity and number of complaints may not correlate with the severity of prolapse that the examiner observes.)
   e. Stress incontinence is common. Involuntary urination with coughing, sneezing, laughing, moving from sitting to standing position, or general movement may occur.
   f. The questions listed in the adult section of this chapter regarding vaginal discharge and pelvic pain are appropriate for the aging woman.
   g. The client should be asked if she has any concerns or information to share about her menopausal phase.

h. If the client is undergoing estrogen therapy, inquire specifically about bleeding episodes, fluid retention, breast enlargement, or pain. Ask the client to evaluate the effects and side effects of the therapy.

3. Clinical strategies
   a. Many clients may assume the lithotomy position with help and support from the examiner. Another individual might be needed to support the client's legs, since they may tire easily when the hip joints remain in abduction for extended periods.

   b. Clients with orthopneic problems will need their head elevated during the examination.

   c. Disabled clients may assume the Sims position for a pelvic examination if they are unable to maintain the dorsolithotomy pose.

   d. Papanicolaou smears should be obtained for aging women with the same frequency as with younger women.

   e. Read the *Clinical strategies* section in the adult section of this chapter for further suggestions regarding client comfort and examination procedures.

## Clinical variations: the geriatric client

| CHARACTERISTIC OR AREA EXAMINED | NORMAL | DEVIATIONS FROM NORMAL |
|---|---|---|
| **1.** External genitalia inspection | | |
| **a.** Hair distribution | Pubic hair thinned, perhaps sparse, often gray | Patchy loss of hair |
| | | Total absence of hair |
| | Parasites absent | Nits, pubic lice |
| **b.** Inguinal mons pubis, skin surface characteristics | Smooth, clear | Scars |
| | | Inguinal swelling, excoriation, lesions, rash |
| **c.** Labia majora surface characteristics | Labial folds flattened or may disappear into surrounding skin | Shrinkage accompanied by inflammation |
| | Decrease in subcutaneous fat in folds usually corresponds to degree of loss of subcutaneous fat elsewhere on client's body | Thickening or induration of small areas |
| | | Maceration, ulceration, lesions, nodules |
| | Symmetrical | Marked asymmetry |
| | Skin appears smooth, often shiny, and paler than in younger adult | |
| **d.** Inner surface of labia majora and labia minora | Shiny, usually dry, paler than in young adult | Inflammation |
| | | Maceration |
| | Fewer folds | Lesions, nodules |
| | Usually symmetrical | Varicosities |
| | | Swelling, thickening |
| | | Induration |
| | | Marked asymmetry |
| **e.** Clitoris size | Slightly smaller than in younger adult | Enlargement |
| | | Marked atrophy |
| **f.** Clitoris surface | Medial aspect covered by prepuce | Inflammation |
| | Pink | |
| **g.** Urethral meatus and immediate surrounding tissue | Irregular opening or slit (relaxed perineal musculature may result in meatus being situated more posteriorly; very near or within vaginal introitus) | Discharge from surrounding glands or urethral opening |
| | | Polyp |
| | | Inflammation |
| | Midline location | Urethral caruncles fairly common, appearing as a bright red nodule near urethral meatus |
| | | Lateral position of meatus |

## Clinical variations: the geriatric client—cont'd

| CHARACTERISTIC OR AREA EXAMINED | NORMAL | DEVIATIONS FROM NORMAL |
|---|---|---|
| h. Vaginal introitus and immediate surrounding tissue | May be smaller (admit only one finger) than younger adult, or multiparous client may manifest gaping introitus with vaginal walls rolling toward opening | Surrounding inflammation<br>Profuse vaginal discharge<br>Swelling<br>Lesions<br>Large rectocele, cystocele, enterocele, or marked uterine prolapse will show mucosal tissue bulging through vaginal orifice |
| i. Perineum surface | Smooth, or episiotomy scar (midline or mediolateral) may be visible | Inflammation, fistula<br>Lesions, mass |
| j. Anus surface | Increased pigmentation and course skin | Scars, skin tags<br>Lesions, inflammation<br>Fissures, lumps<br>Excoriation<br>Hemorrhoids |
| k. External genitalia palpation | Soft, homogeneous<br>Nontender | Irregular, nodular<br>Tender |
|   1. Urethral duct | No discharge from urethral duct<br>Nontender | Discharge*<br>Tenderness |
|   2. Bartholin gland area | No tenderness, no swelling, homogeneous tissue<br>No discharge | Tender, swelling, nodules<br><br>Discharge* |
|   3. Perineum | Thin, rigid<br>Lateral episiotomy scar may be visible<br>Nontender | Paper thin<br><br>Tender |
|   (*Note:* At time of insertion of finger into vaginal orifice, estimate opening and vaginal orifice tone) | Opening may be very narrow and admit one finger only<br>Opening may be very relaxed; client has difficulty squeezing examiner's finger with voluntary vaginal constriction | |
| 2. Insert middle finger and index finger (if possible) into vagina; press posteriorly with firm gradual motion; ask client to strain down or bear down to elicit: | | |
|   a. Bulging | Vaginal wall may roll slightly outward | Bulge appears from anterior wall<br>Bulge appears from posterior wall<br>Uterus emerges at opening (cervix may be visible at opening, or may protrude beyond opening)<br>(*Note:* The cervix is often eroded and hypertrophied with marked uterine prolapse.) |
|   b. Urinary incontinence<br>(*Note:* A speculum with narrow blades may need to be used if client has small introitus.) | No incontinence | Incontinent |
| 3. Internal inspection<br>  a. Cervix | | |
|     1. Color | Paler than in younger woman; color evenly distributed | Inflamed (red) in local areas or generally |

*Prepare a culture of any discharge.

| CHARACTERISTIC OR AREA EXAMINED | NORMAL | DEVIATIONS FROM NORMAL |
|---|---|---|
| | Symmetrical, circumscribed erythema surrounding os may indicate normal condition of exposed columnar epithelium; however, beginning examiners should consider any reddened appearance a problem for consultation | Markedly pale<br>Cyanotic<br>Erythema, especially if patchy or if borders irregular around os |
| 2. Position | Midline<br>Cervix and os may be pointed in anterior or posterior direction<br>Cervix protrudes less into vaginal tube; may be flush against back of vaginal wall<br>Surrounding fornices diminish or may disappear | Situated laterally<br><br>Projection of over 3 cm (1¼ inches) into vaginal tube |
| 3. Size | Cervix decreases in size with aging | Over 4 cm (1½ inches) in diameter |
| 4. Surface | Smooth; may appear paler than in younger woman<br>Occasional visible squamocolumnar junction (symmetrical reddened circle around os)<br>Nabothian cysts common (smooth, round, yellowish raised areas) | Reddened granular area around os (especially asymmetrical), friable tissue<br>Red patches, lesions<br>Strawberry spots<br>White patches |
| 5. Os | Often very narrow or stenosed; in some instances may be obliterated | Absence of os should be reported as problem<br>(*Note:* If secretions from uterus are trapped by nonfunctional os, the uterus may be enlarged and tender on palpation.) |
| 6. Cervical discharge | Often scanty; if present, should be clear or slightly opaque and odorless | Odor foul<br>Colored (yellowish, greenish, gray)<br>Also note odor of stale urine<br>Bloody discharge |
| **b.** Vagina | Length of tube shortens with aging | |
| 1. Color | Appears paler than in younger women | Reddened<br>Lesions<br>Pallor (associated with anemia) |
| 2. Surface | Less moisture<br>Smooth (rugae diminish with aging)<br>Shiny | Leukoplakia<br>Dried<br>Lesions, cracks, petechiae<br>Bleeding |
| 3. Consistency | Smooth, homogeneous | Nodular<br>Swollen |
| 4. Secretions | If present, should be clear or slightly opaque<br>Odorless | Thick, curdy, frothy<br>Gray, greenish, yellowish<br>Foul odor |
| 5. Amount of secretion | May be absent or sparse | Profuse |
| **4.** Bimanual examination | | |
| **a.** Vaginal wall surface<br>(*Note:* Examiner may be able to insert one finger only.) | Smooth, homogeneous<br>Nontender | Nodular<br>Tender |
| **b.** Cervix | Cervical protrusion into vaginal vault diminishes<br>Cervix may be flush against back of vault | |

## Clinical variations: the geriatric client—cont'd

| CHARACTERISTIC OR AREA EXAMINED | NORMAL | DEVIATIONS FROM NORMAL |
|---|---|---|
| | In some instances examiner may not be able to palpate cervix | |
| 1. Size | Diminished | Enlarged |
| 2. Contour | Evenly rounded, may be slightly ovoid | Irregular in shape |
| 3. Consistency and surface | Firm (like tip of nose) | Soft, nodular, or hard |
| | Smooth | |
| 4. Mobility | Cervix remains mobile, but mobility may be less noticeable if protrusion into vaginal vault greatly diminished | Immobile, fixed, or discomfort associated with movement |
| | Movement should not cause discomfort | |
| 5. Location | Midline | Laterally displaced |
| 6. Patency of os | Os may be smaller but should be palpable | Stenosis of os may be normal finding; however, beginning examiners should report this as problem |
| 7. Fornices surrounding cervix | Diminish (may disappear) with aging; if palpable, should be pliable, smooth, and nontender | Irregular or nodular surface, tender on palpation |
| c. Uterus | Greatly diminishes in size; most often not palpable at all | Enlarged |
| | If body of uterus palpated with internal hand, should be smooth, firm, freely movable, and nontender | Nodular, irregular, hardened, or indurated areas; tender on palpation |
| | | Fixed |
| d. Ovaries | Atrophy with age and rarely palpable in aging women | Marked tenderness in adnexal area |
| | Fallopian tubes not palpable | Nodulation or mass palpated |
| | | Pulsations |
| | | Ascites and pleural fluid accumulation sometimes associated with adnexal masses |
| 5. Rectovaginal examination | | |
| a. Palpable characteristics | Rectal wall should feel smooth and homogeneous | Nodular, thickened |
| | Nontender | Tender |
| | Rectovaginal septum should feel thin, smooth, and pliable | Pouching on anterior rectal wall |
| | Uterine body rarely palpated, and posterior fornix difficult to locate | Any palpated mass abnormal |
| | Anal sphincter tone may be somewhat diminished but should be nontender | Uterus bulging into rectal wall |
| | | Anal sphincter manifesting no tone |

**Cognitive
self-assessment**

Match the lettered structures with the corresponding numbered label.
1.  _L_  Anus
2.  _F_  Clitoris
3.  _C_  Labia minora
4.  _K_  Perineum
5.  _H_  Urethral meatus
6.  _A_  Prepuce
7.  _E_  Mons pubis
8.  _I_  Vaginal introitus
9.  _B_  Opening of Skene gland
10.  _G_  Labia majora
11.  _D_  Vestibule
12.  _J_  Bartholin gland

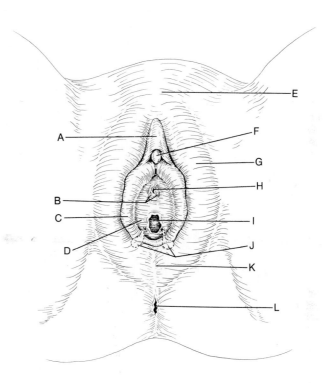

13. Which of the following statements is/are true?
    ☐ a.  The labia majora extend from the mons pubis to the fourchette.
    ☑ b.  The labia minora are darker in color and thinner than the majora.
    ☐ c.  The visible part of the clitoris is normally no more than 2 cm long and 1 cm wide.
    ☑ d.  The perforated hymen can leave visible rounded fragments at the introital margins.
    ☐ e.  The perineum usually feels thicker and more flexible in a nulliparous woman.
    ☐ f.  all except c
    ☐ g.  b and e
    ☒ h.  all except a
    ☐ i.  a, c, and e

14. Which of the following statements is/are true?
    ☒ a. Bartholin glands are lateral and slightly posterior to the vaginal orifice.
    ☒ b. Bartholin glands are usually not visible but can be palpated.
    ☒ c. Skene ducts are located in the paraurethral area.
    ☐ d. When Skene ducts are "milked," they usually exude a small amount of clear discharge.
    ☒ e. A visible discharge from Bartholin glands should be considered abnormal.
    ☐ f. all except e
    ☐ g. a, c, and e
    ☒ h. all the above
    ☐ i. all except d
    ☐ j. b and d

15. Which of the following statements is/are true about preparation of the client for a pelvic examination?
    ☐ a. A vinegar douche administered the night before a scheduled pelvic examination is usually recommended.
    ☐ b. Demonstrating the instruments used for a pelvic examination before using them generally increases anxiety on the part of teenage clients.
    ☒ c. Covering the client's knees with the drape while she is in lithotomy position maintains the illusion that she is "decently" covered.
    ☒ d. If the client breathes deeply and slowly through her mouth and concentrates on the breathing rhythm, she is more likely to relax.
    ☒ e. If a disabled client cannot assume or maintain the lithotomy position, the Sims position can be used.
    ☐ f. a and d
    ☐ g. b, d, and e
    ☒ h. c, d, and e
    ☐ i. all except e

Match the lettered structures shown at the top of p. 391 with the corresponding numbered label.
16. __D__ Uterus (isthmus)
17. __G__ Introitus
18. __B__ Ovary
19. __H__ Rectum
20. __K__ Cervix
21. __C__ Uterus (fundus)
22. __M__ Perineum
23. __F__ Urethra
24. __A__ Fallopian tube
25. __L__ Vagina
26. __I__ Rectouterine pouch
27. __E__ Bladder
28. __J__ Fornix

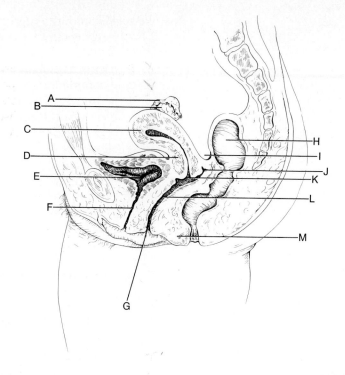

29. Which of the following statements is/are true?
    - ☒ a. The vagina inclines posteriorly at about a 45-degree angle with the vertical plane of the body.
    - ☒ b. The anterior vaginal wall is more sensitive to pressure than the posterior wall.
    - ☒ c. Vaginal discharge is normally odorless.
    - ☐ d. A whitish, creamy vaginal discharge should be considered abnormal.
    - ☒ e. The vaginal surface often appears thinner and paler in an elderly client.
    - ☐ f. a, b, and c
    - ☐ g. c, d, and e
    - ☐ h. all except c
    - ☐ i. all the above
    - ☐ j. all except d

30. Which of the following statements is/are true about normal deviation of findings related to pelvic examination?
    - ☒ a. The cervix softens in the fourth to sixth week of pregnancy.
    - ☒ b. The cervix usually appears bluish or purplish in early pregnancy.
    - ☒ c. The multiparous cervical os is slitlike in appearance.
    - ☒ d. The uterus's size is decreased in an elderly client.
    - ☒ e. Vaginal mucosa may become increasingly friable with aging.
    - ☒ f. all the above
    - ☐ g. all except e
    - ☐ h. a, c, and e
    - ☐ i. b, c, and d

31. Retroversion of the uterus:
    - [ ] a. rarely occurs
    - [x] b. is a tilting backward of the entire uterus
    - [ ] c. occurs with aging
    - [x] d. when marked, may permit palpation of the fundus through the rectum
    - [x] e. results in the cervix facing more anteriorly in the vagina
    - [x] f. b, d, and e
    - [ ] g. all except c
    - [ ] h. all except a
    - [ ] i. b, c, and d

32. Anteflexion of the uterus:
    - [ ] a. results in the cervix facing more posteriorly in the vagina
    - [x] b. results in easy palpation of the fundus
    - [ ] c. is a tilting forward of the entire uterus
    - [ ] d. occurs with aging
    - [ ] e. may permit palpation of the fundus through the rectum
    - [ ] f. all except e
    - [ ] g. a, b, and c
    - [ ] h. c and d
    - [ ] i. b and c

33. A normal cervix:
    - [x] a. is covered by a smooth, pink epithelium
    - [ ] b. is a granular, vascular membrane
    - [x] c. has an os with a slitlike appearance after childbirth
    - [ ] d. is immobile
    - [x] e. feels firm, like the tip of your nose
    - [ ] f. all except a
    - [ ] g. a, c, and e
    - [ ] h. b, d, and e
    - [ ] i. all except b
    - [ ] j. a and d

34. When you use the vaginal speculum:
    - [x] a. it is usually warmed and lubricated with water
    - [ ] b. a commercial lubricant should be used at all times
    - [ ] c. on insertion, exert pressure against the anterior wall to avoid client discomfort
    - [ ] d. the blades are vertical on initial insertion
    - [ ] e. on insertion the blades are partially open to permit viewing of the vaginal wall
    - [ ] f. all except e
    - [ ] g. all except d
    - [ ] h. a, c, and d
    - [ ] i. b and e

35. During bimanual palpation, the normal uterus:
    - [ ] a. is immobile
    - [ ] b. feels spongy at the fundus
    - [x] c. is usually 5 to 8 cm long
    - [x] d. feels firm
    - [ ] e. feels nodular
    - [ ] f. all except b
    - [ ] g. a and d
    - [ ] h. a, b, and c
    - [x] i. c and d

36. Which of the following statements is/are true about normal palpable findings during a bimanual examination?
    ☒ a. The cervix is freely movable (1 to 2 cm in each direction) when manipulated by the examiner's fingers.
    ☐ b. The normal cervical os is closed and will not admit a fingertip.
    ☒ c. Approximately 85% of uteri are in an anteposition and can be palpated anteriorly.
    ☒ d. Normal ovaries are 4 to 6 cm, firm to touch, and movable.
    ☒ e. Round ligaments are sometimes palpated as cordlike structures
    ☐ f. a, d, and e
    ☐ g. b and c
    ☐ h. all except b
    ☐ i. b, c, and d
37. The rectovaginal examination is performed:
    ☒ a. to confirm the uterine position
    ☒ b. to reassess adnexal areas
    ☒ c. to palpate the rectovaginal cul-de-sac and septum
    ☒ d. to palpate the rectal wall
    ☒ e. to assess anal sphincter tone
    ☐ f. all except c
    ☐ g. all the above
    ☐ h. d and e
    ☐ i. a, c, and d
    ☐ j. all except b

Mark each statement "T" or "F."
38. __T__ The labia may appear somewhat shriveled in a normal multiparous woman.
39. __F__ Skene ducts are often normally somewhat tender when palpated (or milked).
40. __F__ Bartholin gland openings are usually visible.
41. __F__ The perineum usually feels thinner and more rigid in a nulliparous woman.
42. __T__ The squamocolumnar junction may occasionally be visible on a normal cervix.
43. __T__ A normal cervix should extend (project) no more than 3 cm into the vaginal vault.

**PEDIATRIC QUESTIONS**

Mark each statement "T" or "F."
44. __T__ By age 13 years all girls should start to develop pubic hair.
45. __F__ All teens should have a speculum examination by age 16.
46. __T__ The hymen must be perforated for the adolescent to menstruate.
47. __T__ The best method to examine the external genitalia of a 2-year-old is to have the child on the parent's lap.
48. __T__ Perineal irritation in the preschool child is commonly caused by the use of bubble bath.
49. __F__ The labia majora in the infant are more prominent than the labia minora.

**GERIATRIC QUESTIONS**

50. Common genital findings in the aging female are:
    ☐ a. A flaccid, boggy uterus that can usually be palpated in the anterior rectal wall
    ☒ b. diminished vaginal secretions
    ☐ c. Increased protrusion of the cervix into the vaginal vault, resulting in deep fornices surrounding the cervix
    ☒ d. paler appearing vaginal walls
    ☒ e. flatter labia majora and diminished skinfolds
    ☐ f. all the above
    ☐ g. b, d, and e
    ☐ h. a, c, and e
    ☐ i. all except b
    ☐ j. none of the above

51. Sexual functioning of the elderly female:
    ☐ a. usually ceases after age 65 years
    ☐ b. is not usually advisable if the client has osteoarthritis or cardiac disease
    ☒ c. may be consciously relinquished by the individual
    ☐ d. should be rigorously promoted by the practitioner
    ☐ e. none of the above

52. Vulvitis may occur because of:
    ☒ a. poor nutrition
    ☒ b. poor hygiene practices
    ☒ c. urinary incontinence
    ☐ d. excess vaginal secretions
    ☒ e. obesity
    ☐ f. all the above
    ☐ g. none of the above
    ☐ h. all except d
    ☐ i. b and c

## SUGGESTED READINGS
### General

Bates, B.: A guide to physical examination, ed. 3, Philadelphia, 1983, J.B. Lippincott Co., pp. 273-295.

Malasanos, L., and others: Health assessment, ed. 2, St. Louis, 1981, The C.V. Mosby Co., pp. 397-417.

Martin, L.L.: Health care of women, Philadelphia, 1978, J.B. Lippincott Co., pp. 29-56, 201-218.

Patient assessment: examination of the female pelvis, part 1, Am. J. Nurs. **78**(10), 1978.

Patient assessment: examination of the female pelvis, part 2, Am. J. Nurs. **78**(11), 1978.

Prior, J.A., Silberstein, J.S., and Stang, J.M.: Physical diagnosis: the history and examination of the patient, ed. 6, St. Louis, 1981, The C.V. Mosby Co., pp. 345-364.

Walker, K., Hall, W.D., and Hurst, J.W., editors: Clinical methods, vol. 1, Boston, 1976, Butterworths, Inc., pp. 223-263, 272-281.

### Pediatric

Alexander, M., and Brown, M.S.: Pediatric history taking and physical diagnosis for nurses, ed. 2, New York, 1979, McGraw-Hill Book Co., pp. 261-279.

Barness, L.: Manual of pediatric physical diagnosis, ed. 5, Chicago, 1981, Year Book Medical Publishers, Inc., pp. 156-158.

Daniel, W.A., Jr.: Adolescents in health and disease, St. Louis, 1977, The C.V. Mosby Co., pp. 27-41, 132-150.

Huffman, J.W.: Gynecologic examination of the premenarcheal child, Pediatr. Ann., Dec. 1974, pp. 6-18.

Mager, J.: The pelvic examination: a view from the other end of the table, Ann. Intern. Med. **83**:563-564, 1975.

Marshall, W.A., and Tanner, J.M.: Variations in pattern of pubertal changes in girls, Arch. Dis. Child. **44**:291-303, 1969.

Rauh, J., and Brookman, R.R.: Adolescent developmental stages. In Johnson, T.R., Moore, W.M., and Jefferies, J.E., editors: Children are different: developmental physiology, Columbus, Ohio, 1978, Ross Laboratories, pp. 25-30.

### Geriatric

Burnside, I.M., editor: Nursing and the aged, ed. 2, New York, 1981, McGraw-Hill Book Co., pp. 367-372, 375-379.

Carotenuto, R., and Bullock, J.: Physical assessment of the gerontologic client, Philadelphia, 1980, F.A. Davis Co., pp. 113-118.

Griggs, W.: Sex and the elderly, Am. J. Nurs. **78**(8):1352-1354, 1978.

Steinberg, F.U., editor: Care of the geriatric patient, ed. 6, St. Louis, 1983, The C.V. Mosby Co., pp. 381-387.

ASSESSMENT OF THE

# Musculoskeletal system

## VOCABULARY

**abduction**  Movement of the limbs, or the trunk and head, away from the median plane of the body.

**adduction**  Movement of the limbs, or the trunk and head, toward the median plane of the body.

**ankylosis**  Fixation of a joint, often in an abnormal position, usually resulting from destruction of articular cartilage, as in rheumatoid arthritis.

**bunion**  Abnormal prominence on the inner aspect of the first metatarsal head, with bursal formation; results in lateral or valgus displacement of the great toe.

**bursa**  A fibrous fluid-filled sac found between certain tendons and the bones beneath them.

**bursitis**  Inflammation of a bursa.

**carpal tunnel syndrome**  Painful disorder of the wrist and hand induced by compression of the median nerve between the inelastic carpal ligament and other structures within the carpal tunnel.

**circumduction**  Circular movement of a limb.

**clonus**  Spasmodic alternation of muscular contraction and relaxation.

**cogwheel rigidity**  Abnormal motion in the muscle tissues characterized by jerky movements when the muscle is passively stretched.

**crepitus**  Dry, crackling sound or sensation heard or felt as a joint is moved through its range of motion.

**dorsiflexion**  Backward bending or flexion of a joint.

**epicondyle**  Round protuberance above the condyle (at the end of a bone).

**epiphysis**  End of a long bone that is cartilaginous during early childhood and becomes ossified during late childhood.

**extension**  Movement that brings a limb into or toward a straight condition.

**external rotation**  Outward turning of a limb.

**fasciculation**  The localized, uncoordinated, uncontrollable twitching of a single muscle group innervated by a single motor nerve fiber.

**flexion**  Movement that brings a limb into or toward a bent condition.

**gait: stance**  In walking, the resting phase in which the feet, legs, and body are still.

**gait: swing**  In walking, the process of lifting the foot in back, swinging it through, and placing it in front of the other foot.

**gout**  Metabolic disease that is a form of acute arthritis; marked by inflammation of the joints.

**internal rotation**  Inward turning of a limb.

**kyphosis**  Abnormal convexity of the posterior curve of the spine.

**lordosis**  Abnormal anterior concavity of the spine.

**myalgia**  Tenderness or pain in the muscle.

**osteoarthritis**  Form of arthritis in which one or many of the joints undergo degenerative changes.

**plantar flexion**  Extension of the foot so that the forepart is depressed with respect to the position of the ankle.

**pronate**  To turn the forearm so that the palm faces downward or to rotate the leg or foot inward.

**rheumatoid arthritis**  Chronic, destructive collagen disease characterized by inflammation, thickening, and swelling of the joints.

**scoliosis**  Lateral curvature of the spine.

**spondylitis**  Inflammation of one or more of the spinal vertebrae, usually characterized by stiffness and pain.

**sprain**  Traumatic injury to the tendons, muscles, or ligaments around a joint; characteristics are pain, swelling, and discoloration of the skin over the joint.

**strain** Temporary damage to the muscles, usually caused by excessive physical effort.

**subluxation** Partial or incomplete dislocation.

**supinate** To turn the forearm so that the palm faces upward or to rotate the foot and leg outward.

**tendonitis** Inflammation of a tendon.

**tennis elbow** Inflammation of the tissue at the lower end of the hu-

merus at the elbow joint, caused by repetitive flexing of the wrist against resistance; also called *external humeral epicondylitis*.

**valgus** Bending outward.

**varus** Turning inward.

## Overview

Assessment of the musculoskeletal system can be performed on many levels, from gross observations of function to the electrical evaluation of selected muscle fiber groups. For the purpose of this chapter musculoskeletal evaluation is directed toward functional assessment and detection of the presence, location, and extent of dysfunction. Emphasis is placed on observation of gait, symmetry and function of joints, bones, and muscles, and range of motion as it relates to activities of daily living.

## Cognitive objectives

At the end of this chapter the learner will demonstrate knowledge of assessment of the musculoskeletal system by the ability to do the following:

1. State the anatomy and function of a joint.
2. Describe assessment criteria for evaluating joint function.
3. Describe selected methods of evaluating a symptomatic joint, including the drawer test, the McMurray test, and the Thomas test.
4. List the normal range of motion position of the joints to be assessed during a screening examination.
5. Describe a systematic method for evaluating the skeletal system.
6. Explain a systematic method of evaluating muscle function during a screening evaluation using the make/break technique.
7. Describe the normal gait sequence and assessment criteria for evaluating gait functioning.
8. Identify selected characteristics of the pediatric musculoskeletal examination.
9. Identify selected characteristics of the geriatric musculoskeletal examination.

## Clinical objectives

At the end of this chapter the learner will perform a systematic assessment of the musculoskeletal system, demonstrating the ability to do the following:

1. Obtain a health history appropriate to the screening evaluation of the musculoskeletal system. This should include demonstration of knowledge of the client's ability to perform the activities of daily living as well as in-depth investigation of symptoms such as musculoskeletal pain analysis and skeletal, muscle, or joint problems.
2. Demonstrate inspection of the client's musculoskeletal system, including body build, bone structure and contour, symmetry, posture, gait, strength, and coordination.
3. Demonstrate inspection of the client's range of motion of all joints. Communicate an interpretation of findings as related to normal.
4. Demonstrate palpation of the client's musculoskeletal system, noting the following:
   a. Bone structure and contour
   b. Joint stability and characteristics and any deviations from normal
   c. Muscle mass, including hypertrophy or atrophy
5. Demonstrate screening techniques to evaluate muscle strength of the fingers, hands, wrists, triceps, biceps, deltoids, feet, ankles, hips, hamstrings, gluteals, abductors, adductors, quadriceps, and trunk muscle groups.
6. Demonstrate ability to perform special evaluation techniques for the knee, hip, and lower back, including:
   a. Knee-fluid evaluation
   b. Drawer test
   c. McMurray test
   d. Thomas test
   e. Back pain evaluation techniques
7. Summarize results of the assessment with a written description of findings.

## Health history additional to screening history

1. Review the client's employment situation, both past and present. What are the working conditions and risks (regarding lifting or accident proneness) for the musculoskeletal system?

2. To what extent does the client walk or exercise each day?
3. Are there recent weight changes that could have stressed the musculoskeletal system?
4. Inquire regarding the client's ability to perform activities of daily living. (The following questions are arranged according to function. If the interviewer receives a response indicating difficulty, that area should be evaluated further during the physical assessment.)
   a. Eating
      (1) Opening containers
      (2) Cutting meat
      (3) Chewing and swallowing
      (4) Preparing food
      (5) Getting food to mouth
      (6) Measuring and taking medications
   b. Bathing
      (1) Running water and testing temperature
      (2) Undressing self
      (3) Getting into and out of tub or shower
   c. Dressing
      (1) Getting clothes
      (2) Putting on prosthesis
      (3) Putting on clothes
      (4) Using zippers
      (5) Buckling
      (6) Tying
      (7) Buttoning
      (8) Putting on shoes (shoelaces)
   d. Grooming
      (1) Washing hair
      (2) Brushing hair
      (3) Brushing teeth
      (4) Shaving
      (5) Grooming nails
      (6) Applying makeup
      (7) Washing clothes
   e. Elimination
      (1) Bowel routine
      (2) Bladder routine
   f. Activity (consider safety factor)
      (1) Walking
      (2) Getting into and out of chair
      (3) Getting into and out of bed
      (4) Transferring
      (5) Turning
   g. Communication
      (1) Speech
      (2) Telephone
5. Often clients complain of musculoskeletal problems. The following outline details the symptoms analysis profile for the complaint of *pain*. This profile may be slightly adapted to collect information about any client with a musculoskeletal complaint. Following the detailed pain analysis profile are numerous other musculoskeletal complaints. Accompanying each of the items listed are important evaluative components. These components may be added to or may replace certain components of the pain analysis profile.
   a. Pain
      (1) When was the client last well?
         (a) When did *this type* of pain start occurring?
         (b) How long has the client been bothered with musculoskeletal pain in general?
      (2) Date of current problem onset
      (3) Character of specific complaint
         (a) Pressure sensation
         (b) Stiffness
         (c) Numb, tingling sensation
         (d) Single area, multiple areas
         (e) Sharp versus dull or shooting pain
         (f) If radiation of pain occurs, note to where (hips, buttocks or legs, unilateral vs. bilateral)
      (4) Nature of onset
         (a) Slow (over several weeks, days, hours)
         (b) Abrupt (over several minutes)
      (5) Client's hunch of precipitating factors
         (a) Recent injury
         (b) Recent strenuous activity, exercise, lifting
         (c) Sudden movement
         (d) Stress
      (6) Course of problem
         (a) Comes and goes
         (b) Becoming progressively worse or better
         (c) Relieved by medication, rest, exercise, etc.
      (7) Location of problem
         (a) Anatomical location
         (b) Unilateral versus bilateral
      (8) Relation to other entities
         (a) Clumsiness
         (b) Weakness
         (c) Paralysis
         (d) Anesthesia (hypoesthesia, hyperesthesia)
         (e) Gastroenterological complaints (ulcer disease, pancreatitis, bowel problems, biliary colic)
         (f) Gynecological complaints (e.g., endometriosis)
         (g) Urological complaints (calculi, prostatic disease)

       (h) Chills
       (i) Fever
       (j) General malaise
       (k) Stiffness
    (9) Patterns
       (a) Worse with movement or better with activity
       (b) Worse following coughing or defecation
       (c) Worse in AM or PM (gets better or worse as day progresses)
       (d) Worse following exercise or specific movements
       (e) Worse when riding in car
       (f) Episodes of problem getting closer together and worse
       (g) Episodes of problem getting closer together but not worse
    (10) Efforts to treat
       (a) Exercise program
       (b) Weight reduction program
       (c) Rest
       (d) Medications
       (e) Physician evaluation
    (11) How does pain interfere with client's activities of daily living?
  b. Gait difficulty
    (1) Clumsiness
    (2) Weakness
    (3) Client unaware of position in space
    (4) Pain
    (5) Stiffness
    (6) Systemic difficulty such as dizziness or vision problem
  c. Voluntary muscle complaints
    (1) Muscle weakness or fatigue
    (2) Stiffness
    (3) Pain
    (4) Wasting (atrophy)
    (5) Paralysis
    (6) Tremor
    (7) Tic
    (8) Cogwheel movement
    (9) Spasms
    (10) Aching muscles
    (11) Muscle hypertrophy
  d. Skeletal complaints
    (1) Recent fractures
    (2) Abnormalities in skeletal contour
    (3) Absence of or change of movements in a part
    (4) Crepitus
    (5) Pain with movement
    (6) Ecchymosis or hematoma of injured part

  e. Joint complaints
    (1) Recent injury (explore event in detail, including direction joint was stressed)
    (2) Change in contour or size of joint
    (3) Limitations of joint motion
    (4) Swelling or redness of skin around joint
    (5) Local pain or ache that increases with muscle contraction

6. Any client complaining of vague or generalized musculoskeletal complaints should be questioned in detail regarding history of both self and family, social history, personal psychological history; a detailed review of systems should be carried out.

7. Any client with a musculoskeletal complaint should be questioned regarding activities of daily living and occupational history. Both areas should include questions about the type of work or activity (present and past), working conditions, injury proneness, and safety precautions.

8. As well as evaluating clients with complaints or injuries, the practitioner must develop a profile to identify clients at risk and intervene with preventive education techniques. Although the following is not an inclusive list, it represents the type of risk profile data that should be collected regarding the musculoskeletal system.
  a. Client who exercises, jogs, plays tennis, etc. only sporadically or less than twice a week
  b. Athlete playing contact sports without a structured conditioning program
  c. Participation in athletics without proper supportive or protective equipment
  d. Occupation requiring lifting of awkward or heavy items
  e. Occupation requiring operation of press machines or equipment such as farm machinery that could catch clothing or limbs, causing crushing or mutilating injury
  f. Client overweight for height and body build
  g. Family history of arthritis or musculoskeletal diseases
  h. Pregnancy
  i. Client with poor eyesight or unsafe environment (such as throw rugs or darkened stairway)
  j. Client with systemic complaint such as dizziness, light-headedness, or difficulty determining body position in space
  k. Any client unable to perform activities of daily living

## Clinical guidelines

Before assessment of the musculoskeletal system, the practitioner must study and memorize several things: (1) the anatomy of the skeletal system and the names of the bones to be assessed, (2) the anatomy and normal range and degree of motion of the joints to be assessed, and (3) the major muscle groups to be evaluated and the anticipated normal response to each group. It is assumed that the student is knowledgeable in these areas.

Because of the vast complexity of assessment of the musculoskeletal system, an integrated body-region approach will be used. During examination of each region, the bones, joints, and muscles will be evaluated. This should save the examiner time as well as provide a more integrated assessment of each region.

| THE STUDENT WILL: | TO IDENTIFY: | |
| --- | --- | --- |
| | NORMAL | DEVIATIONS FROM NORMAL |
| **1.** Have goniometer at hand (if ranges of motion are to be measured) (*Note:* For musculoskeletal assessment, client should be undressed to underpants only or underpants and bra and gown.) | | |
| **2.** Observe client walking into room (Fig. 14-1) | Gait smooth, coordinated, rhythmic Walks with ease, arms extended to sides, standing erect; gaze straight forward | Walks with difficulty or with assistance Fasciculations, tremors |

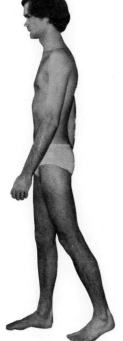

**FIG. 14-1.** Inspect client's gait.

**3.** Measure client's height and weight    (See Tables 2-1 and 2-2.)

# Clinical guidelines—cont'd

|  | TO IDENTIFY: | |
|---|---|---|
| **THE STUDENT WILL:** | **NORMAL** | **DEVIATIONS FROM NORMAL** |

**Trunk**

**1.** Observe client standing erect (front, back, and side) (Fig. 14-2)

Stands erect
Symmetry of body parts
Straight spine
Normal spine curvature: cervical spine concave; thoracic spine convex; lumbar spine concave
Knees in direct straight line between hips and ankles
Feet flat on floor pointing directly forward

Asymmetry
Unable to maintain straight posture
Lateral spine curvature
Asymmetry in height of shoulders or iliac crest
Lordosis or kyphosis, varus or valgus deformity
Medial or lateral rotation of feet

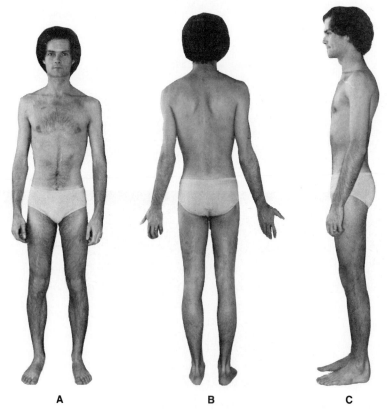

A                          B                          C

**FIG. 14-2. A,** Anterior inspection. **B,** Posterior inspection. **C,** Lateral inspection.

| | TO IDENTIFY: | |
|---|---|---|
| **THE STUDENT WILL:** | **NORMAL** | **DEVIATIONS FROM NORMAL** |
| **2.** With client standing, observe spine from posterior as client bends from waist to touch toes; note range of motion and symmetry (Fig. 14-3) | Straight spine<br>Iliac crests to equal height<br>Shoulders of equal height<br>Convexity of thoracic spine | Lateral deviation of spine<br>Asymmetry of shoulder height ("razor back" deformity) (Fig. 14-4) |

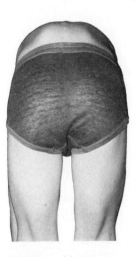

**FIG. 14-3.** Inspect shoulder and hip symmetry and spine straightness during forward bending.

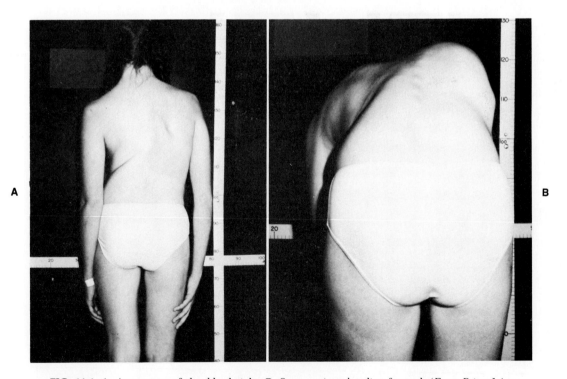

**FIG. 14-4. A,** Asymmetry of shoulder height. **B,** Same patient, bending forward. (From Prior, J.A., and Silberstein, J.S.: Physical diagnosis: the history and examination of the patient, ed. 5, St. Louis, 1977, The C.V. Mosby Co.)

## Clinical guidelines—cont'd

|  | TO IDENTIFY: | |
|---|---|---|
| **THE STUDENT WILL:** | **NORMAL** | **DEVIATIONS FROM NORMAL** |
| **3.** Observe client hyperextending spine (Fig. 14-5) | 30° hyperextension from neutral position | Unable to hyperextend without losing balance, or pain with hyperextension |

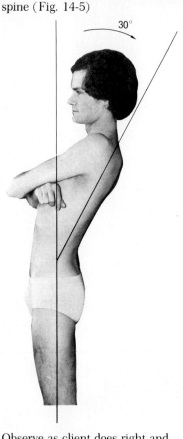

30°

FIG. 14-5. Hyperextension of the spine.

|  |  | |
|---|---|---|
| **4.** Observe as client does right and left lateral bending; may be necessary to stabilize client's pelvis (Fig. 14-6) | 35° flexion both ways from midline position | Decreased flexion degree or pain with bending |

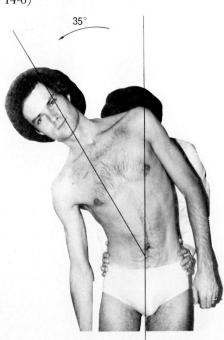

35°

FIG. 14-6. Lateral bending of the spine.

| | TO IDENTIFY: | |
| --- | --- | --- |
| **THE STUDENT WILL:** | **NORMAL** | **DEVIATIONS FROM NORMAL** |
| 5. Observe as client rotates upper trunk (stabilize pelvis) to right and left (Fig. 14-7) | 30° rotation in both directions from direct forward position | Decreased rotation capability<br>Rotation with discomfort |

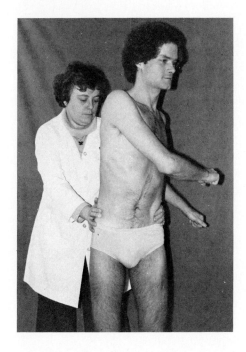

**FIG. 14-7.** Functional testing of trunk rotation; examiner stabilizes client's hips.

| | | |
| --- | --- | --- |
| 6. Palpate along spinal processes and paravertebral muscles; may be helpful to have client hunch shoulders forward and slightly flex (Fig. 14-8) | Straight spine<br>Nontender | Curvature of spine<br>Tenderness<br>Spasm of paravertebral muscles |

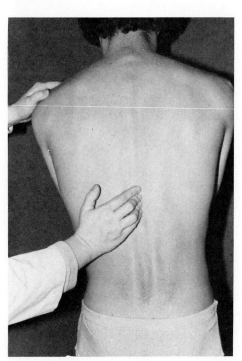

**FIG. 14-8.** Palpation of vertebral column.

## Clinical guidelines—cont'd

| THE STUDENT WILL: | TO IDENTIFY: | |
| --- | --- | --- |
| | **NORMAL** | **DEVIATIONS FROM NORMAL** |

**Gait**

1. Have client walk across room and back; observe for rhythm and smoothness

| | | |
| --- | --- | --- |
| a. Gait phase | Conformity; ability to follow gait sequencing of both stance and swing | Pain or discomfort with gait |
| b. Cadence | Symmetry of gait | Unsteady |
| | Regular smooth rhythm | Jerky |
| c. Stride length | Symmetry in length of leg swing | Asymmetry or irregularity |
| d. Trunk posture | Smooth swaying related to gait phase | Irregular or jerky |
| e. Arm swing | Smooth, symmetrical | Jerky, asymmetrical, or unrelated to gait |

**Head and neck**

| | | |
| --- | --- | --- |
| 1. With client sitting on examination table, observe musculature of face and neck | Symmetrical appearance | Asymmetry |
| | | Atrophy or hypertrophy of muscles |
| 2. Palpate each temporomandibular joint just anterior to tragus of ear while client opens and closes mouth (Fig. 14-9) | Smooth movement of mandible | Pain, limited range of motion, or crepitus of temporomandibular joint |

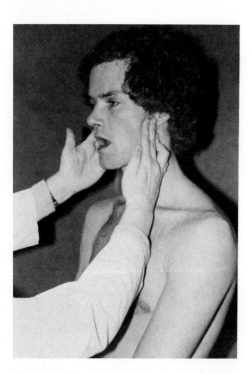

**FIG. 14-9.** Palpation of temporomandibular joint.

| THE STUDENT WILL: | TO IDENTIFY: | |
| --- | --- | --- |
| | NORMAL | DEVIATIONS FROM NORMAL |
| **3.** Move around behind client; inspect and palpate posterior neck, cervical spine, paravertebral, and trapezius muscles | Locate landmarks C7 and T1<br>Nontender cervical spine | Tenderness<br>Nodules<br>Muscular spasm |
| **4.** Evaluate range of motion of neck by asking client to: | | |
|   **a.** Flex chin to chest | 45° from midline | Limited or painful range of motion |
|   **b.** Extend head | 55° from midline | Crepitus of cervical spine |
|   **c.** Laterally bend neck to right and left | 40° each way from midline | |
|   **d.** Rotate chin to shoulders right and left | 70° from midline | |
| **5.** Evaluate neck muscle strength | | |
|   **a.** Have client flex chin to chest; instruct client to maintain position while examiner tries to manually force head upright (Fig. 14-10) | With reasonable strength, unable to force head upright | Able to break muscular flexion before anticipated point |
|   **b.** Have client hyperextend head; instruct client to maintain position while examiner tries to manually force head upright (Fig. 14-11) | With reasonable strength, unable to force head upright | Able to break muscular flexion before anticipated point |

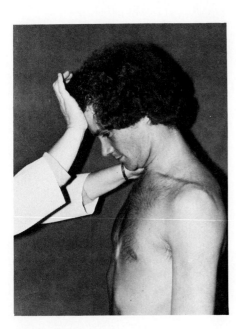

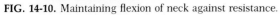

**FIG. 14-10.** Maintaining flexion of neck against resistance.

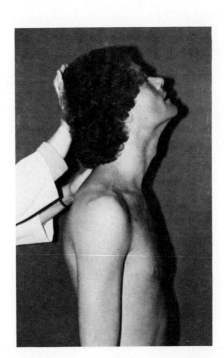

**FIG. 14-11.** Maintaining hyperextension of neck against resistance.

## Clinical guidelines—cont'd

| THE STUDENT WILL: | TO IDENTIFY: | |
| --- | --- | --- |
| | NORMAL | DEVIATIONS FROM NORMAL |

**Hands and wrists**

1. Observe and palpate hands and wrists, including joints

Smoothness; no swelling or deformities noted

Fingers able to maintain full extension

Irregular finger contour
Swelling
Deformities (Fig. 14-12, *A*)
Tenderness (Fig. 14-12, *B*)
Muscular atrophy
Heberden nodes (Fig. 14-12, *C*)

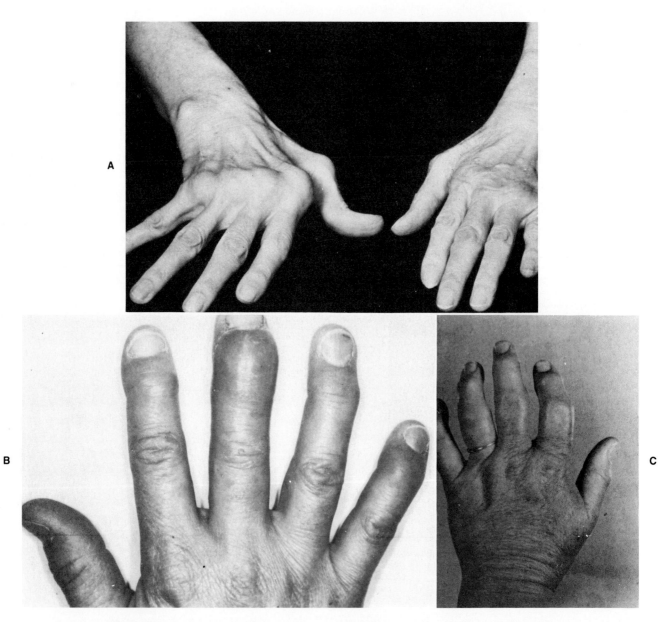

**FIG. 14-12. A,** Unilateral ulnar deviation of metacarpophalangeal joints of right hand secondary to rheumatoid arthritis. **B,** Inflammatory synovitis of distal joint of middle finger. **C,** Heberden nodules in osteoarthritis of the hand. (From Prior, J.A., Silberstein, J.S., and Stang, J.M.: Physical diagnosis: the history and examination of the patient, ed. 6, St. Louis, 1981, The C.V. Mosby Co.

| THE STUDENT WILL: | TO IDENTIFY: | |
| --- | --- | --- |
| | NORMAL | DEVIATIONS FROM NORMAL |
| 2. Observe muscular function and range of motion of fingers and hands; instruct client to: | | |
|   **a.** Extend and spread fingers of both hands (Fig. 14-13, *A*) | Symmetrical response<br>Smooth movement without complaints of discomfort<br>Full flexion and extension | Asymmetrical response<br>Pain on movement |
|   **b.** Make fist with thumb across fingers (Fig. 14-13, *B*) | | |
|   **c.** Grip examiner's first two fingers (Fig. 14-13, *C*) | Bilaterally equal response<br>Tight grip | Unequal response<br>Decreased response |

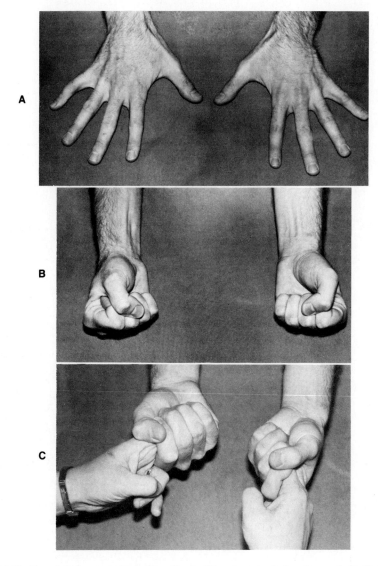

**FIG. 14-13.** Functional assessment of hands. **A,** Fingers extended and spread. **B,** Fist formation. **C,** Hand grip.

## Clinical guidelines—cont'd

| THE STUDENT WILL: | TO IDENTIFY: | |
| --- | --- | --- |
| | NORMAL | DEVIATIONS FROM NORMAL |
| **3.** Observe range of motion of wrist (Fig. 14-14) | | |
|   **a.** Radial deviation *(A)* | 20° movement from central position | Pain with movement |
| | | Decreased movement |
|   **b.** Ulnar deviation *(B)* | 55° movement from central position | |
|   **c.** Extension *(C)* | 70° movement from central position | |
|   **d.** Flexion *(D)* | 90° movement from central position | |

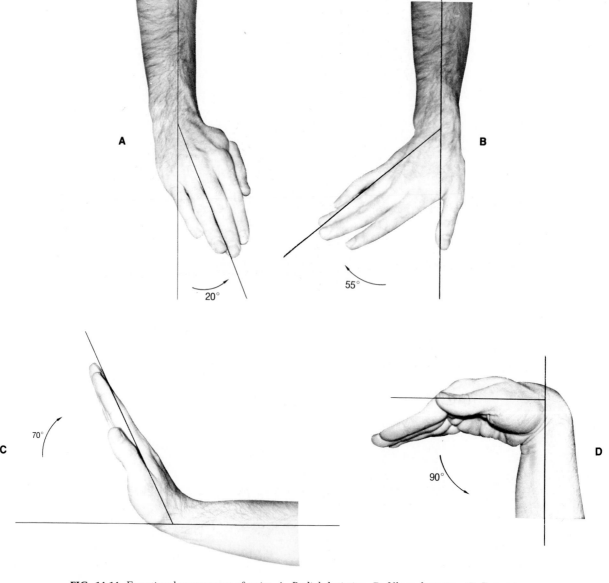

**FIG. 14-14.** Functional assessment of wrist. **A,** Radial deviation. **B,** Ulnar deviation. **C,** Extension. **D,** Flexion.

| THE STUDENT WILL: | TO IDENTIFY: | |
| --- | --- | --- |
| | NORMAL | DEVIATIONS FROM NORMAL |
| **4.** Evaluate wrist strength; instruct client to maintain position against examiner's force by using make/break technique (see *Clinical strategies* for full explanation) | | |
|    **a.** Client flexes wrist; examiner attempts to straighten wrist by grasping client's hand and extending hand to position on a straight plane from client's forearm (Fig. 14-15, *A*) | Bilaterally strong<br>Unable to break position | Asymmetrical response<br>Able to easily break position |
|    **b.** Client extends wrist; examiner grasps client's hand and attempts to flex hand to a position on a straight plane from client's forearm (Fig. 14-15, *B*) | Bilaterally strong<br>Unable to break position | Asymmetrical response<br>Able to easily break position |

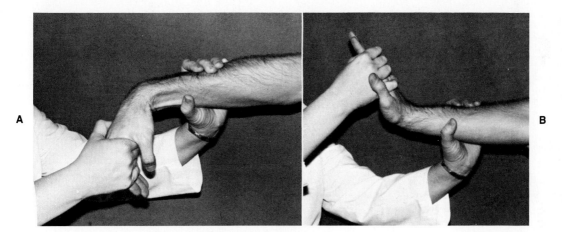

**FIG. 14-15. A,** Maintaining flexed position of wrist against resistance. **B,** Maintaining hyperextended position of wrist against resistance.

## Elbows

| | | |
| --- | --- | --- |
| **1.** Flex client's arm and support; inspect and palpate elbow, including: | | |
|    **a.** Extensor surface of ulna | Skin intact | Swelling |
|    **b.** Olecranon process | Smooth | Inflammation |
|    **c.** Groove on either side of olecranon | Surface nontender without nodules or discomfort | General tenderness<br>Subcutaneous nodules<br>Point tenderness |
|    **d.** Lateral epicondyle | | |
|    **e.** Epitrochlear nodes (palpate lateral groove between biceps and triceps muscle) | Lymph nodes not palpable | Lymph nodes palpated |

## Clinical guidelines—cont'd

| | TO IDENTIFY: | |
|---|---|---|
| THE STUDENT WILL: | NORMAL | DEVIATIONS FROM NORMAL |
| **2.** Evaluate range of motion | | |
|    **a.** Ask client to bend and extend elbow (Fig. 14-16) | 160° full movement<br>Bilaterally equal<br>No discomfort | Limited range of motion<br>Asymmetrical movement<br>Pain at elbow |

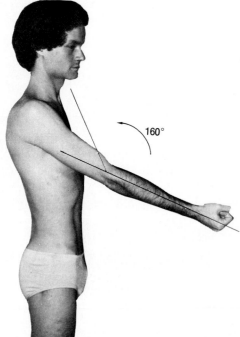

**FIG. 14-16.** Functional assessment of elbow extension.

| | | |
|---|---|---|
|    **b.** Bend client's elbow to 90° angle from shoulder; have client pronate and supinate forearm (Fig. 14-17) | 90° each direction<br>Bilaterally equal<br>No discomfort | Limited range of motion<br>Asymmetrical movement<br>Pain at elbow |

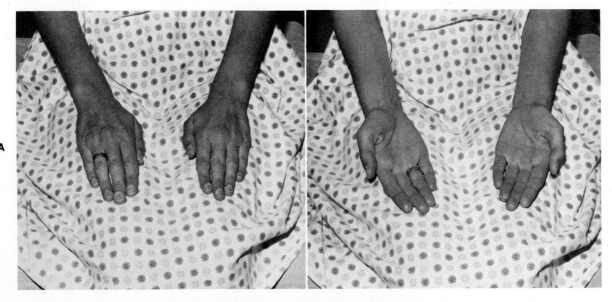

**FIG. 14-17.** Pronation (**A**) and supination (**B**) of forearms and hands.

| THE STUDENT WILL: | TO IDENTIFY: NORMAL | DEVIATIONS FROM NORMAL |
|---|---|---|
| **Shoulders** | | |
| **1.** Inspect shoulders, including shoulder girdle and acromioclavicular junction | Intact<br>Smooth and regular<br>Bilaterally symmetrical | Redness<br>Swelling<br>Nodules |
| **2.** Palpate shoulders, including sternoclavicular joint, acromioclavicular joint, shoulder in general, humerus, and biceps groove | Nontender<br>Smooth and regular<br>Bilaterally symmetrical | Tender, painful<br>Swelling |
| **3.** Evaluate range of motion of shoulders | | |
|    **a.** Client extends arms straight up beside head (Fig. 14-18, *A*) | 180° from resting neutral position<br>Bilaterally equal<br>No discomfort | Limited range of motion<br>Pain with movement<br>Crepitations with movement<br>Asymmetry |
|    **b.** Client hyperextends arm backward (Fig. 14-18, *B*) | 50°<br>Bilaterally equal<br>No discomfort | Limited range of motion<br>Pain with movement<br>Crepitations with movement<br>Asymmetry |

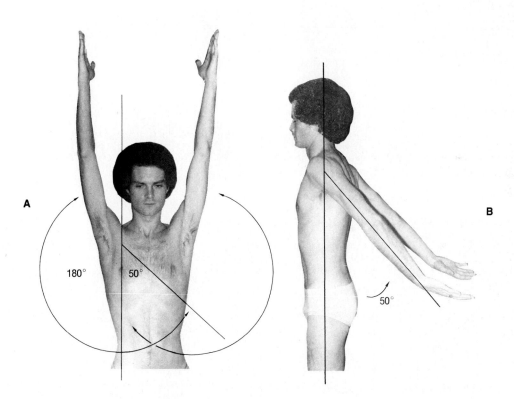

**FIG. 14-18. A,** Abduction and adduction. **B,** Hyperextension of shoulders.

## Clinical guidelines—cont'd

| THE STUDENT WILL: | TO IDENTIFY: | |
| --- | --- | --- |
| | **NORMAL** | **DEVIATIONS FROM NORMAL** |
| **c.** External (outward or lateral) rotation: client starts in abducted location with arms extended directly forward from shoulder, then places hands behind head with elbows out (Fig. 14-18, C) | 90° Bilaterally equal No discomfort | Limited range of motion Pain with movement Crepitations with movement Asymmetry |
| **d.** Internal (inward or medial) rotation: client starts with forearms extended in abducted location, then places hands behind small of back (Fig. 14-18, D) | 90° Bilaterally equal No discomfort | Limited range of motion Pain with movement Crepitations with movement Asymmetry |

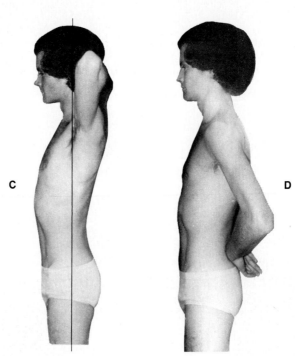

**FIG. 14-18, cont'd. C,** External rotation. **D,** Internal rotation.

### Arm muscles

(Using make/break technique)

| | | |
| --- | --- | --- |
| **1.** Deltoids: client holds arms up while examiner attempts to push them down (Fig. 14-19) | Bilaterally strong Unable to break position | Symmetrically unequal Weak response Pain during technique Muscular spasm |

| THE STUDENT WILL: | TO IDENTIFY: | |
|---|---|---|
| | NORMAL | DEVIATIONS FROM NORMAL |

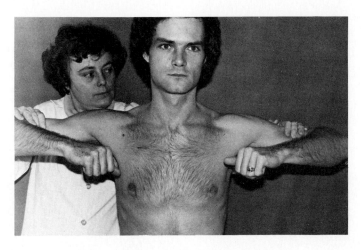

FIG. 14-19. Testing deltoid strength against resistance.

| | | |
|---|---|---|
| **2.** Biceps: client tries to flex arm into fighting position while examiner tries to extend forearm (Fig. 14-20) | Bilaterally strong<br>Unable to break position | Symmetrically unequal<br>Weak response<br>Pain during technique<br>Muscular spasm |
| **3.** Triceps: client tries to straighten forearm while examiner attempts to flex forearm (Fig. 14-21) | Bilaterally strong<br>Unable to break position | Symmetrically unequal<br>Weak response<br>Pain during technique<br>Muscular spasm |

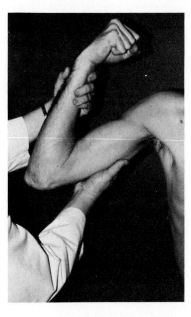

FIG. 14-20. Testing bicep strength against resistance.

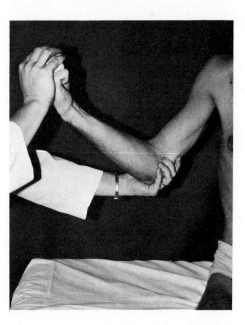

FIG. 14-21. Maintaining extended position of forearm against resistance.

## Clinical guidelines—cont'd

| THE STUDENT WILL: | TO IDENTIFY: | |
| --- | --- | --- |
| | NORMAL | DEVIATIONS FROM NORMAL |

**Feet and ankles**

| THE STUDENT WILL: | NORMAL | DEVIATIONS FROM NORMAL |
| --- | --- | --- |
| **1.** Inspect feet and ankles with client lying down | Smoothness; no swelling or deformities noted | Inflammation |
| | Toes maintain extended and straight position | Swelling over any joint |
| | Toenails intact and neatly trimmed | Gout (Fig. 14-22, *A*) |
| | Feet maintain straight position | Medial deviation of toes (Fig. 14-22, *B*) |
| | | Hallux valgus (Fig. 14-22, *C*) |
| | | Clawtoes (Fig. 14-22, *D*) |
| | | Hammer toes |
| | | Calluses |

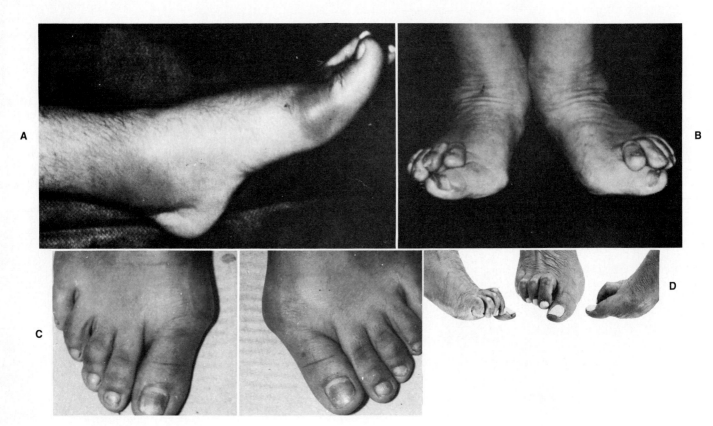

**FIG. 14-22. A,** Inflammatory response of acute gout of the great toe. **B,** Medial deviation of the great toes. **C,** Hallux valgus. **D,** Clawtoes. (**A** and **B** from Prior, J.A., Silberstein, J.S., and Stang, J.M.: Physical diagnosis: the history and examination of the patient, ed. 6, St. Louis, 1981, The C.V. Mosby Co.; **C** from American Academy of Orthopaedic surgeons: Instructional course lectures, vol. 22, St. Louis, 1973, The C.V. Mosby Co.; **D** from Mann, R.A., editor: DuVries' surgery of the foot, ed. 4, St. Louis, 1978, The C.V. Mosby Co.)

| THE STUDENT WILL: | TO IDENTIFY: | |
| --- | --- | --- |
| | NORMAL | DEVIATIONS FROM NORMAL |
| **2.** Palpate feet and ankles | Smooth<br>Nontender | Tenderness (diffuse vs. pinpoint)<br>Swelling<br>Inflammation<br>Ulcerations<br>Nodules |
| **3.** Evaluate range of motion of feet and ankles<br>  **a.** Client dorsiflexes and plantar flexes foot (Fig. 14-23) | Dorsiflexion 20° from midline position<br>Plantar flexion 45° from midline position<br>Bilaterally equal<br>No discomfort | Limited range of motion<br>Pain with movement<br>Crepitations<br>Asymmetry |

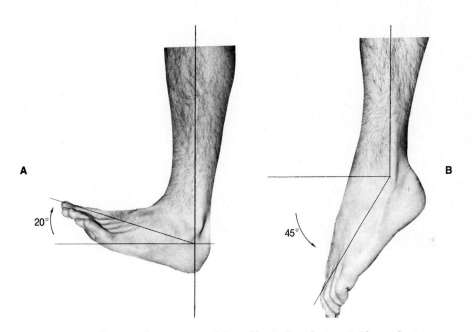

**FIG. 14-23.** Functional assessment of the ankle. **A,** Dorsiflexion. **B,** Plantar flexion.

## Clinical guidelines—cont'd

| THE STUDENT WILL: | TO IDENTIFY: | |
| --- | --- | --- |
| | NORMAL | DEVIATIONS FROM NORMAL |
| **b.** Inversion and eversion of foot (stabilize heel) (Fig. 14-24) | Inversion 30° from midline position<br>Eversion 20° from midline position<br>Bilaterally equal<br>No discomfort | Limited range of motion<br>Pain with movement<br>Crepitations<br>Asymmetry |
| **c.** Flexion and extension of toes | Active movement without discomfort | Painful movement |

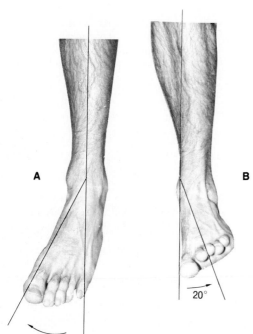

**FIG. 14-24.** Functional assessment of the ankle. **A,** Inversion. **B,** Eversion.

| | | |
| --- | --- | --- |
| **4.** Evaluate muscles of foot and ankle by make/break technique | | |
| **a.** Client is instructed to flex foot upward and maintain position; examiner presses down on big toe (Fig. 14-25) | Bilaterally strong<br>Unable to break position | Unequal<br>Weak response<br>Pain during technique |

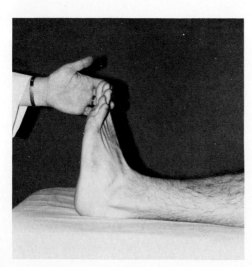

**FIG. 14-25.** Dorsiflexion of the foot against resistance.

| THE STUDENT WILL: | TO IDENTIFY: | |
| --- | --- | --- |
| | NORMAL | DEVIATIONS FROM NORMAL |

**Knee**

1. Inspect knees; note alignment and characteristics

Symmetrical
Smooth
Hollowness present adjacent to and above patella

Swelling
Bowlegged
Knock-kneed
Thickness
Bogginess
Inflammation

2. Palpate knees
   a. Palpate suprapatellar pouch on each side of quadriceps (Fig. 14-26, *A* and *B*)

Smooth, nontender

Bogginess
Thickening
Tenderness
Pain

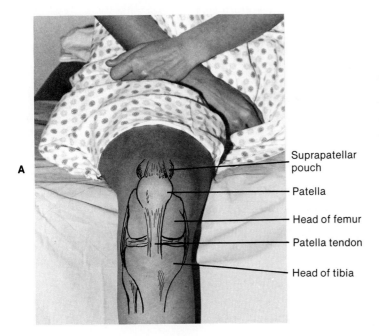
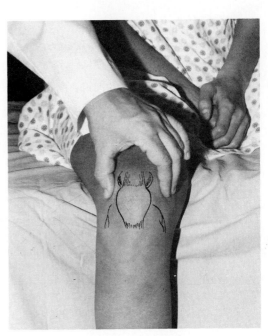

Suprapatellar pouch

Patella

Head of femur

Patella tendon

Head of tibia

**FIG. 14-26. A,** Anatomical structures of the knee. **B,** Palpation of suprapatellar pouch.

## Clinical guidelines—cont'd

| THE STUDENT WILL: | TO IDENTIFY: | |
| --- | --- | --- |
| | NORMAL | DEVIATIONS FROM NORMAL |

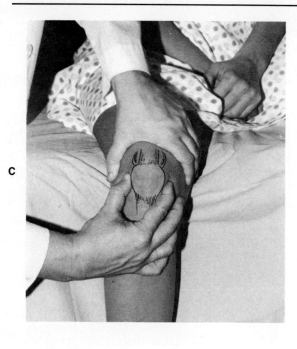

C

**FIG. 14-26, cont'd. C,** Stabilize suprapatellar pouch and palpate each side of patella and over tibiofemoral joint space.

| THE STUDENT WILL: | NORMAL | DEVIATIONS FROM NORMAL |
| --- | --- | --- |
| **b.** Compress suprapatellar pouch with one hand; palpate each side of patella and over tibiofemoral joint space (Fig. 14-26, C) | Smooth, nontender | Bogginess<br>Thickening<br>Tenderness<br>Pain |
| **c.** Palpate popliteal space | Smooth, nontender | Tenderness, redness<br>Nodules and swelling |
| **3.** Evaluate range of motion of knees by asking client to flex knees (Fig. 14-27)<br>May postpone until hip range of motion is evaluated) | 130° from straight extended position<br>No discomfort or difficulty | Decreased range of motion<br>Pain with movement<br>Crepitations |

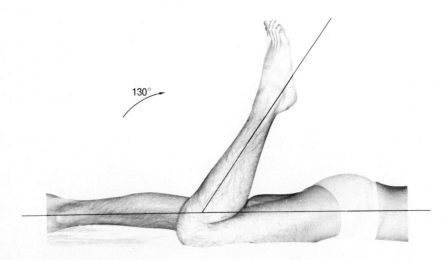

130°

**FIG. 14-27.** Evaluating knee flexion.

| THE STUDENT WILL: | TO IDENTIFY: | |
| --- | --- | --- |
| | NORMAL | DEVIATIONS FROM NORMAL |

### Hips and pelvis

**1.** With patient lying down, inspect and palpate hips for position and stability (Fig. 14-28)

Bilaterally symmetrical
Stable and painless with palpation

Painful hip area (diffuse vs. pinpoint tenderness)
Crepitations

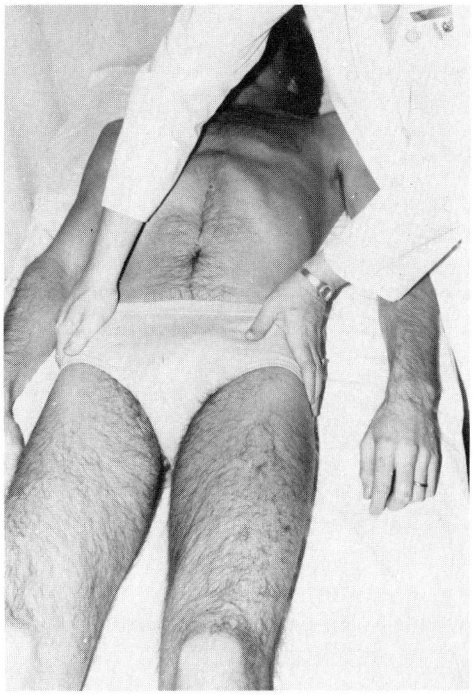

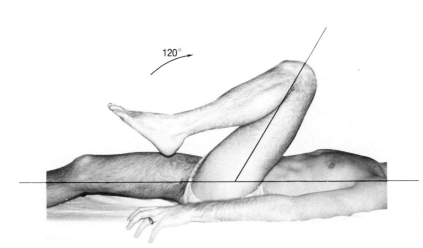

**FIG. 14-28.** Evaluating pelvic stability.

**2.** Evaluate range of motion of hip
  **a.** Instruct client to alternately pull each knee up to chest (Fig. 14-29)

120° from straight extended position

Limited range of motion
Pain or discomfort with movement
Flexion of opposite thigh
Crepitations

120°

**FIG. 14-29.** Evaluating hip flexion.

## Clinical guidelines—cont'd

| THE STUDENT WILL: | TO IDENTIFY: | |
| --- | --- | --- |
| | NORMAL | DEVIATIONS FROM NORMAL |
| **b.** Instruct client to flex hip as far as possible without bending knee (Fig. 14-30) | 90° from straight extended position | Limited range of motion<br>Pain or discomfort with movement<br>Crepitations |

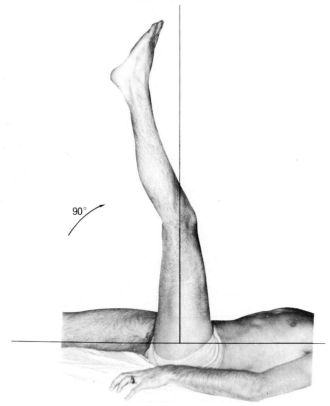

FIG. 14-30. Evaluating hip flexion with leg extended.

| | | |
| --- | --- | --- |
| **c.** Instruct client to place foot on opposite patella; press knee down laterally (external hip rotation) (Patrick test) (Fig. 14-31) | 40° from straight midline position | Limited range of motion<br>Pain or discomfort with movement<br>Crepitations |

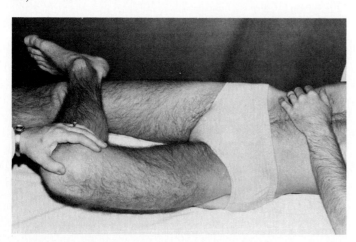

FIG. 14-31. Evaluating external rotation of hip.

| THE STUDENT WILL: | TO IDENTIFY: | |
| --- | --- | --- |
| | NORMAL | DEVIATIONS FROM NORMAL |
| **d.** Instruct client to flex knee and turn medially (or inward); examiner pulls heel laterally (or outward) (internal hip rotation) (Fig. 14-32) | 40° from straight midline position | Limited range of motion<br>Pain or discomfort with movement<br>Crepitations |

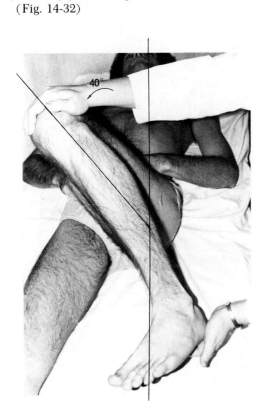

**FIG. 14-32.** Internal hip rotation.

### Leg, hip, and pelvis muscles

(Using make/break technique)

| | | |
| --- | --- | --- |
| **1.** Hip strength: client in supine position attempts to raise legs while examiner tries to hold them down; evaluate one leg at a time | Bilaterally strong<br>Unable to break position | Symmetrically unequal<br>Weak response<br>Pain during technique |

## Clinical guidelines—cont'd

| THE STUDENT WILL: | TO IDENTIFY: | |
| --- | --- | --- |
| | NORMAL | DEVIATIONS FROM NORMAL |
| 2. Hamstrings, gluteals, abductors, and adductors: instruct client to sit and alternately cross legs (Fig. 14-33) | Able to perform<br>Bilaterally equal and without difficulty | Unable to perform<br>Performs with pain or great difficulty |

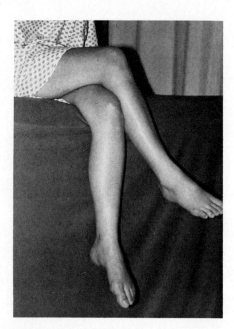

**FIG. 14-33.** Assessment of adductors and hamstring.

| | | |
| --- | --- | --- |
| 3. Quadriceps: client extends leg at knee; examiner attempts to flex knee (Fig. 14-34) | Bilaterally strong<br>Unable to flex knee | Symmetrically unequal<br>Weak response<br>Pain during technique |

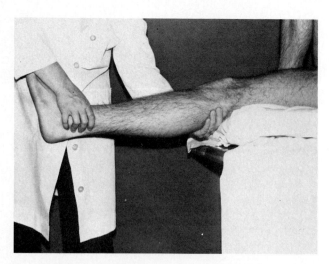

**FIG. 14-34.** Maintaining extended position of anterior thigh muscles against resistance.

| THE STUDENT WILL: | TO IDENTIFY: | |
| --- | --- | --- |
| | NORMAL | DEVIATIONS FROM NORMAL |
| **4.** Hamstrings: client tries to bend knee while examiner attempts to straighten knee (Fig. 14-35) | Bilaterally strong<br>Unable to flex knee | Symmetrically unequal<br>Weak response<br>Pain during technique |

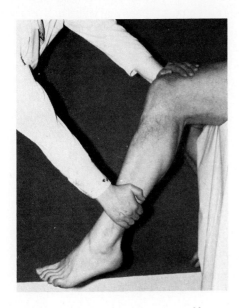

**FIG. 14-35.** Maintaining flexed position of hamstring against resistance.

**Special techniques**

1. Knee evaluation
   **a.** Fluid within knee joint
      1. Palpate patella against femur with leg in full extension; tap on one side of joint
   **b.** Drawer test (to evaluate intactness of cruciate ligaments): client in supine position, knee flexed at right angle; examiner sits on client's foot, thus fixing it on examining table
      1. Instruct client to relax muscle in flexed leg

| | | |
| --- | --- | --- |
| | No fluid waves or bulging on opposite side of joint | Fluid waves palpable on opposite side of joint |

## Clinical guidelines—cont'd

| | TO IDENTIFY: | |
|---|---|---|
| **THE STUDENT WILL:** | **NORMAL** | **DEVIATIONS FROM NORMAL** |
| 2. Press head of tibia forward or backward with both hands (Fig. 14-36) | Unable to displace its position | Tibia can be pulled anteriorly from under femur (indicates injury to anterior cruciate ligament)<br><br>Tibia can be pushed posteriorly from under femur (indicates injury to posterior cruciate ligament) |

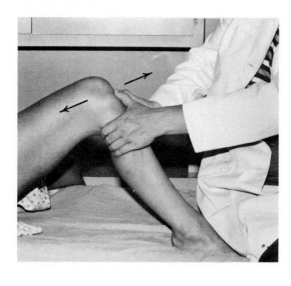

**FIG. 14-36.** Performing drawer test.

| | | |
|---|---|---|
| c. McMurray test (to evaluate presence of damaged or torn meniscus): client is supine with knees and hips strongly flexed toward chest | | |
| 1. Stabilize one hand on client's knee with thumb and index finger on either side of joint space; with other hand, grasp client's heel; with both hands, externally rotate knee and abduct leg at same time (Fig. 14-37) | Stable knee<br>No discomfort | Positive findings: pain, clicking feeling, or inability to extend lower leg |

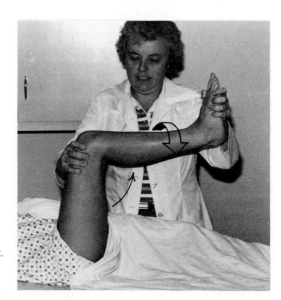

**FIG. 14-37.** Performing McMurray test.

| | TO IDENTIFY: | |
|---|---|---|
| **THE STUDENT WILL:** | **NORMAL** | **DEVIATIONS FROM NORMAL** |

**2.** Hip evaluation

   **a.** Thomas test (to evaluate for flexion contractures of hip): client supine

      1. Instruct client to pull one knee up toward chest as far as possible

| | | |
|---|---|---|
| | Easy flexion<br>Opposite leg remains flat on table (Fig. 14-38, *A*) | Opposite leg and hip flex in response to flexing leg<br>Note degree of flexion (Fig. 14-38, *B*) |

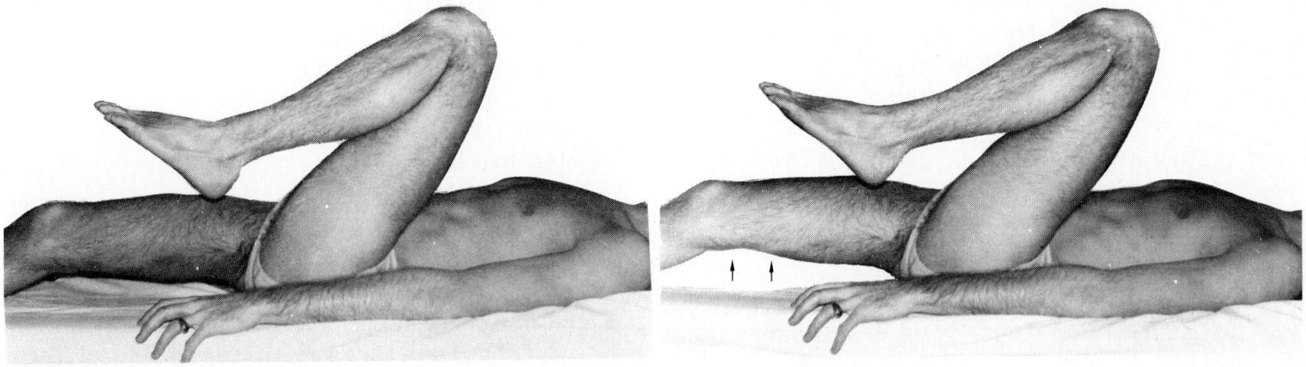

**FIG. 14-38.** Thomas test. **A,** Negative. **B,** Positive.

**3.** Low back pain evaluation

   **a.** Four specific areas of assessment

      1. Observe curvature of lumbar region

      2. Observe trunk positioning

      3. Palpate erector muscles of spine

      4. Evaluate range of motion of lumbar spine

| | | |
|---|---|---|
| | Lumbar lordosis: concavity of lumbar region | Reversal or flattening of lumbar curvature |
| | Upright trunk position | Slightly flexed back<br>Slight lateral bending of trunk |
| | Muscle not in spasm<br>Nontender muscles | Muscle spasms of erector group<br>Tender |
| | | Limited, difficult, or painful range of motion |

   **b.** Laségue sign, or sciatic stretch test (to evaluate low back pain arising from nerve root irritation): client supine

      1. Perform single and alternating straight leg raising

| | | |
|---|---|---|
| | Tightness may be felt, but should be no pain | Pain felt with elevation of leg; then flex knee: pain should be gone as leg further raised |

   **c.** Evaluation of lumbar disc injury

      1. Observe client supine and perform alternating straight leg raising

| | | |
|---|---|---|
| | Tightness may be felt, but should be no pain | Pain felt with elevation of leg<br>Dorsiflexion of foot causes feeling of pressure in lumbosacral area |

## Clinical strategies

1. Assessment of the musculoskeletal system should begin as the client enters the examination room. Use that time to observe ambulatory capabilities and body posturing.

2. Assessment of the musculoskeletal system involves an individual evaluation of bone stability, joint function, and muscle strength and function. The clinical guidelines describe in detail what the examiner must do, as well as the anticipated response. It is essential that the examiner *continuously* keep in mind *what* bones, muscles, or joints are being evaluated as well as the *normal* anticipated response.

3. Many clients complain of vague aches or muscular weakness. The examiner must thoroughly explore the complaint as well as perform a systematic evaluation. In addition, the examiner should watch how the client moves, postures, rises from a sitting position, takes off a coat, and so on.

4. A key consideration when evaluating the musculoskeletal system is symmetry.

5. The client must be undressed. This means shoes and socks, too.

6. It does not matter whether the examination sequence is from the top down or vice versa, but a method of client assessment must be developed and maintained every time a client is evaluated.

7. How much and what type of musculoskeletal assessment each client requires will be individually determined. A young athlete who comes to see the examiner for a college physical will require a basic screening evaluation, whereas a 67-year-old chronically ill woman will require a more thorough assessment. Many times the data collection and early inspection of the client's ability to ambulate, sit, and undress are keys for determining the necessary extent of the assessment.

8. It should be remembered that the practitioner's purpose in collecting data about the musculoskeletal system is to assess the client's functional capabilities, including activities of daily living. If the examiner isolates areas of distress or injury, the client should be referred to the physician for differential diagnosis.

9. While performing extremity evaluation, the examiner should incorporate the assessment of the skin, peripheral vascular system, and neurological system.

10. If the examiner notes a difference in muscle size or in arm or leg diameter or length, a measurement should be recorded. A circumference or length difference of more than 1 cm should be considered abnormal. The examiner *must* be careful to measure from the same spot bilaterally.

11. The technique for measuring the range of motion of a joint follows:
    a. Start with joint in fully extended position.
    b. When the joint is flexed as much as possible, the angle is measured. This is recorded as the angle of greatest flexion (AGF).

12. Although normal flexion angles of joints have been identified in this text, the examiner should realize that there are many deviations from these angles that are considered normal for various individuals of different ages. It is most important that the examiner compare one side of the client's body to the other when measuring angles and considering abnormal findings.

13. Many techniques can be used to measure muscle strength, from actual number scoring to evaluation of minimal or severe weakness. We have used the make/break screening technique to grossly evaluate the client's ability to make and maintain a flexed position while the examiner attempts to break the position. When using this technique, the examiner instructs the client to flex the limb or muscle group being tested and to maintain that position. Then the examiner exerts a steady, gentle retraction against the client's flexed position. The retraction should last 2 to 3 seconds for each position tested. The examiner should apply the same degree of retraction strength against each position being tested.

Although the results will be interpreted subjectively, the examiner will, with practice, determine what an abnormal response is for his or her own strength.

An absolute baseline of muscle testing involves the client's ability to move the limbs or trunk against gravity (e.g., lifting the arm up in the air). Any client who has difficulty moving the trunk or limbs against gravity should be referred for further evaluation.

---

### SAMPLE RECORDING

Muscular development and skeletal structure bilaterally equal, normal for age. No joint deformities, tenderness, or crepitations. Full active range of motion without pain. Normal spinal curve without deformity. No spinal tenderness on palpation. Adequate muscle tone and strength bilaterally.

## History and clinical strategies: the pediatric client

1. Assessment of the child's musculoskeletal system can range from a basic functional screening examination to an extensive joint-by-joint evaluation. The extent of the actual evaluation should be determined for each individual child, based on subjective data as well as gross objective assessment. An active and coordinated toddler who demonstrates basic gross and fine motor functioning appropriate for age will require a less extensive musculoskeletal assessment than a 7-year-old complaining of joint pains and generalized weakness.

2. To subjectively evaluate motor functioning appropriate for age, the examiner must be aware of normal values. Table 14-1 details the sequencing of motor development and approximate age of achievement. The practitioner should consider this sequence when collecting data base information. Any child who lags behind in two or more areas at any given age should be carefully evaluated. Although it is unrealistic to believe that all children develop at the normal rate, nonmastery of these criteria should serve as red flags indicating necessity of a thorough physical evaluation. Conversely, an active, playful, and maturing child who is on or ahead of schedule will need a less detailed evaluation. Some of the values in Table 14-1 have been extracted from the Denver Developmental Screening Test (DDST). Children who appear to be lagging behind in musculoskeletal development may be screened more closely through tests such as the DDST.

*Text continued on p. 447.*

**TABLE 14-1.** Normal age and sequence of motor development in children

| AGE | FINE MOTOR | GROSS MOTOR |
|---|---|---|
| 4 weeks (1 month) | Following with eyes to midline | Turns head to side<br>Keeps knees tucked under abdomen (Fig. 14-39)<br>When pulled to sitting position, has gross head lag and rounded swayed back (Fig. 14-40) |

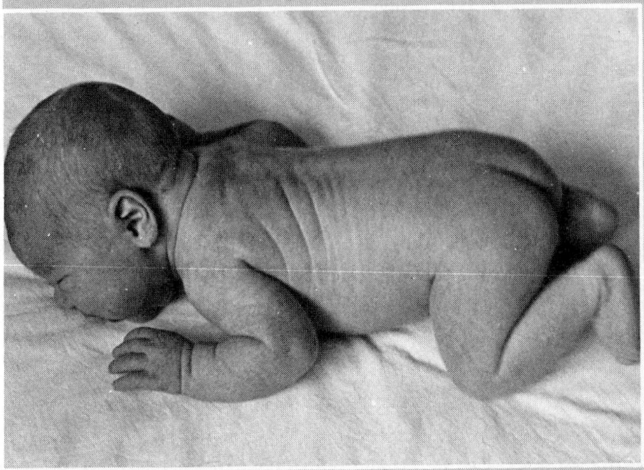

FIG. 14-39. (From Whaley, L.F., and Wong, D.L.: Nursing care of infants and children, ed. 2, St. Louis, 1983, The C.V. Mosby Co.)

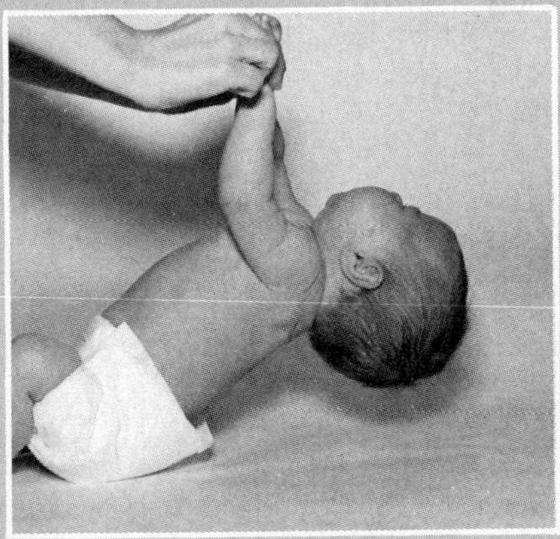

FIG. 14-40. (From Whaley, L.F., and Wong, D.L.: Nursing care of infants and children, ed. 2, St. Louis, 1983, The C.V. Mosby Co.)

Data from Frankenburg, W.K., and Dodds, J.B.: Denver Developmental Screening Test, Denver, 1969, University of Colorado Medical Center.

*Continued.*

**TABLE 14-1.** Normal age and sequence of motor development in children—cont'd

| AGE | FINE MOTOR | GROSS MOTOR |
|-----|-----------|-------------|
| 8 weeks (2 months) | Follows objects well; may not follow past midline (major developmental milestone) | Holds head in same plane as rest of body (Fig. 14-41) Can raise head and maintain position; looks downward |

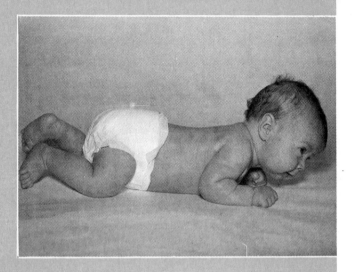

**FIG. 14-41.** (From Whaley, L.F., and Wong, D.L.: Nursing care of infants and children, ed. 2, St. Louis, 1983, The C.V. Mosby Co.)

| AGE | FINE MOTOR | GROSS MOTOR |
|-----|-----------|-------------|
| 12 weeks (3 months) | Follows past midline (Fig. 14-42) When in supine position, puts hands together; will hold hands in front of face | Raises head to 45° angle Maintains posture; looks around with head May turn from prone to side position When pulled into sitting position, shows only slight head lag (Fig. 14-43) |

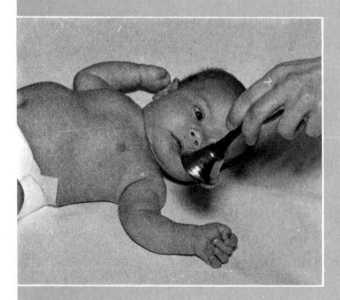

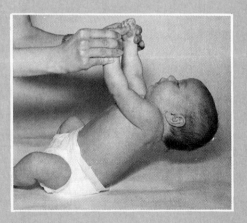

**FIG. 14-42.** (From Whaley, L.F., and Wong, D.L.: Nursing care of infants and children, ed. 2, St. Louis, 1983, The C.V. Mosby Co.)

**FIG. 14-43.** (From Whaley, L.F., and Wong, D.L.: Nursing care of infants and children, ed. 2, St. Louis, 1983, The C.V. Mosby Co.)

**TABLE 14-1.** Normal age and sequence of motor development in children—cont'd

| AGE | FINE MOTOR | GROSS MOTOR |
| --- | --- | --- |
| 16 weeks (4 months) | Grasps rattle (Fig. 14-44)<br>Plays with hands together | Actively lifts head up and looks around (Fig. 14-45)<br>Will roll from prone to supine position<br>When pulled to sitting position, no longer has head lag (Fig. 14-46)<br>When held in standing position, attempts to maintain some weight support |

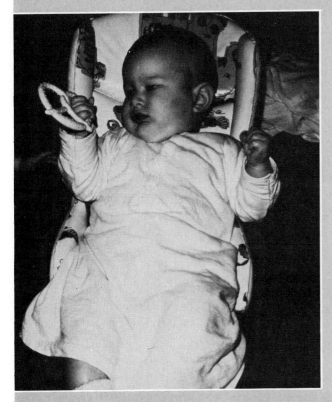

**FIG. 14-44.** (From Bailey, R.A., and Burton E.C.: The dynamic self: activities to enhance infant development, St. Louis, 1982, The C.V. Mosby Co.)

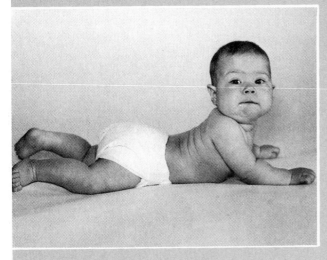

**FIG. 14-45.** (From Whaley, L.F., and Wong, D.L.: Nursing care of infants and children, ed. 2, St. Louis, 1983, The C.V. Mosby Co.)

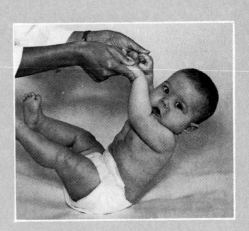

**FIG. 14-46.** (From Whaley, L.F., and Wong, D.L.: Nursing care of infants and children, ed. 2, St. Louis, 1983, The C.V. Mosby Co.)

*Continued.*

**TABLE 14-1.** Normal age and sequence of motor development in children—cont'd

| AGE | FINE MOTOR | GROSS MOTOR |
|---|---|---|
| 20 weeks (5 months) | Can reach and pick up object<br>May play with toes (Fig. 14-47) | Able to push up from prone position and maintain weight on forearms (Fig. 14-48)<br>Rolls from prone to supine and back to prone<br>Maintains straight back when in sitting position (Fig. 14-49) |

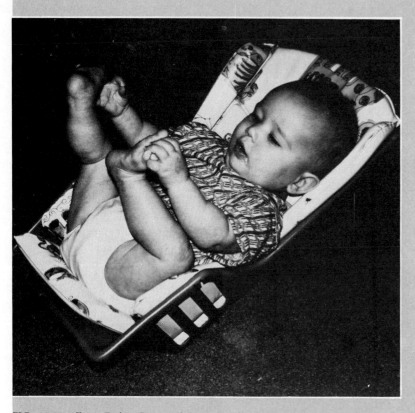

FIG. 14-47. (From Bailey, R.A., and Burton, E.C.: The dynamic self: activities to enhance infant development, St. Louis, 1982, The C.V. Mosby Co.)

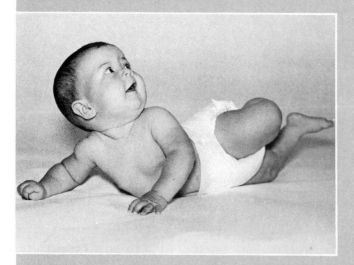

FIG. 14-48. (From Whaley, L.F., and Wong, D.L.: Nursing care of infants and children, ed. 2, St. Louis, 1983, The C.V. Mosby Co.)

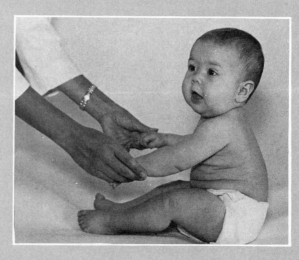

FIG. 14-49. (From Whaley, L.F., and Wong, D.L.: Nursing care of infants and children, ed. 2, St. Louis, 1983, The C.V. Mosby Co.)

**TABLE 14-1.** Normal age and sequence of motor development in children—cont'd

| AGE | FINE MOTOR | GROSS MOTOR |
|---|---|---|
| 24 weeks (6 months) | Will hold spoon or rattle<br>Will drop object and reach for second offered object | Begins to raise abdomen off table<br>Sits, but posture still shaky<br>May sit with legs apart and hands (arms straight) as prop between legs (Fig. 14-50)<br>Supports almost full weight when pulled to standing position |
| 28 weeks (7 months) | Can transfer object, one hand to another<br>Grasps objects in each hand | Sits alone; still uses hands for support<br>When held in standing position bounces (Fig. 14-51)<br>Pulls feet to mouth |

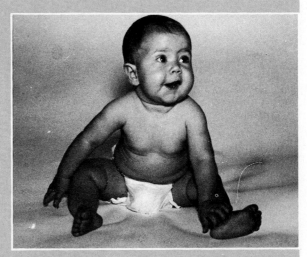

**FIG. 14-50.** (From Whaley, L.F., and Wong, D.L.: Nursing care of infants and children, ed. 2, St. Louis, 1983, The C.V. Mosby Co.)

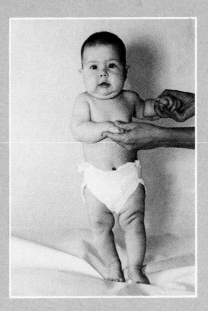

**FIG. 14-51.** (From Whaley, L.F., and Wong, D.L.: Nursing care of infants and children, ed. 2, St. Louis, 1983, The C.V. Mosby Co.)

*Continued.*

**TABLE 14-1.** Normal age and sequence of motor development in children—cont'd

| AGE | FINE MOTOR | GROSS MOTOR |
|---|---|---|
| 32 weeks (8 months) | Beginning thumb-finger grasping (Fig. 14-52) | Sits securely without support (major developmental milestone) (Fig. 14-53) |

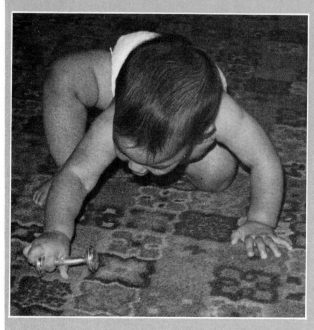

FIG. 14-52.(From Whaley, L.F., and Wong, D.L.: Nursing care of infants and children, ed. 2, St. Louis, 1983, The C.V. Mosby Co.)

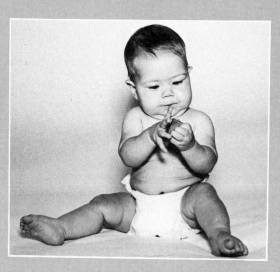

FIG. 14-53.(From Whaley, L.F., and Wong, D.L.: Nursing care of infants and children, ed. 2, St. Louis, 1983, The C.V. Mosby Co.)

| AGE | FINE MOTOR | GROSS MOTOR |
|---|---|---|
| 36 weeks (9 months) | Continued development of thumb-finger grasp<br><br>May bang objects together | Steady sitting; can lean forward and still maintain position<br>Begins creeping (abdomen off floor) (Fig. 14-54)<br>Can stand holding onto stabilizing object when placed in that position; still may not be able to pull self into standing position |

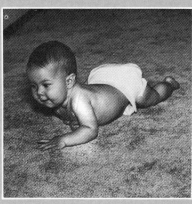

FIG. 14-54. (From Whaley, L.F., and Wong, D.L.: Nursing care of infants and children, ed. 2, St. Louis, 1983, The C.V. Mosby Co.)

**TABLE 14-1.** Normal age and sequence of motor development in children—cont'd

| AGE | FINE MOTOR | GROSS MOTOR |
|---|---|---|
| 40 weeks (10 months) | Practices picking up small objects (Fig. 14-55)<br>Points with one finger<br>Will offer toys to people but unable to let go of object | Can pull self into standing position; unable to let self down again (Fig. 14-56) |

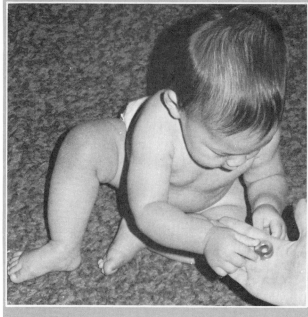

FIG. 14-55. (From Whaley, L.F., and Wong, D.L.: Nursing care of infants and children, ed. 2, St. Louis, 1983, The C.V. Mosby Co.)

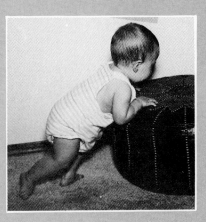

FIG. 14-56. (From Whaley, L.F., and Wong, D.L.: Nursing care of infants and children, ed. 2, St. Louis, 1983, The C.V. Mosby Co.)

| AGE | FINE MOTOR | GROSS MOTOR |
|---|---|---|
| 44 weeks (11 months) | | Moves about room holding onto objects (Fig. 14-57) |

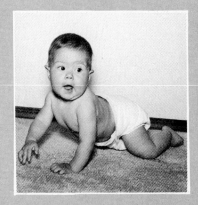

FIG. 14-57. (From Whaley, L.F., and Wong, D.L.: Nursing care of infants and children, ed. 2, St. Louis, 1983, The C.V. Mosby Co.)

*Continued.*

**TABLE 14-1.** Normal age and sequence of motor development in children—cont'd

| AGE | FINE MOTOR | GROSS MOTOR |
|---|---|---|
| | | Preparing to walk independently, wide-base stance (Fig. 14-58)<br>Stands securely, holding on with one hand |

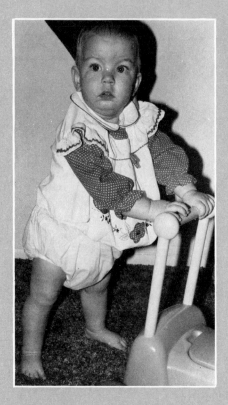

FIG. 14-58

| | | |
|---|---|---|
| 48 weeks (12 months) | May hold cup and spoon and feed self fairly well with practice (Fig. 14-59) | Able to twist and turn and maintain posture<br>Able to sit from standing position |

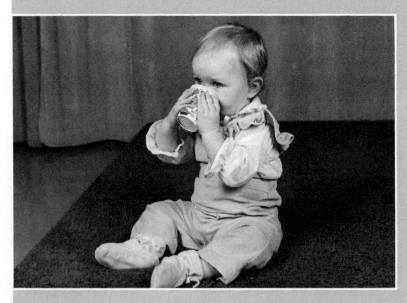

**FIG. 14-59.** (From The baby checkup book by Sheila Hillman. Copyright © 1982 by Hillman Press. By permission of Bantam Books, Inc. All rights reserved.)

**TABLE 14-1.** Normal age and sequence of motor development in children—cont'd

| AGE | FINE MOTOR | GROSS MOTOR |
| --- | --- | --- |

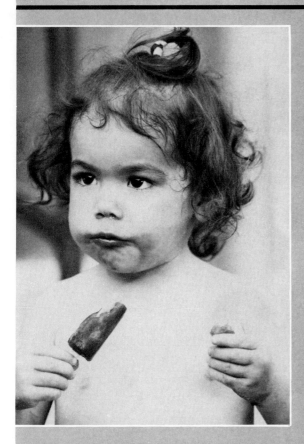

FIG. 14-70. (From Powell, M.L.: Assessment and management of developmental changes and problems in children, ed. 2, St. Louis, 1981, The C.V. Mosby Co.)

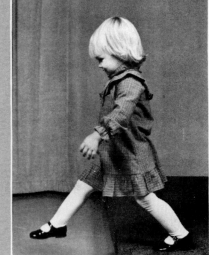

FIG. 14-71. (From The baby checkup book by Sheila Hillman. Copyright © 1982 by Hillman Press. By permission of Bantam Books, Inc. All rights reserved.)

*Continued.*

**TABLE 14-1.** Normal age and sequence of motor development in children—cont'd

| AGE | FINE MOTOR | GROSS MOTOR |
| --- | --- | --- |
| 3 years | Can unbutton front buttons<br>Copies vertical line within 30°<br>Copies "O"<br>Able to build eight-cube tower (Fig. 14-72) | Walks upstairs, alternating feet on steps<br>Walks downstairs, two feet on each step<br>Pedals tricycle<br>Jumps in place<br>Able to perform broad jump |
| 4 years | Able to copy "+"<br>Picks longer line three out of three times | Walks downstairs, alternating feet on steps<br>(Fig. 14-73) |

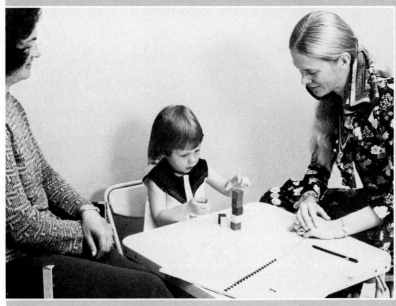

**FIG. 14-72.** (From Powell, M.L.: Assessment and management of developmental changes and problems in children, ed. 2, St. Louis, 1981, The C.V. Mosby Co.)

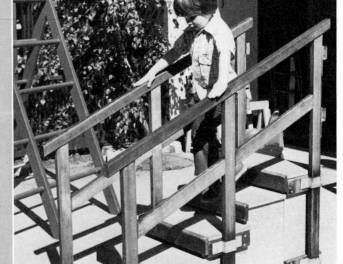

**FIG. 14-73.** (From Powell, M.L.: Assessment and management of developmental changes and problems in children, ed. 2, St. Louis, 1981, The C.V. Mosby Co.)

**TABLE 14-1.** Normal age and sequence of motor development in children—cont'd

| AGE | FINE MOTOR | GROSS MOTOR |
|---|---|---|
| | Draws a stick man (Fig. 14-74) | Able to button large front buttons<br>Able to balance on one foot for approximately 5 seconds (Fig. 14-75) |

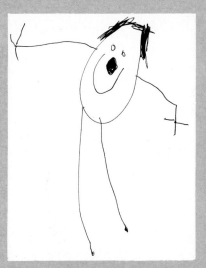

**FIG. 14-74**

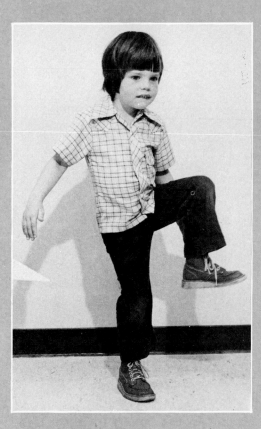

**FIG. 14-75.** (From Powell, M.L.: Assessment and management of developmental changes and problems in children, ed. 2, St. Louis, 1981, The C.V. Mosby Co.)

*Continued.*

**TABLE 14-1.** Normal age and sequence of motor development in children—cont'd

| AGE | FINE MOTOR | GROSS MOTOR |
|---|---|---|
| 5 years | Able to dress self with minimal assistance (Fig. 14-76)<br>Able to draw three-part human figure<br>Draws ☐ following demonstration<br>Colors within lines | Hops on one foot<br>Catches ball bounced to child two out of three times<br>Able to demonstrate heel-toe walking |

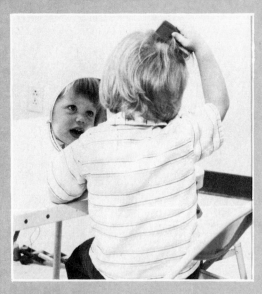

**FIG. 14-76.** (From Powell, M.L.: Assessment and management of developmental changes and problems in children, ed. 2, St. Louis, 1981, The C.V. Mosby Co.)

| AGE | FINE MOTOR | GROSS MOTOR |
|---|---|---|
| 6 years | Copies ☐<br>Draws six-part human figure (Fig. 14-77)<br>Printing skills increase | Jumps, tumbles, skips, hops<br>Able to walk straight line<br>Able to skip rope with practice<br>Able to ride two-wheel bicycle<br>Able to demonstrate heel-toe backward walking |

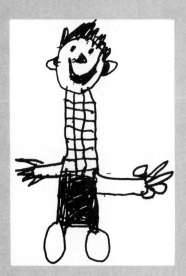

**FIG. 14-77**

**TABLE 14-1.** Normal age and sequence of motor development in children—cont'd

| AGE | FINE MOTOR | GROSS MOTOR |
|---|---|---|
| 7 years | Able to read small print<br>Able to print well (Fig. 14-78)<br>Able to write in script with practice (Fig. 14-79) | Able to play hopscotch and to skip well<br>Running, climbing abilities becoming more co-ordinated |

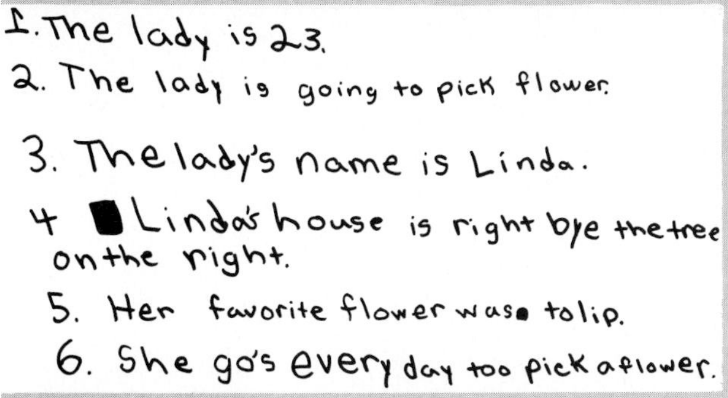

1. The lady is 23.
2. The lady is going to pick flower.
3. The lady's name is Linda.
4. ■ Linda's house is right bye the tree on the right.
5. Her favorite flower was a tolip.
6. She go's every day too pick a flower.

FIG. 14-78

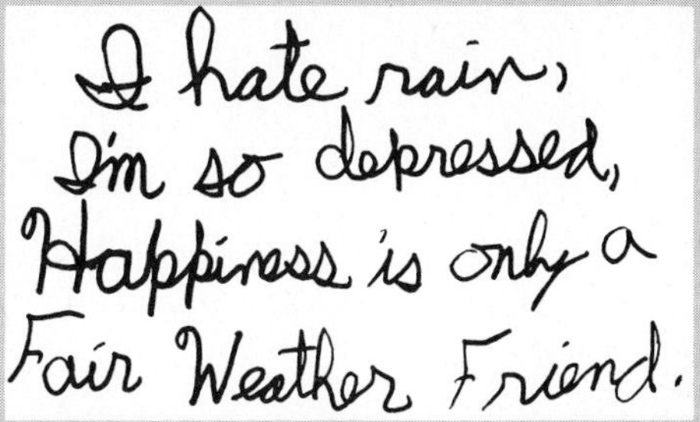

I hate rain,
I'm so depressed,
Happiness is only a
Fair Weather Friend.

FIG. 14-79

| 8 years | Handwriting skills show maturity | Movements become more graceful (Fig. 14-80) |

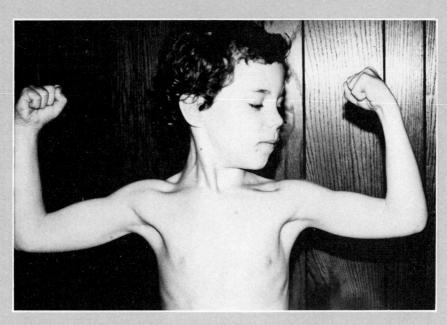

**FIG. 14-80.** Assessing the musculoskeletal system of a cooperative 7-year-old.

*Continued.*

**TABLE 14-1.** Normal age and sequence of motor development in children—cont'd

| AGE | FINE MOTOR | GROSS MOTOR |
|---|---|---|
| 9 years | Writing and drawing skills continue to show maturity and less awkwardness (Fig. 14-81) | Development of hand-eye coordination; assists with playing baseball, basketball, soccer (Fig. 14-82) |

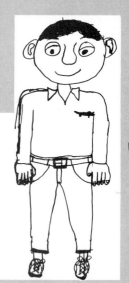

B

A

I'm getting a higher bunk bed.
I'm getting a bigger bike.
I'm getting to cross Connecticut Ave.
     all by my self if I like.
I'm getting to help do dishes.
I'm getting to weed the yard.
I'm getting to think that 11
     could be hard.

**FIG. 14-81**

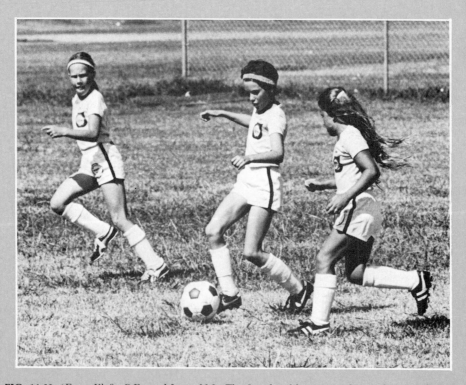

**FIG. 14-82.** (From Klafs, C.E., and Lyon, M.J.: The female athlete: a coach's guide to conditioning and training, ed. 2, St. Louis, 1978, The C.V. Mosby Co.)

**TABLE 14-1.** Normal age and sequence of motor development in children—cont'd

| AGE | FINE MOTOR | GROSS MOTOR |
|---|---|---|
| 10 years | | Girls taller than boys<br>Continued sports and coordinated activities (Fig. 14-83)<br>Physically more active |

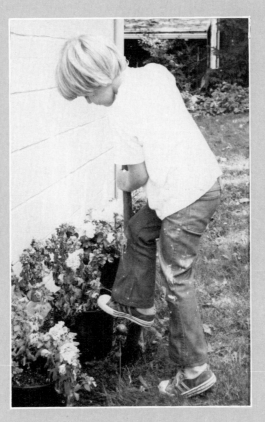

**FIG. 14-83.** (From Powell, M.L.: Assessment and management of developmental changes and problems in children, ed. 2, St. Louis, 1981, The C.V. Mosby Co.)

| | | |
|---|---|---|
| 11 years | | May appear awkward because of preadolescent growth spurt<br>May do less well in sports |

*Continued.*

**TABLE 14-1.** Normal age and sequence of motor development in children—cont'd

| AGE | FINE MOTOR | GROSS MOTOR |
|---|---|---|
| 12 years | | Growth spurt begins<br>Coordination decreases (Fig. 14-84) |

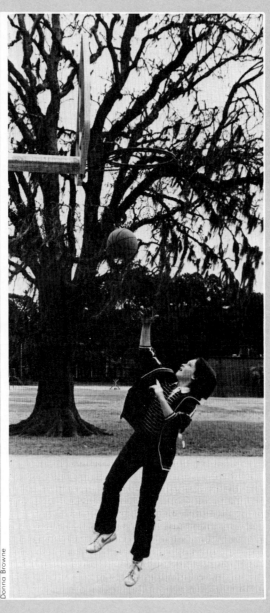

**FIG. 14-84.** (From Godow, A.G.: Human sexuality, St. Louis, 1982, The C.V. Mosby Co.)

| AGE | FINE MOTOR | GROSS MOTOR |
|---|---|---|
| 13 years | | Continues to have coordination difficulty<br>Poor posture may become problem |

3. The approach used to examine the musculoskeletal system in the child will vary greatly, depending on the child's age.

   a. Up to 6 months (Fig. 14-85). Assessment should be done with the child undressed to the diaper and supine on the examining table or the parent's lap. Although the examiner should observe the symmetry and overall kicking and wiggling movement of the child, the actual palpation and joint and muscle evaluation is done with the child's passive participation. As the child becomes older, the examiner must position the child in a way that facilitates the evaluation. For example, place a 4-month-old in a prone position to evaluate his ability to push up on hands and roll from a prone to a supine position; place in a standing position to evaluate muscle strength of the legs.

   b. Six months to 1 year (Fig. 14-60). Approach the child slowly. Start the evaluation by playing with his fingers and toes. As the child becomes accustomed to your touching, slowly move from distal limb evaluation to neck, hip, and spine evaluation. Much can be observed about the child's musculoskeletal and neurological systems by watching the child sitting and playing with hands and feet. If the examiner charges toward the child and frightens him, the child may stiffen up, cry, or decide not to cooperate. An inaccurate musculoskeletal evaluation will follow.

   c. One to 3 years (Fig. 14-86). The examiner should let the toddler show off a little: watch him walk, play with blocks, and climb onto the examining table. Much can be learned about the development and functioning of the musculoskeletal system through observation.

      Once the child is situated for the examination, the examiner should again start with the hands and feet. To evaluate the child's range of motion and ability to follow directions, a game of imitation might follow: instruct the child to "Do as I do"; if that does not work, games such as catching and kicking a ball, building a tower of blocks, and playing peek-a-boo may facilitate the examination.

      Although much of the assessment can be done by playing and watching, techniques such as hip examination require specific manipulations that must be working into the total physical evaluation.

   d. Three to 6 years (Fig. 14-87). A slow, "let's play" approach is still helpful for the unsure preschooler. The examiner should watch the child undress and climb onto the examination table. The child should be ready to play hopping

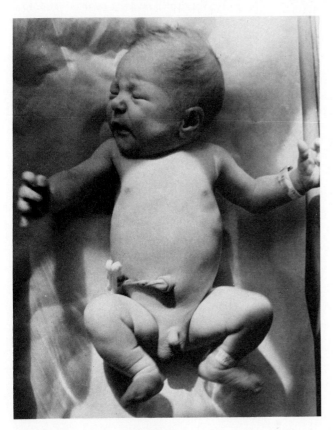

**FIG. 14-85.** Make a general observation of the musculoskeletal system of the neonate.

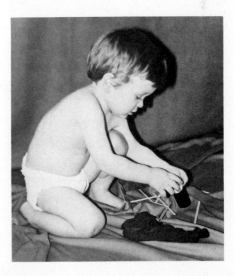

**FIG. 14-86.** Make a general observation of the musculoskeletal system of the toddler.

games and jumping, squatting, and bending exercises that will facilitate the physical evaluation. The challenge for the examiner with this age child is to invent techniques that will evoke cooperation from the child. Sometimes a game of "Simon Says" works. For example, "Simon says keep your arm as stiff as a tree and don't let me push it down."

e. Over age 6 years (Fig. 14-80). These children should be ready to fully cooperate with the examiner. The degree of cooperation will usually depend on how the examiner approaches the child. The brisk examiner may get less cooperation and fewer data than will the examiner who takes a few minutes to play with the child, watch him write his name, and demonstrate how strong he is by allowing him to show off his muscles and squeeze the examiner's hand.

4. Many parents may express concern that their children have foot problems. Following are some principles of foot evaluation:

a. Examine the foot for complete range of motion.
b. Do not limit the evaluation to the foot only; also evaluate for stability, deformity, and range of motion of the knee, hip, and spine.
c. Palpate the underside of the foot to evaluate for deformities of the forefoot or the hindfoot.
d. Observe for tibial torsion or bowing.
e. Observe the older infant or child walking without shoes. (Note that a cold floor on bare feet may distort the child's gait.)
f. Observe for muscular weakness or asymmetry.
g. Inspect the child's shoes for evidence of abnormal wear. Normal heel-toe gait wears the shoes more on the outer border of the heel and the inner border of the toe. Toddlers will normally wear down the medial edge of the shoe first.
h. Inspect the child's shoes for size and general fit.
   (1) High shoes that cover the ankle are necessary only if the child walks out of low-cut shoes. The ankles are not supported by high shoes, nor is the support necessary.
   (2) Shoes should be long enough to allow the thumb to be pressed between the end of the big toe and the end of the shoe while the child maintains a weight-bearing position.
i. Evaluation for flat feet
   (1) Before a child begins to walk, the foot does not actually have any arch.
   (2) When a child first begins to stand, the feet normaly pronate slightly inward (Fig. 14-88). The child assumes a wide-base stance, and the weight line normally falls toward the inner side of the foot.

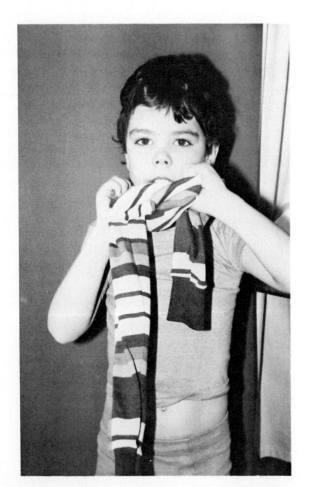

**FIG. 14-87.** Make a general observation of the musculoskeletal system of the preschooler.

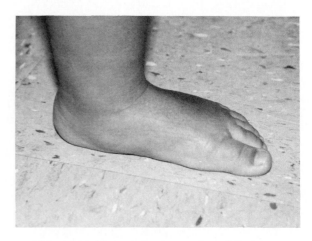

**FIG. 14-88.** Normal pronation of a toddler's foot.

(3) Between 12 and 30 months the arch strengthens, and the weight bearing falls more directly with the middle of the foot (Fig. 14-89).

(4) Any child older than 30 months whose feet maintain a pronated medial position in which the medial border of the foot becomes prominent should be referred for further evaluation.

j. Evaluation for pigeon toes

(1) Many children may demonstrate inward bending of the foot (either of the ankle or toes), the tibia (tibial torsion), or the femur (femoral torsion).

(2) If the examiner notes any inward bending of any of these areas, the child should be referred for further evaluation.

k. Evaluation of toe walking. Babies and older children may demonstrate toeing downward or toe-walking techniques. Toe walking may be normal, or it may be found in children with spastic

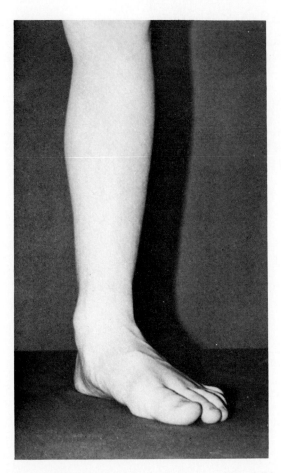

**FIG. 14-89.** Normal arch of a foot in an older child.

diseases, congenital shortening of the Achilles tendon, early muscular dystrophy, or infantile autism. The examiner should manually dorsiflex the child's foot to evaluate the stretchability of the Achilles tendon. Any child with a tight or shortened Achilles tendon (dorsiflexion less than 20 degrees) should be referred. Likewise, any child demonstrating other musculoskeletal or neurological problems should be referred.

5. Children may complain of muscular aches and pains. Although a thorough history and physical evaluation are mandatory, the examiner must also be aware of normal "growing pains." Boys between 11 and 18 years and girls between 9 and 16 years experience rapid growth spurts. At times the skeletal system grows faster than the muscular system; therefore the children may feel discomfort in their limbs.

6. Curvature of the spine is a common finding in children, particularly during puberty. There are two types of scoliosis:

a. Functional: This is the most frequency type found in young children. The spine is curved when the child stands, but if the child bends over to touch his toes, the curvature disappears.

b. Idiopathic: The spine remains curved when the child is sitting as well as bending forward.

There is pelvic tilt, and there may be a shortened leg. Even though all children must be evaluated for lateral spinal bending, teenagers are at high risk. Teenage girls (12 to 13 years old) are at highest risk to show development of scoliosis. Any child with noted spinal curvature should be referred for further evaluation. Most studies have shown that the approximate time of spinal curvature development is the same time that pubic hair develops. Each child deserves a careful inspection and palpation of the spine.

7. Hip evaluation for possible congenital hip dislocation (Ortolanis test)

a. Problem is found more in girls than boys.

b. Parent may report difficulty diapering the child.

c. Infant should be checked at every visit from newborn stage until about 2½ years of age.

d. Technique (Fig. 14-90)

(1) Baby supine, knees brought to 90-degree angle with back

(2) Examiner's hands on knees, index finger along lateral thigh to feel click vibration if present

(3) Knees brought up, then flexed laterally; a newborn's knees should almost lie flat on bed (160° to 175°)

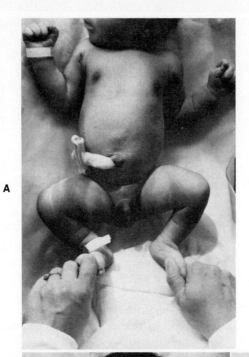

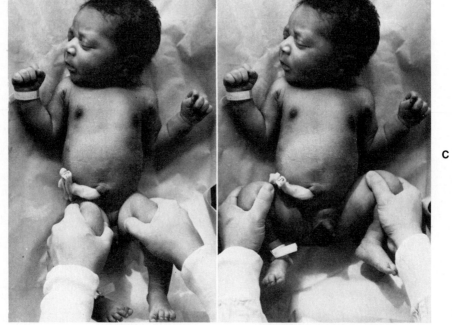

**FIG. 14-90.** Ortolanis test. **A,** Initial observation of symmetry. **B,** Hips flexed at 90-degree angle. **C,** Hips externally rotated.

e. Abnormal findings
  (1) Pop, click, or snap during manipulation technique
  (2) Bilaterally unequal response
  (3) Sudden cry of pain during procedure
8. Hip and knee evaluation for teenage boys, who are at risk for two specific types of skeletal problems:
  a. Slipped capital femoral epiphysis. Even though this is a hip injury, the boy will usually have pain in the knee or lateral distal thigh. Many times an injury precipitated by an activity such as jumping off an object will precede. Any boy with these complaints should be referred. Objective assessment data include the following:
    (1) Deep palpation to the hip causes pain and tenderness.
    (2) There is increased pain with abduction, internal or external rotation, or flexion of the hip.
    (3) In severe cases the examiner may see a shortening of the affected leg caused by muscle spasm and upward displacement of the femoral head.
  b. Osgood-Schlatter disease. The boy will usually complaint that his knee hurts. Although no specific injury may precede, an increase in running or jumping will aggravate the pain. Any teenage boy with this complaint should be referred. Objective assessment data include the following:
    (1) Specific location of pain by one finger will not be at the knee itself but at a point inferior to the knee, on the head of the tibia.
    (2) Inspection of the area will reveal a slight elevation.
    (3) Tapping the area with the knuckles will cause pain.

Although Osgood-Schlatter disease has traditionally been referred to as the disease of the young athletic teenage male, many orthopedists believe that as more girls become active in athletics there will be a greater incidence of the disease among females.

## Clinical variations: the pediatric client

The clinical guidelines for the musculoskeletal system of children vary greatly, depending on the age of the child, his cooperation, and his motor development. The examiner will spend a great deal of time developing routines for examining different ages. The guidelines and motor development sequence presented here represent normal findings for children of various ages.

Special techniques for evaluation of feet and shoes, muscle aches and pains, scoliosis, and hips have been discussed under *Clinical strategies*. These must be incorporated into the following guidelines.

To use the guidelines, the examiner must know the developmental norms for the age of the child being examined and have the cleverness to collect these data during the examination. If the examiner does not have the cooperation of the child, an inaccurate evaluation will result.

By age 6 years a child should be able to fully cooperate with the examiner. Evaluation of a child less than 6 years of age will probably not require following the guidelines in order. Instead, the examiner must watch the child walk, climb, play patty-cake, jump, and skip to gather the necessary data. Other more specific suggestions, such as "kiss your knee" or "touch your toes," will aid specific joint and muscle evaluation.

## Clinical variations: the pediatric client—cont'd

| CHARACTERISTIC OR AREA EXAMINED | NORMAL | DEVIATIONS FROM NORMAL |
| --- | --- | --- |
| 1. Weighing and measuring child | (See Figs. 14-91 and 14-92.) | |

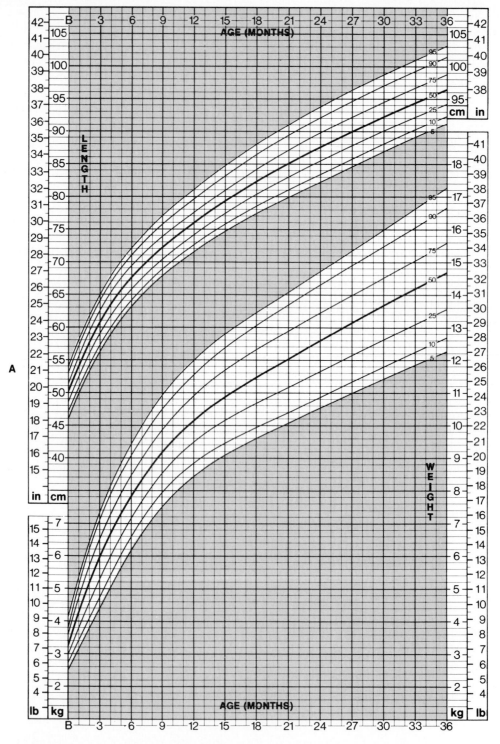

FIG. 14-91. **A,** Boys: birth to age 36 months—physical growth (length, weight), National Center for Health Statistics percentiles. (Adapted from Hamill, P.V.V., and others: Am. J. Clin. Nutr. **32:**607-629, 1979. Data from the Fels Research Institute, Wright State University School of Medicine, Yellow Springs, Ohio. Provided as a service of Ross Laboratories, 1980.)

| CHARACTERISTIC<br>OR AREA EXAMINED | NORMAL | DEVIATIONS FROM NORMAL |
|---|---|---|

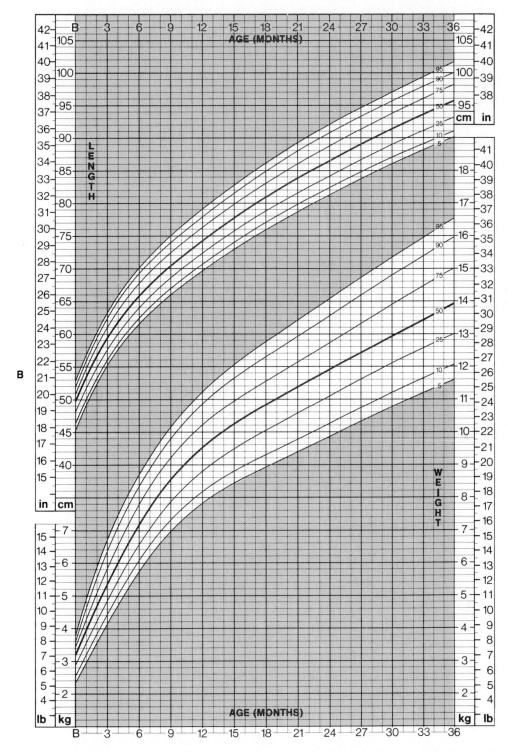

**FIG. 14-91, cont'd. B,** Girls: birth to age 36 months—physical growth (length, weight), National Center for Health Statistics percentiles. (Adapted from Hamill, P.V.V., and others: Am. J. Clin. Nutr. **32:**607-629, 1979. Data from the Fels Research Institute, Wright State University School of Medicine, Yellow Springs, Ohio. Provided as a service of Ross Laboratories, 1980.)

# Clinical variations: the pediatric client—cont'd

| CHARACTERISTIC OR AREA EXAMINED | NORMAL | DEVIATIONS FROM NORMAL |
|---|---|---|

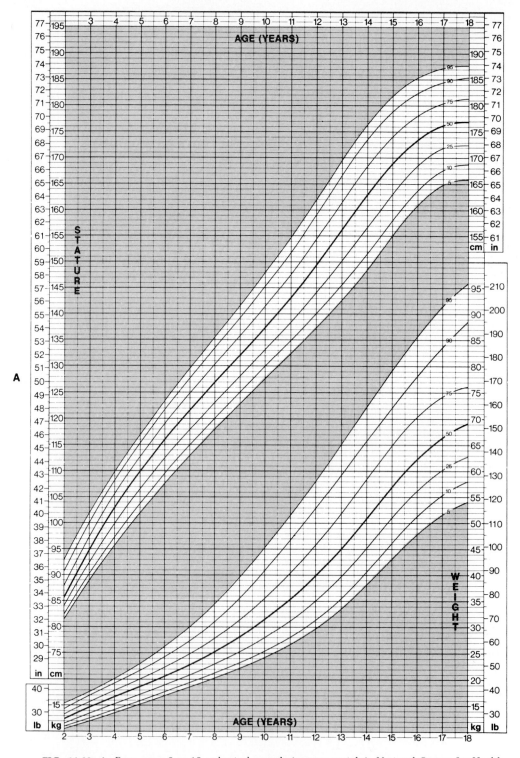

**FIG. 14-92. A,** Boys: ages 2 to 18—physical growth (stature, weight). National Center for Health Statistics percentiles. (Adapted from Hamill, P.V.V., and others: Am. J. Clin. Nutr. **32:**607-629, 1979. Data from the Fels Research Institute, Wright State University School of Medicine, Yellow Springs, Ohio. Provided as a service of Ross Laboratories, 1980.)

| CHARACTERISTIC<br>OR AREA EXAMINED | NORMAL | DEVIATIONS FROM NORMAL |
|---|---|---|

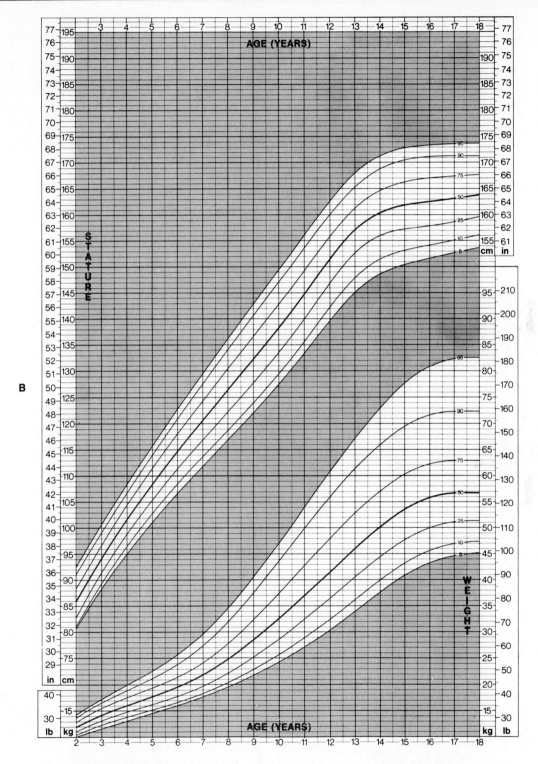

**FIG. 14-92, cont'd. B,** Girls: ages 2 to 18—physical growth (stature, weight), National Center for Health Statistics percentiles. (Adapted from Hamill, P.V.V., and others: Am. . Clin. Nutr. **32:**607-629, 1979. Data from the Fels Research Institute, Wright State University School of Medicine, Yellow Springs, Ohio. Provided as service of Ross Laboratories, 1980.)

## Clinical variations: the pediatric client—cont'd

| CHARACTERISTIC OR AREA EXAMINED | NORMAL | DEVIATIONS FROM NORMAL |
|---|---|---|
| **2.** Trunk (child lying or standing)<br>   **a.** Spine | Spine straight<br>Newborn: convex (Fig. 14-93)<br>3 to 4 months: cervical curve develops as child holds head up | |

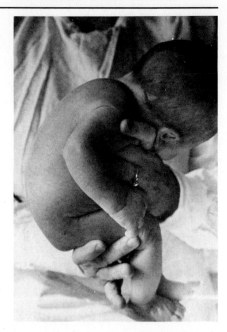

FIG. 14-93. Normal convex curvature of newborn's spine.

12 to 18 months: lumbar curve develops as child learns to walk (Fig. 14-94)

Lumbar lordosis in toddlers

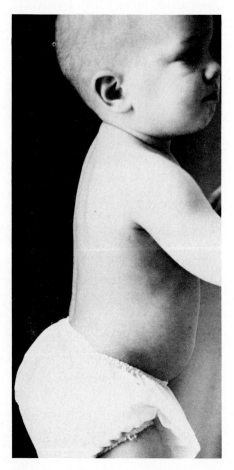

FIG. 14-94. Normal lumbar curvature of toddler's spine.

| CHARACTERISTIC OR AREA EXAMINED | NORMAL | DEVIATIONS FROM NORMAL |
|---|---|---|
| **FIG. 14-95.** Adult curvature in school-age child. | Beyond 18 months: cervical spine concave; thoracic spine convex, but less than that of adult; lumbar spine concave, like that of adult (Fig. 14-95)<br>No dimpling or bulges along spine<br>Black children may more frequently show lordosis | Dimpling or bulges along spine, or thickening<br>Lumbar lordosis in children over 6 years<br>Curved spine either in standing or bent-over position |
| 1. Bending to touch toes | Straight spine, both in upright and bending position<br>Iliac crests of equal height<br>Shoulders equal height<br>Convexity of thoracic spine | Functional vs. idiopathic scoliosis (see *Clinical strategies*)<br>Unequal iliac crests in either standing or bent-over position |
| 2. Hyperextension | 30° hyperextension from neutral position | Unable to hyperextend without losing balance, or pain with hyperextension |
| 3. Lateral bending | 35° flexion both ways from midline position | Decreased flexion degree, or pain with bending |
| 4. Lateral rotation | 30° rotation in both directions from direction forward position | Decreased rotation capability<br>Rotation with discomfort |
| 5. Spinal process palpation | Straight spine<br>Nontender | Curvature of spine<br>Tenderness<br>Spasm of paravertebral muscles |
| **3.** Gait | Newly walking babies and toddlers have wide stance and wide-waddle gait pattern, which tends to disappear by approximately 2 to 2½ years (Fig. 14-58) | Unsteady or jerky<br>Pain or discomfort<br>Irregular or jerky trunk posturing<br>Asymmetrical or jerky arm swing unrelated to gait |

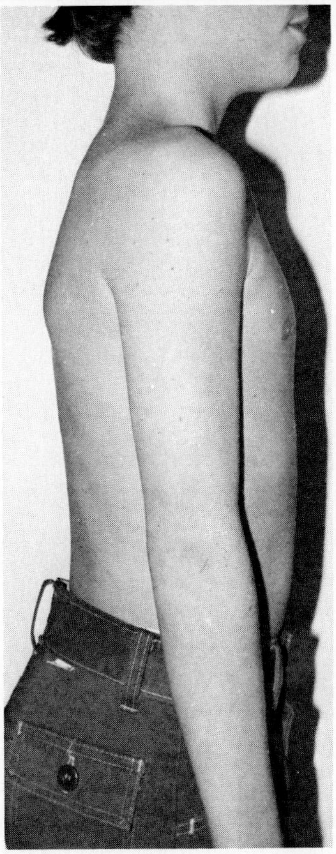

## Clinical variations: the pediatric client—cont'd

| CHARACTERISTIC OR AREA EXAMINED | NORMAL | DEVIATIONS FROM NORMAL |
|---|---|---|
| | Gait should become progressively stronger, steadier, and smoother as child matures; any deviation from this, or history of increasing falls or balance problems, should be considered abnormal (also evaluate shoes; see *Clinical strategies*)<br>Smooth, regular gait with symmetrical arm swing | |
| **4.** Head and neck | | |
| **a.** Musculature | Symmetrical appearance | Asymmetry<br>Atrophy or hypertrophy of muscles |
| **b.** Temporomandibular joint | Smooth movement of mandible | Pain, limited range of motion, or crepitus of temporomandibular joint |
| **c.** Posterior neck | Locating landmarks may be difficult in small child because of short neck and excess baby fat<br>Locate C7, T1, nontender cervical spine | Tenderness, spasms<br>Nodules |
| **d.** Range of motion of neck | | |
| 1. Chin flexion | 45° from midline | Limited or painful range of motion |
| 2. Head extension | 55° from midline | Crepitus of cervical spine |
| 3. Lateral bending | 40° each way from midline | |
| 4. Rotation of shin to shoulders | 70° from midline | |
| **e.** Muscle strength of back | | |
| 1. Chin flexion, position maintenance | With reasonable strength, unable to force head upright | Able to break muscular flexion before anticipated point |
| 2. Head hyperextension, position maintenance | With reasonable strength, unable to force head upright | Able to break muscular flexion before anticipated point |
| **5.** Hands and wrists | Smoothness; no swelling or deformities noted<br>Fingers able to maintain full extension position | Irregular finger contour<br>Swelling<br>Deformities<br>Tenderness<br>Muscular atrophy<br>Heberden nodes<br>Long spider or short clubbed fingers |
| **a.** Range of motion of fingers and wrists | | |
| 1. Finger extension | Symmetrical response<br>Smooth movements without complaints of discomfort<br>Full flexion and extension | Asymmetrical response<br>Pain on movement |
| 2. Fist | Bilaterally equal response | Unequal response<br>Decreased response |
| 3. Grip | Tight grip | Pain with movement |
| 4. Radial deviation | 20° | Decreased movement |
| 5. Ulnar deviation | 55° | |
| 6. Extension | 70° | |
| 7. Flexion | 90° | |
| **b.** Wrist strength | | |
| 1. Wrist flexion, position maintenance | Bilaterally strong<br>Unable to break position* | Asymmetrical response<br>Able to easily break position |
| 2. Wrist extension, position maintenance | Bilaterally strong<br>Unable to break position | Asymmetrical response<br>Able to easily break position |

*Throughout pediatric guidelines, according to resistance appropriate for age.

| CHARACTERISTIC OR AREA EXAMINED | NORMAL | DEVIATIONS FROM NORMAL |
|---|---|---|
| **6.** Elbows | | |
|   **a.** Palpation | Skin intact | Swelling |
| | Smooth | Inflammation |
| | Surface nontender, without nodules or discomfort | General tenderness |
| | | Subcutaneous nodules |
| | Lymph nodes not palpable | Point tenderness |
| | | Lymph nodes palpated |
|   **b.** Range of motion | | |
|     1. Extension and flexion | 160° full movement | Limited range of motion |
| | Bilaterally equal | Asymmetrical movement |
| | No discomfort | Pain at elbow |
|     2. Pronation and supination | 90° each direction | Limited range of motion |
| | Bilaterally equal | Asymmetrical movement |
| | No discomfort | Pain at elbow |
| **7.** Shoulders | | |
|   **a.** Inspection | Intactness | Redness |
| | Skin smooth and regular | Swelling |
| | Bilaterally symmetrical | Nodules |
|   **b.** Palpation | Nontender | Tender, painful |
| | Smooth and regular | Swelling |
| | Bilaterally symmetrical | |
|   **c.** Range of motion | | |
|     1. Extension | 180° from resting neutral position | Limited range of motion |
| | Bilaterally equal | Pain with movement |
| | No discomfort | Crepitations with movement |
| | | Asymmetry |
|     2. Hyperextension | 50° | Limited range of motion |
| | Bilaterally equal | Pain with movement |
| | No discomfort | Crepitations with movement |
| | | Asymmetry |
|     3. External rotation | 90° | Limited range of motion |
| | Bilaterally equal | Pain with movement |
| | No discomfort | Crepitations with movement |
| | | Asymmetry |
|     4. Internal rotation | 90° | Limited range of motion |
| | Bilaterally equal | Pain with movement |
| | No discomfort | Crepitations with movement |
| | | Asymmetry |
| **8.** Arm muscles: use make/break technique | | |
|   **a.** Deltoids | Bilaterally strong | Symmetrically unequal |
| | Unable to break position | Weak response |
| | | Pain during technique |
| | | Muscular spasm |
|   **b.** Biceps | Bilaterally strong | Symmetrically unequal |
| | Unable to break position | Weak response |
| | | Pain during technique |
| | | Muscular spasm |
|   **c.** Triceps | Bilaterally strong | Symmetrically unequal |
| | Unable to break position | Weak response |
| | | Pain during technique |
| | | Muscular spasm |

## Clinical variations: the pediatric client—cont'd

| CHARACTERISTIC OR AREA EXAMINED | NORMAL | DEVIATIONS FROM NORMAL |
|---|---|---|
| **9.** Shoulder muscles: lift infant under arms | Infant able to maintain position on examiner's hands (Fig. 14-96) | If muscles weak, child will slip through examiner's hands |

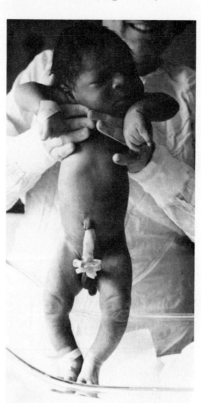

**FIG. 14-96.** Newborn shoulder muscle assessment.

| CHARACTERISTIC OR AREA EXAMINED | NORMAL | DEVIATIONS FROM NORMAL |
|---|---|---|
| **10.** Feet and ankles | | |
|    **a.** Inspection | Smoothness; no swelling or deformities noted | Inward or lateral deviation of feet or toes, tight Achilles tendons |
| | Toes maintain extended and straight position | Flat feet |
| | Toenails intact and neatly trimmed | |
| | Feet maintain straight position | |
| | (See *Clinical strategies* for additional observation criteria.) | |
|    **b.** Palpation | Smooth | Tenderness: diffuse vs. point |
| | Nontender | Swelling |
| | | Inflammation |
| | | Nodules |
|    **c.** Range of motion | | |
|       1. Dorsiflexion and plantar flexion | Dorsiflexion 20° from midline position | Dorsiflexion less than 20° because of tight tendon |
| | Plantar flexion 45° from midline position | Limited range of motion |
| | Bilaterally equal | Pain with movement |
| | No discomfort | Crepitations |
|       (Instruct child to stand on toes.) | | Asymmetry |
|       2. Inversion | Inversion 30° from midline position | Inversion or eversion when foot at rest |
|       3. Eversion | Eversion 20° from midline position | Limited range of motion |
| | Bilaterally equal | Pain with movement |
| | No discomfort | Asymmetry |

| CHARACTERISTIC OR AREA EXAMINED | NORMAL | DEVIATIONS FROM NORMAL |
|---|---|---|
| **d.** Muscular evaluation: maintain dorsiflexed position against opposite pull | Bilaterally strong<br>Unable to break position | Unequal<br>Weak response<br>Pain during technique |
| **11.** Knee | Knees in direct straight line between hip, ankle, great toe | Deviation of line so that it maintains position of hip, knee, ankle, fourth or fifth toe<br>Rotation of feet or lower legs (see *Clinical strategies*) |
| | Valgum: medial malleolus > 2.5 cm (1 inch) apart with knees touching; normal for children 2 to 3½ years old (may be present and normal in some children up to 12 years) (Fig. 14-97)<br>Varum: medial malleolus touching, knees > 2.5 cm (1 inch) apart; needs further evaluation for tibial torsion (may be normal until 18 months to 2 years of age) | May be seen with systemic diseases such as polio, rickets, syphilis |
| | Smooth, symmetrical | Swelling, thickness<br>Inflammation<br>Inflamed, painful joints in black children may be sign of sickle cell anemia<br>Enlargement of tibial tubercles in teenage boys may be sign of Osgood-Schlatter disease |

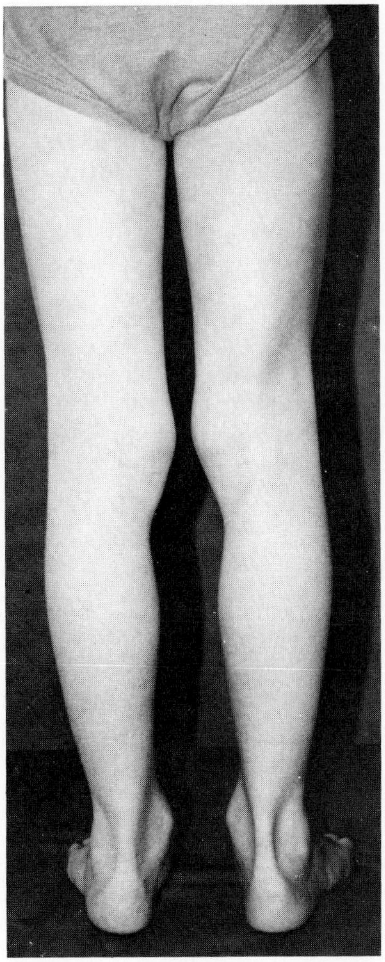

FIG. 14-97. School-age child: normal valgum position.

| CHARACTERISTIC OR AREA EXAMINED | NORMAL | DEVIATIONS FROM NORMAL |
|---|---|---|
| **a.** Palpation of knees and popliteal space | Smooth, nontender | Bogginess<br>Thickening<br>Tenderness, redness<br>Painful<br>Nodules and swelling |
| **b.** Range of motion evaluation | 130° from straight extended position<br>No discomfort or difficulty | Decreased range of motion<br>Pain with movement<br>Crepitations |

## Clinical variations: the pediatric client—cont'd

| CHARACTERISTIC OR AREA EXAMINED | NORMAL | DEVIATIONS FROM NORMAL |
|---|---|---|
| **12.** Hips and pelvis | | |
| **a.** Inspection and palpation | | |
| 1. Babies to 3 years | Gluteal folds bilaterally equal<br>No click, snap, or dislocation felt<br>Hip rotation of 160° to 175° bilaterally equal | Difference in height of gluteal folds<br>Click, snap felt<br>Unequal range of motion<br>Sudden cry during procedure |
| 2. Children over 3 years: use adult technique to evaluate | | |
| a. Knee to chest | 120° from straight extended position | Limited range of motion<br>Pain or discomfort with movement<br>Flexion of opposite thigh<br>Crepitations |
| b. Hip flexion without bending knee | 90° from straight extended position | Limited range of motion<br>Pain or discomfort with movement<br>Crepitations |
| c. External rotation | 40° from straight midline position | Limited range of motion<br>Pain or discomfort with movement<br>Crepitations<br>In teenage boys with slipped femoral epiphysis: much pain with external rotation or abduction of hip |
| d. Internal rotation | 40° from straight midline position | Limited range of motion<br>Pain or discomfort with movement<br>Crepitations |
| **b.** Muscular evaluation | | |
| 1. Hips | | |
| a. Flexion against examiner's pushing | Bilaterally strong<br>Unable to break position | Symmetrically unequal<br>Weak response<br>Pain during technique |
| 2. Hamstring | | |
| a. Leg crossing | Able to perform<br>Bilaterally equal and without difficulty | Unable to perform<br>Performs with pain or great difficulty |
| b. Bending of knee against examiner's pushing | Bilaterally strong<br>Unable to flex knee | Symmetrically unequal<br>Weak response<br>Pain during technique |
| 3. Quadriceps | | |
| a. Extension of lower leg against examiner's pushing | Bilaterally strong<br>Unable to flex knee | Symmetrically unequal<br>Weak response<br>Pain during technique |

# History and clinical strategies: the geriatric client

1. The normal aging process is accompanied by numerous musculoskeletal changes:
   a. Decrease in bone mass, which results in increased vulnerability to stress in weight-bearing areas and predisposes to fractures
   b. Thinning (possibly collapse) of intervertebral discs
   c. Calcificaton within cartilage and ligaments
   d. Less elastic tendons
   e. Decrease in muscle mass, tone, and strength (however, at age 60 the decrease usually does not exceed a 10% to 20% loss)
      (1) Less ability to perform intense, sudden exercise
      (2) Decreased endurance with exercise (less ability to hold isometric contractions)
      (3) Decreased agility
2. Risk factors. As with all other aging changes, these alterations occur at different rates in different individuals. The changes are gradual and not often presented as a complaint. The rate of change is greatly affected by a number of variables or risk factors.
   a. General physical health of client
      (1) Decreased respiratory capacity and reserve
      (2) Diminished circulatory supply
      (3) Arthritic changes accompanied by symptoms
      (4) Neurogenic disorders affecting voluntary muscle response or sensory alterations
      (5) Other physical changes that are accompanied by symptoms that interfere with body function or fitness: pain, diminished vision, fatigue, and weakness
   b. Obesity
   c. Immobility, either short term (2 to 3 weeks) related to injury or episodic illness, or long term
   d. Sedentary life-style (a hypokinetic state can perpetuate itself)
   e. Depression
   f. Inadequate nutrition and/or fluid intake
   g. Mind-altering drugs (e.g., tranquilizers, sedatives, alcohol)
   h. Fear of falling
   i. Confusion or altered mental state (inattentiveness)

   All the variables mentioned contribute to reduced physical activity, which in turn promotes and hastens the changes associated with the aging musculoskeletal system.
3. Presenting symptoms related to musculoskeletal problems:

a. The major symptoms to inquire about are listed in the geriatric data base in Chapter 2 (p. 46). These complaints relate to the following:
   (1) General feeling of well-being
   (2) Muscle function
   (3) Joint and bone function and appearance
   (4) Extremity function
   (5) Back and spine function
   (6) Gait
   (7) Sleeping patterns
b. Further details about symptom analysis are offered in the adult section of this chapter:
   (1) Pain
   (2) Gait difficulty
   (3) Voluntary muscle function complaints
   (4) Skeletal complaints
   (5) Joint complaints
c. Symptoms that should be explored in detail follow:
   (1) Weakness
      (a) Onset sudden or slow?
      (b) Isolated to a specific body part or generalized (e.g., difficulty swallowing, lid drooping, unilateral weakness, or weakness in feet, ankles, hands)?
      (c) Associated with any particular activity (e.g., stair climbing [how many], rising from a chair, walking on level ground)?
      (d) Does weakness occur at onset of activity or after activity has been sustained (how long or how much)?
      (e) Associated symptoms (e.g., dizziness, "black-outs," numbness or tingling, pain, tics or fasciculations, tremors, shortness of breath)
      (f) Associated stiffness of joints, spasms, or muscle tension (do these symptoms occur at night?)
      (g) Associated weight gain or loss
      (h) Associated mood or mental changes
      (i) Medications being taken
   (2) "Restless" legs (usually at night)
      (a) Associated symptoms of back pain, muscle cramps in legs, numbness or coldness of extremities?
      (b) How is this relieved?
   (3) History of injuries, falls (inquire specifically about all accidents, minor "spills," or injuries that are recent; client may not be aware that a pattern of increased stumbling, falls, or limited agility is emerging if injuries are not obvious or incapacitating)
   (4) Decrease in height (ask client to estimate number of inches over last few years; last year)

4. Osteoarthritis is described as a universal aging process that is usually noninflammatory and involves deterioration and abrasions of the articular cartilage and possibly formation of new bone at the joint surfaces. The examiner must determine whether joint and bone changes are creating symptoms or signs that alter the physical functioning of the client. It is estimated that 50% of individuals over age 60 years and 78% of those over age 78 years manifest signs or symptoms related to arthritis.
   a. Risk factors
      (1) Advancing age
      (2) History of excessive use of a given joint (or group of joints)
      (3) Obesity
      (4) Family history of arthritis (especially with involvement of hands and fingers)
      (5) History of injuries to a given joint (or group of joints)
      (6) History of joint abnormalities (e.g., laxness of ligaments)
   b. Joints most frequently involved with symptomatic arthritic changes are weight-bearing areas:
      (1) Knees
         (a) Client frequently notices crepitation. (*Note:* Crepitation can also be heard or palpated in normal joints.)
         (b) Pain, stiffness, and/or joint enlargement may be evident.
         (c) Quadriceps may atrophy because of disuse resulting from pain.
      (2) Hips
         (a) Pain may be local or referred to buttock or inner aspect of thigh.
         (b) Hip may be held in partially flexed and adducted position.
         (c) Hip extension and rotation are diminished.
      (3) Spine (cervical and lumbar areas most frequently affected)
         (a) Cervical crepitation on movement is noticed by client. Weakness, numbness, or sensory changes may be noticed in upper arm, forearm, and thumb and fingers. "Black-out" spells occasionally occur with neck rotation.
         (b) Spinal changes may result in stiffness, loss of lordotic curve, or exaggerated kyphosis.
      (4) Fingers
         (a) May manifest outward changes, especially distal joint enlargement or node formation (Fig. 14-98).
         (b) Range of motion may be limited because of pain.
         (c) Interosseous spaces may be atrophied as a result of decrease in use of fingers and hands.
      (5) Shoulders: pain experienced on movement, especially abduction.
      (6) Ribs: arthritis changes in the costovertebral joint may produce localized pain on palpation or referred pain to chest wall.
   c. Symptoms are often increased by weather changes or prolonged immobility.
   d. Temporary relief is often completely or partially provided by rest, heat application, or analgesics. (*Note:* Heat application can be a risk if the client

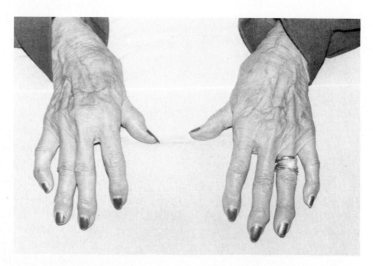

**FIG. 14-98.** Distal joint deformities associated with osteoarthritis.

does not check temperature of water or heating device; the client's sensitivity to heat may be impaired. Also, gastrointestinal complaints may result from frequent use of some analgesics.)

5. Osteoporosis is described as a decrease in mass and density of the skeleton, affecting approximately 29% of the aging female population and 18% of aging males.* Involvement is more intense in the long bones and vertebral column.
   a. Risk factors
      (1) Postmenopausal state
      (2) Immobility
      (3) Cushing syndrome
      (4) Advanced diverticulitis (interferes with calcium absorption)
      (5) Hyperthyroidism (increased bone resorption)
      (6) History of limited calcium dietary intake
      (7) Heparin
      (8) Diabetes mellitus
   b. Symptoms are often absent or mild; vague discomfort in back is experienced.
   c. Vulnerability to fractures (of spine, femur, and pelvis) is greatly increased.
   d. Loss of height occurs as a result of kyphotic changes and vertebral fractures.
   e. Point tenderness of the spine is a signal of acute vertebral problems.
6. If the examiner is confronted with a client who is disabled or incapacitated with discomfort or reduced function, the need for safety and performance of activities of daily living should be assessed. Detailed questions regarding activities of daily living are offered on p. 27 in Chapter 1, and inquiries and concerns for safety are described on p. 32 of Chapter 1.
7. Physical assessment. The aging client who is not afflicted with illness or athritic changes should be able to participate in the musculoskeletal assessment as it is described in the adult section of this chapter. Normal range of motion of joints and muscular strength and tone should be the same as with the younger adult. Even if muscular strength is reduced by 10% to 20%, the client should be able to sustain the opposition of the examiner in the testing for muscular strength. The following general patterns may be noted.
   a. Response to examiner commands may be slower.

b. General muscle bulk may be reduced. The arms and legs may appear thinner and flabby.
c. *Note:* Many "normal" clients (including young adults) cannot touch their toes as they bend forward from the waist.)

8. Early signs of musculoskeletal deviations. As physical disability and/or advanced aging changes encroach on the elderly client, the response to musculoskeletal physical assessment manifests an increasing number of deviations from normal findings. Some of the early (or more subtle) signs are:
   a. Posture (stance) (Fig. 14-99). The appearance is one of general flexion (any or all of these signs may be evident).
      (1) Head and neck thrust forward
      (2) Dorsal kyphosis or kyphoscoliosis
      (3) Flexion at the elbow and wrist
      (4) Hips slightly flexed
      (5) Knees flexed
      (6) Broad stance (feet spread farther apart)
   b. Gait should be carefully evaluated in *all* clients. They should be permitted to wear shoes.
      (1) Gait phases

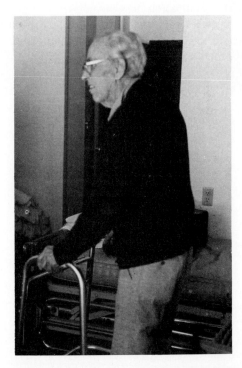

**FIG. 14-99.** Posture (stance) featuring head and neck thrust forward, dorsal kyphosis, hip flexion, and knees slightly flexed.

*Smith, R.W., Jr., Eyler, W.R., and Melinger, R.C.: On the incidence of senile osteoporosis, Ann. Intern. Med. **52:**773, 1960.

(a) Heel strike (Fig. 14-100). Dorsiflexors that normally decelerate the foot before striking may be weakened. The flat of the foot strikes the floor. The client may lift the leg farther off the floor with each step.

(b) Foot at midstance; other foot is pushing off (Fig. 14-101). Weakened quadriceps may not be able to stabilize the knee while the foot is bearing weight. Lateral and anteroposterior hip stability may not be maintained if gluteus muscles are weakened.

(c) Foot is pushing off (Fig. 14-102). Weakened gastrocnemius and soleus unable to elevate the body to permit the other foot to swing freely.

(d) Swing phase (Fig. 14-103). Swing may be shortened, foot may be lifted farther off the ground (marching style), or foot may just fall or slide forward (shuffling pattern).

(2) Arms may be held out to assist with balance or move in a rowing motion.

(3) Arm movement may be limited or absent.

(4) Normal vertical body motions that accompany push-off and stance phases tend to diminish.

(5) Upper torso may sway from side to side to assist with maintaining balance.

(6) Feet may be farther apart (broadened base to maintain balance).

(7) Steps may be uneven or tottering.

(8) Shortened step and shuffling propulsive gait with limited arm movement are associated with parkinsonism.

(9) Individuals who are weak or unsteady watch their feet as they walk.

c. Range of motion
(1) Most often limited because of pain (client stops movement abruptly).
(2) Weight-bearing joints (knees, hips, and lumbar spine) are frequently affected. Joints that are frequently used (cervical spine, shoulder, elbow, and fingers) may have limited range or pain associated with movement.
(3) Loss of full spinal range of motion, particularly in the lumbar area.

d. Muscle appearance and function
(1) Muscle wasting may be evident near immobile joints or in extremities that have limited motion (e.g., deep interosseous spaces often appear in severely arthritic hands).
(2) Mild bilateral muscle weakness (particularly of lower extremities) may not be noticed by the examiner during the opposition testing. Careful evaluation of gait and stair climbing may reveal more subtle weaknesses.

9. Functional testing for activities of daily living. The examiner will be assessing many elderly clients who have permanent muscle or joint function loss or other altered health states that contribute to diminished physical ability. Beyond the assessment of body parts for functional capacity, the examiner needs to assess the client's ability to move about and to perform essential functions at home. The client often compensates for weakened muscle groups by altering posture or assisting movement with other body parts or special devices (e.g., cane, walker). The following assessment tests the ability and combination of major muscle groups to perform vital activities of daily living.

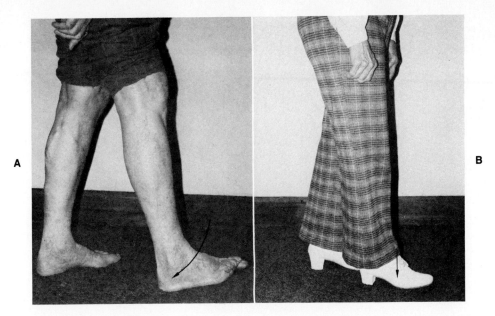

FIG. 14-100. **A,** Right foot demonstrating normal heel strike; left foot is bearing weight. **B,** Weakened dorsiflexors allow flat of right foot rather than heel to strike the floor.

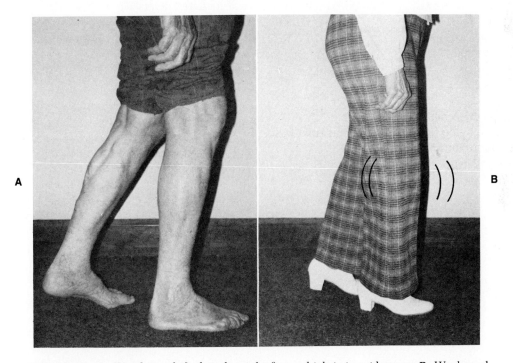

FIG. 14-101. **A,** Weight is shifted to the right foot, which is in midstance. **B,** Weakened right leg is wobbly while bearing weight (midstance phase). A weakened or painful leg or foot results in a shortened stride, since that weight can be shifted quickly back to the other foot.

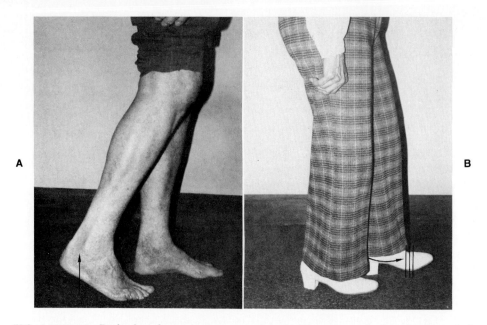

FIG. 14-102. **A,** Right foot demonstrates normal body lift at the end of push phase; left leg has swung free to a new step position. **B,** Weakened right leg is unable to lift the body sufficiently to permit left foot to swing freely.

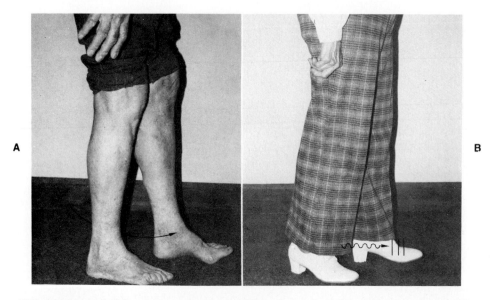

FIG. 14-103. **A,** Left leg demonstrates normal free swing. **B,** Left leg demonstrates shuffle-forward rather than free swing. Stride is shortened.

## Clinical variations: the geriatric client

| THE EXAMINER WILL OBSERVE: | COMMENTS |
| --- | --- |
| **1.** Client rising from lying to sitting position (Fig. 14-104) | Often rolls to one side and pushes with arms to raise to elbow position<br>Grabbing siderail or adjacent table may help client to pull up to full sitting position |

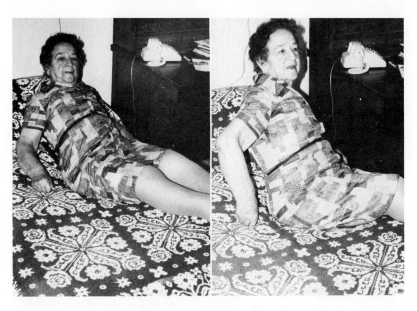

**FIG. 14-104**

| | |
| --- | --- |
| **2.** Client rising from chair to standing position (Fig. 14-105) | May supplement weakened leg muscles by pushing with arms (*Note:* Chairs without arms provide no support for clients who need to push away to rise to a standing position.)<br>Upper torso thrusts forward before body rises; feet spread far apart to provide broad support base |

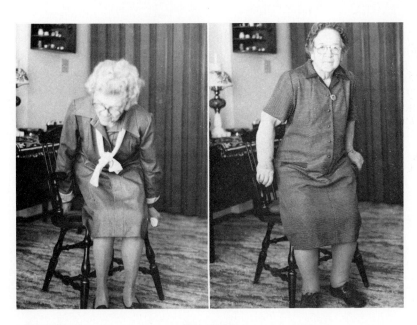

**FIG. 14-105**

## Clinical variations: the geriatric client—cont'd

| THE EXAMINER WILL OBSERVE: | COMMENTS |
|---|---|
| **3.** Client walking (Fig. 14-106) | Note heel strike, midstance, push-off, swing phase, arm motion, and upper trunk motion<br>(See comments about gait phases on p. 404) |

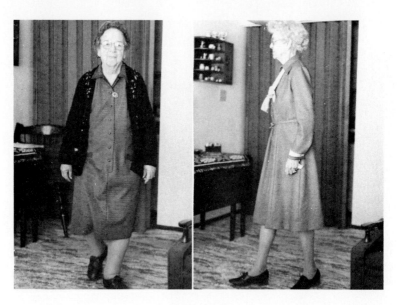

FIG. 14-106

| | |
|---|---|
| **4.** Client climbing step (Fig. 14-107) | May use favorite leg (stronger one) to climb stair<br>Will usually hold handrail for balance and may pull body up and forward with that arm |

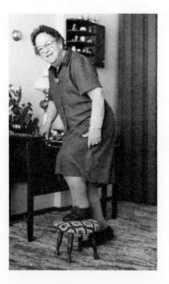

FIG. 14-107

| THE EXAMINER WILL OBSERVE: | COMMENTS |
|---|---|
| **5.** Client descending step (Fig. 14-108) | Often descends steps sideways, lowering weaker leg first and holding rail with both hands<br>If unsteady or insecure, client often watches feet while lowering and standing on them |

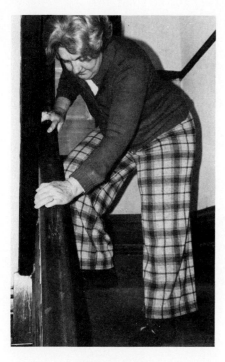

**FIG. 14-108**

| | |
|---|---|
| **6.** Client picking up item from floor (Fig. 14-109) | Grasps or leans on table or handrail for support while lowering body; one hand may be firmly supported on thigh to assist in lowering and in elevating upper torso to standing position; client may avoid bending knees and stoop from waist |

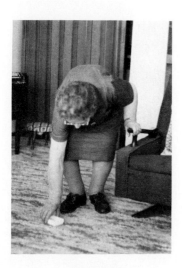

**FIG. 14-109**

## Clinical variations: the geriatric client—cont'd

| THE EXAMINER WILL OBSERVE: | COMMENTS |
| --- | --- |
| 7. Client tying shoes while seated (Fig. 14-110) | Tests for manual dexterity and flexibility of spine<br>Client may use footstool to reduce need for spinal flexion |

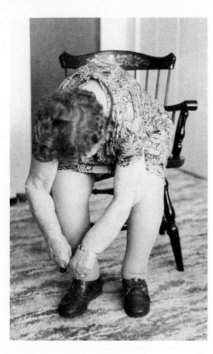

FIG. 14-111

| | |
| --- | --- |
| 8. Client putting on and pulling up trousers (or stockings) (Fig. 14-111) | Clothing often pulled over feet while client seated; final act of pulling up clothing demonstrates shoulder and upper arm strength |

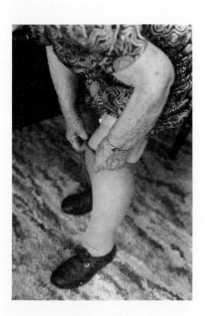

FIG. 14-110

| THE EXAMINER WILL OBSERVE: | COMMENTS |
|---|---|
| **9.** Client puttting on sweater or jacket (Fig. 14-112) | Often applies first sleeve to weaker arm or shoulder; may use internal or external shoulder rotation to reach remaining sleeve and to thrust arm into it |

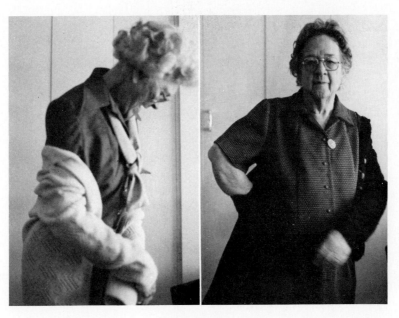

**FIG. 14-112**

| | |
|---|---|
| **10.** Client zipping dress in back (Fig. 14-113) (or fastening brassiere) | Some individuals discard all garments that fasten in back; others find someone else to zip them up<br>This maneuver tests ability to rotate shoulders |

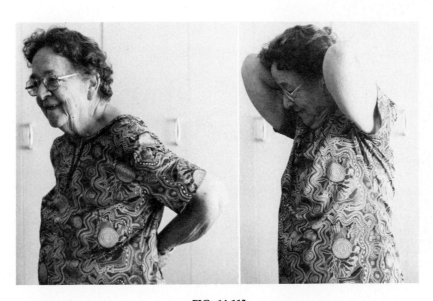

**FIG. 14-113**

## Clinical variations: the geriatric client—cont'd

| THE EXAMINER WILL OBSERVE: | COMMENTS |
|---|---|
| **11.** Client combing hair in back and at sides (Fig. 14-114) | Shows ability to grasp and maneuver brush or comb, wrist flexion, and shoulder rotation <br><br> Some clients will turn back of head toward comb to accommodate diminished external shoulder rotation |

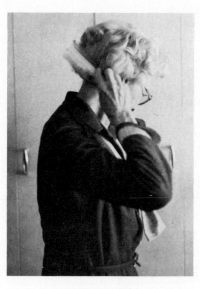

**FIG. 14-114**

| | |
|---|---|
| **12.** Client pushing chair away from table (while seated in chair) (Fig. 14-115) | Demonstrates upper arm, shoulder, lower arm strength, and wrist motion; some clients will rise to standing position and ease chair out with torso |

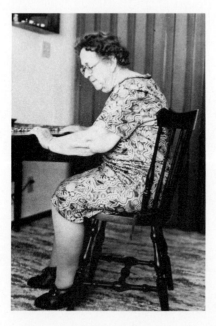

**FIG. 14-115**

| THE EXAMINER WILL OBSERVE: | COMMENTS |
| --- | --- |

**13.** Client buttoning button, writing name, picking up paper from table (Fig. 14-116) (*Note:* Tooth brushing can be used to show a combination of manual dexterity, grip strength, wrist range of motion, and strength of forearm.)

Shows manual dexterity and finger-thumb opposition

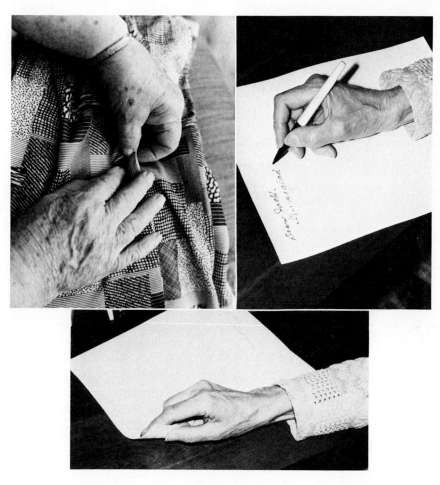

**FIG. 14-116**

**Cognitive
self-assessment**

Mark each statement "T" or "F."

1. _____ The two articulating surfaces of a joint are cartilage.
2. _____ It is important to examine muscles both during relaxation and during contraction.
3. _____ *Varus* is a term used to describe an angular deviation of an extremity.
4. _____ Another name for kyphosis is swayback.
5. _____ Where there is muscle disease, the tendon stretch reflex is greatly altered.
6. _____ As the client ages, decreased muscle strength is caused by an increased amount of collagen in the muscle tissue, followed by fibrosis of the connective tissue.
7. _____ The kind of arthritis that occurs many times with the aging process is called rheumatoid arthritis.
8. _____ The normal lumbar curve is convex.
9. _____ The straight leg raise test is generally a good test to use in evaluation of a disc problem.
10. _____ The curvature seen in scoliosis is considered to be a varus deformity.

Match the definitions in column B with the terms in Column A.

| Column A | Column B |
|---|---|
| 11. _____ Supination | a. Potential space, often filled with fluid, for decreasing friction between two layers that move on each other |
| 12. _____ Pronation | |
| 13. _____ Eversion | |
| 14. _____ Inversion | b. To move toward the medial line |
| 15. _____ Abduction | c. Rounded protuberance at the end of a bone |
| 16. _____ Adduction | d. Position of the hand in which the palmar surface faces upward |
| 17. _____ Condyle | |
| 18. _____ Bursa | e. Turning inward toward the median |
| 19. _____ Varus | f. Turning out and away from the median |
| 20. _____ Valgus | g. Bending outward |
| | h. Bending inward |
| | i. Position of the hand in which the palmar surface faces downward |
| | j. Movement of the part away from the midline |

21. Which of the following musculoskeletal problems does *not* involve the joint?
    □ a. Sprain
    □ b. Rheumatoid arthritis
    □ c. Bursitis
    □ d. Tendonitis
    □ e. Gout

22. Having the client bend forward to touch his toes is done:
    □ a. to check spinal range of motion
    □ b. with the examiner standing in front of the client
    □ c. to make spinal deformities easier to detect
    □ d. with the examiner standing behind the client
    □ e. to evaluate balance
    □ f. a, c, and e
    □ g. a, b, and c
    □ h. a, c, and d
    □ i. b, c, and e
    □ j. all the above

23. The muscle wasting and decreasing muscle strength in an older adult results from:
    ☐ a. the muscle tissues collecting increased amounts of collagen
    ☐ b. stenosis of the muscle fibers
    ☐ c. fibrosis of connective tissue
    ☐ d. decompensation of muscle mass caused by arteriosclerosis
    ☐ e. a, b, and d
    ☐ f. b and d
    ☐ g. a and c
    ☐ h. all the above

24. Susan Mulligan, a 24-year-old pregnant client, comes to you because of a repeated "charley horse" in her right leg. Which of the following techniques would you recommend to her for stopping the muscle cramp? (Select the *best* answer.)
    ☐ a. Massage the leg.
    ☐ b. Plantar flex the right foot.
    ☐ c. Dorsiflex the right foot.
    ☐ d. Elevate the leg from the hip.

25. Which of the following is not part of a joint?
    ☐ a. Synovial membrane
    ☐ b. Bone
    ☐ c. Ligament
    ☐ d. Capsule
    ☐ e. Muscle

26. For which *one* of the following clients would a measurement of muscle mass be most important?
    ☐ a. Routine physical of a 46-year-old with a 20-year history of polio and resulting crippling of the right side
    ☐ b. An 18-year-old football player who "sprained" his ankle 2 hours ago
    ☐ c. A 30-year-old man who just had a cast removed from his right leg following a motorcycle-related injury 6 weeks ago
    ☐ d. A 58-year-old man who has had a right-sided paralysis for 2 weeks secondary to a stroke
    ☐ e. A 24-year-old pregnant woman with a 4-day history of fluid retention

27. Gait evaluation is an important part of musculoskeletal assessment. Which of the following should be included in the client's gait evaluation?
    ☐ a. Phase
    ☐ b. Cadence
    ☐ c. Stride length
    ☐ d. Trunk posture
    ☐ e. Pelvic posture
    ☐ f. Arm swing
    ☐ g. all except e
    ☐ h. all except b
    ☐ i. all except a
    ☐ j. all except f
    ☐ k. all the above

28. Painless nodules commonly found around the tendon sheaths of the wrist are:
    - ☐ a. ganglia
    - ☐ b. fovea
    - ☐ c. tophi
    - ☐ d. tenalgia
    - ☐ e. rheumatoid nodules

29. The best instruction you can offer to a client who wants to know what to do in case of a muscle cramp is:
    - ☐ a. tell him to stretch the muscle fibers of the cramping muscle by placing the limb in a position that will stretch the affected muscle
    - ☐ b. rub the area vigorously until the cramp goes away
    - ☐ c. apply ice to the cramping muscle
    - ☐ d. apply heat to the cramping muscle
    - ☐ e. none of the above

30. Basic evaluation of the musculoskeletal system of an asymptomatic adult should at minimum include:
    - ☐ a. assessment of activities of daily living
    - ☐ b. gait
    - ☐ c. spinal curvature
    - ☐ d. joint evaluation
    - ☐ e. tissue evaluation around joints
    - ☐ f. muscle mass evaluation
    - ☐ g. muscle strength evaluation (make/break technique)
    - ☐ h. all the above
    - ☐ i. all except e
    - ☐ j. all except f
    - ☐ k. all except g
    - ☐ l. all except c

**PEDIATRIC QUESTIONS**

31. The normal spinal curvature of the child is different from that of the adult. Identify the *correct* curvature from the following descriptions.
    - ☐ a. The thoracic convexity is decreased and the lumbar concavity is increased.
    - ☐ b. The thoracic concavity is decreased and the lumbar convexity is increased.
    - ☐ c. The thoracic convexity is increased and the lumbar concavity is decreased.
    - ☐ d. The thoracic concavity is increased and the lumbar convexity is decreased.

32. Much of the skeletal makeup of the small child is cartilaginous tissue. Ossification of most bones occurs by _____ of age.
    - ☐ a. 8 months
    - ☐ b. 2 years
    - ☐ c. 5 years
    - ☐ d. 8 years
    - ☐ e. 12 years

33. A parent brings an 18-month-old child for evaluation because the child has "flat feet." All the following statements are true except one. Identify the *false* statement.
    - ☐ a. When a child begins to stand, his feet normally pronate inward.
    - ☐ b. The flap of skin that makes the child's feet appear flat is actually adipose tissue and will disappear as the child grows older.
    - ☐ c. There is no such thing as flat feet in children.
    - ☐ d. Before the weight-bearing period there really is no medial arch of the foot.
    - ☐ e. When the child assumes a wide-base stance, the weight line normally falls on the medial aspect of the foot, giving the appearance that the child has flat feet.

34. Which of the following children should be referred because of a lag in motor development?
    - ☐ a. Four-month-old Kara, who is unable to sit by herself
    - ☐ b. Eight-month-old William, who is unable to roll from prone to supine position and back to prone position
    - ☐ c. Nine-month-old Ryan, who is unable to pull himself into a standing position
    - ☐ d. Two-year-old Lynn, who is unable to build a four-block tower
    - ☐ e. Jason, age $3\frac{1}{2}$ years, who is unable to skip

35. Behaviors for evaluating the gross motor development of 3-year-old Stephen are:
    - ☐ a. able to jump in place
    - ☐ b. able to walk up stairs, alternating feet on steps
    - ☐ c. able to walk down stairs, two feet on each step
    - ☐ d. pedals a tricycle
    - ☐ e. able to walk a straight line, one foot in front of other
    - ☐ f. all the above
    - ☐ g. all except c
    - ☐ h. all except e
    - ☐ i. a, b, and e
    - ☐ j. c, d, and e

36. Certain orthopedic conditions are typically associated with pubertal growth. When developing a routine for evaluating the musculoskeletal system of both teenage boys and girls, thorough emphasis should be placed on:
    - ☐ a. evaluation of the hands
    - ☐ b. evaluation of the knees
    - ☐ c. evaluation of the ankles
    - ☐ d. evaluation of the spine
    - ☐ e. evaluation of the hips
    - ☐ f. none of the above
    - ☐ g. all except a
    - ☐ h. b, c, and e
    - ☐ i. b, d, and e
    - ☐ j. all the above

37. By the time an individual is 70 years old:
    - ☐ a. he usually manifests a 50% loss of muscle strength
    - ☐ b. arthritis of the hip and knee joints are symptomatic
    - ☐ c. he often manifests a longer endurance rate with isometric contractions
    - ☐ d. none of the above

38. Some of the risk factors associated with diminished physical functioning in elderly individuals are:
    - ☐ a. sedentary life style
    - ☐ b. altered mental state
    - ☐ c. obesity
    - ☐ d. pain
    - ☐ e. diminished circulatory supply to body parts
    - ☐ f. a, d, and e
    - ☐ g. a, b, and c
    - ☐ h. all the above
    - ☐ i. a, c, and d

39. Early or mild weakness of lower extremities:
    - ☐ a. is usually easily validated with make/break assessment procedures
    - ☐ b. is always unilateral
    - ☐ c. may be identified by asking the client to climb a step
    - ☐ d. none of the above

40. The joints most commonly involved with symptomatic arthritis are:
    - ☐ a. wrists
    - ☐ b. knees
    - ☐ c. hips
    - ☐ d. ankles
    - ☐ e. lumbar spine
    - ☐ f. b, c, and e
    - ☐ g. b, c, and d
    - ☐ h. a, d, and e
    - ☐ i. all the above

41. In a normally functioning gait:
    - ☐ a. the gluteus maximus helps to stabilize the hip while one foot is in stance position
    - ☐ b. the tibial dorsiflexors decelerate the foot as it approaches heel strike
    - ☐ c. the upper torso often sways from side to side to maintain balance
    - ☐ d. none of the above
    - ☐ e. a and b

## SUGGESTED READINGS

### General

Bates, B.: A guide to physical examination, ed. 3, Philadelphia, 1983, J.B. Lippincott Co., pp. 324-369.

Debrunner, H.U.: Orthopaedic diagnosis, Chicago, 1982, Year Book Medical Publishers, Inc.

DeGowin, E., and DeGowin, R.: Bedside diagnostic examination, ed. 3, New York, 1976, Macmillan Publishing Co., Inc.

Judge, R.D., and Zuidema, G., editors: Methods of clinical examination: a physiologic approach, Boston, 1974, Little, Brown & Co., pp. 285-305.

Malasanos, L., and others: Health assessment, ed. 2, St. Louis, 1981, The C.V. Mosby Co., pp. 443-517.

Nordmark, M.T., and Rohweder, A.W.: Scientific foundations of nursing, ed. 3, Philadelphia, 1975, J.B. Lippincott Co., pp. 187-220.

Norkin, C., and Levangie, P.: Joint structure and function, Philadelphia, 1983, F.A. Davis Co.

Piercey, M.L.: Assessment of low back pain, Nurse Pract. **1**(4):18-21, 1976.

Prior, J.A., Silberstein, J.S., and Stang, J.M.: Physical diagnosis: the history and examination of the patient, ed. 6, St. Louis, 1981, The C.V. Mosby Co., pp. 429-463.

### Pediatric

Alexander, M., and Brown, M.S.: Pediatric history taking and physical diagnosis for nurses, ed. 2, New York, 1979, McGraw-Hill Book Co., pp. 283-319.

Barness, L.: Manual of pediatric physical diagnosis, ed. 5, Chicago, 1981, Year Book Medical Publishers, Inc., pp. 167-192.

Coley, I.L.: Pediatric assessment of self-care activities, St. Louis, 1978, The C.V. Mosby Co.

Daniel, W.A., Jr.: Adolescents in health and disease, St. Louis, 1977, The C.V. MOsby Co., pp. 363-377.

DeAngelis, C.: Basic pediatrics for the primary health care provider, Boston, 1975, Little, Brown & Co., pp. 57-60, 86-93, 231-237.

Frankenburg, W.K., and others: The newly abbreviated and revised Denver Developmental Screening Test, J. Pediatr. **99**(6):995-999, 1981.

McMillan, J., Nieburg, P., and Oski, F.: The whole pediatrician catalog, Philadelphia, Philadelphia, 1977, W.B. Saunders Co., pp. 38-42.

Pillitteri, A.: Nursing care of the growing fmaily: a child health text, Boston, 1977, Little, Brown & Co., pp. 128-139, 166-168, 191-193, 219-223.

Powell, M.L.: Assessment and management of developmental changes and problems in children, ed. 2, St. Louis, 1981, The C.V. Mosby Co.

Whaley, L.F., and Wong, D.L.: Nursing care of infants and children, ed. 2, St. Louis, 1983, The C.V. Mosby Co., pp. 223-226, 417-433.

### Geriatric

Andriola, M.J.: When an elderly patient complains of weakness . . ., Geriatrics **33**(6):79-84, 1978.

Caird, F.I., and Judge, T.G.: Assessment of the elderly patient, London, 1977, Pitman Medical Publishing Co., Ltd., pp. 65-86.

Carotenuto, R., and Bullock, J.: Physical assessment of the gerontologic client, Philadelphia, 1980, F.A. Davis Co., pp. 121-125.

Cohen, S.B.: Arthritis—but what sort? Geriatrics **37**((12):49-56, 1982.

Eliopoulos, C.: Gerontological nursing, New York, 1979, Harper & Row, Publishers, Inc., pp. 196-206.

Gilmore, R.L.: Recognizing problems of the aging spine, Geriatrics **35**(11):83-92, 1980.

Reich, M.L.: Arthritis: avoiding diagnostic pitfalls, Geriatrics **37**(6):46-54, 1982.

Steinberg, F.U., editor: Care of the geriatric patinet, ed. 6, St. Louis, 1983, The C.V. Mosby Co., pp. 47-73; 143-153, 530-561.

Woodruff, D.S., and Birren, J.: Aging: scientific perspectives and social issues, New York, 1975, D. Van Nostrand Co., pp. 257-276.

ASSESSMENT OF THE

# Neurological system

## VOCABULARY

**ageusia** Absence or impairment of the sense of taste.

**anesthesia** Partial or complete loss of sensation.

**anosmia** Absence or impairment of the sense of smell.

**aphasia** Absence or impairment of the ability to communicate through speech.

**ataxia** Inability to coordinate muscular movement.

**athetosis** Condition in which there are slow, irregular involuntary movements in the upper extremities, especially the hands and fingers.

**cerebellar system** Receives sensory and motor input and coordinates muscular activity; also helps to maintain posture and equilibrium.

**clonus** Abnormal pattern of neuromuscular functioning characterized by rapidly alternating involuntary contraction and relaxation of skeletal muscles.

**dura mater** Tough, fibrous connective tissue that lies directly beneath the periosteum of the cranium.

**dysesthesia** Sensation of something crawling on the skin or of pricks of pins and needles.

**dysmetria** An inability to fix the range of movement in a muscular activity.

**dyssynergia** Failure of muscular coordination. Also known as *ataxia*.

**extrapyramidal system** The motor pathways lying outside the pyramidal tract that help to maintain muscle tone and to control body movements such as walking; includes nerve pathways between the cerebral cortex, basal ganglia, brain stem, and the spinal cord.

**fasciculation** A localized uncontrollable twitching of one muscle group that is innervated by a single motor nerve.

**graphesthesia** Ability to recognize symbols, numbers, or letters traced on the skin.

**hyperesthesia** An abnormally increased sensitivity to sensory stimuli such as touch or pain.

**hyperkinesis** Hyperactivity or excessive muscular activity.

**hypoesthesia** Decreased or dulled sensitivity to stimulation.

**hyposmia** Defective sense of smell.

**kinesthetic sensation** Ability to detect the position of a body part when it is moved through space.

**lower motor neurons** Nerve cells that originate in the anterior horn cells of the spinal column and travel to innervate the skeletal muscle fibers. Injury or disease of this area will result in decreased muscle tone, reflexes, or strength.

**myoclonus** Twitching or clonic spasm of a muscle group.

**paresthesia** Abnormal sensation such as numbness or a tingling feeling.

**proprioception** Awareness of posture, movement, and changes in equilibrium.

**pyramidal tract** Bundle of upper motor neurons that coordinate voluntary movements originating in the motor cortex of the brain; nerve fibers travel through the brain stem and the spinal cord, where they synapse with anterior horn cells; responsible for the coordinated response of voluntary movements; also called *corticospinal tract*.

**Romberg test** Evaluates an individual's ability to maintain a given position when standing erect with feet together and eyes closed.

**spasticity** Increased tone or contractions of muscles causing stiff and awkward movements; seen with upper motor neuron lesions.

**stereognosis** Ability to recognize objects by the sense of touch.

**tic** Spasmodic muscular contraction most commonly involving the face, head, neck, or shoulder muscles.

**tremor** A continuous involuntary trembling movement of a part or parts of the body.

**two-point discrimination** Ability to identify being touched by two sharp objects simultaneously.

**upper motor neurons** Nerve cells that originate in the cerebral cortex and project downward; make up the corticobulbar and pyramidal tracts and end in the anterior horn of the spinal cord; responsible for fine and discrete conscious movements.

**vertigo** The sensation of moving around in space (subjective vertigo) or of objects moving about oneself (objective vertigo); results in disturbance of the individual's equilibrium.

## Overview

Although the techniques of the neurological examination are fairly easy to implement, the interpretation of findings is complex. The examiner is challenged to understand the physiological interpretations of the elicited responses during neurological testing. References for response interpretations are listed under the suggested readings for this chapter.

Assessment of the neurological system may range from a basic screening of function to a highly detailed and lengthy process. This chapter details the process for performing a *screening* neurological examination for asymptomatic clients. The examination evaluates six major areas:

1. Mental assessment and speech patterns
2. Cranial nerves
3. Proprioception and cerebellar function
4. Muscular function
5. Sensory function
6. Reflex function

If the examiner identifies abnormalities in any of the findings, a more detailed evaluation and referral are warranted.

## Cognitive objectives

At the end of this chapter the learner will demonstrate knowledge of assessment of the neurological system by the ability to do the following.

1. Apply the terms in the vocabulary list.
2. List each of the 12 cranial nerves and define the tests used to assess their integrity and the normal and abnormal responses.
3. List the functions of the cerebellum and define the tests used to assess its integrity and the normal and abnormal responses.
4. Describe the differences between the upper and lower motor neurons.
5. Describe the differences between the pyramidal and extrapyramidal tracts and define the tests used to assess their integrity and the normal and abnormal responses.

6. List the sensory modalities usually tested during a screening neurological examination and discuss the normal and abnormal responses.
7. List the deep tendon reflexes examined during a neurological examination, the site of stimulus, and normal and abnormal responses.
8. Describe the evaluation techniques and the significance of the Babinski reflex and clonus.
9. Explain the relationship of a reflex arc and a deep tendon reflex.
10. Identify selected characteristics of the pediatric neurological examination.
11. Identify selected characteristics of the geriatric neurological examination.

## Clinical objectives

At the end of this chapter the learner will perform a systematic assessment of the neurological system, demonstrating the ability to do the following:

1. Obtain a health history appropriate to the screening evaluation of the neurological system.
2. Demonstrate testing of the cranial nerves.
3. Demonstrate testing methods to evaluate the intactness of the proprioception and cerebellar systems.
   a. Use two techniques to evaluate general intactness.
   b. Use two techniques to evaluate upper extremity intactness.
   c. Use one method to evaluate lower extremity intactness.
4. Demonstrate testing methods to evaluate the intactness of sensation, including:
   a. Light touch sensation
   b. Painful sensation
   c. Vibratory sensation
5. Demonstrate one method for evaluating cortical and discriminatory forms of sensation.
6. Demonstrate testing of the deep tendon reflexes, including biceps, triceps, brachioradialis, patellar, and Achilles reflexes.

7. Demonstrate testing of pathological reflexes, including Babinski response, and the test for ankle clonus.
8. Summarize results of the assessment with a written description of findings.

## Health history additional to screening history

1. Any positive finding collected during the screening history should be further explored to describe its characteristics as well as its relation to the client's ability to function. For example, if a client complains of shooting pains in the right leg, the examiner should describe (a) the characteristics of the leg pain (symptom analysis) and (b) how that leg pain interferes with activities of daily living.
2. Complaints such as weakness, nervousness, tremors, or tics should be fully investigated regarding symptom analysis as well as how they interfere with the client's ability to maintain activities of daily living.
3. Clients with complaints of balance problems need further questioning to determine how that problem is precipitated (i.e., position, time of day, activity related, etc.).
4. The term *convulsions* has many meanings. If the client gives this complaint, in-depth data must be collected to document what this term means to the client. Note the following:

a. What happens to the client's eyes during a convulsion?
b. Parts of the body involved?
c. Muscles flaccid versus stiff, tense versus twitching?
d. How long does this last?
e. How many times during past day, week, month, year, years?
f. Current medications?
g. Cause?
h. Interference with activities of daily living, driving, occupation?

5. Head injury and headache history profiles are discussed under *Health history* in Chapter 4.
6. For the client complaining of pain associated with the neurological system, symptom analysis should be performed. The following may be helpful in evaluating the characteristics of that pain:
a. Quality of pain: dull ache, throbbing, sharp or stabbing, burning, pressing, stinging, cramping, gnawing, pricking, shooting
b. Associated manifestation: crying, decreased activities, sweating, muscle rigidity or tremor, impaired mental processes or concentration
7. Objective data can be collected during the history session by noting evidence of factors such as abnormalities in speech, language function, memory, emotional status, and judgment.

## Clinical guidelines

| THE STUDENT WILL: | TO IDENTIFY: NORMAL | DEVIATIONS FROM NORMAL |
|---|---|---|
| **1.** Gather equipment necessary to perform the screening neurological examination:<br>a. Penlight<br>b. Tongue blade<br>c. Safety pin<br>d. Tuning fork (200 to 400 cps)<br>e. Cotton wisp<br>f. Percussion hammer<br>g. Odorous materials | | |

| THE STUDENT WILL: | TO IDENTIFY: | |
| --- | --- | --- |
| | NORMAL | DEVIATIONS FROM NORMAL |

**Mental and speech pattern**

(Mental health status has been previously discussed)

1. Speech pattern

   **a.** Assess during data base collection

| | | |
| --- | --- | --- |
| | Client gives information requested | Error in choice of words or syllables |
| | Speech smooth and flowing | Difficulty in articulation: may involve thought process, tongue, or lips |
| | Logical thought process | Slurred speech (tone sounds slurred) |
| | Able to relate past events | Poorly coordinated or irregular speech |
| | Voice tone has inflections | Monotone voice |
| | Strong voice able to increase volume | Weak voice |
| | Clear voice | Nasal tone, rasping or hoarse, whisper voice |
| | | Stuttering |

**Cranial nerves**

1. CN I: olfactory nerve

   **a.** Obtain information through history or instruct client to close eyes and properly identify aromatic substance (coffee, toothpaste, orange, oil of clove) held under the nose (Fig. 15-1); test one nostril at a time

| | | |
| --- | --- | --- |
| | Client correctly identifies item and odor | Unable to smell anything |
| | | Incorrect identification of odor being tested |

2. CN II: optic nerve (Fig. 15-2) (described in Chapter 7)

   **a.** Testing visual acuity

   **b.** Funduscopy examination

   **c.** Visual fields by confrontation

| | | |
| --- | --- | --- |
| | As previously discussed in Chapter 7 | As previously discussed in Chapter 7 |

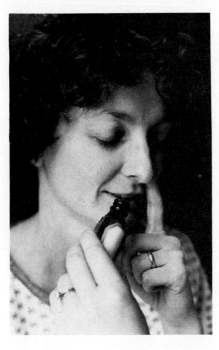

**FIG. 15-1.** Evaluating CN I (olfactory).

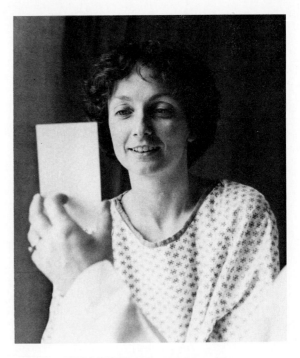

**FIG. 15-2.** Evaluating CN II (optic).

## Clinical guidelines—cont'd

| THE STUDENT WILL: | TO IDENTIFY: | |
| --- | --- | --- |
| | NORMAL | DEVIATIONS FROM NORMAL |
| **3.** CN III: oculomotor nerve (Fig. 15-3) (described in Chapter 7) | As previously discussed in Chapter 7 | As previously described in Chapter 7 |
| **4.** CN IV: trochlear nerve (Fig. 15-4) (described in Chapter 7) | As previously described in Chapter 7 | As previously described in Chapter 7 |

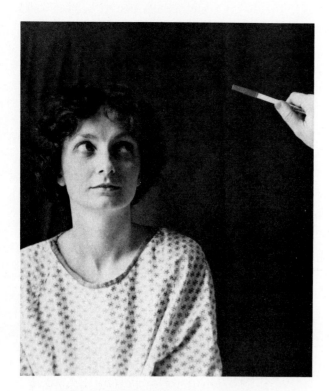

**FIG. 15-3.** Evaluating CN III (oculomotor).

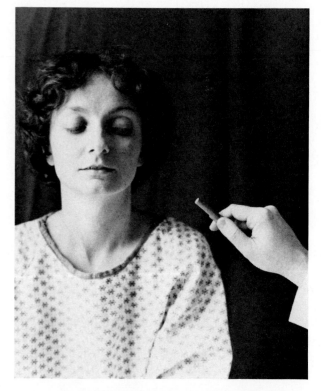

**FIG. 15-4.** Evaluating CN IV (trochlear).

| THE STUDENT WILL: | TO IDENTIFY: | |
| | NORMAL | DEVIATIONS FROM NORMAL |
| --- | --- | --- |
| **5.** CN V: trigeminal nerve<br> **a.** Test *motor* function, instructing client to clench the teeth; then palpate temporal and masseter muscles (Fig. 15-5)<br> **b.** Test *sensory* function with client's eyes closed<br>    1. Light sensation: wipe cotton wisp lightly over client's anterior scalp and paranasal sinuses (Fig. 15-6) | Bilaterally strong muscle contractions<br><br><br><br><br><br>Tickle sensation, equally present over palpated areas | Inequality in muscle contractions<br>Pain with muscle contractions<br>Twitching<br>Asymmetry in movement of jaw<br><br><br>Decreased or unequal sensation |

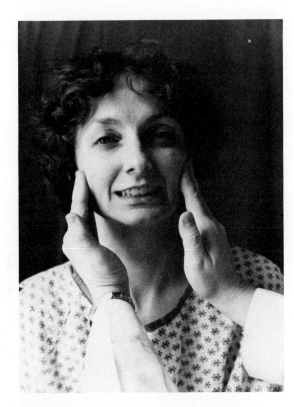

**FIG. 15-5.** Evaluating CN V (trigeminal—motor).

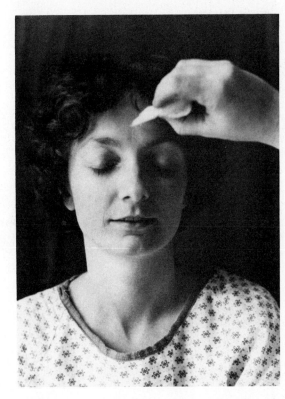

**FIG. 15-6.** Evaluating CN V (trigeminal—light sensory).

## Clinical guidelines—cont'd

| THE STUDENT WILL: | TO IDENTIFY: | |
| | NORMAL | DEVIATIONS FROM NORMAL |
| --- | --- | --- |
| 2. Deep sensation: use alternating blunt and sharp ends of safety pin over client's forehead and paranasal sinus areas (Fig. 15-7) | Able to feel pressure and pain equally throughout<br>Able to differentiate between sharp and dull | Decreased or unequal sensation |
| 3. Corneal reflex: use cotton wisp on cornea; instruct client to look up (approach from side) (Fig. 15-8) | Bilateral blink to corneal touch | No blink (make sure abnormal response not caused by contact lenses) |

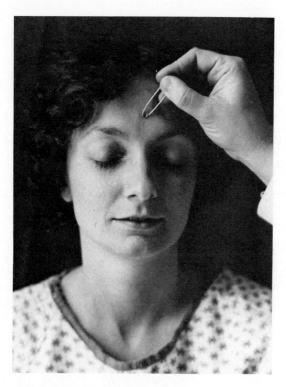

**FIG. 15-7.** Evaluating CN V (trigeminal—deep sensory).

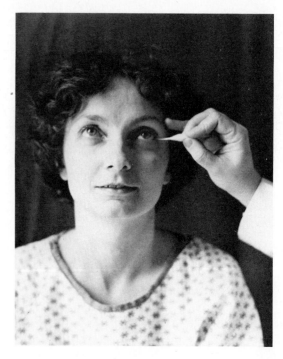

**FIG. 15-8.** Evaluating CN V (trigeminal—corneal reflex).

| | TO IDENTIFY: | |
| THE STUDENT WILL: | NORMAL | DEVIATIONS FROM NORMAL |
| --- | --- | --- |
| **6.** CN VI: abducens nerve (described in Chapter 7) (Fig. 15-9) | As previously described in Chapter 7 | As previously described in Chapter 7 |
| **7.** CN VII: facial nerve | | |
|    **a.** Inspect face both at rest and during conversation | Symmetry of face | Asymmetry, unequal movements, facial weakness<br>Drooping on one side of face or mouth<br>Unable to maintain position until instructed to relax |

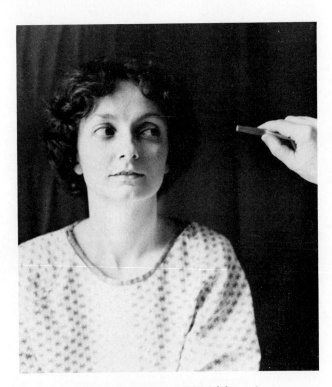

**FIG. 15-9.** Evaluating CN VI (abducens).

# Clinical guidelines—cont'd

| THE STUDENT WILL: | TO IDENTIFY: | |
| --- | --- | --- |
| | **NORMAL** | **DEVIATIONS FROM NORMAL** |

**b.** Instruct client to:
  1. Raise eyebrows
  2. Frown
  3. Close eyes tightly
  4. Show teeth
  5. Smile
  6. Puff out cheeks
  (Fig. 15-10)

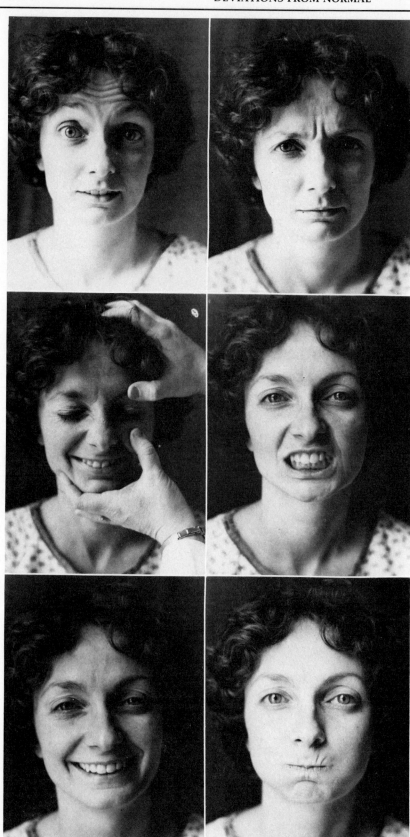

**FIG. 15-10.** Evaluating CN VII (facial).

| THE STUDENT WILL: | TO IDENTIFY: | |
| --- | --- | --- |
| | NORMAL | DEVIATIONS FROM NORMAL |
| c. Evaluate taste over anterior half of tongue (sensory branch of facial nerve) with sugar, salt, lemon juice; instruct client to stick tongue out and leave it out during testing process; use cotton applicator to place small quantity of substance on client's tongue | Able to correctly identify taste | Unable to identify substance<br>Consistently identifies substance incorrectly |
| 8. CN VIII: acoustic nerve (Fig. 15-11); hearing assessment described in Chapter 6 | As previously described in Chapter 6 | As previously described in Chapter 6 |
| 9. CN IX: glossopharyngeal nerve<br>CN X: vagus nerve (tested together) | | |
| a. Instruct client to say "ah" (Fig. 15-12) | Bilaterally equal upward movement of soft palate and uvula<br>Speech smooth<br>Gag will occur | Asymmetry of soft palate movement or tonsillar pillar movement; lateral deviation of uvula<br>Gag reflex absent |
| b. If posterior portion of tongue or pharynx is stimulated: | | |
| 1. Taste: posterior third of tongue (by history) | Able to taste sweet, salt, sour | Unable to differentiate tastes |

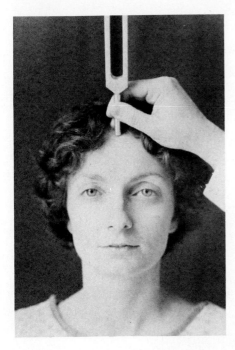

FIG. 15-11. Evaluating CN VIII (acoustic).

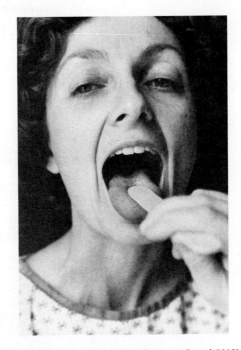

FIG. 15-12. Evaluating CN IX (glossopharyngeal) and CN X (vagus).

## Clinical guidelines—cont'd

| THE STUDENT WILL: | TO IDENTIFY: | |
|---|---|---|
| | NORMAL | DEVIATIONS FROM NORMAL |
| **10.** CN XI: spinal accessory nerve | | |
|     **a.** Instruct client to shrug shoulders upward against examiner's hand (Fig. 15-13, *A*) | Strength and symmetry of contraction of trapezius muscles | Muscle weakness: unilateral, bilateral Pain or discomfort |
|     **b.** Have patient turn head to side against examiner's hand; repeat with other side (Fig. 15-13, *B*) | Observe contraction of opposite sternocleidomastoid muscle; note force of movement against examiner's hand | Unable to maintain contracted muscle position Asymmetry, difficulty of movement |

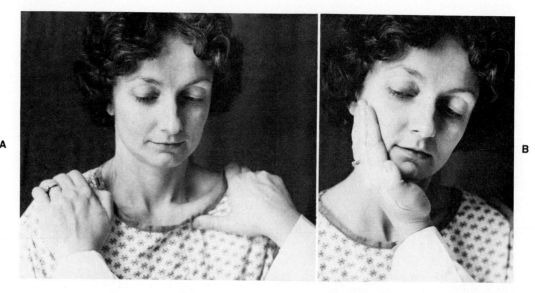

**FIG. 15-13. A,** Evaluating CN XI (spinal accessory). **B,** Evaluating CN XI (spinal accessory).

| | | |
|---|---|---|
| **11.** CN XII: hypoglossal nerve | | |
|     **a.** Motor development of tongue | | |
|         1. Instruct client to stick tongue out and move from side to side (Fig. 15-14) | As previously described in Chapter 5 | As previously described in Chapter 5 |

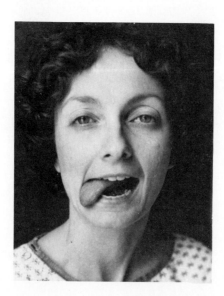

**FIG. 15-14.** Evaluating CN XII (hypoglossal).

| THE STUDENT WILL: | TO IDENTIFY: | |
| | NORMAL | DEVIATIONS FROM NORMAL |

## Proprioception, cerebellar, and motor function

Three areas of coordination and motor function will be evaluated:

1. General function
2. Upper extremity function
3. Lower extremity function

Following are examination techniques for the evaluation of proprioception, cerebellar, and motor functions. For the asymptomatic client the examiner is encouraged to use at least *two* techniques for each area to be assessed. Which two the examiner chooses may depend on the age and overall physical ability of the client. For example, it is not necessary for every client to perform deep knee bends.

Motor function depends on the intactness of three areas:

1. Intact muscles
2. Functioning of the neuromuscular junction
3. Intact cranial and spinal nerves

More specifically, proprioception and cerebellar function depend on the intactness of the upper and lower neurons and the cerebellar system.

The *upper motor neurons* originate in the cerebral cortex and project downward. These neurons make up the corticobulbar tract, which ends in the brain stem, and the corticospinal tract (or pyramidal tract), which ends in the anterior horn of the spinal cord. This tract is responsible for particularly fine and discrete conscious movement.

Malfunctioning within the corticospinal tract will cause a paralysis or spasticity response. Deep tendon reflexes will increase, and the client will experience decreased voluntary functioning of fine motor ability.

The *lower motor neurons* originate in the anterior horn cells of the spinal cord, leave the spinal cord, and travel to and innervate the muscle fibers. Injury or disease affecting the lower motor neurons will result in decreased or absent muscle tone, reflexes, or strength. The examiner will observe local or general muscle wasting and atrophy as well as fasciculations of affected areas.

The *extrapyramidal motor neurons* originate in the cerebral cortex but lie outside the pyramidal or corticospinal tracts. Their function is to help maintain muscle tone and gross body movements such as walking. Clients may have disease of the pyramidal tract and still maintain gross body functioning because of the intactness of the extrapyramidal and lower motor neurons.

If the client is functioning by using the extrapyramidal system, the examiner would expect to find slow or sluggish voluntary movement, slowed coordination, and decrease in fine motor functioning. The reflexes would be normal.

The *proprioception and cerebellar systems* function to maintain posture and balance. Any malfunctioning of this area would impair muscle coordination or the ability to perform movements smoothly. Muscle tone may be decreased, and the examiner may find that following the deep tendon reflex examination the limb tends to "swing."

## Clinical guidelines—cont'd

| THE STUDENT WILL: | TO IDENTIFY: NORMAL | DEVIATIONS FROM NORMAL |
|---|---|---|
| **1.** General (use two for screening of gross motor and balance testing) | | |
| **a.** Assess client's gait function by asking client to walk across room, turn, and walk back | Maintains upright posture; walks unaided, maintaining balance, opposing arm swing | Poor posturing, ataxia, unsteady gait, rigid or no arm movements, wide-base gait, trunk and head held tight, legs bend from hips only, client lurches or reels, scissors gait, steppage gait, staggering gait, parkinsonian gait (stooped posture, flexion at hips, elbows, knees) |
| **b.** Perform Romberg test by asking client to stand with feet together, arms resting at sides, first with eyes open, then with eyes closed (Fig. 15-15) | Slight swaying, but upright posture and foot stance maintained | Unable to maintain foot stance; moves to wider foot base to maintain posture |
| **c.** Instruct client to walk a straight line, placing heel of one foot directly against toes of other foot (Fig. 15-16) | Able to maintain heel-toe walking pattern along straight line | Unable to maintain heel-toe walking pattern Steps to wider-base gait to maintain upright posture |
| **d.** Instruct client to close eyes and stand on one foot and then other (Fig. 15-17) | Able to maintain position for at least 5 seconds | Unable to maintain single-foot balancing for 5 seconds |

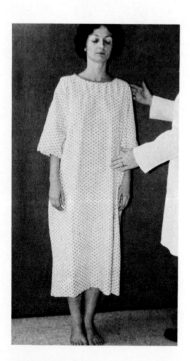

**FIG. 15-15.** Balance testing using Romberg test.

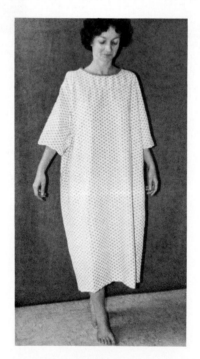

**FIG. 15-16.** Evaluating balance by having client walk a straight line.

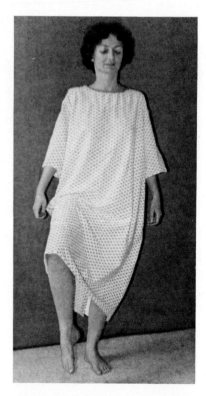

**FIG. 15-17.** One-foot balance testing with eyes closed.

| THE STUDENT WILL: | TO IDENTIFY: | |
| --- | --- | --- |
| | NORMAL | DEVIATIONS FROM NORMAL |
| **e.** Hopping in place: instruct client to first hop on one foot and then other (Fig. 15-18) | Able to follow directions successfully<br>Muscle strength adequate to follow through | Unable to hop or to maintain single-leg balance |
| **f.** Knee bends: instruct client to hold hands outward and perform several shallow or deep knee bends (Fig. 15-19) | Able to follow directions successfully<br>Muscle strength adequate to follow through | Unable to perform activity because of balance difficulty or muscle strength |
| **g.** Walk on toes, then heels | Able to follow directions by walking several steps on toes and then heels<br>May need to use hands to maintain balance | Unable to maintain balance<br>Poor muscle strength<br>Unable to complete activity |

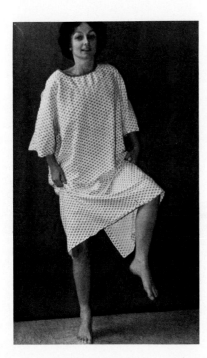

FIG. 15-18. Evaluating balance by having client hop in place.

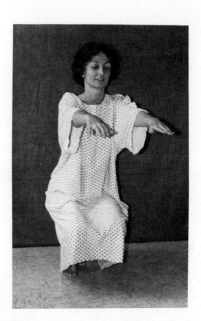

FIG. 15-19. Balance testing by having client perform deep knee bends.

| | | |
| --- | --- | --- |
| **2.** Upper extremity testing (use two for screening of upper extremity and fine motor testing) | | |
| **a.** Using pronation and supination of hands, instruct client to alternately tap knees (do both hands together); use rapid movement (see Fig. 14-17) | Bilaterally equal timing<br>Purposeful movement<br><br>Able to maintain rapid pace | Unequal movement<br>Sloppy or increasingly sloppy movement<br><br>Unable to maintain rapid pace |

## Clinical guidelines—cont'd

| THE STUDENT WILL: | TO IDENTIFY: | |
| --- | --- | --- |
| | NORMAL | DEVIATIONS FROM NORMAL |
| **b.** With arm stretched outward, instruct client to use index fingers to alternately touch nose (eyes closed) rapidly (Fig. 15-20) | Able to repeatedly touch nose<br>Rhythmic response | Sloppy response<br>Misses nose many times<br>Arms unable to maintain testing position, drift downward |

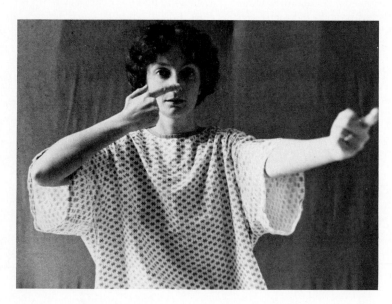

**FIG. 15-20.** Evaluating fine motor function by having client touch nose with alternating hands.

| | | |
| --- | --- | --- |
| **c.** Evaluate client's ability to perform rapid rhythmic alternating movement of fingers (test each hand separately); ask client to touch each finger to thumb, in rapid sequence (Fig. 15-21) | Can rapidly and purposefully touch each finger to thumb | Unable to coordinate fine, discrete, rapid movement |

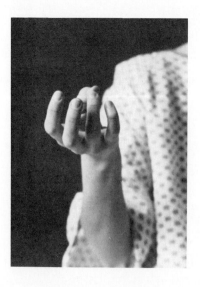

**FIG. 15-21.** Evaluating fine motor function by rapid rhythmic alternating movement of fingers.

| THE STUDENT WILL: | TO IDENTIFY: | |
| --- | --- | --- |
| | NORMAL | DEVIATIONS FROM NORMAL |
| **d.** Instruct client to rapidly move index finger back and forth between client's nose and examiner's finger (approximately 46 cm [18 inches] apart); test one hand at a time (Fig. 15-22) | Able to maintain activity with conscious coordinated effort | Unable to maintain continuous touch with both own nose and examiner's finger<br>Unable to maintain rapid movement<br>Coordination difficulty obvious |

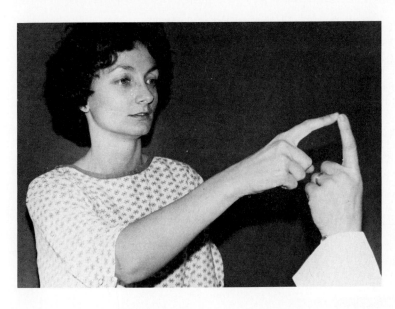

**FIG. 15-22.** Evaluating fine motor function by rapid movement of client's finger between own nose and examiner's finger.

| | | |
| --- | --- | --- |
| **3.** Lower extremity testing for fine motor function | | |
| **a.** Instruct seated client to place heel of one foot just below opposite knee on tibia; then instruct client to run heel down shin to foot; repeat with other foot (Fig. 15-23) | Able to purposefully run heel down opposite shin<br>Bilaterally equal coordination | Unable to coordinate activity<br>Heel keeps moving off shin<br>Unequal responses<br>Tremors or awkwardness |

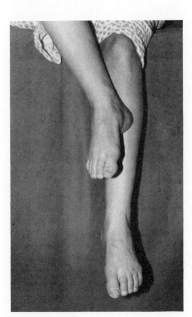

**FIG. 15-23.** Evaluating fine motor function by having client run heel of one foot down tibia of other leg.

# Clinical guidelines—cont'd

| THE STUDENT WILL: | TO IDENTIFY: | |
| --- | --- | --- |
| | NORMAL | DEVIATIONS FROM NORMAL |

## Muscular function

Muscle function and strength testing are discussed in Chapter 14.

## Sensory function

This component of the examination evaluates intactness of the dermatomes and major peripheral nerves. The examiner must have knowledge of normal dermatome areas and the spinal nerves represented as well as the major peripheral nerves and areas of sensation.

The examiner should test the peripheral extremities in several areas for sensation. If sensation is intact, no further extremity evaluation is necessary. If the peripheral sensation is impaired, the examiner should move up the extremities, testing periodically until a level or area of sensation is identified. Beyond the extremities the examiner should also evaluate the forehead, cheeks, and abdomen.

If a deviation is identified, try to map out the area involved.

The examiner must compare bilateral responses in each of the following sensation testing categories.

| THE STUDENT WILL: | NORMAL | DEVIATIONS FROM NORMAL |
| --- | --- | --- |
| **1.** Primary sensory screening | | |
| **a.** Light touch sensation: use cotton wisp to lightly touch each designated area (client's eyes closed) (Fig. 15-24) | Client perceives light sensation<br>Client able to correctly point to spot where touched | Unable to perceive touch<br>Incorrectly identifies touched location<br>Asymmetrical response |

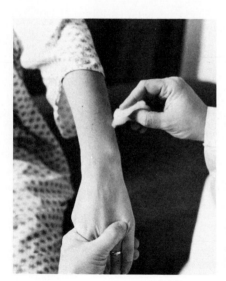

**FIG. 15-24.** Evaluating light sensory function of forearm (eyes closed).

| THE STUDENT WILL: | NORMAL | DEVIATIONS FROM NORMAL |
| --- | --- | --- |
| **b.** Painful sensation: using pointed tip of a pin, lightly prick each designated area (client's eyes closed) (Fig. 15-25); it may be helpful to alternate light and pain sensations to more accurately evaluate client's response | Client perceives pain<br>Client able to correctly point to spot where touched | Unable to perceive pain sensation<br>Incorrectly identifies touched location<br>Asymmetrical response |

| THE STUDENT WILL: | TO IDENTIFY: | |
|---|---|---|
| | NORMAL | DEVIATIONS FROM NORMAL |

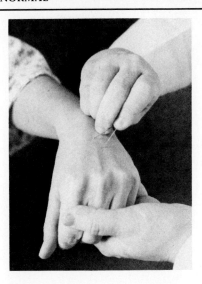

**FIG. 15-25.** Evaluating pain sensation (eyes closed).

| | | |
|---|---|---|
| **c.** Vibration sensation: have client verbalize what is felt when a vibrating tuning fork is placed on a bony area of wrist, ankle, and sternum (Fig. 15-26) | Client feels sense of vibration (decreased sensation may be normal response in order adults) | Unequal or decreased vibratory sensations |

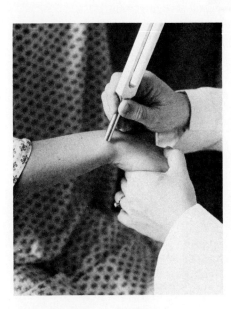

**FIG. 15-26.** Evaluating vibratory sensation over bony prominence.

# Clinical guidelines—cont'd

| THE STUDENT WILL: | TO IDENTIFY: | |
| --- | --- | --- |
| | NORMAL | DEVIATIONS FROM NORMAL |

**2.** Cortical and discriminatory forms of sensation (use one for screening)

**a.** Stereognosis: place small familiar object in client's hand and ask client to identify it (Fig. 15-27) — Appropriate identification — Unable to correctly identify object

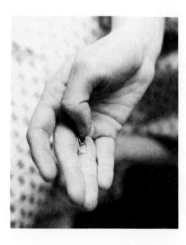

**FIG. 15-27.** Evaluating stereognosis by client's ability to properly identify a familiar object placed in the hand (eyes closed).

**b.** Two-point discrimination: touch selected parts of the body simultaneously with two sharp objects (client's eyes closed); ask client if one or two objects are used (Fig. 15-28)

Can distinguish two-point discrimination
Fingertips: 2.8 mm
Palms: 8 to 12 mm
Chest/forearm: 40 mm
Back: 40 to 70 mm
Upper arm/thigh: 75 mm

Unable to tell two-point discrimination within normal limits

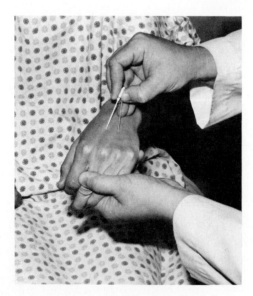

**FIG. 15-28.** Evaluating two-point discrimination of dorsal surface of hand (eyes closed).

| THE STUDENT WILL: | TO IDENTIFY: | |
| | NORMAL | DEVIATIONS FROM NORMAL |
| --- | --- | --- |
| **c.** Graphesthesia: use blunt instrument to draw number or letter on client's hand, back, or other area (client's eyes closed) (Fig. 15-29) | Client able to recognize drawn number or letter | Client unable to distinguish number or letter |

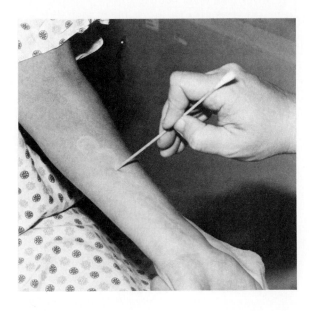

**FIG. 15-29.** Evaluating discriminatory sensation by using graphesthesia (eyes closed).

| | | |
| --- | --- | --- |
| **d.** Kinesthetic sensation: with client's eyes closed, grasp client's finger and move its position (Fig. 15-30) | Client able to describe how finger position has changed | Unable to distinguish position change |

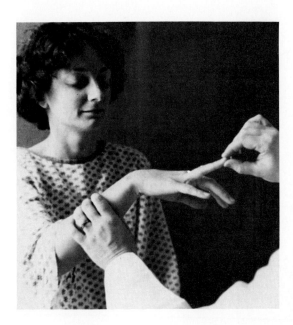

**FIG. 15-30.** Evaluating discriminatory sensation by using kinesthesia (eyes closed).

## Clinical guidelines—cont'd

| | TO IDENTIFY: | |
|---|---|---|
| **THE STUDENT WILL:** | **NORMAL** | **DEVIATIONS FROM NORMAL** |

**Reflex status**

The reflex arc consists of five steps:
1. The receptor cells of the tendon are stimulated.
2. The nerve impulse travels along an afferent or sensory neuron from the receptor cells by means of the dorsal root until it synapses with an anterior horn cell.
3. After the synapse the impulse is transmitted directly or indirectly to an efferent neuron.
4. The impulse travels along the efferent or motor neuron by means of the ventral root until it innervates a skeletal muscle.
5. The skeletal muscle contracts.

During evaluation of the client's reflexes, irritation or disruption to any portion of the reflex arc will result in disruption of the reflex response. This includes the areas previously discussed regarding corticospinal, sensory, or lower motor neuron disturbances. (See *Clinical strategies* for a description of percussion technique and the use of reinforcment.)

Deep tendon reflex responses are commonly scored as follows:
1. 4+ or + + + +: brisk, hyperactive, clonus
2. 3+ or + + +: more brisk than normal but not necessarily indicating disease
3. 2+ or + +: normal
4. 1+ or +: low normal; sluggish response
5. 0: no response

It will take a beginning examiner much practice and working with a preceptor to determine the actual clinical criteria for this scoring. In attempting to elicit an accurate response, the examiner must be confident that the technique being used is correct.

1. Deep tendon reflexes (all are to be tested; client to be seated)

   a. Biceps reflex (tests C5 and C6): client's arm should be partially flexed at elbow, with palms down; examiner places thumb on biceps tendon and strikes reflex hammer on thumb toward tendon (Fig. 15-31)

   | | |
   |---|---|
   | Bilaterally equal response; responds rapidly | Hyperactive or diminished response |
   | Contraction of biceps | Unequal response bilaterally |

**FIG. 15-31.** Tendon of biceps brachialis muscle. (Percuss at arrow.)

| | TO IDENTIFY: | |
|---|---|---|
| **THE STUDENT WILL:** | **NORMAL** | **DEVIATIONS FROM NORMAL** |
| **b.** Triceps tendon (tests C6, C7, and C8): flex client's arm at elbow, palm relaxed at side of body; abduct elbow; strike triceps tendon above elbow (Fig. 15-32) | Extension of elbow and contraction of triceps muscle<br>Bilaterally equal response | Hyperactive or diminished response<br>Unequal response bilaterally |

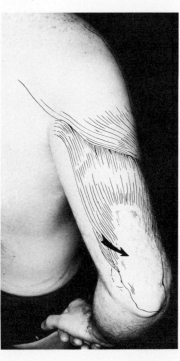

**FIG. 15-32.** Tendon of triceps muscle. (Percuss at arrow.)

| | | |
|---|---|---|
| **c.** Brachioradialis tendon (tests C5 and C6): with client's forearm resting on abdomen or lap (palm down), strike radius 2.5 to 5 cm (1 to 2 inches) above wrist over tendon (Fig. 15-33) | Flexion of elbow and pronation of forearm<br>Bilaterally equal response | Hyperactive or diminished response<br>Unequal response bilaterally |

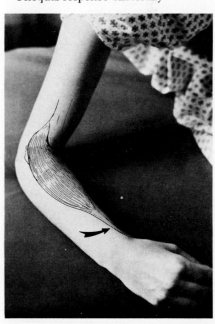

**FIG. 15-33.** Tendon of brachioradialis muscle. (Percuss at arrow.)

## Clinical guidelines—cont'd

| | TO IDENTIFY: | |
| THE STUDENT WILL: | NORMAL | DEVIATIONS FROM NORMAL |
| --- | --- | --- |
| **d.** Abdominal reflexes (tests T8, T9, T10, T11, and T12): with client lying, lightly stroke with sharp instrument both above and below umbilicus in directions as indicated (Fig. 15-34) | Abdominal muscles contract slightly Umbilicus moves slightly toward area of stimulus Bilaterally equal response | Absent or unilateral response |

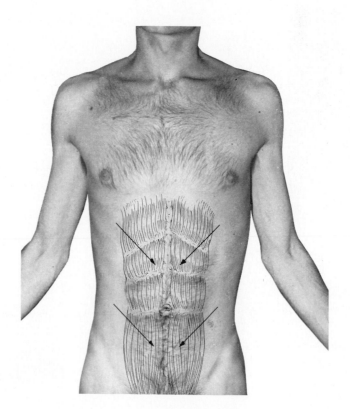

**FIG. 15-34.** Assessment of abdominal reflexes.

| THE STUDENT WILL: | TO IDENTIFY: | |
| --- | --- | --- |
| | NORMAL | DEVIATIONS FROM NORMAL |
| **e.** Knee (patellar) reflex (tests L2, L3, and L4): with client sitting or lying and knee flexed and relaxed, tap patellar tendon just below patella (Fig. 15-35) | Contraction of quadriceps with extension of lower leg from knee<br>Bilaterally equal rsponse | Hyperactive or diminished response<br>Unequal response bilaterally |
| **f.** Ankle (Achilles) reflex (tests S1 and S2): with leg somewhat flexed at knee, dorsiflex ankle; strike Achilles tendon (Fig. 15-36) | Plantar flexion of foot at ankle<br>Bilaterally equal response | Hyperactive or diminished response<br>Unequal response bilaterally |

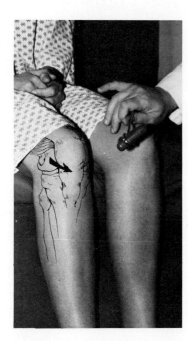

**FIG. 15-35.** Assessment of patellar tendon. (Percuss at arrow.)

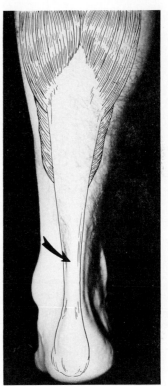

**FIG. 15-36.** Achilles tendon. (Percuss at arrow.)

## Clinical guidelines—cont'd

| | TO IDENTIFY: | |
|---|---|---|
| **THE STUDENT WILL:** | **NORMAL** | **DEVIATIONS FROM NORMAL** |
| **2.** Pathological reflexes | | |
| **a.** Plantar (Babinski) response: using moderately sharp object, stroke lateral aspect of sole from heel to ball of foot, curving medially across ball (Fig. 15-37) | Flexion of great toe, with fanning of other toes | Extension of great toe, with fanning of other toes<br><br>Indicates pyramidal tract disease |

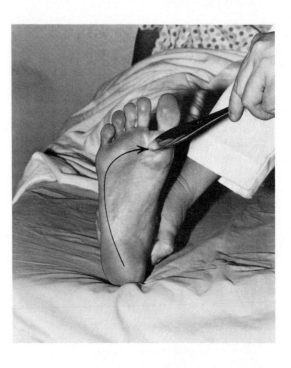

FIG. 15-37. Evaluating for plantar (Babinski) reflex.

| | | |
|---|---|---|
| **b.** Test for ankle clonus (if reflexes are hyperactive): support knee in partly flexed position; with other hand, sharply dorsiflex foot and maintain in flexion (Fig. 15-38) | No movement of foot | Rhythmic oscillations between dorsiflexion and plantar flexion |

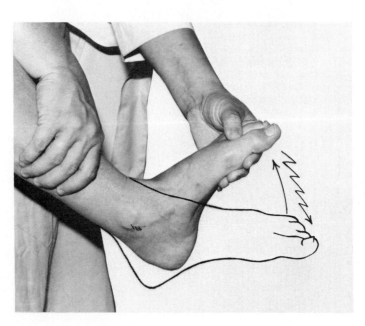

FIG. 15-38. Evaluating for ankle clonus.

## Clinical strategies

1. Symmetry is the key!
2. There are numerous tests to screen the various neurological systems. Which specific set the examiner chooses is up to the individual. There should be consideration of the client's functional ability to understand and follow through. For example, deep knee bends or rapid alternating hand movement would not be appropriate for an older adult with osteoarthritis.
3. The important issue is to provide selected screening exercises in each of the designated areas. To skip a total area of assessment is inappropriate.
4. Develop a *method* to examine the neurological system and stick to that general method every time. This will prevent missing any aspect.
5. The percussion hammer, like all other assessment tools, must be correctly used to obtain the desired response. Following are several strategies:
    a. The client must be relaxed and the extremities loose.
    b. The limb should be positioned so that there is slight tension on the tendon to be evaluated. For example, flex the knee to approximately 90 degrees before testing the patellar tendon.
    c. The examiner should hold the percussion hammer between the thumb and index finger loosely so that, as the examiner taps the desired tendon, the hammer is able to move in a smooth and rapid yet controlled direction.
    d. The action of percussion with a hammer should be just like the percussion used on the thorax or abdomen. The examiner should use a rapid wrist-flick motion to percuss the desired tendon.

The tap should be quick, firm, and well directed. As soon as the tendon is tapped, the examiner should flick the wrist back so that the hammer doesn't remain on the tendon.
    e. Before the actual percussion, the examiner should palpate the desired tendon so that the precise location will be percussed (Fig. 15-39).
6. If the client is heavy, deep tendon reflexes may be very difficult to elicit. The examiner should spend time trying to specifically locate the tendon before striking it with the hammer.
7. If the examiner has difficulty eliciting the deep tendon reflex in a client who shows no signs of neurological dysfunction, several techniques may be tried.
    a. Change the client's position. If the client was sitting, try the technique with the client lying down. Any position may be used, as long as there is slight tension of the muscle or tendon being tested.
    b. If the examiner has difficulty eliciting the deep tendon reflex response of the lower extremity, it may be helpful to use the Jendrassik maneuver of reinforcement. The client locks the fingers together and pulls one hand against the other while the examiner attempts to elicit the lower leg reflexes.
    c. Reinforcement for the upper extremities may include instructing the client to tightly clench the teeth or tighten the muscles in the legs.
    d. If the examiner continues to have difficulty, the percussion technique should be reexamined.
8. Because of the vast complexity of the neurological examination, it must be reemphasized that the clinical guidelines presented in this chapter are meant to be used for well-adult screening. If the examiner is expected to examine a client with neurological dysfunction, there will be a need to gain additional skills.

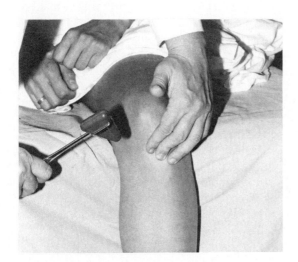

**FIG. 15-39.** Percussing tendon.

### SAMPLE RECORDING

Alert, oriented ×3, CN intact I to XII, coordinated movements and gait, negative Romberg. Cerebellar, sensory, and motor testing intact and bilaterally equal for both upper and lower extremities.
DTR intact, bilaterally equal, neither diminished nor hyperactive.

## History and clinical strategies: the pediatric child

1. The neurological assessment of the child is unlike that of the adult because the central nervous system of babies and very young children is incompletely developed and in fact operates at a subcortical level. The newborn neurological examination reflects brain stem and spinal cord activity. As the child develops, and with increased myelinization and maturation of the neurological system, the examination becomes more like that for the adult client. The clinical guidelines for assessment of the pediatric client have four components: (a) assessment of infants under 1 year of age, (b) assessment of children 1 to 3 years of age, (c) assessment of children over age 3 years, and (d) screening assessment of neurological "soft" signs.

2. The data base history provides evaluative characteristics to accurately assess the maturational and neurological status of the child. In addition to this, the examiner should inquire about the mother's pregnancy when assessing a newborn or infant. Specifically, the mother should be queried regarding history of drug usage, infections, trauma, intoxication, and metabolic disturbances. A careful family history should be gathered regarding seizure disorders or systemic diseases such as muscular dystrophy or cerebral palsy.

3. The parents should be asked if the child has continued to grow and mature normally. Ask how this child's development compares to that of siblings.

4. Has the parent noted any clumsiness, unsteady gait, progressive muscular weakness, or unexplained falling? Describe.

5. Has the child experienced learning or school difficulties associated with attention, interest, activity level, or ability to concentrate?

6. Has the child had a head injury or neurological problems such as seizure, tremor, or weakness in the past? Describe in detail.

7. Has the parent noticed or has the child complained of any problems when going up and down stairs? Is there muscular weakness or weakness when getting up from a lying position on the floor? These are screening questions for muscular dystrophy and should be asked during an examination.

8. The neurological examination, like the musculoskeletal examination, begins as the examiner first meets the child. The examiner should note overall alertness, coordination, and body muscle tone. Observe the child undressing or the parent undressing the child. The examiner should observe for gross floppiness, incoordination, or weakness.

9. In older children, the examiner should evaluate language, as well as adaptive and motor behavior.

10. In younger children the examiner should watch the child at play. Observe the infant lying on the examination table or sitting in the parent's lap. Observe the toddler moving around the room, taking off shoes, and using a pincer grip. Observations should include purposefulness of movements, symmetry, and motor tone.

11. The examiner must get a general impression of the child's abilities and responsiveness.

12. Even for young children there must be some structure to neurological assessment. Although the examiner must be alert to neurological function and maturational development throughout the examination, there must be a designated time for actual reflex testing, motor tone evaluation, and cerebellar functioning. When the examiner incorporates these techniques does not matter. We recommend placing them in the middle of the examination. Although they are not considered intrusive procedures, such as the ear and throat examination, their successful evaluation is dependent on the full cooperation and enthusiasm of the child.

13. The Denver Developmental Screening Test (DDST) (Fig. 15-40, *A* and *B*) or the Denver Developmental Screening Test Revised (DDST-R) (Fig. 15-41) should be used to evaluate the personal/social, fine motor/adaptive, language, and gross motor functioning of all children from 1 month through 6 years. These evaluations are meant to uncover "red flags" that indicate lags in the child's development. The DDST-R was released in 1981. The purpose of this new shortened version is to collect screening data without the lengthy procedure required by the DDST. The examiner is encouraged to use the DDST-R first and then progress to the full DDST for those children who require a more extensive evaluation. The directions and equipment for using either of the DDST forms are extremely important in attaining valid and reliable results. The box on p. 512 provides an overview of the procedures. Every examiner should become familiar with these and other similar screening tests, such as the Goodenough Draw-a-Person test (see box on p. 513), and incorporate them into practice on a regular basis.

*Text continued on p. 514.*

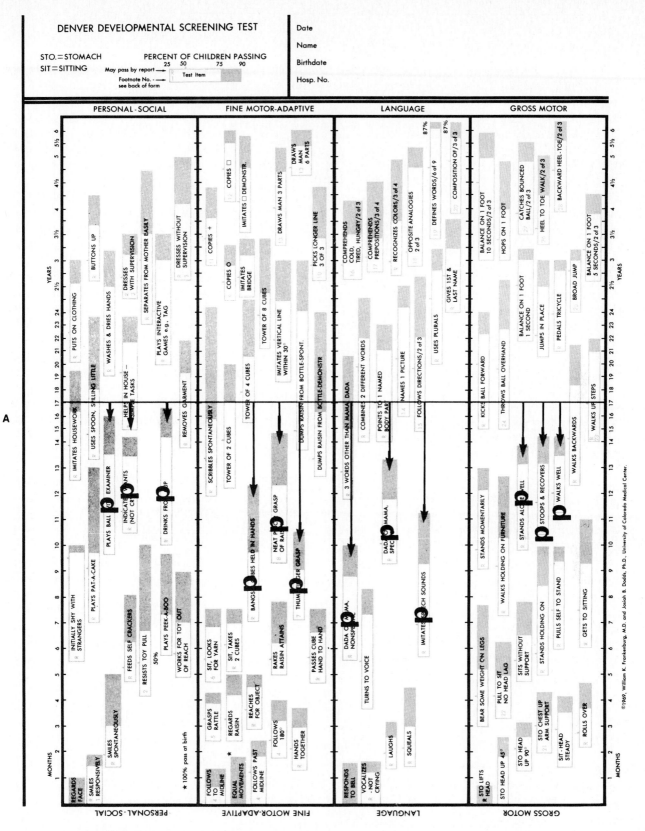

**FIG. 15-40. A,** Denver Developmental Screening Test (DDST). (From Frankenburg, W.K., Sciarillo, W., and Burgess, D.: J. Pediatr. **99**(6):995-999, 1981.)                *Continued.*

DATE

NAME

DIRECTIONS

BIRTHDATE

HOSP. NO.

1. Try to get child to smile by smiling, talking or waving to him.  Do not touch him.
2. When child is playing with toy, pull it away from him.  Pass if he resists.
3. Child does not have to be able to tie shoes or button in the back.
4. Move yarn slowly in an arc from one side to the other, about 6" above child's face.
   Pass if eyes follow 90° to midline.  (Past midline; 180°)
5. Pass if child grasps rattle when it is touched to the backs or tips of fingers.
6. Pass if child continues to look where yarn disappeared or tries to see where it went.  Yarn
   should be dropped quickly from sight from tester's hand without arm movement.
7. Pass if child picks up raisin with any part of thumb and a finger.
8. Pass if child picks up raisin with the ends of thumb and index finger using an over hand
   approach.

9. Pass any en-
   closed form.
   Fail continuous
   round motions.

10. Which line is longer?
    (Not bigger.)  Turn
    paper upside down and
    repeat.  (3/3 or 5/6)

11. Pass any
    crossing
    lines.

12. Have child copy
    first.  If failed,
    demonstrate

When giving items 9, 11 and 12, do not name the forms.  Do not demonstrate 9 and 11.

13. When scoring, each pair (2 arms, 2 legs, etc.) counts as one part.
14. Point to picture and have child name it.  (No credit is given for sounds only.)

15. Tell child to:  Give block to Mommie; put block on table; put block on floor.  Pass 2 of 3.
    (Do not help child by pointing, moving head or eyes.)
16. Ask child:  What do you do when you are cold? ..hungry? ..tired?  Pass 2 of 3.
17. Tell child to:  Put block on table; under table; in front of chair, behind chair.
    Pass 3 of 4.  (Do not help child by pointing, moving head or eyes.)
18. Ask child:  If fire is hot, ice is ?; Mother is a woman, Dad is a ?; a horse is big, a
    mouse is ?.  Pass 2 of 3.
19. Ask child:  What is a ball?  ..lake? ..desk? ..house? ..banana? ..curtain? ..ceiling?
    ..hedge? ..pavement?  Pass if defined in terms of use, shape, what it is made of or general
    category (such as banana is fruit, not just yellow).  Pass 6 of 9.
20. Ask child:  What is a spoon made of? ..a shoe made of? ..a door made of?  (No other objects
    may be substituted.)  Pass 3 of 3.
21. When placed on stomach, child lifts chest off table with support of forearms and/or hands.
22. When child is on back, grasp his hands and pull him to sitting.  Pass if head does not hang back.
23. Child may use wall or rail only, not person.  May not crawl.
24. Child must throw ball overhand 3 feet to within arm's reach of tester.
25. Child must perform standing broad jump over width of test sheet.  (8-1/2 inches)
26. Tell child to walk forward,          heel within 1 inch of toe.
    Tester may demonstrate.  Child must walk 4 consecutive steps, 2 out of 3 trials.
27. Bounce ball to child who should stand 3 feet away from tester.  Child must catch ball with
    hands, not arms, 2 out of 3 trials.
28. Tell child to walk backward,          toe within 1 inch of heel.
    Tester may demonstrate.  Child must walk 4 consecutive steps, 2 out of 3 trials.

DATE AND BEHAVIORAL OBSERVATIONS (how child feels at time of test, relation to tester, attention
span, verbal behavior, self-confidence, etc,):

B

**FIG. 15-40, cont'd. B,** Directions for Denver Developmental Screening Test. (From W.K. Frankenburg and J.B. Dobbs, University of Colorado Medical Center, 1969.

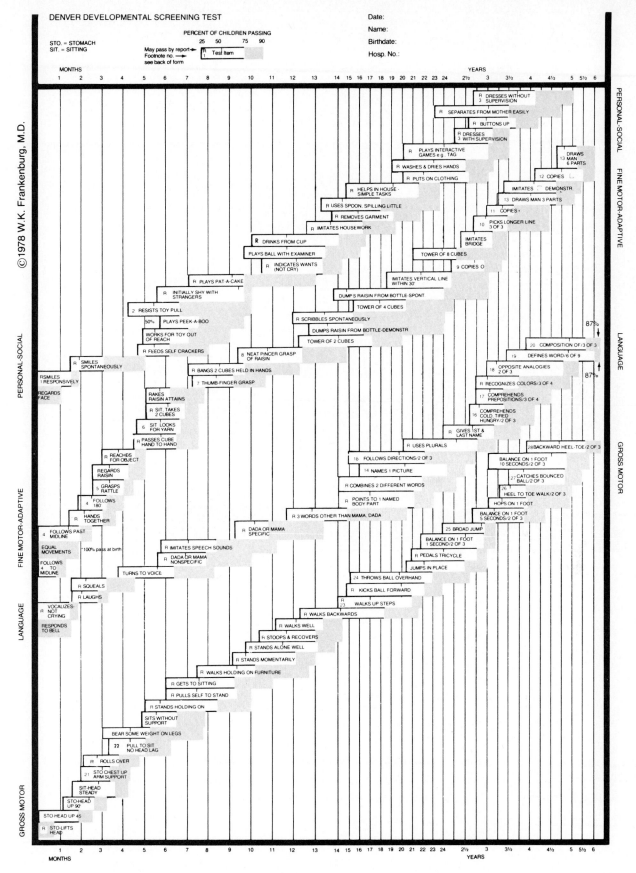

**FIG. 15-41.** Denver Developmental Screening Test Revised (DDST-R). (From Frankenburg, W.K., Sciarillo, W., and Burgess, D.: J. Pediatr. **99**(6):995-999, 1981.)

## DENVER DEVELOPMENTAL SCREENING TESTS

### Denver Developmental Screening Test (DDST)

*Overview:* This test is composed of four major categories: personal/social, fine motor/adaptive, language, and gross motor.

*Use:* Children from ages 1 month through 6 years. The tool was development for potential evaluation every month through 24 months, then every 6 months until age 6 years.

*Limitations:* Frankenburg and associates [J. Pediatr. **99**(6):995-999, 1981] report that one weakness of the DDST is in terms of predictive validity with lower socioeconomic groups.

*Procedures:* The DDST takes approximately 30 minutes to administer. The examiner should use a regulated DDST kit and follow the procedure manual exactly.* According to the instructions, items are scored "P" for pass, "F" for fail, and "R" for refusal. *Fail* is used to designate any item not passed by the child being tested that is passed by 90% of all children of the same age. If it is determined that the child is not performing in his typical behavior, the DDST should be repeated at a later date.

### Denver Developmental Screening Test Revised (DDST-R)

*Overview:* This test is composed of the same four categories (above) as the DDST.

*Use:* Same as for the DDST.

*Limitations:* Same as for the DDST.

*Procedures:* The DDST-R should take between 15 and 20 minutes to administer. The examiner should use a regulated DDST-R kit and follow the procedure manual exactly.* According to the instructions, only the items passed are scored. *Fail* is considered similar to the same designation in the DDST. Subsequent testing of the child requires administering only those items not previously scored with a "P" that are to the left of the child's age line.

*DDST and DDST-R kits and instruction manuals are available from LADOCA Publishing Foundation, E. Fifty-first and Lincoln St., Denver, Colo. 80216.

## GOODENOUGH DRAW-A-PERSON TEST

*Purpose:* This screening test assesses mental or intellectual development in children from 3 to 10 years of age.

*Instructions:* The child is seated at a table and given a pencil with an eraser and an piece of paper. The examiner should tell the child to "draw the best picture of a man or a person that you can draw." No other instructions should be given. The child should then be left alone and given as much time as needed to draw the picture.

*Scoring:* Using the scoring criteria listed below, give one (1) point for each item in the drawing. Each point equals 3 months. The number of points are then converted to months and/or years. The final score in months or years is approximately equal to the child's mental age.

*IQ:* The child's IQ may be approximated by the following method: Divide the child's calculated mental age (determined by the Goodenough test) by his or her real chronologic age and then multiply that number by 100. This will given an approximate IQ.

### Scoring criteria

1. Head present
2. Legs present
3. Arms present
4. Trunk present
5. Trunk longer than broad
6. Shoulder indicated
7. Both arms and legs attached to trunk
8. Legs and arms attached to trunk at proper level
9. Neck present
10. Outline of neck continuous with that of head or trunk or both
11. Eyes present
12. Nose present
13. Mouth present
14. Both nose and mouth in two dimensions; two lips shown
15. Nostrils indicated
16. Hair shown
17. Hair on more than circumference of head, non-transparent, better than scribble
18. Clothing present
19. Two articles of clothing, nontransparent
20. Entire clothing with sleeves and trousers shown, nontransparent
21. Four or more articles of clothing definitely indicated
22. Costume complete without incongruities
23. Fingers shown
24. Correct number of fingers
25. Fingers in two dimensions, length greater than breadth, angle subtended not greater than 180 degrees
26. Opposition of thumbs shown
27. Hands shown distinct from fingers and arms
28. Arm joints shown (elbow or shoulder or both)
29. Head in proportion
30. Arms in proportion
31. Legs in proportion
32. Feet in proportion
33. Arms and legs in two dimensions
34. Heel shown
35. Lines somewhat controlled
36. Lines well controlled
37. Head outline well controlled
38. Trunk outline well controlled
39. Outline of arms and legs well controlled
40. Outline of features well controlled
41. Ears present
42. Ears present in correct position
43. Eyebrows or lashes present
44. Pupil shown
45. Proportion of eyes correct
46. Glance directed to front in profile drawing
47. Both chin and forehead shown
48. Projection of chin shown
49. Profile with not more than one error
50. Correct profile

Data from Goodenough, F.L.: Measurement of intelligence by drawings, New York, 1926, World Book Co.

14. Table 15-1 lists the milestones associated with normal neurological development. Note that the find and gross motor criteria are the same as listed in Chapter 14, on assessment of the musculoskeletal system. These criteria reflect items tested by the Denver Developmental Screening Test.

15. Table 15-2 lists "red flags," or warning signs, to determine whether the child's neurological development is lagging. Although every expert would agree that children mature at different rates, norms for lag limits must be developed. If the examiner encounters a child who seems to have difficulty, special attention should be given to a thorough neurological examination, implementation of the Denver Developmental Screening Test or similar tool, and, finally, referral to a physician.

16. As with the adult examination, the following clinical guidelines reflect screening procedures for the healthy child. If the child shows significant signs of neurological difficulty, referral and in-depth evaluation are warranted.

**TABLE 15-1.** Normal developmental milestones*

| AGE | FINE MOTOR | GROSS MOTOR | SOCIAL/ADAPTIVE | LANGUAGE |
|---|---|---|---|---|
| 1 month | Follows with eyes to midline | Turns head to side<br>Keeps knees tucked under abdomen<br>When pulled to sitting position has gross head lag and rounded swayed back | Regards face | Responds to bell |
| 2 months | Follows objects well; may not follow past midline (major developmental milestone | Holds head in same plane as rest of body<br>Can raise head and maintain position; looks downward | Smiles responsively | Vocalizes (not crying) |
| 3 months | Follows past midline<br>When in supine position puts hands together; will hold hands in front of face | Raises head to 45° angle<br>Maintains posture<br>Looks around with head<br>May turn from prone to side position<br>When pulled into sitting position shows only slight head lag | | Laughs |
| 4 months | Grasps rattle<br>Plays with hands together | Actively lifts head up and looks around<br>Will roll from prone to supine position<br>When pulled to sitting position no longer has head lag<br>When held in standing position attempts to maintain some weight support | | Squeals |
| 5 months | Can reach and pick up object<br>May play with toes | Able to push up from prone position and maintain weight on forearms<br>Rolls from prone to supine and back to prone<br>Maintains straight back when in sitting position | Smiles spontaneously | |

Data from Frankenburg, W.K., Sciarillo, W., and Burgess, D.: J. Pediatr. **99**(6):995-999, 1981.
*For more specific data, see *Clinical guidelines* and Figs. 15-40 and 15-41.

**TABLE 15-1.** Normal developmental milestones—cont'd

| AGE | FINE MOTOR | GROSS MOTOR | SOCIAL/ADAPTIVE | LANGUAGE |
|---|---|---|---|---|
| 6 months | Will hold spoon or rattle<br>Will drop object and reach for second offered object | Begins to raise abdomen off table<br>Sits, but posture still shaky<br>May sit with legs apart; holds arms straight as prop between legs<br>Supports almost full weight when pulled to standing position | | |
| 7 months | Can transfer object, one hand to other<br>Grasps objects in each hand | Sits alone; still uses hands for support<br>When held in standing position bounces<br>Puts feet to mouth | | |
| 8 months | Beginning thumb-finger grasping | Sits securely without support (major developmental milestone) | Feeds self crackers | Turns to voice |
| 9 months | Continued development of thumb-finger grasp<br>May bang objects together | Steady sitting; can lean forward and still maintain position<br>Begins creeping (abdomen off floor)<br>Can stand holding onto stabilizing object when placed in that position; still may not be able to pull self into standing position | | |
| 10 months | Practices picking up small objects<br>Points with one finger<br>Will offer toys to people but unable to let go of objects | Can pull self into standing position; unable to let self down again | Plays peek-a-boo | |
| 11 months | | Moves about room holding onto objects<br>Preparing to walk independently, wide-base stance<br>Stands securely, holding on with one hand | | Imitates speech sound |
| 12 months (1 year) | May hold cup and spoon and feed self fairly well with practice<br>Can offer toys and release them | Able to twist and turn and maintain posture<br>Able to sit from standing position<br>May stand alone at least momentarily | | "Dada" or "mama" specific |
| 14 months | | Plays pat-a-cake | | |
| 15 months | Can put raisins into bottle<br>Will take off shoes and pull toys | Walks alone well<br>Able to seat self in chair | | |
| 16 months | | Plays ball with examiner | | |
| 18 months | Holds crayon<br>Scribbles spontaneously (major developmental milestone) | May walk up and down stairs holding hand<br>May show running ability | | |

*Continued.*

**TABLE 15-1.** Normal developmental milestones—cont'd

| AGE | FINE MOTOR | GROSS MOTOR | SOCIAL/ADAPTIVE | LANGUAGE |
|---|---|---|---|---|
| 20 months | | Imitates housework | Three words other than "mama" or "dada" | |
| 24 months (2 years) | Able to turn doorknob<br>Able to take off shoes and socks<br>Able to build two-block tower<br>Dumps raisins from bottle following demonstration | May walk up stairs by self, two feet on each step<br>Able to walk backward<br>Able to kick ball | Uses spoon | |
| 28 months | | | Combines two words | |
| 30 months (2½ years) | Able to build four-block tower<br>Scribbling techniques continue<br>Feeding self with increased neatness<br>Dumps raisins from bottle spontaneously | Able to jump from object<br>Walking becomes more stable, wide-base gait decreases<br>Throws ball overhanded | | |
| 36 months (3 years) | Can unbutton front buttons<br>Copies vertical lines within 30°<br>Copies 0<br>Able to build eight-cube tower | Walks upstairs, alternating feet on steps<br>Walks down stairs, two feet on each step<br>Pedals tricycle<br>Jumps in place<br>Able to perform broad jump | Pulls on shoes | Follows two or three simple directions |
| 48 months (4 years) | Able to copy +<br>Picks longer line three out of three times | Walks down stairs, alternating feet on steps<br>Able to button large front buttons<br>Able to balance on one foot for approximately 5 seconds | Dresses with supervision | Gives first and last name |
| 60 months (5 years) | Able to dress self with minimal assistance<br>Able to draw three-part human figure<br>Draws □ following demonstration<br>Colors within lines | Hops on one foot<br>Catches ball bounced to child two out of three times<br>Able to demonstrate heel-toe walking | Dresses without supervision | Recognizes three colors |

**TABLE 15-2** Developmental lag warning signs*

| AGE | GENERAL | HEARING AND SPEECH | VISION | ARMS | LEGS |
|---|---|---|---|---|---|
| 6 weeks | Tremors, asymmetry, or jerky spastic movements | Does not respond to loud noise by startle reflex<br>High-pitched cry | Failure to follow or fix at 22 to 30.5 cm (9-inch to 12-inch) distance | Excessive head lag on pulling to sitting position | Immobility<br>Continued limb extension |
| 6 months | No smiling<br>Jerky or spastic movements<br>Does not seem to recognize parent | Failure to turn toward sound<br>Does not laugh or squeal | Failure to fix or follow both near and distance objects | Failure to keep head steady when pulled to sitting position<br>Persistent fisting<br>Preference, one hand<br>Fails to push up or roll over | Increased adductor tone<br>Increased reflexes<br>Clonus |
| 10 months | Lack of imitation<br>Does not reach for toy<br>Not attempting to feed self or put things in own mouth | Does not babble<br>Does not imitate speech sounds | Displays squint or nystagmus | Abnormal hand posture<br>Failure to pass cube from one hand to other | Absence of weight bearing while held<br>Failure to sit without support |
| 18 months | Absence of constructive play<br>Persistence of drooling<br>Indicates wants only by crying | Lack of words, specifically "mama" or "dada" | Any apparent visual defect | No finger-thumb (pincer) grip<br>Does not bang blocks together | Unable to stand bearing weight without support |
| 2 years | Does not play peek-a-boo<br>Not drinking from cup<br>Failure to concentrate | Absence of words other than "mama" and "dada" | Failure to match toys | Does not attempt building with blocks<br>Tremor or ataxia | Unable to walk without aid |

Modified from Wood, B., editor: A pediatric vade-mecum, London, England, 1974, Lloyd-Luke (Medical Books) Ltd.
*See also Table 15-3.

# Clinical variations: the pediatric client
### THE INFANT (NEWBORN TO 12 MONTHS)

In assessing the infant the examiner is primarily concerned with three factors:
1. Reflex pattern and development
2. Motor skills development
3. Behavioral and socialization development

The infant develops greatly during the first year of life. In fact, there is more neurological maturation during the first year than in any other. The examiner must closely evaluate this development month by month. The infant should be assessed by the DDST as well as according to the following clinical guidelines.

| CHARACTERISTIC OR AREA EXAMINED | NORMAL | DEVIATIONS FROM NORMAL |
|---|---|---|
| **1.** Mental assessment | Appears quiet, content<br>Eyes open<br>Recognizes face of significant other<br>Smiles responsively (after 2 months) | Fretful, tense<br>Tremors or spastic movements |
| **2.** Speech | Cry loud and possibly angry<br>Cooing after 3 months<br>Babbles after 4 months<br>One or two words (mama, dada) after 9 months | High pitched, shrill<br>Penetrating cry |
| **3.** Cranial nerves: unable to directly test; observe child's functioning, involving at least partial intactness of following cranial nerves: | | |
|   **a.** CN III, IV, VI | Follows movement with eyes<br>Matures from 1 month onward | Response not shown at time appropriate for age |
|   **b.** CN V | Rooting reflex, sucking reflex | Asymmetry of response<br>Asymmetry of face during response |
|   **c.** CN VII | Wrinkles forehead, smiles after 2 months | Spastic or movement with tremor |
|   **d.** CN VIII | Moro reflex to loud noise<br>Turns head toward sound | |
|   **e.** CN IX, X | Swallowing, gag reflex | |
|   **f.** CN XII | Evaluated as infant sucks and swallows | |

| CHARACTERISTIC OR AREA EXAMINED | NORMAL | DEVIATIONS FROM NORMAL |
|---|---|---|
| 4. Proprioception, cerebellar, and motor function | Observe infant for spontaneous activity, symmetry, and smoothness of movement<br>Ease and passiveness during swallowing<br>Fine and gross motor development as detailed in Chapter 14 (see also Table 15-1)<br>Gradual purposeful movement after age 2 months | Spasticity, tremors, jerky movements<br>Frequent choking or difficulty with sucking<br>Unable to achieve developmental milestones<br>Any child in question should be evaluated by DDST |
| 5. Sensory function<br>a. Light touch<br>b. Pain | Not normally tested<br>Responds by withdrawal of all limbs and crying<br>After 8 months may withdraw only limb tested | <br>Withdrawal of limited limbs, asymmetrical withdrawal, no withdrawal |
| c. Vibratory<br>d. Discriminatory | Not normally tested<br>Not normally tested | |
| 6. Muscular function (muscle tone)<br>a. General observation | Symmetry; limbs semiflexed and slightly abducted (see Fig. 14-85) | Frog position: hips in abduction (almost flat to table) with hips externally rotated<br>Opisthotonos: infant prone, maintains back positions with neck hyperextended<br>Hand-over-head position<br>Any asymmetry or spasticity of movement |
|  | Meaningful grasping after age 3 months | Persistence of fisted hand beyond 3 months |
| b. Evaluation by pulling infant to sitting position using wrists (pull-to-sit maneuver) | Newborn will hold head at 45° angle or less until at upright sitting position; then head will flop forward<br>By 4 months head should remain in line with body and should no longer flop forward | <br><br>Head flop beyond 4 months |
| c. Range of motion | Able to easily perform range of motion techniques as described in Chapter 14 | Spastic muscular response<br>Marked resistance to range of motion attempt<br>Quick spastic response when limbs released |
| 7. Reflex testing: deep tendon reflexes not normally tested; more important to evaluate infant responses, some of the most common of which are detailed in Table 15-3 | Patellar reflex present at birth, followed by Achilles and brachial triceps reflex present by 6 months | If reflexes continue beyond expected disappearance age, examiner should become suspicious |

**TABLE 15-3.** Infantile reflexes

| REFLEX | TECHNIQUE FOR EVALUATION | APPEARANCE AGE | DISAPPEARANCE AGE | NORMAL RESPONSE |
|---|---|---|---|---|
| **Reflexes to evaluate position and movement** | | | | |
| Moro (Fig. 15-42) | Startle infant by making loud noise, jarring examination surface, or slightly raising infant off examination surface and letting him fall quickly back onto examining table | Birth | 1 to 4 months | Infant abducts and extends arms and legs; index finger and thumb assume **C** position; then infant pulls both arms and legs up against trunk as if trying to protect self |
| Tonic neck (Fig. 15-43) | Infant supine; rotate head to side so that chin is over shoulder | Birth to 6 weeks | 4 to 6 months | Arm and leg on side to which head turns extends; opposite arm and leg flex; infant assumes fencing position (some normal infants may never show this reflex) |

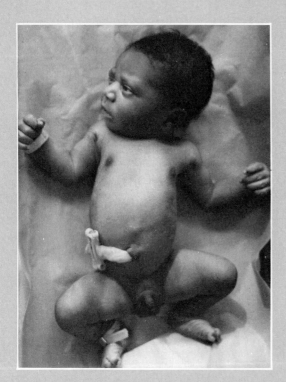

**FIG. 15-42**

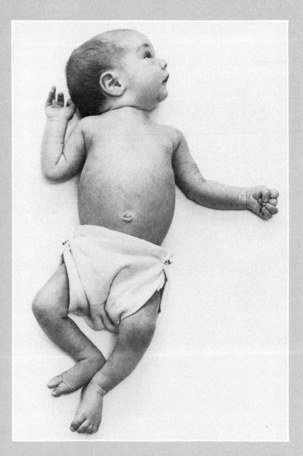

**FIG. 15-43.** (From Jensen, J., Benson, R., and Bobak, I.: Maternity care: the nurse and the family, St. Louis, 1977, The C.V. Mosby Co.)

relieve symptoms or alleviate stress is important. Self-medication, self-imposed immobility, use of alcohol, social withdrawal, and denial are examples of new behaviors that might be uncovered with a careful history.

2. The neurological screening examination described in the adult section of this chapter can be used with the majority of elderly clients. The major variations in the aging client's responses to the examination follow:
   a. Responses to the examiner's commands may be carried out more slowly.
   b. The senses of smell and taste may be diminished.
   c. Deep tendon reflexes may be slightly diminished (especially the ankle jerk); however, absence or exaggeration of any of the deep tendon reflexes should be reported as a problem.
   d. The vibratory sensation in both feet and ankles may be diminished; however, full sensation should be reported at midcalf. (*Note:* This finding should be reported as a problem by beginning practitioners.)

3. Neurological assessment of the elderly individual becomes complicated when the client is disabled by other problems. Diminished vision or hearing, arthritis, confusion or disorientation, or cardiorespiratory problems may be accompanied by fatigue, weakness, inattentiveness, or other symptoms that mask neurological deficits. Symptoms related to other illnesses may prevent the client from going through the motions of an examination. It might be helpful to conduct the examination over two or three sessions to avoid client fatigue. The beginning practitioner will have to seek advice from a preceptor regarding decisions about which functions are important for the client to complete if the client is greatly disabled.

4. Following are some major physical signs for which the examiner should be alert:
   a. Facial asymmetry, drooping of the side of the mouth (flat nasolabial fold), asymmetrical wrinkling on forehead, drooling at side of mouth, or tongue fasciculation (while at rest in the mouth). If any are apparent, ask the client to swallow a sip of water. The observer should be alert for coughing, sputtering, dribbling, or fluid remaining in the mouth after the swallow.
   b. Weakness of extremities (unilateral or symmetrical response); note the following:
      (1) Extent of range of motion and strength to opposition
      (2) Accompanying muscle atrophy
      (3) Sensory responses to pain, touch, vibration, and temperature
      (4) Reflexes (normal, present, absent, hyperactive, or diminished)
      (5) Comparison of weakened side to other side in all areas of assessment
   c. Gait disturbances (see geriatric section in Chapter 14 for details to observe)
   d. Tremors. Some authors state that mild head tremors are normal for elderly individuals; however, the examiner should report all tremors for consultation.
      (1) Anxiety or hyperthyroidism tremors are often fine, rapid, and irregular. Facial tics or twitching may be present. Tremors usually increase with action and decrease with relaxation. Excessive perspiration may be apparent.
      (2) Parkinsonian tremors are slower and occur at rest. The "pill-rolling" pattern of thumb and opposing fingers may be evident. All body movements are slowed or diminished.
      (3) Cerebellar tremors vary in rate and are usually intention tremors.
      (4) Essential tremors (or those associated with aging) occur at a moderate rate and frequently involve the jaw, tongue, or entire head. The head may move up and down or laterally. The tremors disappear on relaxation and are usually not disabling; there is no accompanying rigidity. There may be a familial history of such tremors. The tremors may begin in middle age and continue at the same level of severity throughout the remainder of life.
      (5) Metabolic tremors involve a flapping motion of the wrist, which suddenly drops and then returns to the original position. The client is usually very ill and manifests numerous other signs.
   e. Mental acuity alteration (see Chapter 2 for specific behaviors to assess).
   f. Labile emotional responses (specific behaviors listed in Chapter 2).

5. Stroke. This is a word commonly used by professional and lay people to describe a sudden neurological deficit that results in a variety of signs, including paralysis or weakness of body parts. The cause of the problem is usually vascular, but the effects are neurological and are therefore described in this chapter. Strokes are often classified in terms of stages of appearance or severity:

a. Transient ischemial attacks are neurological deficits with acute onset and limited duration (5 to 20 minutes). A variety of symptoms or signs might be manifested. Dizziness, confusion, unilateral weakness or numbness, and aphasia are some of the complaints. These episodes often leave few or no aftereffects and sometimes precede a stroke. The frequency and severity of these "spells" or "attacks" vary greatly among individuals.

b. Reversible ischemic neurological deficit is similar to the transient attacks, except that the signs and symptoms linger for several days before disappearing.

c. Stroke-in-evolution is a slowly progressive focal deficit occurring and accumulating in a step-by-step or stuttering fashion over a period of days or weeks. Signs and symptoms become more apparent over this period of time.

d. The onset of signs and symptoms of a completed stroke are abrupt and become stabilized (over a period of days or weeks or years).

6. Risk factors associated with strokes
   a. Family history of strokes or vascular disease
   b. Client history of hypertension
   c. Cardiac enlargement
   d. History of myocardial infarction or angina pectoris
   e. Congestive heart failure
   f. Diabetes mellitus
   g. History of peripheral vascular disease
   h. History of transient ischemial attacks

## Cognitive self-assessment

1. The cranial nerves are outside the brain and spinal cord. Therefore the cranial nerves are part of the:
   ☐ a. central nervous system
   ☐ b. peripheral nervous system

2. Every reflex arc pathway includes:
   ☐ a. a receptor
   ☐ b. an efferent fiber
   ☐ c. an afferent fiber
   ☐ d. a muscle or gland
   ☐ e. a brainstem
   ☐ f. all except c
   ☐ g. all except a
   ☐ h. all except e
   ☐ i. all the above

3. While examining a client's patellar reflexes, you get no response. One method you can use to aid you in getting a response is to:
   ☐ a. have client cross legs, and test the patellar reflexes one at a time
   ☐ b. have client dorsiflex feet
   ☐ c. have client lock fingers together and pull one hand against the other
   ☐ d. have client place both hands under the knees to add more tension on the patellar ligaments

4. A deep tendon reflex _____ dependent on an intact motor nerve fiber.
   ☐ a. is
   ☐ b. is not

5. Extension of the elbow is the normal response of the _____ reflex.
   ☐ a. triceps
   ☐ b. biceps

6. _____ of the great toe is a normal response to the plantar reflex.
   ☐ a. Flexion
   ☐ b. Extension

7. Which of the following is *not* part of a screening neurological assessment?
   - ☐ a. Mental status
   - ☐ b. Proprioception and cerebellar function
   - ☐ c. Cranial nerve evaluation
   - ☐ d. Sensory evaluation
   - ☐ e. Deep tendon reflexes
   - ☐ f. b and e
   - ☐ g. none of the above

8. A function of the cerebellum is integration of muscle contractions for maintenance of posture. Characteristics of a client with a "cerebellar gait" are:
   - ☐ a. walking with a wide gait
   - ☐ b. trunk and head held rigidly
   - ☐ c. the legs bent at the hip
   - ☐ d. the arms held outward to maintain balance
   - ☐ e. most walking takes place on the balls and toes of the feet, with no heel strike
   - ☐ f. none of the above
   - ☐ g. a, c, d, and e
   - ☐ h. b, d, and e
   - ☐ i. a, b, and c
   - ☐ j. all the above

9. In assessing the client's proprioceptive or cerebellar function, which of the following tests *are* appropriate?
   - ☐ a. Instruct client to pat his leg as fast as he can with his hand.
   - ☐ b. Instruct client to spread fingers as far as possible and to resist the examiner's attempt to squeeze them together.
   - ☐ c. Instruct client to do a deep knee bend.
   - ☐ d. Instruct client to take the heel of one foot and run it down the opposite shin.
   - ☐ e. Instruct client to close his eyes. The examiner grasps the index finger of the client's hand and changes its position (e.g., up or down). The client then describes how the position was changed.
   - ☐ f. none of the above
   - ☐ g. b, d, and e
   - ☐ h. b, c, and e
   - ☐ i. a, c, and d
   - ☐ j. a, b, and c

10. When performing a screening evaluation of sensory function, it is only necessary to evaluate the following areas:
    - ☐ a. lateral aspect of upper thighs
    - ☐ b. inner aspect of upper arms
    - ☐ c. dorsal or palmar surface of hands
    - ☐ d. bottom or dorsal surface of feet
    - ☐ e. upper middle aspect of back
    - ☐ f. all the above
    - ☐ g. a, b, and e
    - ☐ h. a and b
    - ☐ i. c, d, and e
    - ☐ j. c and d

11. Sensory function testing techniques include:
    ☐ a. pain sensation
    ☐ b. light touch sensation
    ☐ c. temperature identification
    ☐ d. vibration evaluation
    ☐ e. position sense
    ☐ f. stereognosis
    ☐ g. all the above
    ☐ h. all except a
    ☐ i. all except c
    ☐ j. all except e
    ☐ k. all except f

Mark each statement "T" or "F."

12. _____ The Romberg test involves asking the patient to stand with feet together and arms outstretched, with eyes open and then closed.

13. _____ The cerebellum receives both sensory and motor input, coordinates muscular activity, and maintains equilibrium.

14. _____ The examiner should compare sensitivity in the proximal and distal portions of the extremities.

Match the definitions in column A with the terms in column B.

| Column A | Column B |
|---|---|
| 15. _____ Continuous rapid twitching of a muscle without movement of the limb | a. tic |
| 16. _____ An involuntary, rhythmic, rapid back-and-forth movement of a limb | b. myoclonus |
| 17. _____ An occasional twitch of a shoulder or a group of facial muscles | c. chorea |
| 18. _____ Strong involuntary jerks of the body that occur at irregular intervals | d. fasciculation |
| 19. _____ A hiccup is an example | e. tremor |

Match the cranial nerves in column A with the anticipated motor action of that nerve in column B.

| Column A | Column B |
|---|---|
| 20. _____ CN V | a. Muscles of the face, including those around eyes and mouth |
| 21. _____ CN VIII | b. Movement of the tongue |
| 22. _____ CN X | c. Temporal and masseter muscles and lateral jaw movement |
| 23. _____ CN XII | d. Ability to swallow |
| | e. Hearing and balance |

Testing of the deep tendon reflexes is a rather simple mechanical process. The significance of testing, however, reflects intactness of the neurological system from the tendon to the motor nerve in the spinal cord. Match each reflex in column A with the motor nerve it evaluates in column B.

| Column A | Column B |
|---|---|
| 24. _____ Biceps reflex | a. C7, C8 |
| 25. _____ Triceps reflex | b. L4, L5, S1, S2 |
| 26. _____ Knee reflex | c. L2, L3, L4 |
| 27. _____ Ankle reflex | d. C5, C6 |
| 28. _____ Plantar response | e. S1, S2 |

**PEDIATRIC QUESTIONS**

29. It is possible to partially evaluate cranial nerve function by which of the following ages?
   - ☐ a. 2 months
   - ☐ b. 8 months
   - ☐ c. 3 years
   - ☐ d. 6 years
   - ☐ e. 8 years

30. The correct response to the Moro reflex is which of the following?
   - ☐ a. The arm and leg on the side to which the head turns extend; the opposite arm and leg flex
   - ☐ b. The infant grasps the examiner's hand, and the toes flex downward.
   - ☐ c. The infant paces in place, alternately lifting each leg
   - ☐ d. The infant responds with rapid abduction of both arms and legs; the index finger and thumb assume a C position.
   - ☐ e. The infant grasps the examiner's hands, the infant's legs abduct and the toes fan outward.

31. The sucking reflex disappears by approximately which of the following ages?
   - ☐ a. 8 months
   - ☐ b. 12 months
   - ☐ c. 16 months
   - ☐ d. 24 months
   - ☐ e. 30 months

32. The examiner should expect a child to feed himself crackers or cookies by which of the following ages?
   - ☐ a. 4 months
   - ☐ b. 6 months
   - ☐ c. 8 months
   - ☐ d. 10 months
   - ☐ e. 12 months

33. Which of the following definitions best defines neurological "soft signs"?
   - ☐ a. Objective signs that are present because of an open portion of the spinal column
   - ☐ b. Objective findings of babies before mature development of their neurological systems
   - ☐ c. Objective signs found in hyperactive children
   - ☐ d. Objective signs associated with vague complaints such as clumsiness, motor overload, or mirroring of extremity movements
   - ☐ e. There is no such term

**GERIATRIC QUESTIONS**

34. Neurological signs associated with the normal aging process might include:
    - ☐ a. diminution or absence of ankle jerk response
    - ☐ b. ptosis
    - ☐ c. fasciculations of the tongue
    - ☐ d. all of the above
    - ☐ e. none of the above
35. Transient ischemial attacks:
    - ☐ a. may occur in the form of black-out spells
    - ☐ b. may affect speech ability
    - ☐ c. all the above
    - ☐ e. none of the above
36. Risk factors associated with strokes might include:
    - ☐ a. a history of nervousness
    - ☐ b. a history of transient ischemial attacks
    - ☐ c. a history of hypothyroidism
    - ☐ d. all of the above
    - ☐ e. none of the above

## SUGGESTED READINGS
### General

Adams, V.M.: Principles of neurology, ed. 2, New York, 1981, McGraw-Hill Book Co.

Bates, B.: A guide to physical examination, ed. 3, Philadelphia, 1983, J.B. Lippincott, pp. 370-427.

DeMeyer, W.: Technique of the neurological examination: a programmed text, ed. 3, New York, 1980, McGraw-Hill Book Co.

Essentials of the neurological examination, Philadelphia, 1974, SmithKline Corporation.

Judge, R.D., and Zuidema, G., editors: Methods of clnical examination: a physiologic approach, Boston, 1974, Little, Brown & Co., pp. 341-366.

Malasanos, L., and others: Health assessment, ed. 2, St. Louis, 1981, The C.V. Mosby Co.

Patient assessment: neurological examination, I, Programmed instruction, Am. J. Nurs. 75:9, 1975.

Patient assessment: neurological examination, II, Programmed instruction, Am. J. Nurs. 75:11, 1975.

Patient assessment: neurological examination, III, Programmed instruction, Am. J. Nurs. 76:4, 1976.

Prior, J.A., Silberstein, J.S., and Stang, J.M.: Physical diagnosis: the history and examination of the patient, ed. 6, St. Louis, 1981, The C.V. Mosby Co.

Van Allen, M.W.: Pictorial manual of neurologic tests: a guide to the performance and interpretation of the neurologic examination, Chicago, ed. 2, 1981, Year Book Medical Publishers.

Walleck, C.: Neurological assessment for nurses: a part of nursing process, Neurosurg. Nurs. 10:13-16, 1978.

### Pediatrics

Alexander, M., and Brown, M.S.: Pediatric history taking and physical diagnosis for nurses, ed. 2, New York, 1979, McGraw-Hill Book Co., pp. 320-381.

Barness, L.: Manual of pediatric physical diagnosis, ed. 5, Chicago, 1981, Year Book Medical Publishers, Inc. pp. 193-208.

Frankenburg, W.K., Dick, N.P., and Carland, J.: Development of preschool-aged children of different social and ethnic groups: implications for developmental screening, J. Pediatr. 87(7):125-232, 1975.

Frankenburg, W.K., and others: The newly abbreviated and revised Denver Developmental Screening Test, J. Pediatr. 99(6):995-999, 1981.

Goodenough, F.L.: Measurement of intelligence by drawings, New York, 1926, World Book Co.

Hayes, J.S.: The McCarthy scales of children's abilities: their usefulness in developmental assessment, Pediatr. Nurs. 7:35-37, 1981.

Hughes, J.: Synopsis of pediatrics, ed. 5, St. Louis, 1980, The C.V. Mosby Co., pp. 718-720.

Johnson, T.: Children are different. In Johnson, T.R., Moore, W.M., and Jeffries, J.E., editors: Developmental philosophy, ed. 2, Columbus, Ohio, 1978, Ross Laboratories, p. 34.

McMillan, J., Nieburg, P., and Oski, F.: The whole pediatrician catalog, Philadelphia, 1977, W.B. Saunders Co., pp. 74-75, 319-322.

O'Pray, M.: Developmental screening tools: using them effectively, Matern. Child Nurs. J. 5(2):126-130, 1980.

Pillitteri, A.: Nursing care of the growing family: a child health text, Boston, 1977, Little, Brown & Co., pp. 37-41.

Whaley, L.F., and Wong, D.L.: Nursing care of infants and children, ed. 2, St. Louis, 1983, The C.V. Mosby Co., 226-238.

### Geriatric

Caird, F.I., and Judge, T.G.: Assessment of the elderly patient, London, 1977, Pitman Publishing Ltd., pp. 48-52, 65-86.

Carotenuto, R., and Bullock, J.: Physical assessment of the gerontologic client, Philadelphia, 1980, F.A. Davis Co., pp. 127-139.

Granacher, R.P.: The neurologic examination in geriatric psychiatry, Psychosomatics 22(6):485-499, 1981.

Ross, G.S., and Klassen, A.: The stroke syndrome. I. Pathogenesis, Hosp. Med. 9(3):7-37, 1973.

Ross, G.S., and Klassen, A.: The stroke syndrome. II. Clinical and diagnostic aspects, Hosp. Med. 9(4):58-81, 1973.

Steinberg, Franz U., editor: Care of the geriatric patient, ed. 6, St. Louis, 1983, The C.V. Mosby Co., pp. 462-481.

# 16

# Physical examination integration format

The purpose of this chapter is to discuss the integration of the total physical examination. Throughout, the description of the assessment techniques has been abbreviated. The examiner is referred to the individual chapters for a detailed description. The clinical information has been divided to show the following:

1. The examination format
2. The assessment techniques
3. The systems involved in the assessment procedure
4. Important strategies

At the end of this detailed description is a summary of the pediatric variations and suggested approaches for the pediatric client.

## Equipment for physical examination

| | |
|---|---|
| Eye examination charts | Writing surface for examiner |
| Ophthalmoscope | |
| Otoscope with pneumatic bulb | Patient examination gown |
| Stethoscope | Vaginal speculum (for female clients) |
| Tongue blades | |
| Penlight | Pap smear materials |
| 4 × 4-inch gauze pads | Percussion hammer |
| Examination gloves | Tuning fork |
| Cotton applicator sticks | Odorous material |
| Lubricant | Cotton balls |
| Drape sheet | Sharp and dull testing instruments |
| Gooseneck light | |
| Examination table with stirrups | Ruler |

## Data base history

This should be a time for the examiner to get to know and develop a profile about the client. This profile should be synthesized and provide the examiner with a framework for approaching the client during the physical assessment.

1. Major concern of client. The examiner must decide whether to examine that area first or whether to wait and examine it during the normal sequence.
2. General approach to the client. The examiner will get to know the client during preparation of the rather lengthy data base. Although the examiner may decide to maintain a systematic and progressive physical examination approach, the client's personality and individual preferences should be incorporated. For example, if the client states that he becomes short of breath when he lies flat, the examiner may decide to keep the head of the examining table up a little and to keep the recumbent period to a minimum.
3. Major areas needing special attention. Many times the examination simply confirms what the examiner already knows. Therefore the examiner should bring to the physical assessment session a "problem list" of areas needing special in-depth evaluation.

## Integrated physical assessment

1. The physical examination of each client should begin as the examiner first meets the client. Assessment of objective data should continue throughout the subjective data base collection period.

During the initial introductory period, collect

data by watching the client walk down the hall, come into the examination room, take off and hang up his coat, shake hands with the examiner, sit down on a chair in the office or examination room, and carry on all introductory conversation.

The examiner may identify areas with obvious difficulties or deviations. Areas requiring primary assessment follow:

a. Gait: difficulty walking, use of assisting devices
b. Stiffness, weakness
c. Difficulty standing, sitting, rising from sitting position
d. Difficulty taking off coat or hanging it up
e. Obvious musculoskeletal deformities
f. General affect
g. Appearance of interest and involvement
h. Eye contact with examiner
i. Speech pattern or difficulties
j. Dress and posture
k. Overview of mental alertness, orientation, and thought process integrity
l. Tremors or motor difficulties
m. Obvious eye problem or blindness
n. Corrective lenses
o. Difficulty hearing
p. Use of assisting devices
q. Obvious shortness of breath; posture that would facilitate breathing
r. Cyanosis, pale or flushed appearance
s. Language problem or foreign language speaker
t. Cultural orientation
u. Significant others accompanying client
v. Obesity or emaciation
w. Malnourishment

2. After the initial assessment and data base collection the client should be prepared for the physical assessment.
   a. Instruct client to empty bladder (collect specimen if desired)
   b. Instruct client to remove all clothing (including shoes, socks, bra, and underpants) put on gown, and sit on chair in examination room.

To perform the examination, the approach to body systems must be fragmented for two purposes: (a) to accommodate a regional physical assessment approach and (b) to coordinate client and examiner positions during the assessment process.

Following the assessment the examiner must reunite the body systems for the actual physical assessment write-up. The examiner should not feel compelled to follow the stated outline; the goal should be to develop an individualized routine.

## Clinical guidelines for physical examination integration

| PROCEDURE OR FORMAT | ASSESSMENT TO INCLUDE | BODY PART OR SYSTEM INVOLVED | CLINICAL STRATEGIES FOR ADULTS AND GERIATRIC CLIENTS |
|---|---|---|---|
| 1. Assess vital functions and other baseline measurements: client should be in gown and seated on end of examination table or in chair | Temperature<br>Blood pressure (both arms)<br>Radial pulse<br>Respirations<br>Height<br>Weight | Cardiovascular<br>Thorax and lungs | If deviation from normal discovered, reevaluate when associated system assessed |
| | Vision testing<br>  Snellen chart<br>  External eye function | Visual<br>Neurological—CN II (optic nerve) | |
| **Client is seated**<br>2. Examine client's hands | Skin surface characteristics<br>Temperature and moisture of hands<br>Characteristics of nails<br>Clubbing | Integumentary<br><br><br>Cardiovascular<br>Respiratory | Both examiner and client will be at ease if examiner starts with client's hands |

| PROCEDURE OR FORMAT | ASSESSMENT TO INCLUDE | BODY PART OR SYSTEM INVOLVED | CLINICAL STRATEGIES FOR ADULTS AND GERIATRIC CLIENTS |
|---|---|---|---|
| | Skeletal characteristics and/or deformities of fingers and hands | Musculoskeletal | Fine motor neurological assessment may be included at this point; others find it more convenient to perform neurological assessment as a clustered procedure toward end of evaluation period |
| | Range of motion and motor strength of fingers and hands | | |
| | Muscle wasting | | |
| | Asymmetry | | |
| **3.** Examine client's arms from hands to shoulders | Skin surface characteristics | Integumentary | Examine each arm separately |
| | Muscle wasting | Musculoskeletal | |
| | Asymmetry | | |
| | Radial pulses: compare one arm to other | Cardiovascular | May have already been done during vital sign evaluation |
| | Range of motion and motor strength of wrists, elbows, forearms, upper arm, shoulders | Musculoskeletal Neurological | Note that, again, neurological assessment has been delayed |
| | | | Use make/break techniques |
| | Palpation of epitrochlear lymph nodes | Lymphatic | |
| **4.** Examine client's head and neck | Facial characteristics and symmetry | Head and neck Neurological | Observe head and neck, taking in as much information as possible |
| | Skin surface characteristics | Integumentary | Do not be tempted to touch until after thorough observation |
| | Symmetry and external characteristics of eyes and ears | | |
| | Hair characteristics: texture, distribution, quantity | | |
| | Palpation of hair and scalp | | Palpate thoroughly; do not be intimidated by hair spray or dirty hair (may need to wash hands before progressing) |
| | Palpation of facial bones | Musculoskeletal | |
| | Client opens and closes mouth for evaluation of temporomanidbular joint | Neurological—CN V (trigeminal nerve) | |
| | Clenching teeth | | |
| | Palpation of sinus regions | | |
| | Client clenches eye tight, wrinkles forehead, smiles, sticks out tongue, and puffs out cheeks | Neurological—CN VII, XII (facial, hypoglossal nerves) | Very straightforward |
| | | | Provide client with step-by-step instructions |
| | Eye and near-vision assessment | Visual | |
| | External eye examination: eyebrows, eyelids, eyelashes, surface characteristics, lacrimal apparatus, corneal surface, anterior chamber, iris | | |
| | Near-vision screening and eye function: pupillary response, accommodation, cover-uncover test | Neurological—CN II, III (optic, oculomotor nerves) | |

## Clinical guidelines for physical examination integration—cont'd

| PROCEDURE OR FORMAT | ASSESSMENT TO INCLUDE | BODY PART OR SYSTEM INVOLVED | CLINICAL STRATEGIES FOR ADULTS AND GERIATRIC CLIENTS |
|---|---|---|---|
| | Extraocular eye movements; vision field testing | Neurological—CN III, IV, VI, (oculomotor, trochlear, abducens nerves) | |
| | Internal eye examination: red reflex, disc, cup margins, vessels, retinal surface, vitreous | | Room must be darkened; should have small amount of secondary light<br>Remember to instruct client to focus on single object at distance |
| | Ear and hearing assessment<br>External ear examination: alignment, surface characteristics, external canal | Ear and auditory | |
| | Use ticking watch to evaluate hearing | Neurological—CN VIII (acoustic nerve) | Room must be quiet |
| | Otoscope examination: characteristics of external canal, cerumen, eardrum (landmarks, deformities, inflammation) | | Use largest speculum that will fit into canal; if necessary, review technique guidelines for using otoscope |
| | Rinne and Weber tests | Auditory and neurological—CN VIII (acoustic nerve) | |
| | Nasal examination: note structure, septum position; use nasal speculum to evaluate patency, turbinates, meatuses | Nose, mouth, and oropharynx | Even though uncomfortable, should be part of every thorough assessment |
| | Evaluation of sense of smell | Neurological—CN I (olfactory nerve) | |
| | Mouth examination: inspect gingivobuccal fornices, buccal mucosa, and gums | Nose, mouth, and oropharynx | |
| | Inspection of teeth: number, color, surface characteristics | | If client has dentures, they should be removed |
| | Inspection and palpation of tongue: symmetry, movement, color, surface characteristics | | |
| | Inspection of floor of mouth: color, surface characteristics | | |
| | Inspection of hard and soft palates: color, surface characteristics | | |
| | Inspection of oropharynx: note mouth odor, anteroposterior pillars, uvula, tonsils, posterior pharynx | | |
| | Evaluation of gag reflex | Neurological—CN IX, X (glossopharyngeal, vagus nerves) | |

| PROCEDURE OR FORMAT | ASSESSMENT TO INCLUDE | BODY PART OR SYSTEM INVOLVED | CLINICAL STRATEGIES FOR ADULTS AND GERIATRIC CLIENTS |
|---|---|---|---|
| | Evaluation of range of motion of head and neck: instruct client to swing shoulders upward against examiner's resistance; head movement positions, neck flexion, extension, ear-to-shoulder flexion, chin-to-shoulder rotation | Musculoskeletal Neurological—CN XI (accessory nerve) | |
| | Observation of symmetry and smoothness of neck and thyroid | | Client's gown should be lowered slightly so that examiner may fully inspect neck |
| | Palpation of carotid pulses Observation for jugular venous distention | Cardiovascular | |
| | Palpation of trachea, thyroid (isthmus and lobes), lymph nodes (preauricular, postauricular, occipital, tonsillar, submaxillary, submental, superficial cervical chain, posterior cervical, deep cervical chain, and supraclavicular) | Lymphatic | Client may need drink of water to facilitate swallowing during thyroid evaluation |
| | Completion of assessment of cranial nerves: use cotton swab to evaluate light sensation to forehead, cheeks, chin (trigeminal nerve sensory tract) | Neurological—CN V (trigeminal nerve) | Client should be instructed to close eyes and identify where and when light touch felt |
| **5.** Assess posterior chest: examination moves behind client; client seated; gown to waist for men; gown removed but pulled up to cover breasts for women | Observation of posterior chest: symmetry of shoulders, muscular development, scapular placement, spine straightness, posture | Musculoskeletal | |
| | Observation of skin: intactness, color, lesions | Integumentary | |
| | Observation of respiratory movement: excursion, quality, depth, and rhythm of respirations | Thorax and lungs | |
| | Palpation of posterior chest: evaluate muscles and bone structure, palpate excursion of chest expansion; palpate down vertebral column; note straightness | Musculoskeletal Thorax and lungs | |
| | Palpation of posterior chest for fremitus | | Palpate with base of fingers while client says "how now brown cow" or "ninety-nine" |

## Clinical guidelines for physical examination integration—cont'd

| PROCEDURE OR FORMAT | ASSESSMENT TO INCLUDE | BODY PART OR SYSTEM INVOLVED | CLINICAL STRATEGIES FOR ADULTS AND GERIATRIC CLIENTS |
|---|---|---|---|
| | Percussion of posterior chest for resonance, respiratory excursion | Thorax and lungs | During excursion evaluation, demonstrate to client how to take deep breath and hold it<br>Measure amount of excursion with ruler |
| | Percussion with fist along costovertebral angle for kidney tenderness | Genitourinary | |
| | Inspection, bilateral palpation, and percussion along lateral axillary chest walls | Thorax and lungs | |
| | Auscultation of posterior and axillary chest walls for breath sounds; note quality of sounds heard and presence of adventitious sounds | Thorax and lungs | Instruct client to breathe deeply by mouth |
| **6.** Assess anterior chest: move around to front of client; client should lower gown to waist | Inspection of: skin color, intactness, presence of lesions, muscular symmetry, bilaterally similar bone structure | Integumentary<br>Musculoskeletal | |
| | Observation of chest wall for pulsations or heaving | Cardiovascular | |
| | Observation of movement during respirations | Thorax and lungs | |
| | Observation of client's ease with respirations, posture, pursing lips | | |
| | **Female breasts:** Note size, symmetry, contour, moles or nevi, breast or nipple deviation, dimpling, or lesions; evaluate range of motion of shoulders and regularity of breast tissue during various movements:<br>1. Client's arms extended over head<br>2. Client's arm behind head<br>3. Client's hands behind small of back<br>4. Client's hands pushed tightly against each other at shoulder level<br>5. Client leaning over slightly so that breasts hang away from chest wall; note symmetry and pull on suspensory ligaments | Musculoskeletal<br>Breast | It would be helpful to explain to client basically what she will be expected to do and why, before actual examination; may help to alleviate client anxiety as well as facilitate active participation<br>During examination, it may be helpful to provide discussion as to what is being observed; breast self-examination instruction should follow at some point to reiterate these and other aspects of breast examination |

| PROCEDURE OR FORMAT | ASSESSMENT TO INCLUDE | BODY PART OR SYSTEM INVOLVED | CLINICAL STRATEGIES FOR ADULTS AND GERIATRIC CLIENTS |
|---|---|---|---|
| | **Male breasts:** Note size, symmetry, breast enlargement, nipple discharge, or lesions | | |
| | **All clients:** Palpation of anterior chest wall for stability, crepitations, muscular or skeletal tenderness | Musculoskeletal | |
| | Palpation of precordium for thrills, heaves, pulsations | Cardiovascular | Be sure to evaluate chest while client is sitting upright and then leaning forward |
| | Palpation of left chest wall to locate point of maximum impulse (PMI) | | |
| | Palpation of chest wall for fremitus, as with posterior chest | Thorax and lungs | |
| | Percussion of anterior chest for resonance | Thorax and lungs | If examiner has difficulty percussing woman's anterior chest because of large breasts, percuss downward until breast tissue reached; then postpone continued percussion until client lies down |
| | **For female clients:** Palpation of breasts, including all four quadrants, tail of breast, and areolar area; note firmness, tissue qualities, lumps, areas of thickness, or tenderness | Breast | Client should be comfortably seated with arms resting at side |
| | Palpation of nipples; note elasticity, tissue characteristics, discharge | | As before, discuss what is being done so that client can incorporate similar techniques into breast self-examination |
| | **All clients:** Palpation of lymph nodes associated with lymphatic drainage of breast, including supraclavicular and infraclavicular, central, lateral, axillary, pectoral, subscapular, scapular, brachial, intermediate, and internal mammary areas | Lymphatic | |
| | **For male clients:** Palpation of breast; note swelling or presence of excessive tissue or lumps, nipple discharge, or lesions | | |
| | **All clients:** Auscultation of breath sounds of anterior chest from apex to base; note quality, rate, type, presence of adventitious sounds | Thorax and lungs | Instruct client to breathe deeply through mouth |

## Clinical guidelines for physical examination integration—cont'd

| PROCEDURE OR FORMAT | ASSESSMENT TO INCLUDE | BODY PART OR SYSTEM INVOLVED | CLINICAL STRATEGIES FOR ADULTS AND GERIATRIC CLIENTS |
|---|---|---|---|
| | Auscultation of heart: aortic area, pulmonary area, Erb point, tricuspid area, apical area, note rate, rhythm, location, intensity, frequency, timing, and splitting of $S_1$, $S_2$, $S_3$, $S_4$ murmurs | Cardiovascular | Examiner must decide whether to start at apical area and work upward or start at aortic area and work downward. Examiner should develop routine method of procedure<br>If examining large-breasted woman, part of auscultatory evaluation may be deferred until client lying down |
| **Client is assisted to lying or low Fowler position** | | | |
| 7. Assess anterior chest in recumbent position | Inspection of jugular venous pressure for height seen above sternal angle | Cardiovascular | Be sure to extend footrest for client's legs<br>See *Clinical strategies,* (Chapter 9), for cardiovascular examination techniques to measure jugular venous pressure |
| | **Female breast inspection:** Symmetry, contour, venous pattern, skin color, areolar area (note size, shape, surface characteristics), nipples (note direction, size, shape, color, surface characteristics, possible crusting) | Breasts | Provide drape for legs and abdomen<br>Place towel under back of side to be evaluated<br>Instruct client to abduct arm overhead<br>Explain procedures to client as performed |
| | **Female breast palpation:** Note firmness, tissue qualities, lumps, areas of thickness, or tenderness; aoreolar and nipple area (note elasticity, tissue characteristics, discharge) | | Following breast palpation, may take time to teach client to palpate own breasts |
| | **All clients:** Palpation of anterior chest wall for cardiac movements or thrills, heaves, pulsations | Cardiovascular | |
| | Auscultation of heart: aortic area, pulmonary area, Erb point, tricuspid area, apical area; note $S_1$, $S_2$, $S_3$, $S_4$ murmurs (location, rate, rhythm, intensity, frequency, timing, splitting); turn client slightly to left side; repeat assessment of these areas | Cardiovascular | Examination with client lying on left side may not need to be done for all clients |
| 8. Assess abdomen: provide chest drape for females; expose abdomen from pubis to epigastric region | Observation of skin characteristics from pubis to midchest region; note scars, lesions, vascularity, bulges, navel | Integumentary | Client should be comfortably positioned with pillow under head and knees slightly flexed to relax abdominal muscles |

| PROCEDURE OR FORMAT | ASSESSMENT TO INCLUDE | BODY PART OR SYSTEM INVOLVED | CLINICAL STRATEGIES FOR ADULTS AND GERIATRIC CLIENTS |
|---|---|---|---|
| | Observation of abdominal contour | Abdominal | |
| | Observation of movement of abdomen, peristalsis, pulsations | Gastrointestinal Cardiovascular | |
| | Auscultation of abdomen (all quadrants); note bowel sounds, bruits, venous hums | Gastrointestinal Cardiovascular | |
| | Percussion of abdomen (all quadrants) and epigastric region for tone | Gastrointestinal | |
| | Percussion of upper and lower liver borders and estimation of liver span | | Liver percussion should occur at midclavicular line |
| | Percussion of left midaxillary line for splenic dullness | | |
| | Light palpation of all four quadrants; note tenderness, guarding, masses | | Allow client to become accustomed to examiner's hands |
| | Deep palpation of all four quadrants; note tenderness, guarding masses | | Gently but firmly move palpation deeper and deeper until examiner convinced that abdomen sufficiently assessed |
| | Deep palpation of right costal margin for liver border | | Examiner must decide whether to use one-hand or two-hand approach |
| | Deep palpation of left costal margin for splenic border | | |
| | Deep palpation of abdomen for right and left kidneys | | |
| | Deep palpation of midline epigastric area for aortic pulsation | Cardiovascular | Tenderness in epigastric area normal |
| | Testing abdominal reflexes with pointed instrument | Neurological | |
| | Client raises head for evaluation of flexion and strength of abdominal muscles | Musculoskeletal | Note use of arms or hands to assist; older client may have difficulty with this technique |
| | Light palpation of inguinal region for lymph nodes, femoral pulses, and bulges that may be associated with hernia | Lymphatic Cardiovascular Abdominal | |
| 9. Assess lower limbs and hips: client is lying; abdomen and chest should be draped | Inspection of client's feet and legs for skin characteristics, vascular sufficiency, pulses; note deformities of toes, feet, nails, ankles, legs | Integumentary Cardiovascular, peripheral vascular Musculoskeletal | |
| | Palpation of feet and lower legs; note temperature, pulses, tenderness, deformities | Cardiovascular Musculoskeletal | |

## Clinical guidelines for physical examination integration—cont'd

| PROCEDURE OR FORMAT | ASSESSMENT TO INCLUDE | BODY PART OR SYSTEM INVOLVED | CLINICAL STRATEGIES FOR ADULTS AND GERIATRIC CLIENTS |
|---|---|---|---|
| | Range of motion and motor strength of toes, feet, ankles, and knees | Musculoskeletal Neurological | Motor strength testing may be postponed until patient seated |
| | Range of motion and motor strength of hips | | |
| | Palpation of hips for stability | | |
| **10.** Assess genitalia, pelvic region, and rectum: client is lying and adequately draped | **For males:** Inspection and palpation of external genitalia, including pubic hair, penis and scrotum, testes, epididymides, and vas deferens; inspect sacrococcygeal and perianal areas and anus for surface characteristics (with client lying on left side with right hip and knee flexed) | Genitourinary | If mass in scrotal sac suspected, transilluminate |
| | Palpation of anus, rectum, and prostate gland with gloved finger | | Lubricate finger and slowly insert; wait for sphincter to relax before advancing finger |
| | Note characteristics of stool when gloved finger removed | Gastrointestinal | |
| | **For females** (client should be lying in lithotomy position): Inspection and palpation of external genitalia, including pubic hair, labia, clitoris, urethral and vaginal orifices, perineal and perianal area and anus for surface characteristics | Genitourinary | |
| | Insertion of vaginal speculum and inspection of surface characteristics of vagina and cervix | | |
| | Collection of Pap smear and culture specimen | | |
| | Bimanual palpation to assess form, size, and characteristics of vagina, cervix, uterus, adnexa | | Lubricate first two fingers of gloved hand to be inserted internally; other hand should be positioned on abdomen directly above internal hand |
| | Vaginal-rectal examination to assess rectovaginal septum and pouch, surface characteristics, broad ligament tenderness | | When examination completed, client should be offered tissue for drying of genital area |
| | Rectal examination to assess anal sphincter tone, surface characteristics (anal culture may be obtained) | | |
| | Note characteristics of stool when gloved finger removed | Gastrointestinal | |

| PROCEDURE OR FORMAT | ASSESSMENT TO INCLUDE | BODY PART OR SYSTEM INVOLVED | CLINICAL STRATEGIES FOR ADULTS AND GERIATRIC CLIENTS |
|---|---|---|---|
| **Client is seated** | | | |
| **11.** Assess neurological system: assist client to sitting position; should have gown on and be draped across lap | Observation of client moving from lying to sitting position; note use of muscles, ease of movement, and co-ordination | Neurological Musculoskeletal | |
| | Testing sensory function of neurological system by using light and deep (dull and sharp) sensation of forehead, paranasal sinus area, hands, lower arms, feet, lower legs | Neurological (sensory function): CN V (trigeminal nerve) | Client's eyes should be closed; instruct client to either point to or verbally report area that has been touched Alternate light, dull, and pinprick sensations Test bilaterally |
| | Bilateral testing and comparison of vibratory sensations of ankle, wrist, sternum | | |
| | Testing two-point discrimination of palms, thigh, back | Cortical, discriminatory sensory of neurological system | |
| | Testing stereognosis or graphesthesia | | |
| | Testing fine motor functioning and coordination of upper extremities by instructing client to perform at least two of following: 1. Alternating pronation and supination of forearm 2. Touching nose with alternating index fingers 3. Rapidly alternating finger movements to thumb 4. Rapid movement of index finger between nose and examiner's finger | Proprioception and cerebellar function of neurological system | Perform technique bilaterally and compare responses |
| | Testing and bilaterally comparing fine motor functioning and coordination of lower extremities by instructing client to run heel down tibia of opposite leg | | |
| | Alternately crossing legs over knee | Musculoskeletal | |
| | Testing and bilaterally comparing deep tendon reflexes, including: 1. Biceps tendon 2. Triceps tendon 3. Trachioradial tendon 4. Patellar tendon 5. Achilles tendon | Reflex status of neurological system | If client shows any neurological problems, evaluate by Babinski and ankle clonus tests |

## Clinical guidelines for physical examination integration—cont'd

| PROCEDURE OR FORMAT | ASSESSMENT TO INCLUDE | BODY PART OR SYSTEM INVOLVED | CLINICAL STRATEGIES FOR ADULTS AND GERIATRIC CLIENTS |
|---|---|---|---|
| **Client is standing** | | | |
| **12.** Palpate scrotum and inguinal region (male) | Palpation of scrotum and inguinal regions for characteristics and hernias | Genitourinary | Instruct client to bear down or cough during hernia evaluation |
| **13.** Assess neurological and musculoskeletal system | Assessment of client's gait: observe and palpate straightness of client's spine as client stands and bends forward to touch toes | Musculoskeletal Neurological | Elderly clients may not be able to do this |
| | With client's waist stabilized, evaluation by hyperextension, lateral bending, rotation of upper trunk | | |
| | Assessment of proprioception and cerebellar and motor function by using at least two of following:<br>1. Romberg test (eyes closed)<br>2. Walking straight heel-to-toe formation<br>3. Standing on one foot and then other (eyes closed)<br>4. Hopping in place on one foot and then other<br>5. Knee bends | | Client's age and general ability may help define which technique to use<br>Protect client from falling by remaining close and ready to catch him if necessary<br>Elderly clients may not be able to do this |

## Integration of the pediatric examination

The procedure for integrating the pediatric examination will depend entirely on the age and cooperation of the child. By the time the child reaches school age, he should be able to participate fully in a cooperative manner. It is the younger child who will present the challenge. The following format changes should facilitate a thorough assessment.

| AGE AND PREPARATION | PROCEDURES | SYSTEMS INVOLVED |
|---|---|---|
| **1.** Newborn to 6 months: undressed, lying on examination table | 1. Obtain history, highlighting developmental or problem areas<br>2. Check vital signs: temperature, pulse, respiration<br>3. Record weight, length, chest and head circumference<br>4. Observe child lying on examination table; note color, general health, body symmetry, gross motor movement, alertness, gross and fine motor development, language development, social adaptive development, skin characteristics, and response to sound and vision stimulation | Cardiovascular, neurological, musculoskeletal, integumentary, visual, auditory |
| | 5. Examine and manipulate hands, arms, shoulders, feet, legs; note range of motion and tone | Musculoskeletal, neurological |
| | 6. Examine skin over extremities, chest, abdomen, and back | Integumentary, cardiovascular |
| | 7. Auscultate thorax, lungs, heart, abdomen | Thorax, lungs, cardiovascular, gastrointestinal |
| | 8. Palpate and examine external characteristics of head, neck, face, axillary region | Lymphatic, head, neck, visual, auditory, oral, nasal |
| | 9. Palpate thorax, abdomen, and umbilical area | Thorax, abdomen |
| | 10. Observe and palpate external genitalia, inguinal area, and hip stability | Genital, musculoskeletal |
| | 11. Examine eyes with ophthalmoscope | Visual |
| | 12. Examine mouth, teeth (development), tongue, posterior pharynx, nose | Oral, nasal |
| | 13. Examine ears with otoscope | Auditory |

## Integration of the pediatric examination—cont'd

| AGE AND PREPARATION | PROCEDURES | SYSTEMS INVOLVED |
|---|---|---|
| **2.** Six months to 2 years: child in diaper, sitting on parent's lap; examiner's chair should be in front of parent's chair and examiner's knees should touch parent's; during supine examination, child may lie on parent's and examiner's lap | 1. Obtain history highlighting developmental or problem areas | |
| | 2. Perform developmental, social, vision, speech, hearing, and fine and gross motor assessment during play and initial "get acquainted" period | Neurological, visual, speech, auditory, musculoskeletal |
| | 3. Record weight, length, and chest and head circumference (until 18 months) | |
| | 4. Check vital signs, including blood pressure in children over 18 months of age; may be postponed until later if child becomes agitated | |
| | 5. Auscultate lungs and heart | Thorax, cardiovascular |
| | 6. Examine skin over extremities, chest, abdomen, and back | Integumentary, cardiovascular |
| | 7. Examination and manipulate hands, arms, shoulders, feet, legs; note range of motion and tone | Neurological, musculoskeletal |
| | 8. Palpate and examine external characteristics of head, neck, face, axillary region | Lymphatic, head, neck, visual, auditory, oral, nasal |
| | 9. Auscultate abdomen with child in supine position on parent's and examiner's lap | Gastrointestinal |
| | 10. Palpate thorax, abdomen, and umbilical area | Thorax and abdomen |
| | 11. Observe and palpate external genitalia, inguinal area, and hip stability | Genital, musculoskeletal |
| | 12. Examine eyes with ophthalmoscope | Visual |
| | 13. Examination mouth, teeth (development), tongue, posterior pharynx, nose | Oral, nasal |
| | 14. Examine ears with otoscope | Auditory |
| **3.** Two to 4 years: undressed to underpants; may be examined either on parent's lap or examination table; much of assessment may be inform as examiner observes and plays with child | Same as for child from 6 months to 2 years; refer to individual chapter for detailed discussion of strategies | |
| **4.** Four to 6 years: undressed to underpants, sitting on examination table; assessment should move toward adult format; child's developmental immaturity may necessitate that examiner alter various examination techniques to facilitate child's participation and correct response | Same as for child from 6 months to 2 years | |
| **5.** Over 6 years old: in gown on examination table | Same as for adult client | |

## Physical examination write-up

The data base and the information collected during the physical assessment must be organized and documented. The components of the documentation are (1) subjective data base, (2) physical assessment, (3) risk profile, and (4) problem list. Before the actual documentation the examiner must decide whether to record the data on plain paper or on a predesigned form. Each has advantages and disadvantages. We prefer plain paper.

| Advantages | Disadvantages |
|---|---|
| *Plain paper* | |
| Documentation space is not a problem. | The examiner must be organized; if not, rambling and insignificant data may be a problem. |
| Specific data for individual client may be emphasized as necessary. | All examiners in the agency may not use the same format. |
| *Predeveloped form* | |
| Departmental continuity is maintained. | Individual situations may be difficult to emphasize. |
| Data will be easy to locate by other examiners. | Examiner may not have adequate space for documentation. |
| It is a reminder for completeness. | If form was developed before examiner's input, it may not include all data the examiner wants to collect. |
| | Separate forms necessary for pediatric and geriatric clients. |

Once the style of documentation is determined, the examiner must synthesize the client's historical and physical data and record information in the following areas. The examiner is urged to record *what* is observed, heard, percussed, or palpated and to avoid vague and nondescriptive terms such as *normal, negative, good,* or *poor.*

## Documentation format

1. Subjective data base
   a. Biographical data
   b. Reason for visit
   c. Present health status
   d. Current health data: immunizations, allergies, last examination
   e. Past health status: childhood illnesses, serious or chronic illnesses, serious accidents or injuries, hospitalizations, operations, emotional health, obstetrical health
   f. Family history
   g. Review of physiological systems: general, nutritional integumentary, head, eyes, ears, nose, mouth, neck, breast, cardiovascular, respiratory, hematolymphatic, gastrointestinal, urinary, genital, musculoskeletal, central nervous system, endocrine, and allergic and immunological
   h. Psychosocial history: general status, response to illness, significant others, occupational history, educational level, activities of daily living, habits, financial status
   i. Health maintenance efforts: maintenance of self health, health care patterns
   j. Environmental health: general assessment, employment, home, neighborhood, community
2. Physical assessment
   a. Vital statistics: height, weight, temperature, pulse, blood pressure (both arms, lying, sitting, standing)
   b. General statement of appearance
   c. Mental health
   d. Integumentary: skin, nails, body hair
   e. Head and neck: scalp, hair, face, neck, lymph nodes, thyroid, trachea, sinuses
   f. Nose: patency, surface characteristics
   g. Mouth, pharynx: oral cavity characteristics, teeth, tongue, voice, tonsillar area and posterior pharynx
   h. Ear and auditory: external ear, canal, TM characteristics, hearing, Rinne and Weber tests
   i. Eye and visual: external eye characteristics, vision, eye movement, funduscopy
   j. Thorax and lungs: thorax characteristics, breathing pattern and rate, percussion tone, auscultatory characteristics
   k. Cardiovascular: all pulses, blood pressure, extremity circulation, precordium characteristics, heart sounds
   l. Breast: surface characteristics, areolae and nipples, palpation characteristics, lymphatic assessment, breast self-examination assessment
   m. Abdominal, rectal: contour, surface characteristics, bowel sounds, percussion tones, palpation characteristics, liver and spleen, bladder, kidney characteristics, CVA tenderness, hernias, rectal examination findings
   n. Genital
      (1) Female: external genitalia characteristics, internal-cervical, vagina, uterus, adnexa characteristics
      (2) Male: external genitalia characteristics, palpation characteristics of penis and scrotum, inguinal hernia evaluation
   o. Musculoskeletal: muscular development and

strength, skeletal and joint characteristics and symmetry, range of motion

p. Neurological: orientation, intactness of CN I to XII, coordination of fine and gross motor movements and gait, sensory evaluation, reflexes

3. Risk profile: those items from the client's history and physical assessment that might indicate risk to the overall health state. These are potential problems. Examples that may be considered a risk for some clients are detailed in the data base in Chapter 1.

4. Problem list. The problem list should be a synthesis of those items that are currently identified as stressors for the client. The stressors may be physiological, sociological, psychological, or a combination of these. The problems are those items that reduce the client's overall level of health. Once the problems are listed and assigned a priority, it can then be decided which are within the examiner's scope of practice to handle and which must be referred.

It is important for the examiner to cluster subjective and objective data to describe problems. The following unrelated examples demonstrate a holistic approach to problem identification.

a. Weight gain: 18 pounds in past year; exercise limited to game of tennis twice a month; expresses desire to diet but needs direction

b. Short of breath when walking up more than one flight of stairs; moderate edema below midcalf bilaterally; fine rales in lower bases bilaterally

c. Limited range of motion in right shoulder interferes with activities of daily living: dressing, preparing meals

d. Cataracts bilaterally; interfere with reading and driving at night

e. BP 180/120 (right arm) lying, 172/112 (right arm) sitting; retinal A-V ratio appears to be 2/4; arteriolar narrowing

f. Periodic slight urinary incontinence since birth of child 3 years ago; cystocele noted on vaginal examination

g. Complaints of LLQ discomfort for 6 months; cyclic with menses; increased discomfort at ovulation time and just before menses; thickening in left adnexa area; increased tenderness with palpation of left adnexa area; menses regular; pinpoint tenderness on deep palpation in LLQ

h. Smokes one pack of cigarettes a day for past 15 years; deep nonproductive cough for past 5 years, becoming worse; increased breathing difficulty when climbing more than one flight of stairs; decreased breath sounds on right; bilateral rales or rhonchi in base of lungs; slight clearing with cough

i. Death of spouse 2 months ago; since then increased periods of depression, 10-pound weight loss, decreased desire to maintain own health state

# Answers

## Chapter 2

1. i
2. Any of the following are correct:
   a. Client's initial response to examiner
   b. Body appearance
   c. Body movements
   d. Gait
   e. Facial expression
   f. Vocal tones
   g. Speech
   h. Apparel
   i. Grooming
   j. Odors
   k. General mannerisms
3. c
4. d
5. e
6. a
7. b
8. f
9. h

## Chapter 3

| | | |
|---|---|---|
| 1. T | 14. c | 27. d |
| 2. T | 15. d | 28. k |
| 3. T | 16. a | 29. b |
| 4. F | 17. d | 30. h |
| 5. T | 18. g | 31. e |
| 6. T | 19. h | 32. d |
| 7. T | 20. c | 33. i |
| 8. T | 21. f | 34. T |
| 9. T | 22. g | 35. F |
| 10. T | 23. j | 36. F |
| 11. e | 24. a | 37. d |
| 12. b | 25. i | 38. c |
| 13. a | 26. l | 39. e |

## Chapter 4

| | | |
|---|---|---|
| 1. d | 8. e | 15. b |
| 2. c | 9. j | 16. i |
| 3. a | 10. c | 17. f |
| 4. e | 11. d | 18. i |
| 5. c | 12. h | 19. d |
| 6. b | 13. a | 20. g |
| 7. b | 14. g | 21. e |

## Chapter 5

| | | |
|---|---|---|
| 1. i | 10. b | 18. c |
| 2. h | 11. f | 19. c |
| 3. b | 12. i | 20. i |
| 4. b | 13. f | 21. c |
| 5. a | 14. h | 22. d |
| 6. i | 15. i | 23. f |
| 7. d | 16. h | 24. c |
| 8. b | 17. b | 25. f |
| 9. c | | |

## Chapter 6

| | | |
|---|---|---|
| 1. c | 9. j | 16. f |
| 2. a | 10. h | 17. b |
| 3. c | 11. h | 18. d |
| 4. c | 12. F | 19. T |
| 5. i | 13. T | 20. F |
| 6. c | 14. F | 21. T |
| 7. i | 15. F | 22. F |
| 8. j | | |

## Chapter 7

| | | |
|---|---|---|
| 1. h | 12. b | 23. e |
| 2. b | 13. j | 24. d |
| 3. h | 14. i | 25. i |
| 4. g | 15. e | 26. c |
| 5. j | 16. h | 27. i |
| 6. c | 17. i | 28. e |
| 7. b | 18. b | 29. c |
| 8. g | 19. a | 30. b |
| 9. f | 20. j | 31. a |
| 10. f | 21. a | |
| 11. g | 22. e | |

## Chapter 8

| | | |
|---|---|---|
| 1. F | 8. d | 19. e |
| 2. T | 9. j | 20. i |
| 3. T | 10. e | 21. f |
| 4. F | 11. b | 22. c |
| 5. F | 12. d | |
| 6. F | 13. c | |
| 7. >, peripheral lung | 14. a | |
| =, first and second | 15. d | |
| intercostals at | 16. g | |
| sternal border | 17. d | |
| <, over trachea | 18. a | |

## Chapter 9

| | |
|---|---|
| 1. h | 23. a. Superior vena cava |
| 2. i | b. Inferior vena cava |
| 3. g | c. Right atrium |
| 4. b | d. Tricuspid valve |
| 5. f | e. Right ventricle |
| 6. i | f. Pulmonary valve |
| 7. g | g. Pulmonary artery |
| 8. f | h. Pulmonary vein |
| 9. f | i. Aorta |
| 10. i | j. Left atrium |
| 11. g | k. Aortic valve |
| 12. j | l. Mitral valve |
| 13. d | m. Left ventricle |
| 14. f | 24. mitral; tricuspid; |
| 15. h | systole |
| 16. g | 25. aortic; pulmonary; |
| 17. b | diastole |
| 18. a | 26. CAI |
| 19. Amplitude | 27. CAI |
| 20. Contour | 28. CVI |
| 21. Amplitude pattern | 29. CAI |
| 22. Symmetry | 30. CVI |

| | | |
|---|---|---|
| 31. CAI | 40. a | 49. e |
| 32. CAI | 41. b | 50. a |
| 33. a | 42. b | 51. e |
| 34. b | 43. a | 52. d |
| 35. b | 44. a | 53. a |
| 36. a | 45. a | 54. e |
| 37. a | 46. d | 55. h |
| 38. a | 47. c | 56. a |
| 39. b | 48. b | 57. b |

## Chapter 10

| | | |
|---|---|---|
| 1. f | 7. T | 13. T |
| 2. b | 8. F | 14. F |
| 3. c | 9. F | 15. T |
| 4. j | 10. F | 16. F |
| 5. j | 11. F | 17. c |
| 6. F | 12. F | 18. i |

## Chapter 11

1. Student can compare own drawing of major abdominal organs with textbook illustration.
2. Any five of the following are correct:
   a. Client supine with arms on chest or at sides
   b. Small pillow under head
   c. Knees slightly flexed
   d. Warm room
   e. Client draped over breasts and pubis
   f. Examiner's hands warm
   g. Short fingernails
   h. Warm stethoscope
   i. Client breathing slowly through mouth
   j. Examiner explaining procedure

| | | |
|---|---|---|
| 3. c | 11. g | 19. f |
| 4. b | 12. g | 20. i |
| 5. b | 13. c | 21. f |
| 6. d | 14. i | 22. d |
| 7. c | 15. h | 23. e |
| 8. a | 16. h | 24. f |
| 9. a | 17. f | 25. g |
| 10. d | 18. h | 26. e |

## Chapter 12

| | | |
|---|---|---|
| 1. N | 14. A | 27. d |
| 2. G | 15. a | 28. f |
| 3. O | 16. b | 29. e |
| 4. B | 17. b | 30. a |
| 5. H | 18. a | 31. c |
| 6. F | 19. a | 32. b |
| 7. C | 20. c | 33. d |
| 8. L | 21. a | 34. c |
| 9. K | 22. f | 35. i |
| 10. D | 23. b | 36. c |
| 11. J | 24. i | 37. a |
| 12. I | 25. b | 38. i |
| 13. M | 26. g | |

## Chapter 13

| | | |
|---|---|---|
| 1. L | 19. H | 36. h |
| 2. F | 20. K | 37. g |
| 3. C | 21. C | 38. T |
| 4. K | 22. M | 39. F |
| 5. H | 23. F | 40. F |
| 6. A | 24. A | 41. F |
| 7. E | 25. L | 42. T |
| 8. I | 26. I | 43. T |
| 9. B | 27. E | 44. T |
| 10. G | 28. J | 45. F |
| 11. D | 29. j | 46. T |
| 12. J | 30. f | 47. T |
| 13. h | 31. f | 48. T |
| 14. g | 32. b | 49. F |
| 15. h | 33. g | 50. g |
| 16. D | 34. a | 51. c |
| 17. G | 35. i | 52. h |
| 18. B | | |

## Chapter 14

| | | |
|---|---|---|
| 1. T | 15. j | 29. a |
| 2. T | 16. b | 30. j |
| 3. T | 17. c | 31. a |
| 4. F | 18. a | 32. e |
| 5. T | 19. g | 33. c |
| 6. T | 20. h | 34. b |
| 7. F | 21. d | 35. h |
| 8. F | 22. h | 36. i |
| 9. T | 23. g | 37. d |
| 10. F | 24. c | 38. h |
| 11. d | 25. b | 39. c |
| 12. i | 26. d | 40. f |
| 13. f | 27. k | 41. e |
| 14. e | 28. a | |

## Chapter 15

| | | |
|---|---|---|
| 1. b | 13. T | 25. a |
| 2. h | 14. T | 26. c |
| 3. c | 15. d | 27. e |
| 4. a | 16. e | 28. b |
| 5. a | 17. a | 29. a |
| 6. a | 18. c | 30. d |
| 7. g | 19. b | 31. b |
| 8. i | 20. c | 32. c |
| 9. i | 21. e | 33. d |
| 10. j | 22. d | 34. a |
| 11. g | 23. b | 35. d |
| 12. F | 24. d | 36. b |

# The Washington guide to promoting development in the young child

## Motor skills

| EXPECTED TASKS | SUGGESTED ACTIVITIES |
|---|---|
| **1 to 3 months** | |
| 1. Holds head up briefly when prone | 1. Place infant in prone position |
| 2. Head erect and bobbing when supported in sitting position | 2. Support in sitting position with his head erect |
| 3. Head erect and steady in sitting position | 3. Pull infant to sitting position |
| 4. Follows object through all planes | 4. Provide with opportunity to observe people or activity |
| 5. Palmar grasp | 5. Hang bright-colored objects and mobiles within reach across crib |
| 6. Moro reflex | 6. Provide with opportunity to observe objects or people while in sitting position |
| | 7. Use infant seat |
| | 8. Alternate bright shiny objects with dark and light visual patterns |
| **4 to 8 months** | |
| 1. Sits with minimal support, with stable head and back | 1. Pull up to sitting position |
| 2. Sits alone steadily | 2. Provide opportunity to sit supported or alone when head and trunk control are stabilized |
| 3. Plays with hands, which are open most of time | 3. Put bright-colored objects within reach |
| 4. Grasps rattle or bottle with both hands | 4. Give toys or household objects: rattles, teething ring, cloth animals or dolls, 1-inch cubes, plastic objects such as cups, rings, and balls |
| 5. Picks up small objects, for example, cube | 5. Offer small objects such as cereal to improve grasp |
| 6. Transfers toys from one hand to other | 6. Offer a variety of patterns or textures to play with |
| 7. Neck-righting reflex | 7. Use squeak toys |

From Barnard, K.E., and Erickson, M.L.: Teaching children with developmental problems: a family care approach, ed. 2, St. Louis, 1976, The C.V. Mosby Co.

| EXPECTED TASKS | SUGGESTED ACTIVITIES |
|---|---|
| **9 to 12 months** | |
| 1. Rises to sitting position | 1. Provide playpen, allow child to pull himself to standing |
| 2. Creeps or crawls, maybe backward at first | 2. Give opportunity and space to practice creeping and crawling |
| 3. Pulls to standing position | 3. Have child practice moving on knees to improve balance prior to walking |
| 4. Stands alone | 4. Have child use walker or straddle toys |
| 5. Cruises | 5. Play airplane with child; have child practice catching himself while rolling on large ball |
| 6. Uses index finger to poke | 6. Provide with objects such as spoons, plastic bottles, cups, ball, cubes, finger foods, saucepans, and lids |
| 7. Finger-thumb grasp | |
| 8. Parachute reflex | |
| 9. Landau reflex | |
| **13 to 18 months** | |
| 1. Walks a few steps without support | 1. Provide opportunity to practice walking, climbing stairs with help |
| 2. Balanced when walking | 2. Give toys that can be pushed around |
| 3. Walks upstairs with help, creeps downstairs | 3. Supervise activity with paper and large crayons |
| 4. Turns pages of book | 4. Provide toys such as cubes, cups, saucepans, lids, rag dolls, and other soft, cuddly toys |
| | 5. Begin introducing child to swing |
| **19 to 30 months** | |
| 1. Runs | 1. Provide opportunity to practice and develop activities |
| 2. Walks up and down stairs, one at a time (not alternating feet) | 2. Provide pattern for child while he watches and then encourage him to try |
| 3. Imitates vertical strokes | 3. Provide tricycle or similar pedal toys; secure foot on pedal if necessary |
| 4. Imitates building tower of four or more blocks | |
| 5. Throws ball overhand | |
| 6. Jumps in place | |
| 7. Rides tricycle | |
| **31 to 48 months** | |
| 1. Walks downstairs (alternating feet) | 1. Continue with blocks, combining materials, toy cars, and trains |
| 2. Hops on one foot | 2. Provide clay and other manipulating materials |
| 3. Swings and climbs | 3. Give opportunities to swing and climb |
| 4. Balances on one foot for 10 seconds | 4. Provide with activities such as finger painting, chalk, and blackboard |
| 5. Copies circle | |
| 6. Copies cross | |
| 7. Draws persons with three parts | |
| **49 to 52 months** | |
| 1. Balances well | 1. Provide with music and games to synchronize hand and foot, tapping with music, skipping, hopping, and dancing rhythmically to improve coordination. |
| 2. Skips and jumps | |
| 3. Can heel-toe walk | |
| 4. Copies square | |
| 5. Catches bounced ball | |

## Feeding skills

| EXPECTED TASKS | SUGGESTED ACTIVITIES |
|---|---|
| **1 to 3 months**<br>1. Sucking reflex present<br>2. Rooting reflex present<br>3. Ability to swallow pureed foods<br>4. Coordinates sucking, swallowing, and breathing | 1. Consider a change in nipple or posturing if there is difficulty in swallowing<br>2. Hold in comfortable relaxed position while feeding<br>3. Pace feeding tempo to infant's needs |
| **4 to 8 months**<br>1. Tongue used in moving food in mouth<br>2. Hand-to-mouth motions<br>3. Recognizes bottle on sight<br>4. Gums or mouths solid foods<br>5. Feeds self cracker | 1. Give finger foods to develop chewing, stimulate gums, and encourage hand-to-mouth motion (cubes of cheese, bananas, dry toast, bread crust, cookies)<br>2. Encourage upright supported position for feeding<br>3. Promote bottle holding<br>4. Introduce solid foods |
| **9 to 12 months**<br>1. Holds own bottle<br>2. Drinks from cup or glass with assistance<br>3. Finger feeds<br>4. Beginning to hold spoon | 1. Bring child in highchair to table and include in part of or entire meal with family<br>2. Have child in sitting position with trunk and feet supported<br>3. Encourage self-help in feeding; use of table foods<br>4. Offer spoon when interest is indicated<br>5. Introduce cup or plastic glass with small amount of fluid |
| **13 to 18 months**<br>1. Holds cup and handle with digital grasp<br>2. Lifts cup and drinks well<br>3. Beginning to use spoon, may turn bowl down before reaching mouth<br>4. Difficulty in inserting spoon into mouth<br>5. May refuse food | 1. Continue offering finger foods<br>2. Use nontip dishes and cups; dishes should have sides to make filling of spoon easy<br>3. Give opportunity for self-feeding<br>4. Provide fluids between meals rather than having child fill up on fluids at mealtime |
| **19 to 30 months**<br>1. Drinks without spilling<br>2. Holds small glass in one hand<br>3. Inserts spoon in mouth correctly<br>4. Distinguishes between food and inedible material<br>5. Plays with food | 1. Encourage self-feeding with spoon<br>2. Do not rush child<br>3. Serve foods plainly but in attractive servings<br>4. Small servings of food will encourage eating more than large servings |
| **31 to 48 months**<br>1. Pours well from pitcher<br>2. Serves self at table with little spilling<br>3. Rarely needs assistance<br>4. Interest in setting table | 1. Encourage self-help<br>2. Give opportunity for pouring (give rice and pitcher to promote pouring skills)<br>3. Encourage child to help set table<br>4. Have well-defined rules about table manners |
| **49 to 52 months**<br>1. Feeds self well<br>2. Social and talkative during meal | 1. Socialize with child at mealtime<br>2. Have child help with preparation, table setting, and serving<br>3. Include child in conversations at mealtimes by planning special times for him to tell about events, situations, or what he did during the day |

# Sleep

| EXPECTED TASKS | SUGGESTED ACTIVITIES |
|---|---|
| **1 to 3 months**<br>1. Night: 4- to 10-hour intervals<br>2. Naps: frequent<br>3. Longer periods of wakefulness without crying | 1. Provide separate sleeping arrangements away from parents' room<br>2. Reduce noise and light stimulation when placing in bed<br>3. Have room at comfortable temperature with no drafts or extremes in heat<br>4. Reverse position of crib occasionally<br>5. Place infant in different positions from time to time for sleep<br>6. Alternate from back to side to stomach<br>7. Keep crib sides up |
| **4 to 8 months**<br>1. Night: 10 to 12 hours<br>2. Naps: 2 to 3 (1 to 4 hours in duration)<br>3. Night awakenings | 1. Keep crib sides up<br>2. Refrain from taking infant into parents' room if he awakens<br>3. Check to determine if there is cause for awakenings: hunger, teething, pain, cold, wet, noise, or illness<br>4. If a baby-sitter is used, attempt to find some person with whom infant is familiar. Explain bedtime and naptime arrangements |
| **9 to 12 months**<br>1. Night: 12 to 14 hours<br>2. Naps: one to two (1 to 4 hours in duration)<br>3. May begin refusing morning nap | 1. Short crying periods may be source of tension release for child<br>2. Observe for signs of fatigue, irritability, or restlessness if naps are shorter<br>3. Provide familiar person to baby-sit up knows sleep routines |
| **13 to 18 months**<br>1. Night: 10 to 12 hours<br>2. Naps: one in afternoon (1 to 3 hours in duration)<br>3. May awaken during night crying (associated with wetting bed)<br>4. As he becomes more able to move about, he may uncover himself, become cold, and awaken | 1. Night terrors may be terminated by awakening child and offering reassurance<br>2. Check to see that child is covered<br>3. Avoid hazardous devices to keep child covered, including blanket clips, pins, and garments that enclose child to neck |
| **19 to 30 months**<br>1. Night: 10 to 12 hours<br>2. Naps: one (1 to 3 hours in duration)<br>3. Doesn't go to sleep at once—keeps demanding things<br>4. May waken crying if wet or soiled<br>5. May awaken because of environmental change of temperature, change of bed, change of sleeping room, addition of sibling to room, absence of parent from home, hospitalization, trip with family, or relatives visiting | 1. Quiet period of socialization prior to bedtime—reading child book or telling story<br>2. Holding child—talking quietly with him<br>3. Ritualistic behavior may be present; allow child to carry out routine; helps him overcome fear of unexpected or fear of dark; for example, child may wish to arrange toys in certain way<br>4. Explain bedtime ritual to baby-sitter<br>5. Give more reassurance, spend more time before bedtime preparation<br>6. Provide familiar bedtime toys or items<br>7. Allow crying-out period if he is safe, comfortable, and tucked in<br>8. Place in bed before he reaches excessive state of fatigue, excitement, or tiredness<br>9. Eliminate sources of stimulation or fear<br>10. Maintain consistent hour of bedtime |

*Continued.*

## Sleep—cont'd

| EXPECTED TASKS | SUGGESTED ACTIVITIES |
|---|---|
| **31 to 48 months** | |
| 1. Daily range: 10 to 15 hours<br>2. Naps: beginning to disappear<br>3. Prolongs process of going to bed<br>4. Less dependent on taking toys to bed<br>5. May awaken crying from dreams<br>6. May awaken if wet | 1. Television programs may affect ability to go to sleep; avoid violent television programs<br>2. Anxiety about going to bed and desire to stay up with parents—requires limits<br>3. Regularity and consistency important to promote good sleeping habits<br>4. Reassurance—night light or leaving door ajar<br>5. Do not use bedtime or naptime as punishment<br>6. Encourage naps if signs of fatigue or irritability are evidenced |
| **49 to 52 months** | |
| 1. Daily range: 9 to 13 hours<br>2. Naps: rare<br>3. Quieter during sleep | 1. Encourage napping if excessive or strenuous activity occurs and child is overly tired<br>2. Explain to child if baby-sitter will be there after child is asleep |

# Play

| EXPECTED TASKS | SUGGESTED ACTIVITIES |
|---|---|
| **1 to 3 months**<br>1. Quieted when picked up<br>2. Regards face of others | 1. Encourage holding and touching of infant by parent<br>2. Provide with cradle gyms and mobiles, brightly colored, visually interesting objects within arm's distance |
| **4 to 8 months**<br>1. Plays with own body<br>2. Differentiates strangers from family<br>3. Seeks out objects<br>4. Grasps, holds, and manipulates objects<br>5. Repeats activities he enjoys<br>6. Bangs toys or objects together | 1. Begin patty-cake and peekaboo<br>2. Provide for periods of solitary play (playpen)<br>3. Encourage holding and touching of infant by parent<br>4. Provide variety of multicolored and multitextured objects that infant can hold<br>5. Encourage exploration of body parts<br>6. Provide floating toys for bath |
| **9 to 12 months**<br>1. Puts objects in and out of containers<br>2. Examines objects held in hand<br>3. Plays interactive games (peekaboo)<br>4. Extends toy to other person without releasing<br>5. Works to get toy out of reach | 1. Continue parent-infant games<br>2. Give opportunity to place objects in containers and pour out<br>3. Provide large and small objects with which to play<br>4. Encourage interactive play |
| **13 to 18 months**<br>1. Plays by himself—may play near others<br>2. Has preferred toys<br>3. Enjoys walking activities, pulling toys<br>4. Throws and picks up objects, throws again<br>5. Imitates, for example, reading newspaper, sweeping | 1. Introduce to other children even though child may not play with them<br>2. Provide music, books, and magazines<br>3. Encourage imitative activities—helping with dusting, sweeping, stirring |
| **19 to 30 months**<br>1. Parallel play—not interactive but plays alongside another child<br>2. Uses both large and small toys<br>3. Rough-and-tumble play<br>4. Play periods longer than before—interested in manipulative and constructive toys<br>5. Enjoys rhymes and singing (television programs) | 1. Provide with new materials for manipulating and feeling—finger paints, clay, sand, stones, water, and soap<br>Wooden toys—cars and animals<br>Building blocks of various sizes, crayons, and paper<br>Rhythmical tunes and equipment—swing, rocking chair, rocking horse<br>Children's books—short, simple stories with repetition and familiar objects; enjoys simple pictures, brightly colored<br>2. Guide child's hand to actively participate with specific activities, for example, using crayons, hammering |
| **31 to 48 months**<br>1. In playing with others, beginning to interact, sharing toys, taking turns<br>2. Dramatizes, expresses imagination in play<br>3. Combining playthings; more use of constructive materials<br>4. Prefers two or three children to play with; may have special friend | 1. Encourage play with small groups of children<br>2. Encourage imaginative and dramatic play activities<br>3. Music: singing and experimenting with musical instruments<br>4. Group participation in rhymes, dancing by hopping or jumping<br>5. Drawing and painting (seldom recognizable) |
| **49 to 52 months**<br>1. Dramatic play and interest in going on excursions<br>2. Fond of cutting and pasting, creative materials<br>3. Completes most activities | 1. Painting and drawing (objects will be out of proportion; details that are most important to child are drawn largest)<br>2. Encourage printing of numbers and letters<br>3. Clay: making recognizable objects<br>4. Cutting and pasting<br>5. Provide with materials, for example, boxes, chairs, barrels, for building sturdy structures |

# Language

| EXPECTED TASKS | SUGGESTED ACTIVITIES |
|---|---|

**1 to 3 months**

*Receptive abilities*
1. Movement of eyes, respiration rate, or body activity changes when bell is rung too close to child's head
2. Smiles when socially stimulated
3. Has facial, vocal, and generalized bodily responses to faces
4. Reacts differently to adult voices

*Expressive abilities*
1. Makes prelanguage vocalizations that consist of cooing, throaty sounds, for example, gu
2. Makes "pleasure" sounds that consist of soft vowels
3. Makes "sucking" sounds
4. Crying may be differentiated for discomfort, pain, and hunger as reported by parent
5. An "A" sound as in cat is commonly heard in distress crying

**Suggested activities (1 to 3 months):**
1. Observe facial expressions, gestures, bodily postures, and movements when vocalizations are being produced
2. Smile and talk softly in pleasant tone while holding, touching, and handling infant
3. Hold, touch, and interact frequently with infant for pleasure
4. Refrain from letting infant engage in prolonged and incessant crying

**4 to 8 months**

*Receptive abilities*
1. Eyes locate source of sound
2. Responds to "hi, there" by looking up at face that is across and in front of him
3. Head turns to sound of cellophane held and crunched 2 feet away and at a 135-degree angle on either side of head
4. Will turn head to locate sound of "look here" when spoken at a 90-degree angle from head 2 feet away*
5. Turns head to sound of rattle
6. Responds differently to vacuum cleaner, phone, doorbell, or sound of dog barking: may cry, whimper, look toward sound, or parent may report change in body tension
7. Responds by raising arms when parent reaches toward him and says "come up"

*Expressive abilities*
1. Uses different inflectional patterns:

   ah                  ah

         uh
2. Laughs aloud when stimulated
3. Has differential patterns of crying when hungry, in pain, or angry
4. Produces vowel sounds and chained syllables (baba, gugu, didi)
5. Makes "talking sounds" in response to others talking to him
6. Babbles to produce consonant sounds: ba, da, m-m
7. Vocalizes to toys
8. Says "da-da" or "ma-ma" but not specific to presence of parents

**Suggested activities (4 to 8 months):**
1. Engage in smiling eye-to-eye contact while talking to infant
2. Vocalize in response to inflectional patterns and when infant is producing babbling sounds; echo the sounds he makes
3. Observe for subtle communication clues such as eye aversion, struggling to move away, flushing of skin, tension of body, or movement of arms
4. Vocalize with infant during handling, while feeding, bathing, dressing, diapering, bedtime preparation, and holding
5. Stimulate laughing by light tickling
6. Observe infant's reactions to bells, whistles, horns, phones, laughing, singing, talking, music box, noise-making toys, and common household noises
7. While talking to infant, hold in position so that he can see your face
8. Have infant placed at position of eye level while talking to him throughout the day
9. If crying or laughing sounds are not discerned at this stage, report to family physician, pediatrician, public health nurse, or well-child clinic

---

*Do not test for localization of sound by producing sound directly behind infant's head.

| EXPECTED TASKS | SUGGESTED ACTIVITIES |
|---|---|

### 9 to 12 months

*Receptive abilities*
1. Ceases activity when name is pronounced or "no-no" is said
2. Gives toys on request when accompanied by facial and bodily gestures
3. Attends to simple commands

*Expressive abilities*
1. Imitates definite speech sounds such as tongue clicking, lip smacking, or coughing
2. Should have two words that are *specific* for parents: "mama," "dada," or equivalents

1. Gain child's attention when giving simple commands
2. Accompany oral directions with gestures
3. Vocalize with child during feeding, bathing, and playtimes
4. Provide sounds that child can reproduce such as lip smacking and tongue clicking
5. Repeat direction frequently and have child participate in action: open and close the drawer; move arms and legs up and down
6. Have child respond to verbal directions: stand up, sit down, close door, open door, turn around, come here

### 13 to 18 months

*Receptive abilities*
1. Attends to person speaking to child
2. Finds "the baby" in picture when requested, for example, on baby food jar, in magazine, or in storybooks
3. Indicates wants by gestures
4. Looks toward family members or pets when named

*Expressive abilities*
1. Uses three words other than mama and data to denote *specific* objects, persons, or actions
2. Indicates wants by naming object such as cookie

1. Incorporate repetition into daily routine of home
   a. Feeding: name child's food and eating utensils; ask if he is enjoying his dessert; concentrate on reviewing day's events in simple manner
   b. Household duties: mother names each item as she dusts; pronounces word while cooking and preparing foods
   c. Playing: identify toys when using them; explain their function
2. Let child see mouthing of words
3. Encourage verbalization and expression of wants

### 19 to 30 months

*Receptive abilities*
1. Points to one named body part
2. Follows two or three verbal directions that are not accompanied by facial or body gestures, for example, put ball on table, give it to mommy, or put toy in box

*Expressive abilities*
1. Combines two different words, for example, "play ball," "want cookie"
2. Names object in picture, for example, cat, bird, dog, horse, man
3. Refers to self by pronoun rather than by name

1. Continue to present concrete objects with words; talk about activities child is involved with
2. Include child in conversations during mealtimes
3. Encourage speech by having child express wants
4. Incorporate games into bathing routine by having child name and point to body parts
5. As child gains confidence in remembering and using words appropriately, encourage less use of gestures
6. Count and name articles of clothing as they are placed on child
7. Count and name silverware as it is placed on table
8. Sort, match, and name glassware, laundry, cans, vegetables, and fruit with child
9. Have child keep scrapbook and add new picture every day to increase recognition of vocabulary words
10. Spend 15 to 20 minutes per day going through booklets and naming pictures; have child point to pictures as objects are named
11. Help child develop functional core vocabulary to express safety needs and information about neighborhood
12. Whenever possible, use word (for example, paper), show object, have child handle and use it, encourage him to watch your face while you say the words, and suggest that he repeat it; refrain from undue pressure

*Continued.*

# Language—cont'd

| EXPECTED TASKS | SUGGESTED ACTIVITIES |
|---|---|

**31 to 36 months**

*Receptive abilities*
1. Takes turns when asked while playing, eating
2. Attends longer to stories and television programs
3. Demonstrates understanding of two prepositions by carrying-out two commands one at a time, for example, "put the block under the chair"
4. Can follow commands asking for two objects or two actions
5. Demonstrates understanding of concepts of big and little, for example, selects larger of two balls when asked for big one
6. Points to additional body parts

*Expressive abilities*
1. Uses regular plurals, for example, adds "s" to apple, box, orange (does not use irregular plurals, for example, mouse to mice)
2. Gives first and last name
3. Names what he has drawn after scribbling
4. On request, tells you his sex, for example, are you a little boy or a little girl?
5. Can repeat a few rhymes or songs
6. On request, tells what action is going on in picture, for example, the kitten is eating

1. Read stories with familiar content but with more detail: nonsense rhymes, humorous stories
2. Expect child to follow simple commands
3. Give child opportunity to hear and repeat his full name
4. Listen to child's explanation about pictures he draws
5. Encourage child to repeat nursery rhymes by himself and with others
6. Address child by his first name

**37 to 48 months**

1. Expresses appropriate responses when asked what child does when tired, cold, or hungry
2. Tells stories
3. Common expression: I don't know
4. Repeats sentence composed of twelve to thirteen syllables, for example, "I am going when daddy and I are finished playing"
5. Has mastered phonetic sounds of p, k, g, v, tf, d, z, lr, hw, j, kw, l, e, w, qe, and o

1. Provide visual stimuli while reading stories
2. Have child repeat story
3. Arrange trips to zoo, farms, seashore, stores, and movies and discuss with child
4. Give simple explanations in answering questions

**49 to 52 months**

*Receptive abilities*
1. Points to penny, nickel, or dime on request
2. Carries out in order command containing three parts, for example, "pick up the block, put it on the table, and bring the book to me"

*Expressive abilities*
1. Names penny, nickel, or dime on request
2. Replies appropriately to questions such as, "What do you do when you are asleep?"
3. Counts three objects, pointing to each in turn
4. Defines simple words, for example, hat, ball
5. Asks questions
6. Can identify or name four colors

1. Play games in which child names colors
2. Encourage use of please and thank you
3. Encourage social-verbal interactions with other children
4. Encourage correct usage of words
5. Provide puppets or toys with movable parts that child can converse about
6. Provide group activity for child; children may stimulate each other by taking turns naming pictures
7. Allow child to make choices about games, stories, and activities
8. Have child dramatize simple stories
9. Provide child with piggy bank and encourage naming coins as they are handled or dropped into bank

# Discipline

| EXPECTED TASKS | SUGGESTED ACTIVITIES |
|---|---|
| **1 to 3 months** | |
| 1. Draws attention by crying | 1. a. Needs should be identified and met as promptly as possible<br>b. Every bit of fussing should not be interpreted as emergency requiring immediate attention<br>c. Infant should not be ignored and permitted to cry for exhaustive periods |
| 2. Infant desires whatever is pleasant and wishes to avoid unpleasant situations | 2. Begin to present limit of having to wait so that infant can learn that tension and discomfort are bearable for short periods |
| 3. Beginning to "wiggle" around | 3. Place infant on surfaces that have sides to protect him from falling off |
| **4 to 8 months** | |
| 1. Begins to respond to "no-no" | 1. a. Reserve "no-no" for times when it is really needed<br>b. Be consistent with word "no-no" for same activity and event that requires it; be friendly and firm with verbal control of limit setting |
| 2. Infant who is left alone for long periods of time may become bored or fretful; learns that crying and whining result in attention | 2. Make special efforts to attend to infant when he is quiet and amusing himself |
| 3. Beginning to show signs of timidity and fretfulness and may whimper and cry when mother separates from him or when strangers pick him up | 3. a. Gradually introduce strangers into infant's environment<br>b. Refrain from promoting frightening situations with strangers during this stage<br>c. Play hiding games like peekaboo in which mother disappears and reappears<br>d. Allow infant to cling to mother and get used to persons a little at a time<br>e. If baby-sitter is used find person familiar to infant or introduce for brief periods before mother leaves infant in her care<br>f. Encourage gentle handling by mother, father, and siblings. Discourage rough handling, especially by strangers |
| 4. Beginning to grasp objects and bring to mouth, but unable to differentiate safe from hazardous items | 4. a. Provide toys that do not have small detachable parts<br>b. Check frequently for small objects in his line of reach<br>5. When traveling in car, place in car restraint with safety belts securely fastened |
| **9 to 12 months** | |
| 1. Beginning to respond to simple commands, for example, "pick up the ball, put the toy in the box" | 1. a. Avoid setting unreasonable number of limits<br>b. Give simple commands one at a time<br>c. Once limit is set, adhere to it firmly each time and connect it immediately with misbehavior<br>d. Respond with consistency in enforcing rule<br>e. Allow time to conform to request<br>f. Gain child's attention |
| 2. Ready to go places on his own and is trying out newly developing motor capacities (not to be confused with naughtiness, "spoiled," or stubbornness) | 2. a. Begin setting and enforcing limits on where child is allowed to travel and explore<br>b. Remove tempting objects<br>c. Remove sources of danger such as light sockets, protruding pot handles, hanging table covers, sharp objects, and hanging cords |

*Continued.*

# Discipline—cont'd

| EXPECTED TASKS | SUGGESTED ACTIVITIES |
|---|---|
| **9 to 12 months—cont'd** | d. Keep child away from fans, heaters, and certain drawers and do not place vaporizer close to infant's crib |
| | e. Keep high chair at least 2 feet away from working and cooking surfaces in kitchen |
| | f. Use gate to keep child out of kitchen when it is being used |
| | g. Be certain that pans, basins, and tubs of hot water are never left unattended |
| | h. Remove all possible poisons or substances that are not food that can be eaten or drunk off floor, low-level cabinets, and under sink |
| | i. Keep child from objects or surfaces that he may chew, for example, porch rails, windowsills, *repainted* toys or cribs that may contain lead |
| | j. Instruct baby-sitter on all safety items |
| 3. Has emerging desires to look at, handle, and touch objects | 3. a. Experiment with diversionary measures |
| | b. Provide child with own play objects |
| 4. Explores objects by sucking, chewing, and biting | 4. a. Remove household poisons, cosmetics, pins, and buttons that he could put in his mouth |
| | b. Be certain that objects that go into mouth are hygienic |
| | c. Check toys for detachable small parts. |
| 5. Beginning to test reactions to certain parental responses during feeding and may become choosy about food | 5. a. Once problem behaviors are defined, plan to work on changing only one behavior at a time until child behaves or conforms to expectations |
| | b. Be certain that child understands old rules before adding new ones |
| | c. Respond with consistency in enforcing old rules: enforce each time, do not ignore next time |
| | d. Provide regular pattern of mealtimes |
| | e. Refrain from feeding throughout day |
| | f. Allow child to decide what he will eat and how much |
| | g. Introduce new foods gradually over period of time |
| | h. Continue to offer foods that may have been rejected first time |
| | i. Do not force food |
| | j. Refrain from physically punishing child for changes in eating habits |
| 6. Beginning to test reactions to parental responses at bedtime preparation | 6. a. Provide regular time for naps and bedtime |
| | b. Avoid excessive stimulation at bedtime or naptime |
| | c. Ignore fussing and crying once safety and physical needs are satisfied and usual ritual is carried out |
| | d. Keep child in own room |
| | e. Refrain from picking up and rocking and holding if needs seem satisfied |
| **13 to 18 months** | |
| 1. Understands simple commands and requests | 1. a. Begin with one rule; add new ones as appropriate |
| | b. In selecting new rules, choose on the basis of being able to clearly define it to self and child, having it reasonable and enforceable at all times; demand no more than fulfillment of defined expectations |
| | c. Plan decisive limits and plan to give consistent attention to them |

| EXPECTED TASKS | SUGGESTED ACTIVITIES |
|---|---|
| 2. In learning mastery over impulses and self-control, child begins testing out limit setting | 2. a. Immediately correct errors in behavior as they occur<br>b. Use consistent enforcement of short-term rules (which are given as verbal commands) and long-term rules (which pertain to chores and family routines)<br>c. Ignore temper tantrums<br>d. Show child when you approve of his behavior and praise for obedience throughout day |
| 3. With increasing fine motor control, child can manipulate objects that may be hazardous | 3. a. Set limits regarding play with doorknobs and car door handles<br>b. Keep away from open windows; latch screens<br>c. Supervise around pools and ponds or drain or fence them<br>d. Lock cabinets<br>e. Keep open jars and bottles out of reach<br>f. Use gate to protect child from falling down stairs |

**19 to 30 months**

| | |
|---|---|
| 1. Attention span increasing | 1. a. Gain attention before giving simple commands, one at a time; praise for success<br>b. Add new rules as child conforms to old ones<br>c. Refrain from expecting *immediate* obedience |
| 2. Begins simple reasoning—asks question why; may be repetitive | 2. Make special efforts to answer questions; give simple explanations; gauge need for simplicity by number of times act is repeated or question asked |
| 3. Interested in further exploration of environment; may lack physical control | 3. a. Supervise on stair rails and waxed floors<br>b. Set rules about crossing streets and carrying knives, sharp objects, or glass objects<br>c. Have outdoor play area securely fenced or supervised<br>d. When riding in car, secure child safely in approved car restraint<br>e. Keep matches out of reach<br>f. Shield adult tools such as knives, lawnmowers, sharp tools |
| 4. Negativistic behavior is expected; responds more frequently with word "no"; may show more resistance at bedtime preparation and during mealtime | 4. a. Practice consistency in responding to behavior<br>b. Allow more time to conform to expectation |
| 5. Behavior may change if new sibling is introduced into family unit | 5. a. Explain verbally or through play that new child is expected<br>b. Exercise more patience with child<br>c. Set special times aside for parental attention to child<br>d. Allow child to help with special care tasks of new sibling |

**31 to 48 months**

| | |
|---|---|
| 1. Displays more interest in conforming | 1. a. Exercise consistency in parental demands; enforce each time and avoid ignoring behavior next time<br>b. Show concrete approval and give immediate recognition for acceptable behavior<br>c. Refrain from use of threats that produce fearfulness |
| 2. Shows greater understanding when simple reasoning is communicated | 2. a. Give simple explanations; allow child chance to demonstrate understanding by talking about event, situation, or rule<br>b. Eliminate unnecessary and impractical rules<br>c. Refrain from constant verbal reprimands<br>d. Denial of privileges should not be excessive or prolonged |

*Continued.*

## Discipline—cont'd

| EXPECTED TASKS | SUGGESTED ACTIVITIES |
|---|---|
| **31 to 48 months—cont'd** | |
| 3. Will respond to simple commands such as putting toys away | 3. a. Assign simple household tasks that child can carry out each day; show approval for performance and success<br>b. Decide if child is capable of doing what is asked by observing him<br>c. Determine how much time is necessary to complete a chore or activity before expecting maximum performance |
| 4. Displays a greater independence in general activities | 4. a. Be extra cautious about supervising riding tricycles in streets and watching for cars in driveways<br>b. Do not permit dashing into street while playing<br>c. Do not allow child to follow ball into street<br>d. Areas under swings and slides should not be paved<br>e. Provide an imitative model that child can copy, for example, do not jaywalk<br>f. Provide scissors that are blunt tipped |
| **49 to 52 months** | |
| 1. Can be given two or three assignments at one time; will carry out in order<br>2. Complies readily with reasonable, well-defined, and consistent requirements<br>3. Understands reasoning | 1. Give more opportunities to be independent<br>2. Use simple explanations and reasoning<br>3. Ask child to define role if he disobeys<br>4. Have child correct mistakes as they occur<br>5. Do not use punishment without warnings<br>6. Praise for successful performance<br>7. Use gold stars on chart for rewards<br>8. If leaving for social obligation, vacation, or visiting away from home, let child know<br>9. Avoid making promises that cannot be kept<br>10. Avoid bribing, ridicule, shaming, teasing, inflicting pain, using unfavorable comparison with other children, and exhibition of behavior by parents they are trying to stop in child<br>11. Remember that child may be imitating models of behavior set up by parents, brothers, sisters, a neighborhood child, or maybe a television hero<br>12. Recognize that there are stress periods in family or child's life that may result in changes in child's behavior including accidents, illness, moving into new neighborhood, separation from friends, death, divorce, and hospitalization of child or parents (be more patient with child's behavior, give more time to conform, show more approval for mastery of tasks, and exercise consistency in handling problems as they occur) |

# Toilet training

| EXPECTED TASKS | SUGGESTED ACTIVITIES |
|---|---|
| **9 to 12 months** | |
| 1. Beginning to show regular patterns in bladder and bowel elimination<br>2. Has one to two stools daily<br>3. Interval of dryness does not exceed 1 to 2 hours | 1. Watch for clues that indicate child is wet or soiled<br>2. Be sure to change diapers when wet or soiled so that child begins to experience contrast between wetness and dryness |
| **13 to 18 months** | |
| 1. Will have bowel movement if put on toilet at approximate time<br>2. Indicates wet pants | 1. Sit child on toilet or potty chair at regular intervals for short periods of time throughout day<br>2. Praise child for success<br>3. If potty chair is used, it should be located in bathroom<br>4. Training should be started when social disruptions are at minimum<br>5. Respond promptly to signals and clues of child by taking him to bathroom or changing pants<br>6. Use training pants, once toilet training is commenced<br>7. Plan to begin training when disruptions in regular routine are minimized, that is, do not begin on vacation |
| **19 to 30 months** | |
| 1. Anticipates need to eliminate<br>2. Same word for both functions<br>3. Daytime control (occasional accident)<br>4. Requires assistance (reminding, dressing, wiping) | 1. Continue regular intervals of toileting<br>2. Reward success<br>3. Dress in simple clothing that child can manage<br>4. Remind occasionally, particularly after mealtime, juice-time, naptime, and playtime<br>5. Take to bathroom before bedtime<br>6. Bathroom should be convenient to use, easy to open door |
| **31 to 48 months** | |
| 1. Takes responsibility for toilet if clothes are simple<br>2. Continues to verbalize need to go; apt to hold out too long<br>3. May have occasional accident<br>4. Needs help with wiping | 1. May still need reminding<br>2. Dress in simple clothing that child can manage<br>3. Ignore accidents; refrain from shame or ridicule |
| **49 to 52 months** | |
| 1. General independence (anticipates needs, undresses, goes, wipes, washes hands) | 1. Praise child for his accomplishment |

# Dressing

| EXPECTED TASKS | SUGGESTED ACTIVITIES |
|---|---|
| **13 to 18 months** | |
| 1. Cooperates in dressing by extending arm or leg | 1. Encourage child to remove socks and so on after task is initiated for him |
| 2. Removes socks, hat, mittens, shoes | |
| 3. Can unzip zippers | 2. Do not rush child |
| 4. Tries to put shoes on | 3. Have him practice with large buttons and with zippers |
| **19 to 30 months** | |
| 1. Can undress | 1. Provide opportunities to button with extra-large-sized buttons |
| 2. Can remove shoes if laces are untied | |
| 3. Helps dress | 2. Encourage and allow opportunity for self-help in getting drink, removing clothes with help, hand washing, unbuttoning, and so on |
| 4. Tries to unbutton | |
| 5. Pulls on simple clothes | 3. Dress in simple clothing |
| | 4. Provide mirror at height child can observe himself for brushing teeth and so on |
| **31 to 48 months** | |
| 1. Greater interest and ability in dressing | 1. Provide with own dresser drawer |
| 2. Intent on lacing shoes (usually does incorrectly) | 2. Simple garments encourage self-help; do not rush child |
| 3. Does not know back from front | 3. Provide large buttons, zippers, slipover clothing |
| 4. Washes and dries hands, brushes teeth | 3. Self hand washing but help with brushing teeth |
| 5. Can button | 5. Provide regular routine for dressing, either in bathroom or bedroom |
| **49 to 52 months** | |
| 1. Dresses and undresses with care except for tying shoes and buckling belts | 1. Assign regular task of placing clothes in hamper or basket |
| | 2. Continue to use simple clothing |
| 2. May learn to tie shoes | 3. Encourage self-help in dressing and undressing |
| 3. Combs hair with assistance | 4. Allow child to select clothes he will wear |

# Home observation for measurement
# of the environment

**BIRTH TO THREE**

Date of interview _____

Child designee _____
(Name)                                           (Age)    (Sex)    (Ethnicity)

Child's birthday _____ Birth order _____

Mother's name _____ Father's name _____

Address _____

| Categories | Raw scores | Percentile scores |
|---|---|---|
| I. Emotional and verbal responsivity of the mother | _____ | _____ |
| II. Avoidance of restriction and punishment | _____ | _____ |
| III. Organization of physical and temporal environment | _____ | _____ |
| IV. Provision of appropriate play materials | _____ | _____ |
| V. Maternal involvement with child | _____ | _____ |
| VI. Opportunities for variety in daily stimulation | _____ | _____ |
| TOTALS | _____ | _____ |

## I. Emotional and verbal responsivity of mother

| | Yes | No |
|---|---|---|
| 1. Mother spontaneously vocalizes to child at least twice during visit (excluding scolding) | | |
| 2. Mother responds to child's vocalizations with a verbal response. | | |
| 3. Mother tells child the name of some object during visit or says name of person or object in a "teaching" style. | | |
| 4. Mother's speech is distinct, clear, and audible. | | |
| 5. Mother initiates verbal interchanges with observer—asks questions and makes spontaneous comments. | | |
| 6. Mother expresses ideas freely and easily and uses statements of appropriate length for conversation (for example, gives more than brief answers). | | |
| * 7. Mother permits child occasionally to engage in "messy" type of play. | | |
| 8. Mother spontaneously praises child's qualities or behavior twice during visit. | | |
| 9. When speaking of or to the child, mother's voice conveys positive feeling. | | |
| 10. Mother caresses or kisses child at least once during visit. | | |
| 11. Mother shows some positive emotional responses to praise of child offered by visitor. | | |
| SUBSCORE | | |

From Whaley, L.F., and Wong, D.L.: Nursing care of infants and children, ed. 2, St. Louis, 1983, The C.V. Mosby Co. Modified from Caldwell, B.M.: Home observation for measurement of the environment (birth to three), Little Rock, Ark., 1970.
*Items that may require direct questions.

## II. Avoidance of restriction and punishment

| | Yes | No |
|---|---|---|
| 12. Mother does not shout at child during visit. | | |
| 13. Mother does not express overt annoyance with or hostility toward child. | | |
| 14. Mother neither slaps nor spanks child during visit. | | |
| *15. Mother reports that no more than one instance of physical punishment occurred during the past week. | | |
| 16. Mother does not scold or derogate child during visit. | | |
| 17. Mother does not interfere with child's actions or restrict child's movements more than three times during visit. | | |
| 18. At least ten books are present and visible. | | |
| *19. Family has a pet. | | |
| SUBSCORE | | |

## III. Organization of physical and temporal environment

| | Yes | No |
|---|---|---|
| 20. When mother is away, care is provided by one of three regular substitutes. | | |
| 21. Someone takes child into grocery store at least once a week. | | |
| 22. Child gets out of house at least four times a week. | | |
| 23. Child is taken regularly to doctor's office or clinic. | | |
| *24. Child has a special place in which to keep his toys and "treasures." | | |
| 25. Child's play environment appears safe and free of hazards. | | |
| SUBSCORE | | |

## IV. Provision of appropriate play materials

| | Yes | No |
|---|---|---|
| 26. Child has some muscle activity toys or equipment. | | |
| 27. Child has a push or pull toy. | | |
| 28. Child has stroller or walker, kiddie car, scooter or tricycle. | | |
| 29. Mother provides toys or interesting activities for child during interview. | | |
| 30. Provides learning equipment appropriate to age—cuddly toy or role-playing toys. | | |
| 31. Provides learning equipment appropriate to age—mobile, table and chairs, high chair, play pen. | | |
| 32. Provides eye-hand coordination toys—items to go in and out of receptable, fit together toys, beads. | | |
| 33. Provides eye-hand coordination toys that permit combinations—stacking or nesting toys, blocks or building toys. | | |
| 34. Provides toys for literature and music. | | |
| SUBSCORE | | |

## V. Maternal involvement with child

| | Yes | No |
|---|---|---|
| 35. Mother tends to keep child within visual range and to look at him often. | | |
| 36. Mother talks to child while doing her work. | | |
| 37. Mother consciously encourages developmental advance. | | |
| 38. Mother invests "maturing" toys with value via her attention. | | |
| 39. Mother structures child's play periods. | | |
| 40. Mother provides toys that challenge child to develop new skills. | | |
| SUBSCORE | | |

## VI. Opportunities for variety in daily stimulation

| | Yes | No |
|---|---|---|
| 41. Father provides some caretaking every day. | | |
| 42. Mother reads stories at least three times weekly. | | |
| 43. Child eats at least one meal per day with mother and father. | | |
| 44. Family visits or receives visits from relatives. | | |
| 45. Child has three or more books of his own. | | |
| SUBSCORE | | |

*Items that may require direct questions.

## THREE TO SIX

Date of interview _____

Child designee _____
　　　　　　　　(Name)　　　　　　　　　　　　　　　　　(Age)　(Sex)　(Ethnicity)

Child's birthday _____ Birth order _____
Mother's name _____ Father's name _____
Address _____

| *Categories* | Raw scores | Percentile scores |
|---|---|---|
| I. Provisions of stimulation through equipment, toys, and experiences | _____ | _____ |
| II. Stimulation of mature behavior | _____ | _____ |
| III. Provision of stimulating physical and language environment | _____ | _____ |
| IV. Avoidance of restriction and punishment | _____ | _____ |
| V. Pride, affection, and thoughtfulness | _____ | _____ |
| VI. Masculine stimulation | _____ | _____ |
| VII. Independence from parental control | _____ | _____ |
| TOTALS | _____ | |

### I. Provision of stimulation through equipment, toys, and experiences

|  | Yes | No |
|---|---|---|

1-12. The following are present in home and either belong to child subject or he is allowed to play with them:
　　1. Toys to learn colors, sizes, shapes—typewriter, pressouts, play school, peg boards, and so on
　　2. Toy or game facilitating learning letters (blocks with letters, toy typewriter, letter sticks, books about letters)
　　3. Three or more puzzles
　　4. Two toys necessitating some finger and whole hand movements (crayons and coloring books, paper dolls)
　　5. Record player and at least five children's records
　　6. Real or toy muscial instrument (piano, drum, toy xylophone or guitar)
　　7. Toy or game permitting free expression (finger paints, play dough, crayons or paint and paper)
　　8. Toys or game necessitating refined movements (paint by number, dot book, paper dolls, crayons and coloring books)
　　9. Toys to learn animals—books about animals, circus games, animal puzzles and so on
　　10. Toy or game facilitating learning numbers (blocks with numbers, books about numbers, games with numbers)
　　11. Building toys (blocks, tinker toys, Lincoln logs)
　　12. Ten children's books
13. At least 10 books are present and visible in the apartment.
14. Family buys a newspaper daily and reads it.
15. Family subscribes to at least one magazine.
16. Family member has taken child on one outing (picnic, shopping excursion) at least every other week.
17. Child has been taken out to eat in some kind of restaurant three or four times in the past year.
18-20. Child has been taken by a family member to the following within the past year:
　　18. Airport
　　19. A trip more than 50 miles from his home (50 miles radial distance, not total distance)
　　20. A scientific, historical, or art museum
21. Child is taken to grocery store at least once a week.

SUBSCORE

### II. Simulation of mature behavior

|  | Yes | No |
|---|---|---|

22-29. Child is encouraged to learn the following:
　　22. Colors
　　23. Shapes
　　24. Patterned speech (nursery rhymes, prayers, songs, TV commercials, and so on)
　　25. The alphabet
　　26. To tell time
　　27. Spatial relationships (up, down, under, big, little, and so on)
　　28. Numbers
　　29. To read a few words
30. Tries to get child to pick up and put away toys after play session—without help.
31. Child is taught rules of social behavior which involve recognition of rights of others.
32. Parent teaches child some simple manners—to say, "Please," "Thank you," "I'm sorry."
33. Some delay of food gratification is demanded of the child, e.g., not to whine or demand food unless within ½ hour of meal time.

SUBSCORE

From Whaley, L.F., and Wong, D.L.: Nursing care of infants and children, ed. 2, St. Louis, 1983, The C.V. Mosby Co. Modified from Caldwell, B.M.: Home observation for measurement of the environment (three to six), Little Rock, Ark., 1976.

### III. Provision of a stimulating physical and language environment (observation items, except**)

| | Yes | No |
|---|---|---|
| 34. Building has no potentially dangerous structural or health defect (plaster coming down from ceiling, stairway with boards missing, rodents, and so on). | | |
| 35. Child's outside play environment appears safe and free of hazards (no outside play area requires an automatic "No"). | | |
| 36. The interior of the apartment is not dark or perceptibly monotonous. | | |
| 37. House is not overly noisy—television, shouts of children, radio, and so on. | | |
| 38. Neighborhood has trees, grass, birds—is esthetically pleasing. | | |
| 39. There are at least 100 square feet of living space per person in the house. | | |
| 40. In terms of available floor space, the rooms are not overcrowded with furniture. | | |
| 41. All visible rooms of the house are reasonably clean and minimally cluttered. | | |
| *42. Mother uses complex sentence structure and some long words in conversing. | | |
| 43. Mother uses correct grammar and pronunciation. | | |
| 44. Mother's speech is distinct, clear, and audible. | | |
| **45. Family has TV and it is used judiciously, not left on continuously (no TV requires an automatic "No"—any scheduling scores "Yes"). | | |
| SUBSCORE | | |

### IV. Avoidance of restriction and punishment (observation items, except**)

| | Yes | No |
|---|---|---|
| 46. Mother does not scold or derogate child more than once during visit. | | |
| 47. Mother does not use physical restraint, shake, grab, pinch child during visit. | | |
| 48. Mother neither slaps nor spanks child during visit. | | |
| 49. Mother does not express over-annoyance with or hostility toward child—complain, say child is "bad" or won't mind. | | |
| 50. Child is not punished or ridiculed for speech. | | |
| **51. No more than one instance of physical punishment occurred during the past week (accept parental report). | | |
| **52. Child does not get slapped or spanked for spilling food or drink. | | |
| SUBSCORE | | |

### V. Pride, affection, and thoughtfulness (observation items, except**)

| | Yes | No |
|---|---|---|
| **53. Parent turns on special TV program regarded as "good" for children. | | |
| **54. Someone reads stories to child or shows and comments on pictures in magazines five times weekly. | | |
| **55. Parents encourages child to relate experiences or takes time to listen to him relate experiences. | | |
| **56. Parent holds child close ten to fifteen minutes per day, such as during TV, story time, visiting. | | |
| **57. Parent occasionally sings to child, or sings in presence of child. | | |
| **58. Child has a special place in which to keep his toys and "treasures." | | |
| **59. Child's art work is displayed some place in house (anything that child makes). | | |
| 60. Mother introduces interviewer to child. | | |
| 61. Mother converses with child at least twice during visit (scolding and suspicious comments not counted). | | |
| 62. Mother answers child's questions or requests verbally. | | |
| 63. Mother usually responds verbally to child's talking. | | |
| 64. Mother provides toys or interesting activities or in other ways structures situation for child during visit when her attention will be elsewhere. (To score "Yes" mother must make an active guiding gesture or suggestion to structure child's play.) | | |
| 65. Mother spontaneously praises child's qualities or behavior twice during visit. | | |
| 66. When speaking of or to child, mother's voice conveys positive feeling. | | |
| 67. Mother caresses, kisses, or cuddles child at least once during visit. | | |
| 68. Mother sets up situation that allows child to show off during visit. | | |
| SUBSCORE | | |

*Throughout interview this refers to *mother* or other *caregiver* who is present for interview.

## VI. Masculine stimulation

|  | Yes | No |
|---|---|---|

69. Child sees and spends some time with father or father figure four days a week.
70. Child eats at least one meal per day, on most days, with mother (or mother figure) and father (or father figure). (One-parent families get an automatic "No.")
71-73. The following are present in home and either belong to child subject or he is allowed to play with them:
   71. Ride toy (tricycle, scooter, wagon, bike with or without training wheels)
   72. Medium wheel toys—trucks, trains, doll carriage, and so on
   73. Large muscle toy (jump rope, swing, ball, climbing object)

SUBSCORE

## VII. Independence from parental control

|  | Yes | No |
|---|---|---|

74. Child is encouraged to try to dress himself.
75. Child is permitted to choose some of his clothing to be worn except on very special occasions.
76. Child is permitted some choice in lunch or breakfast menu.
77. Parent lets child choose certain favorite food products or brands at grocery store.
78. Child is permitted to go to another house to play without having the caregiver accompany him.
79. Child can express negative feelings without harsh reprisal.
80. Child is permitted to hit parent without harsh reprisal.

SUBSCORE
TOTAL SCORE

# Index

Skin—cont'd
  tumors of, 54, 55
  ulcers of
    open, 57
    in pediatric client, 60
  vascularity of, increased, 56
  velvety smooth, 53
  vesicles on; *see* Vesicles
  wheals in; *see* Wheals
  wrinkling of, 40
    general, 40
    increased, in geriatric client, 71
    localized, 40
  yellow tone of, 52
Skin contact materials, skin problems and, 52
Skin tags
  on anus; *see* Anus, skin tags on
  in geriatric client, 72-73
Skin turgor, 54
  in geriatric client, 70-71
  in pediatric client, 62
  poor, 208, 214
    in geriatric client, 227, 229
    in pediatric client, 222, 223
  tenting associated with, 54
Skinfolds
  hygiene of, in pediatric client, 62
  hyperpigmentation in, 52
  increased, in geriatric client, 71
  inguinal, hygiene of, in geriatric client, 71
  inspection of, 59
  moist, lesions on, in geriatric client, 74
  of obese clients, inspection of, 59
Skull; *see also* Head
  abnormally small, 83
    in geriatric client, 99
  adult, lateral view of, 83
  bulge areas on, in geriatric client, 93
  contour of
    in geriatric client, 99
    in pediatric client, 94
  depressions of, 83
    in geriatric client, 99
  enlarged, 83
    in geriatric client, 99
  infant, anatomical structures of, 95
  inspection of, 83
    in geriatric client, 99
    in pediatric client, 92, 94
  lateral expansion of, in geriatric client, 99
  lumps on, 83
    in geriatric client, 99
  marked protrusions of, 83
    in geriatric client, 99
  palpation of, 83, 92
  protruding mandible of, 83
    in geriatric client, 99
  size of
    in geriatric client, 99
    in pediatric client, 94
Slanting of eyes in Down syndrome in pediatric
      client, 183
Sleep(ing)
  in child, 559-560
  with contact lenses, 160
  difficulty in, 37
  discomfort during, neck pain and, in geriatric
      client, 98
  excessive, for child, 255
  habits of, 32
  headache during, 82
  inability to, depression and, 43

Sleep(ing)—cont'd
  interference of shortness of breath with, in ge-
      riatric client, 263
  knee-chest position during, in pediatric client,
      255
Sleeplessness in geriatric client, 47
Slipped capital femoral epiphysis, 451
Slipped femoral epiphysis in teenage boys, 462
Slipping when trying to rise, 41
Slits cut or worn in shoes, 42
Slouched posture, depression and, 43
Sloughing tissue, infected, erosions or ulcers and,
      in pediatric client, 60
Slow body movements, 41
  depression and, 43
Slow speech, 42
Slumping in chair, 40
Slurred speech, 42, 485
Small clothing, 42
Small skull, abnormally, 83
  in geriatric client, 99
Smear, Papanicolaou; *see* Papanicolaou smear
Smegma, definition of, 339
Smell
  inability to, 485
  sense of, evaluation of, in geriatric client, 127
Smile(ing)
  absent, depression and, 43
  constant, 41
    depression and, 43
  diminished, depression and, 43
  pattern of, marked asymmetry of, in geriatric
      client, 99
  by 2- to 4-year-old child, 46
Smoking, 32, 204
  chronic, in geriatric client, 126
  cigarette, chronic, hearing loss and, in geriatric
      client, 152
  cough and, 204
  eye irritation and, 160
  in geriatric client, 265
  increase in pulse and, in geriatric client, 265
  inflammation of mucosal glands and, in geriatric
      client, 131
  pipe; *see* Pipe smoking
Smooth lymph nodes; *see* Lymphatic nodes,
      smooth, nodular
Smoothness
  of skin, 53
  of teeth, excessive, in pediatric client, 122
  of tongue in geriatric client, 130
Smothering feeling, 246
  in geriatric client, 268
  in pediatric client, 260
Snap
  felt in inspection of hips in pediatric client, 462
  opening; *see* Opening snap
Snellen chart for assessment of eyes, 161, 162-163
  clinical strategies for use of, 173-176
  far-vision errors and, 173
  for pediatric client, 178-179
Soap
  antibacterial, phototoxic reactions and, in geri-
      atric client, 69
  facial care and, 52
  rashes and skin irritations and, in pediatric
      client, 60
  as skin irritant in geriatric client, 69
Soft cervix, 373
  in geriatric client, 388
Soft contact lenses, 160
Soft exudates of retinal background, 172
  in pediatric client, 187

Soft lymph nodes; *see* Lymphatic nodes, soft,
      spongy
Soft murmurs, 251
  in geriatric client, 271
Soft palate
  asymmetry of movement of, 491
  edema of, in pediatric client, 124
  inspection and palpation of, 116-117
    in geriatric client, 131
    in pediatric client, 124
  lesions of, 117
    in geriatric client, 131
    in pediatric client, 124
  patches on, 117
    in geriatric client, 131
    in pediatric client, 124
  petechiae on, 117
    in geriatric client, 131
  reddened, 116
    in geriatric client, 131
    in pediatric client, 124
Soft signs, neurological, screening assessment of,
      in school-age child, 528-529
Soft uterine wall, 376
Soles, scaliness of, in pediatric client, 61
Solid tissue, replacement of normal lung tissue by,
      210
  in geriatric client, 228
Sonorous rhonchus; *see* Rhonchus, sonorous
Sore, pressure, erosions or ulcers and, in pediatric
      client, 60
Sore throat; *see* Throat, sore
Sounds
  adventitious, definition of, 201
  auscultatory; *see* Auscultatory sounds
  breath; *see* Breath sounds
  Korotkoff, definition of, 235
  $S_1$; *see* $S_1$ sound
  $S_2$; *see* $S_2$ sound
  $S_3$; *see* $S_3$ sound
  $S_4$; *see* $S_4$ sound
  unintelligible, 38
Space, orientation in, evaluation of, in pediatric
      client, 529
Sparks, flying, eye injury and, 160
Spasm
  of paravertebral muscles, 403, 405
    in pediatric client, 457, 458
  muscular; *see* Muscular spasm
Spastic gait, 41
Spastic movements in newborn to 12-month-old
      child, 518, 519
Spasticity, definition of, 482
Spatula, wooden, for assessment of female geni-
      tourinary system, 365
Speculum
  insertion of, into ear in pediatric client, 146
  nasal
    broad-tipped, otoscope with, for inspection of
        nose and paranasal sinuses, 107
    insertion of, 108
    inspection of internal nasal cavity with, 108-
        110, 121, 127
    otoscope with, in nasal examination of pedi-
        atric client, 120
    use of, 118
  otoscope with all available sizes of, 145
  placement of, in client's ear, 146
  vaginal, 369-371, 379
    in examination of child, 383
    in examination of menstruating adolescent,
        383
    insertion of, in geriatric client, 386

Tic, 41, 484
  definition of, 482
  of face in geriatric client, 99
Tickle sensation, decreased or unequal, 487
Ticklishness, abdominal examination and, in pediatric client, 322
Tight Achilles tendons in pediatric client, 460
Tight clothing, 42
Tilt, pelvic, idiopathic scoliosis and, in pediatric client, 449
Tilted head; *see* Head, tilted
Time, orientation to, assessment of, 36, 37, 43-44
Tinea; *see* Ringworm
Tinkling, high-pitched bowel sounds; *see* Bowel sounds, high-pitched, tinkling
Tinnitus
  definition of, 136
  in geriatric client, 152
  medical history and, 137
Tiring easily, anxiety and, 43
Tissue
  granulation, increase in, in external ear canal in geriatric client, 153
  growth of, from periphery toward center of cornea; *see* Cornea, tissue growth from periphery toward center of
  healing, scars and, in pediatric client, 60
  sloughing, infected, erosions or ulcers and, in pediatric client, 60
  solid, replacement of normal lung tissue by, 210
    in geriatric client, 228
Tobacco, chewing, geriatric client and, 126
Toddler
  auditory function in, evaluation of, 151
  lumbar curvature of spine of, 456
  musculoskeletal system in, assessment of, 447
  nutritional assessment of, 320
  pot belly profile of, 323
  pronation of foot of, 448
  restraint of, for mouth examination, 118, 119
  scaphoid abdomen in, 323
  undressing of, for assessment of integumentary system, 60
  wide stance of, 524
Toe(s)
  dryness or scaling of skin between, in pediatric client, 61
  extension of, 416
  fanning of, with extrusion of great toe, 506
  fissures or hyperkeratosis association with friction on, in geriatric client, 74
  flexion of, 416
  great, gout of, 414
  hammer, 414
  inspection between, 59
  inward deviations of, in pediatric client, 460
  lateral deviation of, in pediatric client, 460
  medial deviation of, 414
  painful movement of, 416
  pigeon, evaluation for, in pediatric client, 449
  walking on
    balance testing by, 495
    evaluation of, in pediatric client, 449
Toenails
  cutting or clipping, 52
  granular surface of, in geriatric client, 75
  long, 59
  thickening of, associated with fungal infection in geriatric client, 75
  uncut, curled over foot in geriatric client, 75
  yellowish discoloration of, in geriatric client, 75
Toilet training in child, 569

Tone(s)
  vocal, 36, 41
  of voice, monotonous and unvaried, in hearing evaluation of geriatric client, 152
Tongue
  absence of papillae on, 115
    in geriatric client, 130
    in pediatric client, 124
  appearing too large for mouth in pediatric client, 124
  attach farther forward than usual in pediatric client, 124
  color of, 115
    in geriatric client, 130
    in pediatric client, 124
  difficulty in articulation involving, 485
  dorsal surface of, 115
  fasciculation of, 115
    in geriatric client, 130
  fissures of, in pediatric client, 124
  frequent wetting of, anxiety and, 43
  furrows in, in pediatric client, 124
  induration of, 115
    in geriatric client, 130
  inspection and palpation of, 115, 116
    in geriatric client, 130
    in pediatric client, 124
  lateral movement of, 115
    in geriatric client, 130
  lesions on, 115
    in geriatric client, 130
    in pediatric client, 124
  limp, on floor of mouth in geriatric client, 130
  lumps on, 115
    in geriatric client, 130
  motor development of, assessment of, in assessment of cranial nerve XII, 492
  nodules on, 115
    in geriatric client, 130
  posterior portion of, stimulation of, in assessment of cranial nerves IX and X, 491
  protrusion of, in pediatric client, 124
  red strawberry, in pediatric client, scarlet fever and, 124
  redness of, 115
    in geriatric client, 130
    in pediatric client, 124
  smooth, in geriatric client, 130
  surface characteristics of, 115
    in geriatric client, 130
    in pediatric client, 124
  symmetry of, 115
    in geriatric client, 130
    in pediatric client, 124
  texture of, in geriatric client, 130
  unable to advance forward to lips in pediatric client, 124
  unilateral atrophy of, in geriatric client, 130
  ventral surface of, 116
    color of, 116
    in geriatric client, 116
    induration of, in pediatric client, 124
    inspection of, 116
    lesions on, 116
      in geriatric client, 130
      in pediatric client, 124
    lumps on, 116
      in pediatric client, 124
    nodules on, in pediatric client, 124
    normal, 116
    pallor of, 116

Tongue—cont'd
  ventral surface of—cont'd
    patches on, 116
      in geriatric client, 130
      in pediatric client, 124
    redness of, 116
    surface characteristics of, 116
Tongue blade
  for examination of mouth and pharynx, 110, 112
  for neurological examination, 484
  use of, 118
Tongue-tied pediatric client, 124
Tonic neck reflex, 520
  in pediatric client, 93, 96
Tonsil tag in geriatric client, 131
Tonsillar lymph nodes
  lymphatic drainage pattern for, 93
  palpation of, 91
    in geriatric client, 101
    in pediatric client, 97
Tonsillar pillar movement, asymmetry of, 491
Tonsils
  coating on, in pediatric client, 125
  exudate on, in pediatric client, 125
  infection of, recurrent, in pediatric client, 120
  large, in pediatric client, 125
  occluding swallowing or breathing in pediatric client, 125
  pus on, in pediatric client, 125
  reddened, in pediatric client, 125
Tooth brushing; *see* Teeth, brushing of
Tophi
  definition of, 136
  of external ear, 139
    in geriatric client, 153
    in pediatric client, 150
Torsion
  femoral, in pediatric client, 449
  of spermatic cord, definition of, 340
  tibial, in pediatric client, 449
Torso, total absence or paucity of movement of, 41
Torso obesity distribution associated with disease in geriatric client, 70
Tortuous vas deferens, 346
  in pediatric client, 355
Torus palatinus, 117
  definition of, 105
  in geriatric client, 131
Total health data base; *see* Health data base, total
Touch
  inability to perceive, 498
  incorrect identification of location of, 498
  sensation of, light, evaluation of, 498
    in infant, 519
Toxicity
  of heart and hypertension medications in health data base for geriatric client, 29
  increase in rate of carotid artery and, in pediatric client, 258
Toys, stimulation of child through, 573
Trachea
  landmarks of, 88
    in geriatric client, 100
    in pediatric client, 96
  lateral deviation of, 214
    in geriatric client, 229
    in pediatric client, 223
  lateral displacement of, 88
    in geriatric client, 100
    in pediatric client, 96
  location of, 88
    in geriatric client, 100
    in pediatric client, 96